Multiple Sclerosis Immunology

Takashi Yamamura • Bruno Gran
Editors

Multiple Sclerosis Immunology

A Foundation for Current and Future Treatments

Springer

Editors
Takashi Yamamura
Immunology, MS Center
NCNP
Tokyo
Japan

Bruno Gran
Division of Clinical Neurosciences
University of Nottingham School of Medicine
Nottingham
UK

ISBN 978-1-4939-4201-5 ISBN 978-1-4614-7953-6 (eBook)
DOI 10.1007/978-1-4614-7953-6
Springer New York Heidelberg Dordrecht London

Softcover reprint of the hardcover 1st edition 2013

Printed on acid-free paper

Springer is part of Springer Science+Business Media (www.springer.com)

Preface

I was diagnosed with secondary progressive multiple sclerosis (MS) in 1994 at the Queen's Medical Centre in Nottingham. At that time, I was told that there was no treatment available apart from steroids. After being diagnosed, I joined the MS society of Great Britain and Northern Ireland. I became a member of its Research Network, when it was formed with the aim to actively involve people affected by MS in all aspects of the Society's research programme and the communication of research results.

Through the Research Network, I have been involved in reviewing grant applications and as a 'research buddy' to researchers in the field. It is through such scheme that I along with two other network members (also affected by MS) were assigned to Dr Gran's research project investigating the role of Toll-like receptors in the modulation of human regulatory T cells. As a consequence of my involvement in this project, I was asked by Dr Gran to talk on "What people with multiple sclerosis would like from Immunology" at the 2-day conference held in Nottingham in October 2010 entitled 'Multiple Sclerosis Immunology: A foundation for current and future treatments', on which this book is based.

The conference brought together researchers and clinical neurologists from all over the world and gave all those who attended a chance to see where the field of MS research stands and where it is heading. It is an exciting time in MS research as many new treatments, mostly immunotherapies, have either been approved or are in the pipeline. Progress is also being made into understanding how the immune system functions in MS and with greater understanding come new potential treatment targets. A continued dialogue between basic and clinical scientists ensures that translation from bench to treatment is more likely to be effective.

People with MS would obviously ultimately like a cure to be found for this debilitating condition, but most would settle for keeping the disease where it is, stopping its progression. A diagnosis of MS brings with it fear and uncertainty; you never know what symptom will hit you next, how long it will last or if indeed it will resolve. Present disease-modifying treatments reduce the number of relapses and may slow progression. I was very interested that trials on alemtuzumab showed an improvement in disability. Unfortunately, the side effects of the treatment are more severe than those of current treatments. With new treatments come new dilemmas for both patients and neurologists in weighing up the pros and cons. Apart from the work on alemtuzumab presented by Dr Coles, I found the presentations by Prof Yamamura, the keynote speaker, and Prof Constantinescu, Head of Academic Neurology in Nottingham, particularly interesting. The first was a fascinating talk on the potential role of gut flora and the increased incidence of MS in Japan. The second was about the frequent association of MS with other autoimmune conditions.

I recently completed a master's degree in parasitology and studied how helminths produce excretory/secretory molecules, which modulate the immune system in the host and are being investigated as potential treatments in various autoimmune conditions. Recruitment has just started in Nottingham for a clinical trial, in which the immunomodulatory effects of the hookworm *Necator americanus* will be tested for the treatment of MS.

Overall, I feel that what immunology can do for people with MS is to give them hope for the future, that the condition can be managed and the slide into disability staved off indefinitely. I find it very encouraging that so much work is being done in the field of MS.

Manchester, UK — Ms. Rebecca Rushworth

Contents

Contributors

Sofia Abrahamsson Division of Brain Sciences, Faculty of Medicine, Building 560/Burlington Danes, Room E415, Imperial College London, 160 Du Cane Road, London W12 0NN UK
e-mail: s.abrahamsson06@imperial.ac.uk

Stephen M. Anderton Centre for Inflammation Research, Centre for Multiple Sclerosis Research and Centre for Immunity Infection and Evolution, University of Edinburgh, Edinburgh, UK
e-mail: steve.anderton@ed.ac.uk

Bogoljub Ciric Department of Neurology, Thomas Jefferson University, Philadelphia, PA 19107, USA
e-mail: bogoljub.ciric@jefferson.edu

Alasdair Coles Department of Clinical Neurosciences, University of Cambridge, Addenbrooke's Hospital, Box 165, Cambridge, CB2 0QQ, UK
e-mail: ajc1020@medschl.cam.ac.uk

Cris S. Constantinescu Division of Clinical Neurosciences, University of Nottingham; C Floor South Block, Queen's Medical Centre, Nottingham NG7 2UH, UK
e-mail: cris.constantinescu@nottingham.ac.uk

James Crooks Division of Clinical Neurosciences, University of Nottingham; C Floor South Block, Queen's Medical Centre, Nottingham NG7 2UH, UK
e-mail: msxjc1@nottingham.ac.uk

Laura J. Edwards Division of Clinical Neurosciences, University of Nottingham; C Floor South Block, Queen's Medical Centre, Nottingham NG7 2UH, UK
e-mail: ljedwards@doctors.org.uk

Mohamed El-Behi Institut du Cerveau et de la Moelle Epinière, INSERM U975, Paris, France
e-mail: mohamed.elbehi@icm-institute.org

Denise C. Fitzgerald Centre for Infection and Immunity, Queen's University Belfast, Belfast, UK
e-mail: d.fitzgerald@qub.ac.uk

Ferenc Gallyas Department of Biochemistry and Medical Chemistry, University of Pecs Medical School, Pecs, Hungary

Nuclear-Mitochondrial Interactions Research Group, Hungarian Academy of Sciences, Budapest, Hungary
e-mail: ferenc.gallyas@aok.pte.hu

Juan J. García-Vallejo Department of Molecular Cell Biology and Immunology, VU University Medical Center, 7057, 1007 MB Amsterdam, The Netherlands
e-mail: j.garciavallejo@vumc.nl

Barbara B. Gawlik Departments of Neurology and Immunobiology, Yale School of Medicine, New Haven, CT 06520, USA
e-mail: barbara.gawlik@yale.edu

Ralf Gold Department of Neurology, St. Josef-Hospital Bochum, Ruhr-Universität, Bochum, Germany
e-mail: ralf.gold@ruhr-uni-bochum.de

Bruno Gran Division of Clinical Neurosciences, University of Nottingham; C Floor South Block, Queen's Medical Centre, Nottingham NG7 2UH, UK
e-mail: bruno.gran@nottingham.ac.uk

Krista Haanstra Department of Immunobiology, Biomedical Primate Research Centre (BPRC), PO Box 3306, 2280 GH, Rijswijk, The Netherlands
e-mail: haanstra@bprc.nl

David A. Hafler Departments of Neurology and Immunobiology, Yale School of Medicine, New Haven, CT 06520, USA
e-mail: david.hafler@yale.edu

Aiden Haghikia Department of Neurology, St. Josef-Hospital Bochum, Ruhr-Universität, Bochum, Germany
e-mail: aiden.haghikia@ruhr-uni-bochum.de

Nuffield Department of Clinical Neurosciences and MRC Human Immunology Unit,Weatherall Institute of Molecular Medicine, John Radcliffe Hospital, University of Oxford, Oxford, UK

B. A. 't Hart Department of Immunobiology, Biomedical Primate Research Centre (BPRC), PO Box 3306, 2280 GH, Rijswijk, The Netherlands
e-mail: hart@bprc.nl

Department of Medical Physiology, University Medical Centre Groningen, Groningen, The Netherlands

Department of Immunology, Erasmus Medical Center, Rotterdam, The Netherlands

MS center ErasMS, Rotterdam, The Netherlands

Bernhard Hemmer Department of Neurology, Technische Universität München, Klinikum rechts der Isar, Department of Neurology, Ismaninger Strasse 22 Munich, Germany
e-mail: hemmer@tum.de

Rogier Q. Hintzen Department of Neurology, Erasmus MC, Room Ba 4.92, P.O. Box 2040, 3000 CA, Rotterdam, The Netherlands
e-mail: r.hintzen@erasmusmc.nl

Juan M. Ilarregui Department of Molecular Cell Biology and Immunology, V University Medical Center, 7057, 1007 MB Amsterdam, The Netherlands
e-mail: j.ilarregui@vumc.nl

Zsolt Illes Division of Clinical and Experimental Neuroimmunology, Department of Neurology, University of Pecs Medical School, Pecs, Hungary
e-mail: zsolt.illes@rsyd.dk

Clinical Neuroscience MR Research Group, Hungarian Academy of Sciences, University of Pecs, Pecs, Hungary

Department of Neurology and Institute of Clinical Research, University of Southern Denmark, Odense, Denmark

S. Anwar Jagessar Department of Immunobiology, Biomedical Primate Research Centre (BPRC), PO Box 3306, 2280 GH, Rijswijk, The Netherlands
e-mail: jagessar@bprc.nl

Joanne Jones Department of Clinical Neurosciences, University of Cambridge, Addenbrooke's Hospital, Box 165, Cambridge, CB2 0QQ, UK
e-mail: jls53@medschl.cam.ac.uk

Yolanda S. Kap Department of Immunobiology, Biomedical Primate Research Centre (BPRC), PO Box 3306, 2280 GH, Rijswijk, The Netherlands
e-mail: kap@bprc.nl

Department of Immunology, Erasmus Medical Center, Rotterdam, The Netherlands

MS center ErasMS, Rotterdam, The Netherlands

Nicole Kerlero de Rosbo Department of Neurology, Rehabilitation, Ophthalmology, Genetics, Maternal and Child Health, University of Genoa, Italy
e-mail: nicole.kerleroderosbo@unige.it

Nathalie Koning Department of Molecular Cell Biology and Immunology, VU University Medical Center, 7057, 1007 MB Amsterdam, The Netherlands
e-mail: nathaliekoning@gmail.com

Yvette van Kooyk Department of Molecular Cell Biology and Immunology, VU University Medical Center, 7057, 1007 MB Amsterdam, The Netherlands
e-mail: y.vankooyk@vumc.nl

Thomas Korn Klinikum rechts der Isar, Department of Neurology, Technische Universität München, Ismaninger Str. 22, 81675 Munich, Germany
e-mail: korn@lrz.tum.de

Markus C. Kowarik Department of Neurology, Technische Universität München, Klinikum rechts der Isar, Department of Neurology, Ismaninger Strasse 22 Munich, Germany
e-mail: kowarik@lrz.tum.de

Karim L. Kreft Department of Neurology, Erasmus University Medical Centre, Dr. Molewaterplein 50, 3015 GE, Rotterdam, The Netherlands
e-mail: k.kreft@erasmusmc.nl

Vijay K. Kuchroo Brigham & Women's Hospital, Center for Neurologic Diseases, Harvard Medical School, Boston, MA, USA
e-mail: vkuchroo@rics.bwh.harvard.edu

Jon D. Laman Department of Immunology, Erasmus Medical Center, Rotterdam, The Netherlands
e-mail: j.laman@erasmusmc.nl

Hans Lassmann Center for Brain Research, Medical University of Vienna, Vienna, Austria
e-mail: hans.lassmann@meduniwien.ac.at

Laura Lovato Department of Neurology, Rehabilitation, Ophthalmology, Genetics, Maternal and Child Health University of Genoa, Italy
e-mail: lauralovato@hotmail.it

Amy E. Lovett-Racke Department of Microbial Infection and Immunity, The Ohio State University, Columbus, OH 43210, USA
e-mail: amy.lovett-racke@osumc.edu

Ali Manouchehrinia Division of Clinical Neurosciences, University of Nottingham, C Floor, South Block, Queen's Medical Centre, Nottingham NG7 2UH, UK
e-mail: a_mn@hotmail.co.uk

Miriam Mattoscio Division of Brain Sciences, Faculty of Medicine, Building 560/Burlington Danes, Room E415, Imperial College London, 160 Du Cane Road, London W12 0NN UK
e-mail: m.mattoscio@imperial.ac.uk

Julia Y. Mescheriakova Department of Neurology, Erasmus University Medical Centre, Dr. Molewaterplein 50, 3015 GE, Rotterdam, The Netherlands
e-mail: j.mescheriakova@erasmusmc.nl

Manoj K. Mishra Hotchkiss Brain Institute, University of Calgary, 3330 Hospital Drive, Calgary, AB T2N 4N1, Canada
e-mail: mkmishra@ucalgary.ca

Sachiko Miyake Department of Immunology, National Institute of Neuroscience, National Center of Neurology and Psychiatry, Tokyo, Japan
e-mail: miyake@ncnp.go.jp

Paolo A. Muraro Division of Brain Sciences, Faculty of Medicine, Building 560/Burlington Danes, Room E415, Imperial College London, 160 Du Cane Road, London W12 0NN UK
e-mail: p.muraro@imperial.ac.uk

Mukanthu H. Nyirenda Division of Clinical Neurosciences, University of Nottingham, C Floor, South Block, Queen's Medical Centre, Nottingham NG7 2UH, UK

Neuroimmunology Unit, Montreal Neurological Institute, McGill University, Montreal, Quebec H3A 2B4, Canada.
e-mail: mukanthu.nyirenda2@mail.mcgill.ca

Michael K. Racke Department of Neurology, The Ohio State University, Columbus, OH 43210, USA
e-mail: michael.racke@osumc.edu

Abdolmohamad Rostami Department of Neurology, Thomas Jefferson University, Philadelphia, PA 19107, USA
e-mail: a.m.rostami@jefferson.edu

Jun-ichi Satoh Department of Bioinformatics and Molecular Neuropathology, Meiji Pharmaceutical University, 2–522-1 Noshio, Kiyose, Tokyo 204–8588, Japan
e-mail: satoj@my-pharm.ac.jp

Lawrence Steinman Department of Neurology and Neurological Sciences, Stanford University, Stanford, CA 94305, USA
e-mail: steinman@stanford.edu

Beckman Center for Molecular Medicine, 279 Campus Drive, Room B002, Stanford University, Stanford, CA 94305, USA

Antonio Uccelli Department of Neurology, Rehabilitation, Ophthalmology, Genetics, Maternal and Child Health, University of Genoa, Italy
e-mail: auccelli@neurologia.unige.it

Center of Excellence for Biomedical Research, University of Genoa, Italy

Advanced Biotechnology Center, Genoa, Italy

Department of Neurology, Rehabilitation, Ophthalmology, Genetics, Maternal and Child Health (DINOGMI), University of Genoa, Largo Paolo Daneo 3, 16132 Genoa, Italy

Pablo Villoslada Department of Neurology, Center of Neuroimmunology, Institute of Biomedical Research August Pi Sunyer (IDIBAPS)—Hospital Clinic of Barcelona, Villarroel 170, 08036 Barcelona, Spain
e-mail: pvilloslada@clinic.ub.es

Martin S. Weber Department of Neurology, Technische Universität München, Klinikum rechts der Isar, Department of Neurology, Ismaninger Strasse 22 Munich, Germany
e-mail: m.weber@lrz.tu-muenchen.de

Takashi Yamamura Department of Immunology, National Institute of Neuroscience, National Center of Neurology and Psychiatry, Tokyo, Japan
e-mail: yamamura@ncnp.go.jp

V. Wee Yong Hotchkiss Brain Institute, University of Calgary, 3330 Hospital Drive, Calgary, AB T2N 4N1, Canada
e-mail: vyong@ucalgary.ca

List of Abbreviations

APC	Antigen-presenting cell
CLP	Common lymphoid progenitor
CNS	Central nervous system
CSF	Cerebrospinal fluid
DAVID	Database for Annotation, Visualization and Integrated Discovery
DEGs	Differentially expressed genes
DM	Diabetes mellitus
DZ	Dizygotic
EAE	Experimental autoimmune encephalomyelitis
ETP	Early thymic progenitor
GEO	Gene Expression Omnibus
GWA study	Genome-wide association study
HLA	Human leucocyte antigen
HPRD	Human Reference Protein Database
HSC	Hematopoietic stem cell
IBD	Identical by descent
IM	Infectious mononucleosis
IPA	Ingenuity pathways analysis
IMSGC	International Multiple Sclerosis Genetic Consortium
KEGG	Kyoto Encyclopedia of Genes and Genomes
LD	Linkage disequilibrium
miRNA	Micro-ribonucleic acid
MS	Multiple sclerosis
MudPIT	Multidimensional Protein Identification Technology
MZ	Monozygotic
NGS	Next-generation sequencing
OR	Odds ratio
PANTHER	Protein Analysis Through Evolutionary Relationships
PBMC	Peripheral blood mononuclear cells
RA	Rheumatoid arthritis
RISC	RNA-induced silencing complex
RR	Risk ratio
SNP	Single-nucleotide polymorphism
95 % CI	95 % confidence interval

List of Definitions

SNP	Single-nucleotide polymorphism; a single nucleotide variation in a genetic sequence that occurs at appreciable frequency in the population
Tagging SNP	An SNP that can predict other SNPs in the region with small probability of error, because SNPs are physically close to one another and tend to be inherited together
Linkage disequilibrium	The non-random association between two or more alleles such that certain combinations of alleles are more likely to occur together on a chromosome than other combinations of alleles
Synonymous	A substitution of one base for another in an exon of a gene coding for a protein, such that the produced amino acid sequence is not modified
Non-synonymous	A non-synonymous substitution results in a change in amino acid
Allele	An allele is one of two or more versions of a gene. An individual inherits two alleles for each gene, one from each parent. If the two alleles are the same, the individual is homozygous for that gene. If the alleles are different, the individual is heterozygous
Locus	The position that a given gene occupies on a chromosome
Concordance rate	A quantitative statistical expression for the concordance (the occurrence of a given trait in both members of a twin pair) of a given genetic trait, in pairs of twins in genetic studies
Multiplex family	Multicase family with affected individuals present in >1 generation
IBD	Identical by descent; a measure of how many alleles of any gene in each of the two individuals came from the same ancestral chromosome
Familial aggregation	Occurrence of a trait in more members of a family than can be readily accounted for by chance
Missense	Mutation resulting in a codon that codes for a different protein

Chapter 1
Th17 Cells in Autoimmune Inflammation and Demyelination in the Central Nervous System

Vijay K. Kuchroo and Thomas Korn

1.1 Introduction

In 2011, an extensive genome-wide association study (GWAS) was published on genetic loci associated with multiple sclerosis (MS; Sawcer et al. 2011). This most recent GWAS involved the unprecedented number of 9,772 MS cases and 17,376 controls of European descent. In addition to HLA DRB1*15:01 conferring increased risk of developing MS and HLA A*02:01, which is protective, a set of novel non-MHC loci were identified to be associated with an increased risk of developing MS. Most of the non-MHC genes/loci that were linked to susceptibility to MS were immune genes, therefore unequivocally supporting that MS is an immune-mediated disease. The sets of genes nearest to the respective lead SNP comprised cytokines and chemokines and their receptors (CXCR5, IL-2RA, IL-7R, IL-12RB1, IL-22Ra2, IL-12A, IL-12B, IRF8, TNFRSF1A, TNFRSF14, and TNFSF14), costimulatory molecules (CD37, CD40, CD58, CD80, CD86, CLECL1), and signal transduction molecules (CBLB, GPR65, MALT1, RGS1, STAT3, TAGAP, TYK2; Sawcer et al. 2011). The majority of these molecules are crucial for the generation and function of T cells.

Upon contact with antigen, T cells become activated, expand, and acquire various effector and regulatory phenotypes. Many of the MS susceptibility genes encode for products that play a critical role in this differentiation process of naive T cells into T helper effector subsets. For example, IL-12, which is a heterodimer composed of IL-12A (p35) and IL-12B (p40), is an essential differentiation factor for development of IFN-γ producing Th1 cells. On the other hand, IL-12B (p40) is also part of the

T. Korn (✉)
Klinikum rechts der Isar, Department of Neurology, Technische Universität München,
Ismaninger Str. 22, 81675 Munich, Germany
e-mail: korn@lrz.tum.de

V. K. Kuchroo
Brigham & Women's Hospital, Center for Neurologic Diseases,
Harvard Medical School, Boston, MA, USA

T. Yamamura, B. Gran (eds.), *Multiple Sclerosis Immunology*,
DOI 10.1007/978-1-4614-7953-6_1, © Springer Science+Business Media New York 2013

cytokine IL-23, which is a heterodimer composed of IL-12B and IL-23p19. IL-23, which signals via STAT3, is necessary for the development of Th17 cells. Interestingly, IL-23R, which has been genetically linked to psoriasis, ankylosing spondylitis, and inflammatory bowel disease by GWAS (Duerr et al. 2006; Nair et al. 2009), has not yet emerged as a gene linked to MS. Thus, there is an urgent need to integrate the data from GWAS into functionally relevant models to understand the mechanisms by which MS is induced and identify relevant targets that could be exploited for drug development. Working models that consider niche-specific conditions that influence the functional phenotype of T helper cell subsets might be particularly rewarding. In this chapter, we will focus on Th17 cells whose significance for the development of immunopathology in autoimmunity and chronic inflammatory conditions is increasingly being recognized.

1.2 Th17 Cells as a Distinct Lineage of T Helper Cells

The *IL-17A*gene was cloned as *Ctla-8* from a $CD8^+$ T cell hybridoma in 1993 (Rouvier et al. 1993). The IL-17 family of cytokines has six members (A–F) and has been thoroughly reviewed (Iwakura et al. 2011; Kolls and Linden 2004; Weaver et al. 2007). Both IL-17 and IL-17F have inflammatory properties but are different in terms of their biological significance in various anatomical compartments (Yang et al. 2008b), which is likely due to differential expression of the receptors on the target cells. Although IL-17 has long been known to be produced by cells of the innate immune system, it attracted much attention only after it was discovered that a subset of effector $CD4^+$ T helper cells also produced IL-17 (Yao et al. 1995). The idea that IL-17-producing T cells might be a distinct $CD4^+$ T helper cell subset was a major conceptual breakthrough because the paradigm of T helper cell development had thus far been dichotomous comprising only Th1 and Th2 cells (Mosmann et al. 1986; Fig. 1.1). Tim Mosmann and Bob Coffman had shown that a naive $CD4^+$ T cell, upon contact with cognate antigen, becomes activated and adopts a specific phenotype, which is characterized by a set of signature cytokines. For example, Th1 cells produce large amounts of IFN-γ and thus activate macrophages and license them to kill intracellular pathogens such as Listeria (Hsieh et al. 1993). In contrast, Th2 cells produce IL-4 and induce eosinophilic inflammation that is crucial to host defense against parasitic infections (Sokol et al. 2008, 2009). These functional properties have been proven in many experimental models and highlight that the development of a particular T helper effector subset is required to induce a specific type of inflammation "customized" for clearing a specific class of pathogen(s). Later, these T helper subsets were shown to require specific differentiation factors and to express "lineage-specific" transcription factors. Th1 cells are induced by IL-12 and express T-bet as their lineage-specific transcription factor, while Th2 cells are induced by IL-4 and express Gata-3 as a Th2-specific master transcription factor (Murphy and Reiner 2002). Since IL-17 is not expressed by either Th1 or Th2 cells, and since IL-17-producing T cells can be generated in the genetic absence of either T-bet or

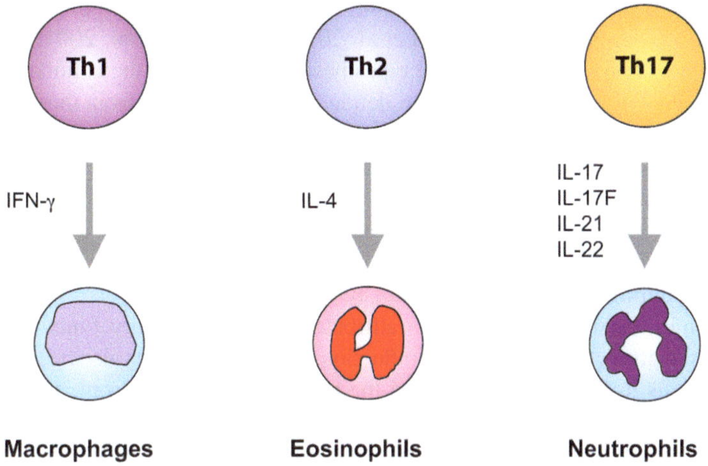

Fig. 1.1 Types of T helper cell-mediated inflammation. Effector functions of Th1- versus Th17-driven immunopathology. Th1, Th2, and Th17 cells have been identified as distinct effector T helper cell lineages. While dysregulated Th2 responses play a role in the pathology of allergic reactions with eosinophils as prototypic responder cells, organ-specific autoimmune diseases such as MS are mediated by Th1 and Th17 cells. IFN-γ, the signature cytokine of Th1 cells induces the upregulation of MHC class II molecules on a variety of immune cell types (but also on astrocytes) and activates macrophages. In contrast, IL-17 unleashes a wide tissue response due to its broad receptor distribution. For example, endothelial cells and astrocytes are activated by IL-17 and produce ELR^+ chemokines (including CXCL1 and CXCL2) that attract neutrophils

Gata-3 transcription factors that are required for the generation of Th1 and Th2 cells, respectively, it was suggested that IL-17-producing T cells might be a lineage distinct from Th1 or Th2 cells (Harrington et al. 2005; Park et al. 2005). This idea was consolidated when ROR-γt was identified to be an indispensable transcription factor in Th17 cells (Ivanov et al. 2006). ROR-γt cooperates with ROR-α, Stat3, and Irf-4 to establish the Th17 program (Brustle et al. 2007; Yang et al. 2007, 2008c). Besides IL-17 (IL-17A), Th17 cells express a set of other cytokines including IL-17F, IL-21, and IL-22 (Korn et al. 2009).

Because of their presence at sites of tissue inflammation and due to production of proinflammatory cytokines, Th17 cells have been implicated in many autoimmune and chronic inflammatory conditions both in animal models and in human diseases. However, it has been difficult to attribute the pathogenicity of Th17 cells to one solitary cytokine that they produce (Haak et al. 2009; Kreymborg et al. 2007; Sonderegger et al. 2008). Yet, IL-17A knockout (KO) mice are relatively resistant to the development of experimental autoimmune encephalomyelitis (EAE; Komiyama et al. 2006) and EAE cannot be induced at all when Th17 responses are not sustained as in IL-23p19 KO mice or in IL-23R KO mice (Awasthi et al. 2009; Cua et al. 2003). Furthermore, GM-CSF KO mice are resistant to EAE and GM-CSF was suggested to be a target of ROR-γt indicating that ROR-γt-driven expression of GM-CSF might define the pathogenicity of T cells in central nervous system (CNS)-directed autoimmunity (Codarri et al. 2011; Hirota et al. 2011; McQualter et al. 2001). However, GM-CSF is produced by many cell types besides T cells and the cellular targets of GM-CSF in autoimmunity are not yet defined. As a conclusion from these studies, it is clear that effector T helper subsets are not functionally equivalent to any individual effector cytokine that they produce and a thorough identification of those (combinations of) factors that make Th17 (and other T cells) pathogenic such that they are able to induce autoimmune tissue inflammation is required. The identification of such factors in pathogenic Th17 cells will provide targets for drug development (see the next section) to prevent and restrain autoimmunopathology.

Although the majority of reports attribute a proinflammatory function to Th17 cells, tissue protective properties or induction of tissue repair has also been attributed to Th17 cells in the liver, the gut, and the heart in models of chronic inflammation (Chang et al. 2006; Sugimoto et al. 2008; Zenewicz et al. 2007). One way to interpret these data is that the proinflammatory and protective functions of Th17 cells are context-dependent, i.e., it might be a result of the anatomical compartment where Th17 cells are generated. Another interpretation of the data is that indeed there are two different subtypes of Th17 cells, one that is pathogenic and another that is nonpathogenic or protective. In order to conceptualize this at a molecular level, it has been very helpful to define various differentiation conditions of Th17 cells in a reductionist but very well-defined setting. Although IL-23, which shares the p40 subunit with IL-12 but has a specific p19 subunit—was initially thought to be the differentiation factor for Th17 cells, it was rapidly recognized that naive T cells did not express the receptor for IL-23 and therefore did not differentiate into Th17 cells upon exposure with IL-23. In 2006, three independent groups discovered that the combination of TGF-β1 and IL-6 was necessary and sufficient to induce IL-17 in naive T cells (Bettelli et al. 2006; Mangan et al. 2006; Veldhoen et al. 2006a). Upon exposure with TGF-β1 and IL-6, naive T cells also start expressing IL-23R and thus become responsive to IL-23 (Zhou et al. 2007). Based on this knowledge, it has been hypothesized that Th17 cells might be different depending on whether or not they have been exposed to IL-23. Although this question has not yet entirely been resolved, it is clear that exposure to IL-23 is required for Th17 cells to attain a pathogenic phenotype (see the next section). The suppression of IL-10 or the induction of IL-7R in precommitted Th17 cells by IL-23 has been suggested to be the mechanism by which IL-23 makes Th17 cells pathogenic (Ghoreschi et al. 2010; McGeachy et al. 2007, 2009). Similar to IL-23, the role of IL-1 in the terminal differentiation of Th17 cells is only partly understood. IL-1R KO mice do not mount productive Th17 responses and IL-23 cannot compensate for this deficit (Sutton et al. 2006). Recent studies show that exposure of naive T cells to IL-1 may induce a functionally distinct subset of Th17 cells that is more proinflammatory than Th17 cells differentiated in the absence of IL-1 (Zielinski et al. 2012). Taken together, emerging data suggest that IL-17-producing T cells may contain distinct subsets that produce different combinations of cytokines together with IL-17 and have distinct functions not only in response to pathogens, but also during autoimmunity and tissue repair.

1.3 Pathogenic and NonPathogenic Th17 cells and Molecular Characteristics that Define Them

Another matter of intense debate has been whether or not TGF-β1 is really required to induce the Th17 differentiation. Although in humans, Th17 differentiation was achieved by IL-6 and IL-23 alone (Acosta-Rodriguez et al. 2007a; Wilson et al. 2007), blockade of TGF-β1 or lack of TGF-β signaling prevented the development of Th17 cells from naive T cells (Li et al. 2007; Veldhoen et al. 2006a, b). In a more recent study, murine naive T cells were differentiated into the Th17 lineage using a cocktail of IL-6 and IL-23 plus IL-1β (Ghoreschi et al. 2010). In these studies, however, endogenous TGF-β (most likely TGF-β3) produced by differentiating Th17 cells was not excluded. Th17 cells that were differentiated without exogenous TGF-β1 had stable expression of ROR-γt and IL-17. However, in contrast to Th17 cells that were induced by TGF-β1 plus IL-6, Th17 cells induced with IL-1β, IL-6 plus IL-23 without addition of exogenous TGF-β resulted in the coexpression of T-bet and these cells were highly pathogenic in inducing EAE upon adoptive transfer into syngeneic animals (Ghoreschi et al. 2010). Yet, another level of complexity was introduced into how Th17 cells are generated in vivo, by the concept that the conditions for the generation of these cells might be different (or distinct subsets of Th17 cells might exist) depending on the site of initial priming of such cells. While gut-derived Th17 cells or antigen-specific Th17 cells that are generated in draining lymph nodes upon subcutaneous immunization require IL-6 for their development, the priming of Th17 cells in the spleen occurs in the genetic absence of IL-6 but might require IL-23 (Hu et al. 2011). It remains to be determined whether these various Th17 cells of distinct compartmental origin can be differentiated on the basis of the cytokines that are required for their differentiation and whether they may attain different effector functions.

The concept of distinct Th17 subsets that differ in their capacity to induce tissue remodeling and repair on one hand and immunopathology on the other hand is intriguing but remains vague as long as there are no markers or functional molecules that define each of these subsets. Recent studies are beginning to shed some light on the inductive events that are required for the generation of different T cell subsets and on their molecular signatures. It is clear that Th17 cells induced by TGF-β1 plus IL-6 do not readily induce EAE upon adoptive transfer unless they have been exposed to IL-23 for prolonged periods of time (Jager et al. 2009). Exposure to IL-23, in addition to suppressing the production of anti-inflammatory cytokines, has now been shown to induce endogenous TGF-β3 in T cells (Lee et al. 2012). Differentiation of T cells with TGF-β3 plus IL-6 induces highly pathogenic Th17 cells that can induce EAE, without any need for exposure to IL-23. Analyzing these different Th17 subsets induced by TGF-β1 plus IL-6 versus TGF-β3 plus IL-6, we have defined a signature of 23 genes that distinguishes pathogenic Th17 cells from nonpathogenic Th17 cells (Lee et al. 2012) (see also Fig. 1.2). Whereas pathogenic Th17 cells coexpress IL-17 together with the transcription factor T-bet and IL-23R, IL-22, and GM-CSF, nonpathogenic Th17 cells express a regulatory module consisting of IL-10 together

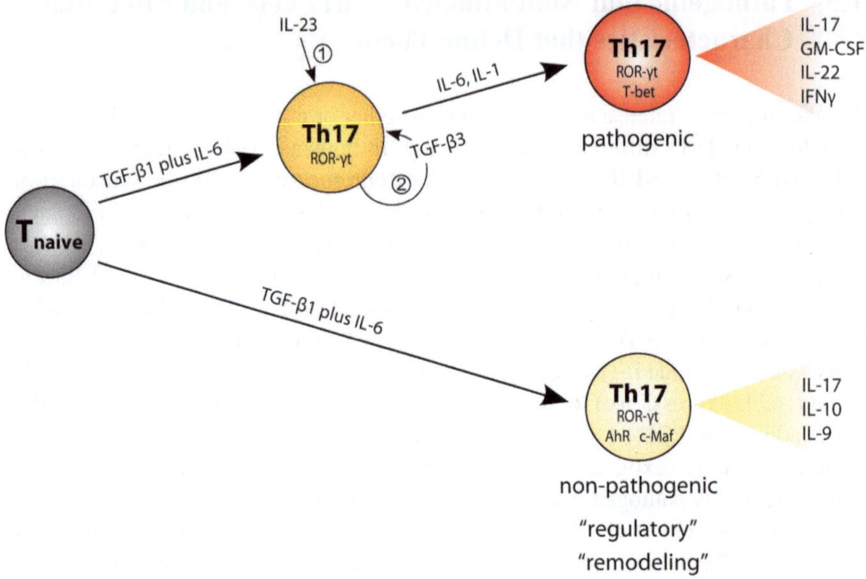

Fig. 1.2 Pathogenic versus nonpathogenic Th17 cells. It is an emerging concept that Th17 cells can be categorized into subsets with distinct effector functions. On a molecular level, exposure to IL-23 confers pathogenic properties to Th17 cells. Notably, when Th17 cells are differentiated by TGF-β1 plus IL-6, they get induced to produce small amounts of TGF-β3. However, IL-23 maintains the production of TGF-β3 in developing Th17 cells (*1*). TGF-β3 acts back on developing Th17 cells (*2*) and, together with IL-6 or IL-1, promotes the development of pathogenic Th17 cells with a distinct expression profile of effector molecules including IL-17, IL-22, GM-CSF, and also T-bet-driven IFN-γ (for details, see text). In contrast, while initiating the Th17 transcriptional program, TGF-β1 plus IL-6 (in the absence of IL-23) result in the induction of an inhibitory module in Th17 cells including IL-10 and the transcription factors AhR and c-Maf

with IL-9, AhR, and c-Maf (Lee et al. 2012). Recent studies with human Th17 cells further support the functional heterogeneity of Th17 cells similar to what has been observed in rodents. One subset of human Th17 cells was shown to coproduce IL-17 and IFN-γ and this subset was found to have specificity for *Candida albicans* antigens. Another subset of human Th17 cells produced IL-17 and IL-10 and was reactive against *Staphylococcus aureus* antigens suggesting that different Th17 subsets may have evolved to clear different types of infections (Zielinski et al. 2012).

1.4 Longevity and Plasticity of Th17 Cells

Since their discovery, it has been a concern that Th17 cells—although necessary for host defense in order to fight certain bacteria and fungi—might be short-lived and not able to mount adequate memory responses. Th17 cells were observed to enter less efficiently into the memory T cell pool than Th1 cells (Pepper et al. 2010).

Yet, Th17 cells are necessary and sufficient for sustained autoimmune responses, chronic inflammation, and antitumor responses. Thus, Th17 responses cannot be short-lived. In an attempt to understand this conundrum, Muranski and colleagues took a sequential profiling approach of transferred Th1 versus Th17 cells (Muranski et al. 2011). Indeed, Th17 cells not only adopt Th1-like features (such as expression of T-bet and production of IFN-γ) in vivo, but also self-renew as IL-17 producers. Therefore, Th17 cells appear to have various developmental stages that are metastable and are subject to a certain degree of plasticity. Th17 cells—perhaps because of their TGF-β-driven developmental history—are not terminally differentiated but appear to have stem cell-like, i.e., self-renewing capacity, and can under specific conditions proceed to terminal effector T cells with Th1-like properties. Using a reporter-/fate-tracking system, complementary results have been reported in EAE (Hirota et al. 2011). Historic IL-17 producers were different from classic Th1 cells in the CNS of EAE mice even though they lost IL-17 production and had turned into IFN-γ (and GM-CSF) producers. On the molecular level, T-bet—once expressed—interacts with Runx-1 to downmodulate the expression of ROR-γt, which might account for the loss of IL-17 production turning Th17 cells into "ex-Th17 cells" (Lazarevic et al. 2011).

Although ex-Th17 cells expressed T-bet and IFN-γ in response to IL-23, specific molecules such as the transcription factor AhR are private to ex-Th17 cells (in relation to classical Th1 cells). Other molecules that belong to the Th17 transcriptional program such as IL-23R, IL-1R, and CCR6 may also persist in reprogrammed Th17 cells. Thus, the homing behavior of reprogrammed Th17 cells and their response to the innate cytokine milieu in the inflamed tissue as well as their mode of cell death and way of regulation by Tregs might be fundamentally different from Th1 cells. Indeed, the contraction of T helper cell populations is an active process and is regulated differentially depending on the compartment (lymphoid tissue versus target tissue) and probably also depending on the effector T cell lineage. Although it has long been known that Th1 cells are very susceptible to Fas-/FasL-induced cell death (Zhang et al. 1997) and Th2 cells to GrzB-mediated apoptosis (Devadas et al. 2006), it remains to be determined whether there is a preferred mode of cell death for Th17 cells. It appears that Th17 cells express high amounts of IL-10Rα and are more susceptible to IL-10- mediated suppression than Th1 or Th2 cells (Huber et al. 2011). It is likely that IL-10, which might be provided by $Foxp3^{+}$ Tregs at the site of inflammation, signals directly into Th17 cells (Chaudhry et al. 2011). However, it is not yet clear whether sensing of IL-10 leads to reprogramming of the inflammatory properties of Th17 cells or triggers their physical attrition.

In general, T helper subsets (or even lineages) might be more plastic than anticipated (Murphy et al. 1996). Upon initial commitment to a specific developmental program, a T cell will become responsive to differentiating cytokines in the ambient milieu. For example, it will be essential whether WSX1 or IL-6Rα will pair with the constitutively expressed gp130 to form a functional IL-27 receptor or a functional IL-6 receptor in this T cell (Stumhofer et al. 2006, 2007). Similarly, expression of IL-23R that pairs with IL-12Rβ1 to form a functional IL-23R or expression of IL-12Rβ2 that also associates with IL-12Rβ1 but builds a functional IL-12 receptor will dictate terminal differentiation or plasticity of a T cell that has already been committed to a developmental program (Lee et al. 2009). Yet, it depends on the lineage commitment how fundamental the fate decisions of a given T cell can be. For example, Th1 cells are relatively stable and cannot easily be reprogrammed while Th2 cells might be switched into a Th1 phenotype in a biased experimental system (Hegazy et al. 2010). Adoptively transferred LCMV-specific Th2 cells can be reprogrammed to express T-bet and produce IFN-γ upon subsequent in vivo infection with LCMV resulting in protective immunity and memory T cells that coexpress T-bet and Gata-3 (Hegazy et al. 2010).

In summary, IL-17 is an early response cytokine that is used as an effector molecule by a series of cells of the innate immune system (Cua and Tato 2010). IL-17 has been adopted by cells of the adaptive immune system and at the moment we are only beginning to understand under which pathophysiologic conditions IL-17 produced by adaptive immune cells plays a role. It has been hypothesized that adaptive immune cell-derived IL-17 might be particularly important in host defense against certain pathogens at epithelial surfaces. Best evidence for this concept comes from studies on $CD4^+$ T cells in the gut where Th17 cells might evolve in response to specific gut microbiota. It is clear that Th17 responses are not short-lived and Th17 memory cells exist although their initial cytokine signature might be modified. There is now a solid basis of evidence that these long-standing Th17 responses might lead to chronic inflammation in the gut and to autoimmunity in the skin or even in the CNS (which is formed by neuroectodermal tissue).

1.5 Th17 Cells and Gut Microbiota

A rediscovered line of research has brought back the attention to the gut microbiome in promoting susceptibility to autoimmunity and chronic inflammation (Honda and Littman 2012) because specific taxa in the gut microbiome can lead to the generation of either proinflammatory Th1 and Th17 cells or Tregs in the gut lamina propria (LP), respectively. Most importantly, mice that were housed germ-free (GF) lacked Th17 cells in the LP of the small intestine and reinstitution of a specific species of bacteria, i.e., segmented filamentous bacteria (SFB), was necessary and sufficient to restore the LP Th17 cell population in the small intestine of GF mice (Ivanov et al. 2009). This observation has raised the possibility that SFB-induced serum amyloid protein A in the terminal ileum, which in turn would activate dendritic cells to produce IL-6 and IL-23, and thus promote the development of Th17 cells that protected the mice from *Citrobacter rodentium* infection (Ivanov et al. 2009). In contrast, clusters IV and XIVa of the genus *Clostridium*—by increasing the amount of available TGF-β—induced the generation of Tregs in the colon LP resulting in resistance to colitis (Atarashi et al. 2011). Polysaccharide A derived from *Bacteroides fragilis* increased the frequency of $Foxp3^+$ Tregs in the mesenteric lymph nodes and enhanced their production of IL-10 in a TLR-2-dependent manner (Round and Mazmanian 2010). These studies suggested that specific proteins or carbohydrate moieties produced by specific members of the gut microbiota promote the generation of proinflammatory

T cells (Th1 or Th17 cells) or regulatory T cells (Foxp3$^+$ Tregs) in the LP, which can be recalled at peripheral sites during infection or inflammation.

It is likely that microbial ligands are sensed by gut-residing dendritic cells or macrophages that translate this input into cytokine signals, which as a consequence, skew T cells into specific functional phenotypes. In addition to bacterial products, ambient homeostatic (or inflammatory) mediators might further condition LP conventional DCs into specific subsets (Coombes and Powrie 2008). In the gut LP, Th17 cell-inducing DCs have been described as CD11c$^+$CD11b$^+$CX3CR1$^+$—a population that also contains macrophages (CD68$^+$CD11c^{low})—while Treg cell- inducing DCs are CD11c^{high}CD103$^+$ (Benson et al. 2007; Coombes et al. 2007; Niess and Adler 2010). In GF mice, the LP is relatively depleted of CX3CR1$^+$ DCs, but not of CD103$^+$ DCs. It is clear that CD103$^+$ DCs can induce Foxp3 expression in conventional T cells by increasing the availability of TGF-β (via αvβ8; Travis et al. 2007) and retinoic acid (RA; Sun et al. 2007). Although CD103$^+$ DCs express retinal dehydrogenases (Aldh1a1 and Aldh1a2), the rate-limiting enzymes for the production of RA, other sources of RA (such as for example intestinal epithelial cells (IEC)) might also be relevant in the gut. In fact, IEC-derived RA is believed to license DCs to adopt a Treg-inducing phenotype in the first place. However, the conditioning process of LP DCs appears to be highly context-dependent because RA in the presence of IL-15 fails to induce tolerogenic DCs, but promotes the production of IL-12p70 by DCs (DePaolo et al. 2011).

Various working hypotheses are being followed to gain insight into the molecular and cellular underpinning of these gut-restricted processes for inflammatory diseases at distal sites such as the joints or the CNS. First, bacterial products, for example, TLR ligands, could induce IL-12 or IL-23 in gut-resident myeloid cells. Spill over of these cytokines would make them available to the systemic compartment. Subsequently, those "distal" tissues that have resident populations of IL-23 receptor-positive cells—as has been shown for the enthesis—would respond to IL-23 by creating a milieu that promotes T cell-driven inflammation. An interesting animal model of inflammatory spondyloarthropathy has been generated based on this idea (Sherlock et al. 2012). Second, specific bacterial products—most likely by activating gut-resident dendritic cells or macrophage populations—would induce either Th17 cells or Tregs in the gut LP that are specific for bacterial antigens. Distal effects of these pathogen (or commensal)-specific LP T cells in peripheral tissues could be due to cross-reactivity with self-antigens. Yet, an alternative scenario has been observed recently (Wu et al. 2010). K/BxN mice develop spontaneous arthritis under regular housing conditions. Arthritis is significantly attenuated under GF conditions, but can be reinstalled upon repopulation of the gut with SFB that restore the LP Th17 compartment. Since arthritis in K/BxN mice is driven by T cell-dependent autoantibodies to glucose-6-phosphate isomerase, distal effects of T cells must be operative. As compared with GF housed mice, regular housed mice have increased frequencies of Th17 cells not only in the LP, but also in the spleen. In this case, splenic Th17 cells are probably gut-derived because they express the gut-homing receptor α4β7. However, their specificity is unclear. Yet, by production of IL-17 that acts directly on B cells, splenic Th17 cells promote the formation of germinal centers resulting in high autoantibody titers and overt clinical disease (Wu et al. 2010). Finally, gut flora-induced, T cell-mediated distal effects might emerge when recirculating self-reactive Th17 cells are directly primed in the intestinal compartment in the first place. Homing of these cells to their target tissues—perhaps preceded by reactivation in draining lymph nodes—might then result in autoimmune pathology (Berer et al. 2011; Krishnamoorthy et al. 2009; Lee et al. 2011b).

1.6 Th17 Cells in EAE

The EAE model has been instrumental in the initial discovery and "validation" of Th17 cells (Langrish et al. 2005). EAE is a model for human MS, but has been extensively exploited in order to investigate T cell-driven pathological events in organ-specific autoimmune diseases (Korn et al. 2010). Similar to other models of organ-specific autoimmunity, EAE was considered as an autoimmune disease induced by Th1 cells. Scientific evidence for this concept came from the fact that EAE can be induced by highly pure in vitro-generated autoreactive T cells that produce IFN-γ (Lafaille et al. 1997). This notion was endorsed by the finding that IFN-γ was found in active EAE lesions and also in MS biopsy material and indeed, when administered as a recombinant drug to MS patients, IFN-γ exacerbated the disease (Panitch et al. 1987; Traugott and Lebon 1988). However, when EAE was induced in IFN-γ KO mice, the KO animals were not resistant to EAE, but instead developed exacerbated disease (Chu et al. 2000; Ferber et al. 1996). Similar findings were obtained with other members of the IFN-γ pathway including IFN-γR KO, TNF KO, Stat1 KO, and IL-12p35 KO mice (Becher et al. 2002; Bettelli et al. 2004; Liu et al. 1998; Willenborg et al. 1996). The conclusion from these genetic models was that EAE can be induced in the absence of bona fide Th1 cells suggesting that this T cell subset might not be sufficient or necessary for the induction of CNS autoimmunity. On the other hand, IL-23p19 mice are completely resistant to EAE (Cua et al. 2003). Since IL-23 is required to stabilize Th17 cells (see above), Th17 cells (instead of Th1 cells) were implicated as the major pathogenic T cell subset in inducing CNS autoimmunity. However, as problematic as was the dismissal of Th1 cells in EAE pathogenesis, equally premature was it to blame the entire pathogenic cascade in EAE on Th17 cells. Indeed, T-bet KO mice are clearly resistant to EAE (Bettelli et al. 2004) and although T-bet is also expressed in non-T cells, its intrinsic role for the development of Th1 cells is well established. Thus, IL-6, IL-23, ROR-γt, and T-bet appear to be essential for the generation of pathogenic T cells and development of EAE (Bettelli et al. 2004; Cua et al. 2003; Ivanov et al. 2006; Samoilova et al. 1998). How can these observations be integrated into a common concept of pathogenic effector T helper cells?

As far as IL-6 is concerned, the best-studied T cell-intrinsic effect of this cytokine is its potency to suppress the expression of Foxp3 and thus to prevent the induction of peripheral Foxp3 Tregs (Bettelli et al. 2006; Korn et al. 2007). This must be a T cell-intrinsic effect since T cell conditional gp130 KO mice have exaggerated frequencies of antigen-specific Tregs upon immunization with MOG in CFA (Korn et al. 2008). At the same time, the frequency of antigen-specific Th17 cells is grossly reduced, which is in line with the in vitro finding that IL-6 plays a pivotal role in regulating the balance between Tregs and Th17 cells (Bettelli et al. 2006).

The role of IL-23 for the generation of encephalitogenic T cells appears to be more complicated. IL-23p19 mice are resistant to EAE (Cua et al. 2003). Th17 cells can be induced in the draining lymph nodes of IL-23- and IL-23R-deficient mice, which is consistent with the idea that IL-23 is not necessary to prime naive T cells into the Th17 lineage. However, Th17 cells are not maintained in the spleens of IL-23R-deficient mice (Awasthi et al. 2009; McGeachy et al. 2009). From these results and due to in vitro experiments where IL-23 stabilizes the expression of IL-17 (Jager et al. 2009; Veldhoen et al. 2006a), it has been suggested that IL-23p19 KO mice are resistant to EAE because they cannot produce a productive Th17 response. However, whether IL-23 "just" stabilizes IL-17 in vivo remains to be determined. Various investigators have proposed T cell-intrinsic effects of IL-23 other than stabilization of the IL-17 locus, including suppression of IL-10, induction of IL-7R, induction of T-bet, and even induction of IFN-γ in precommitted Th17 cells (Hirota et al. 2011; McGeachy et al. 2007, 2009). Work from Casey Weaver's laboratory suggested that Th17 cells start producing IFN-γ when restimulated in the presence of IL-23 and in the absence of TGF-β (Lee et al. 2009). Consistent with this idea, we have detected T-bet as one of the key molecules in the signature of pathogenic Th17 cells. Loss of T-bet but not IFN-γ, largely decreases the ability of Th17 cells to induce EAE. Conversely, exposure of T-bet-deficient autoreactive T cells to TGF-β3 induces these cells to become highly encephalitogenic (see above; Lee et al. 2012). Therefore, TGF-β3 can replace T-bet deficiency in inducing pathogenic Th17 cells.

Although it appears that at a great proportion IL-17-producing $CD4^+$ T helper cells in the target organ are double producers (IL-17 and IFN-γ) or completely turn to the production of IFN-γ, IL-17 itself is still an important effector molecule in promoting tissue inflammation. The receptor for IL-17 (IL-17A) is a heterodimer consisting of IL-17RA and IL-17RC and is expressed on hematopoietic and non-hematopoietic cells including astrocytes (Iwakura et al. 2011) and it is likely that activation of astrocytes by IL-17 is important for early events in neuroinflammation (Kang et al. 2010).

The possibility that different types of T helper effector cells, namely Th1 and Th17 cells are involved in promoting immunopathology in EAE raises the question whether there is a spatial or qualitative difference in the immune reaction that is induced by these types of effector T cells. Several experimental approaches were used to investigate this question. In independent experimental settings, Th1-mediated immunopathology seemed more prevalent in the spinal cord. In contrast, Th17 cells contribute to inducing immunopathology in the brain stem and cerebellum (Stromnes et al. 2008). Since it is not possible (under wild-type conditions) to distinguish between a "classical" Th1 cell and an IFN-γ-producing "Th17" cell, a series of knock-out or conditional knock-out settings were used to confirm whether or not Th1 versus Th17 cells would induce different types of inflammation in the CNS. First, IFN-γR KO recipients of encephalitogenic wild-type T cells develop prominent brain stem inflammation, suggesting that the inability to sense IFN-γ is a susceptibility factor for supraspinal parts of the CNS, but not the spinal cord (Lees et al. 2008;

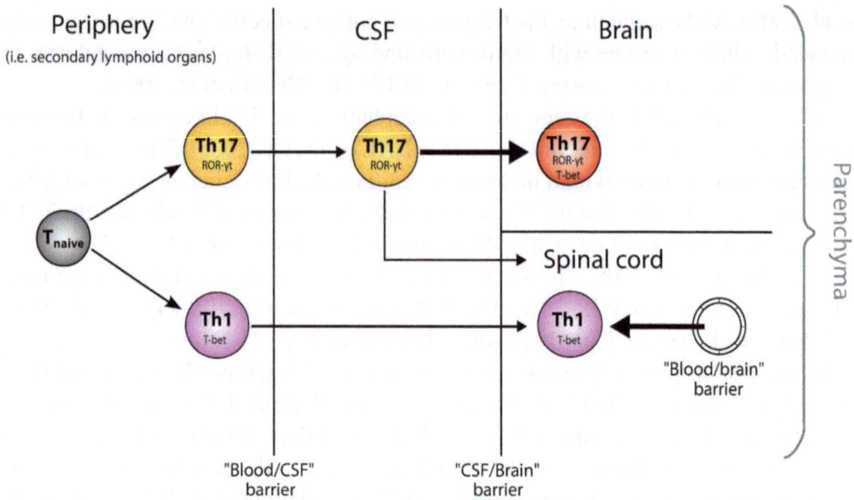

Fig. 1.3 Compartmentalized inflammation in the CNS. CNS entry routes and plasticity of T helper cells across different compartments. Simplified scheme representing the differential pathways of effector T cells as correlated with their functional phenotype. Naive T cells are primed in peripheral organs (e.g. lymph nodes, spleen) and thereby driven into functional effector subsets via master transcription factors according to the encompassed inflammatory milieu. In CNS-directed autoimmunity, Th1 (*purple*) and Th17 cells (*orange*) were recognized as the major infiltrating subsets, albeit differential entry routes as well as properties of lineage plasticity are under debate. Entry from the periphery (*left* panel) into the CNS parenchyma (*right* panel) might be facilitated indirectly via the CSF (*central* panel) and directly via the CNS vasculature. Distinct effector T helper cell subsets might use different entry routes and might thus be targeted to topologically distinct parts of the CNS, e.g., brain versus spinal cord. Concomitantly, the entry might be linked to cellular plasticity of the subsets in situ. "Pathogenic" Th17 cells (*red*) were reported to also express T-bet and produce IFN-γ when recruited to the CNS parenchyma (for details, see text)

Wensky et al. 2005). Second, distinct autoantigenic epitopes might be presented in different parts of the CNS leading to specific and qualitatively (i.e., IFN-γ versus IL-17 promoting) distinct T cell reactions (Stromnes et al. 2008). Third, since the integrin expression on Th1 versus Th17 cells is different, these effector T cell subsets might be guided to distinct parts of the CNS. For example, Th17 cells are able to enter supraspinal parts of the CNS but not the spinal cord in an α4 integrin-independent manner, while Th1 cells are essentially dependent on the expression of α4 to invade into the spinal cord (Rothhammer et al. 2011). In another report (Reboldi et al. 2009), CCR6, which is preferentially but not exclusively expressed on Th17 cells, was shown to guide Th17 cells (but not Th1 cells) to the plexus epithelium via CCL20, which is highly expressed by epithelial cells of the choroid plexus and astrocytes (Meares et al. 2012). Thus, Th17 cells may be exquisitely suited to cross the blood/CSF barrier and enter into the subarachnoid space, which is highly relevant for immune surveillance on one hand, but may also be the compartment where autoimmune reactions build up that later target the CNS parenchyma (Brown and Sawchenko 2007); (Fig. 1.3). Th1 cells and Th17 cells may not only have different ports of entry into the CNS and produce different types of pathology within the

CNS, but may also be different in their potency to promote B cell responses within the target tissue (Mitsdoerffer et al. 2010) and the formation of ectopic lymphoid follicles (Peters et al. 2011). Th17 cells—by virtue of expressing IL-17 and a unique cell surface molecule called podoplanin—have the propensity to promote the formation of ectopic lymphoid structures in the meningeal space (Peters et al. 2011). Lymphoid follicles have also been identified in certain MS patients (perhaps with more aggressive disease courses; Howell et al. 2011; Magliozzi et al. 2007; 2010; Serafini et al. 2004). However, it remains to be determined whether the formation of lymphoid follicle-like structures is associated with enhanced Th17 responses in humans as well.

1.7 Th17 Cells in MS

Th17 cells have been identified in human MS tissue (Montes et al. 2009). Early reports suggested that IL-17 transcripts might be overrepresented in chronic MS lesions (Lock et al. 2002). Later, it was found that IL-17-expressing immune cells, $CD4^+$ T cells and $CD8^+$ T cells, were located within the inflammatory infiltrate of MS lesions (Tzartos et al. 2008). IL-17 mRNA-containing mononuclear cells were increased in blood and CSF of MS patients (Matusevicius et al. 1999) and IL-17-producing $CD4^+$ T cells were overrepresented in the peripheral blood mononuclear cells (PBMCs) of MS patients by epigenetic profiling (Janson et al. 2011). Upon treatment of MS patients with fingolimod, central memory (i.e., $CCR7^+CD45RA^-$) IL-17-producing T helper cells were preferentially reduced (Mehling et al. 2010). Since fingolimod, which is a functional antagonist of the S1P1 receptor, is an approved drug in MS (Kappos et al. 2010), it has—by analogy—been suggested that Th17-type T cells contribute in promoting inflammation in human MS. Only recently it was shown that Th17 clones prevail in the CSF of active MS patients (Brucklacher-Waldert et al. 2009). It might be due to their production of IL-17 and IL-22 that human Th17 cells have the capacity to cross the blood CSF barrier (Kebir et al. 2007). When human Th17 cells subsequently infiltrate into the CNS parenchyma, they coexpress T-bet and IFN-γ representing a phenotype quite similar to what has been reported for pathogenic Th17 cells in mice (Kebir et al. 2009; see above).

In humans, a similar molecular machinery as in mice is operational for the development of Th17 cells (Manel et al. 2008; Paulos et al. 2010; Yang et al. 2008a). A series of surface markers have been identified for human Th17 cells. First, the capacity of $CD4^+$ T helper cells to produce IL-17 is associated with the coexpression of CCR6 and CCR4 (Acosta-Rodriguez et al. 2007b). Within inflamed tissues (particularly in chronic inflammatory bowel disease, but also in joints of rheumatoid arthritis patients), IL-17-producing T helper cells (as well as $CD8^+$ T cells) are entirely comprised within the $CD26^+$ and $CD161^+$ compartment and similar to CCR6, CD161 has been hypothesized to be a homing molecule for inflamed tissues (Cosmi et al. 2008). Based on these observations, it is likely that the significance of Th17 cells is equally well explained by their specific effector functions as by their preferred recruitment to distinct anatomical or functional niches during inflammatory reactions. Th17 cells exhibit very distinct homing properties to epithelial (and perhaps neuroectodermal) tissues. The idea of a niche-specific operational mode of the adaptive immune response is an emerging concept and here, Th17 cells might serve as an example. In the CNS, an increasing number of reports suggests that Th17 cells induce a different lesion topography as opposed to Th1 cells (Kroenke et al. 2008; Reboldi et al. 2009; Rothhammer et al. 2011; Stromnes et al. 2008). Even more, in neuromyelitis optica where the immune response is particularly pronounced at the CSF/glia limitans interface, a Th17 type of response might be pathogenetically relevant because granulocytes are found and IL-6 and IL-17 are elevated in the CSF of these patients as compared with individuals with MS (Chihara et al. 2011; Ishizu et al. 2005; Uzawa et al. 2009). This idea does not refute the assumption that in NMO, anti-AQP4 antibodies contribute to the pathology (Bennett et al. 2009; Bradl et al. 2009), but rather highlights the concept that in order for these NMO-IgG antibodies to unfold their effector functions at the glia limitans of the spinal cord and the optic nerve, a niche-specific—and perhaps Th17-dominated—immune response is required (Carlson et al. 2008; Kivisakk et al. 2009).

In summary, human Th17 cells are probably directly involved in the generation of MS lesions. Similar to what has been observed in murine EAE—human Th17 cells are most likely plastic and coproduce IFN-γ, but have very distinct properties from classic Th1 cells.

1.8 Therapeutic Interventions Targeting Th17 cells

Recent studies on Th1- or Th17-dependent immunopathology in MS and EAE suggest that our knowledge on T cell biology may not only form the basis for the development of new therapeutic interventions in CNS-specific autoimmunity (see below), but may also help us to better stratify patients for already established MS therapeutics. For example, when comparing Th1 versus Th17 cell-induced adoptive transfer EAE, it had been suggested that the Th1-driven disease process was responsive to IFN-β treatment, while IFN-β was inefficient or even worsened the clinical disease in Th17-induced EAE (Axtell et al. 2010). Although IFN-β suppressed the generation of Th17 cells from PBMCs in vitro (perhaps through induction of IL-27; Durelli et al. 2009), it still exacerbated Th17-induced EAE because under conditions of a Th17-driven disease process, IFN-β failed to induce IL-10 in T cells—a process, which is mainly dependent on IFN-γ signaling into APCs. In this in vivo model, IFN-β and IFN-γ most likely cooperated to induce IL-27 in APCs, which in turn induced IL-10 and suppressed IL-17 in T cells (Axtell et al. 2010). This regulatory loop appeared to fail in the absence of sufficient IFN-γ signaling. Indeed, clinical experience with a subset of human MS patients and patients with neuromyelitis optica where the inflammatory process—at least phenomenologically—is driven by neuroantigen-specific Th17 responses supports the idea that IFN-β is inappropriate in this scenario and may even worsen the disease (Kim et al. 2012; Palace et al. 2010). This appears to be also true for a specific subset of MS patients. Yet, there is an ongoing debate whether the measurement of IL-17F in the serum of MS patients before treatment could serve as a biomarker to decide whether or not IFN-β therapy would be efficient. Low serum levels of IL-7 and high levels of IL-17F were proposed to identify potential nonresponders to IFN-β treatment (Lee et al. 2011a). However, this finding was not reproduced in a much larger and well-defined cohort of patients from the dose–response trial of IFN-β1a (Avonex; Bushnell et al. 2012). Since Th17 cells produce a panel of cytokines and also induce a number of effector molecules from the target tissue, it might not be advisable to segment patients on the basis of single cytokines in the serum, which may not reliably reflect the disease process emerging in the CNS.

As a result of the growing understanding of the development and effector functions of Th17 cells, more specific agents that target the IL-23/IL-17 axis are being developed for MS. For example, a phase II study to assess the efficacy of a monoclonal neutralizing antibody to IL-17A (AIN457, secukinumab) on the reduction of MRI activity in relapsing remitting MS has just been completed and will now be followed by a larger phase II trial. Anti-IL-17 treatment—either with a monoclonal antibody to IL-17A (ixekizumab) or a monoclonal antibody to IL-17RA (brodalumab)—proved extremely efficient in psoriasis (Leonardi et al. 2012; Papp et al. 2012) without giving any safety concerns. Notably, while IL-17 is a very prominent effector molecule in skin inflammation that is not only produced by Th17 cells, but also by dermal-derived γδ T cells and innate immune cells (Korn and Petermann 2012; Pantelyushin et al. 2012), the network of effector cytokines in MS (and EAE) is likely to be more complicated, especially since Th17 cells acquire the ability to produce other cytokines once they infiltrate the CNS. In particular, the plasticity of Th17 cells—once recruited to the CNS—is a factor that should be taken into consideration. Yet, based on the data from mouse models and known effector functions of IL-17A, it is anticipated that anti-IL-17 therapy will also be efficacious in MS. It has been quite disappointing, though, that treatment of MS patients with a monoclonal antibody to the p40 subunit, which is common to both IL-12 and IL-23, failed to halt the inflammatory process as measured by gadolinium enhancement in the brain (Segal et al. 2008). However, anti-p40—by virtue of suppressing both Th1 and Th17 cells—might not be equivalent to suppressing just Th17 cells. The fact that IL-12 has the capacity to promote the production of anti-inflammatory IL-10 in T cells under certain circumstances (Jankovic et al. 2007) raises the possibility that IL-12 (in contrast to IL-23, which suppresses the induction of IL-10) might acquire immunomodulatory functions in the course of an inflammatory reaction.

1.9 Concluding Remarks

The investigation of T cell development and T cell fate decisions in vivo will be a highly urgent project in the coming years in order to understand the immunopathology of chronic inflammation and autoimmunity. Here, model diseases such as EAE can be very insightful when the appropriate questions are being asked. Indeed, unexpected findings in the EAE model kept spurring progress in our understanding of T helper cell biology and development of CNS autoimmune disease. Although it is unlikely that a sole pathogenic effector cytokine is entirely responsible for inducing EAE (or

MS), it might well be possible to identify "pathogenic effector programs" within T helper cells that may be driven by transcription factors such as Stat3, Ror-γt, or T-bet. Furthermore, it is an inappropriate oversimplification to exclusively allot the expression of these transcription factors to just one T cell subset. For example, Th17 cells are able to express the Th1 transcription factor T-bet upon sensing particular cytokine cues in the target organ and only then take on highly proinflammatory effector functions (Hegazy et al. 2010; Hirota et al. 2011).

The development of proinflammatory effector T cell responses has several checkpoints. Early during the response—perhaps during T cell priming in secondary lymphoid tissue or in the gut—the availability of IL-6 might dictate whether a pathogenic or a regulatory adaptive T cell response is triggered (Bettelli et al. 2006; Korn et al. 2007). In contrast, a late checkpoint might be the decision whether a proinflammatory response will be transient or sustained. Here, the responsiveness of T cells to IL-23 whose receptor is not expressed on naive T cells but on effector T cells that are committed to the Th17 lineage, will determine the acquisition of sustained proinflammatory effector functions. The response to IL-23 may no longer be exclusively associated with the expression of a pure "Th17" gene program, but may also include the induction of IFN-γ and GM-CSF in Th17 cells. Interestingly, classically committed Th1 cells that keep sensing IL-12 together with sustained TCR stimulation switch on downmodulatory programs and start producing IL-10, which limits their ability to induce inflammation (Berghmans et al. 2006; Chang et al. 2007; Gabrysova et al. 2009; Jankovic et al. 2007; Kemp et al. 2010).

It will be important to understand the molecular mechanism of these late checkpoints in order to identify molecules that can be therapeutically targeted in autoimmune diseases such as MS where the initial steps of T cell commitment have already occurred when the diagnosis is made. At the present state of knowledge, we anticipate that the disease process in MS is dependent on Th17 cells and will be partly dependent on the cytokine IL-17 itself. Yet, when developing compounds for clinical use, it is crucial to consider that targeting effector Th17 cells in general is not going to be equivalent to targeting one solitary effector cytokine of Th17 cells.

Acknowledgments We would like to thank Christopher Sie for helping to prepare the figures and Meike Mitsdörffer for discussing and proof-reading the manuscript. Thomas Korn is recipient of a Heisenberg grant and other grants from the Deutsche Forschungsgemeinschaft (KO 2964/3-2, KO 2964/4-2, and KO 2964/5-1). The authors have no conflicting financial interests.

References

Acosta-Rodriguez EV, Napolitani G, Lanzavecchia A, Sallusto F (2007a) Interleukins 1beta and 6 but not transforming growth factor-beta are essential for the differentiation of interleukin 17-producing human T helper cells. Nat Immunol 8:942–949

Acosta-Rodriguez EV, Rivino L, Geginat J, Jarrossay D, Gattorno M, Lanzavecchia A, Sallusto F, Napolitani G (2007b) Surface phenotype and antigenic specificity of human interleukin 17-producing T helper memory cells. Nat Immunol 8:639–646

Atarashi K, Tanoue T, Shima T, Imaoka A, Kuwahara T, Momose Y, Cheng G, Yamasaki S, Saito T, Ohba Y, Taniguchi T, Takeda K, Hori S, Ivanov II, Umesaki Y, Itoh K, Honda K (2011) Induction of colonic regulatory T cells by indigenous *Clostridium* species. Science 331:337–341

Awasthi A, Riol-Blanco L, Jager A, Korn T, Pot C, Galileos G, Bettelli E, Kuchroo VK, Oukka M (2009) Cutting edge: IL-23 receptor gfp reporter mice reveal distinct populations of IL-17-producing cells. J Immunol 182:5904–5908

Axtell RC, Jong BA de, Boniface K, Voort LF van der, Bhat R, Sarno P De, Naves R, Han M, Zhong F, Castellanos JG, Mair R, Christakos A, Kolkowitz I, Katz L, Killestein J, Polman CH, Waal Malefyt R de, Steinman L, Raman C (2010) T helper type 1 and 17 cells determine efficacy of interferon-beta in multiple sclerosis and experimental encephalomyelitis. Nat Med 16:406–412

Becher B, Durell BG, Noelle RJ (2002) Experimental autoimmune encephalitis and inflammation in the absence of interleukin-12. J Clin Invest 110:493–497

Bennett JL, Lam C, Kalluri SR, Saikali P, Bautista K, Dupree C, Glogowska M, Case D, Antel JP, Owens GP, Gilden D, Nessler S, Stadelmann C, Hemmer B (2009) Intrathecal pathogenic anti-aquaporin-4 antibodies in early neuromyelitis optica. Ann Neurol 66:617–629

Benson MJ, Pino-Lagos K, Rosemblatt M, Noelle RJ (2007) All-trans retinoic acid mediates enhanced T reg cell growth, differentiation, and gut homing in the face of high levels of co-stimulation. J Exp Med 204:1765–1774

Berer K, Mues M, Koutrolos M, Rasbi ZA, Boziki M, Johner C, Wekerle H, Krishnamoorthy G (2011) Commensal microbiota and myelin autoantigen cooperate to trigger autoimmune demyelination. Nature 479:538–541

Berghmans N, Dillen C, Heremans H (2006) Exogenous IL-12 suppresses experimental autoimmune encephalomyelitis (EAE) by tuning IL-10 and IL-5 levels in an IFN-gamma-dependent way. J Neuroimmunol 176:63–75

Bettelli E, Sullivan B, Szabo SJ, Sobel RA, Glimcher LH, Kuchroo VK (2004) Loss of T-bet, but not STAT1, prevents the development of experimental autoimmune encephalomyelitis. J Exp Med 200:79–87

Bettelli E, Carrier Y, Gao W, Korn T, Strom TB, Oukka M, Weiner HL, Kuchroo VK (2006) Reciprocal developmental pathways for the generation of pathogenic effector TH17 and regulatory T cells. Nature 441:235–238

Bradl M, Misu T, Takahashi T, Watanabe M, Mader S, Reindl M, Adzemovic M, Bauer J, Berger T, Fujihara K, Itoyama Y, Lassmann H (2009) Neuromyelitis optica: pathogenicity of patient immunoglobulin in vivo. Ann Neurol 66:630–643

Brown DA, Sawchenko PE (2007) Time course and distribution of inflammatory and neurodegenerative events suggest structural bases for the pathogenesis of experimental autoimmune encephalomyelitis. J Comp Neurol 502:236–260

Brucklacher-Waldert V, Stuerner K, Kolster M, Wolthausen J, Tolosa E (2009) Phenotypical and functional characterization of T helper 17 cells in multiple sclerosis. Brain 132:3329–3341

Brustle A, Heink S, Huber M, Rosenplanter C, Stadelmann C, Yu P, Arpaia E, Mak TW, Kamradt T, Lohoff M (2007) The development of inflammatory T(H)-17 cells requires interferon-regulatory factor 4. Nat Immunol 8:958–966

Bushnell SE, Zhao Z, Stebbins CC, Cadavid D, Buko AM, Whalley ET, Davis JA, Versage EM, Richert JR, Axtell RC, Steinman L, Medori R. (2012) Serum IL-17 F does not predict poor response to IM IFNbeta-1a in relapsing-remitting MS. Neurology 79:531–537

Carlson T, Kroenke M, Rao P, Lane TE, Segal B (2008) The Th17-ELR+ CXC chemokine pathway is essential for the development of central nervous system autoimmune disease. J Exp Med 205:811–823

Chang H, Hanawa H, Liu H, Yoshida T, Hayashi M, Watanabe R, Abe S, Toba K, Yoshida K, Elnaggar R, Minagawa S, Okura Y, Kato K, Kodama M, Maruyama H, Miyazaki J, Aizawa Y (2006) Hydrodynamic-based delivery of an interleukin-22-Ig fusion gene ameliorates experimental autoimmune myocarditis in rats. J Immunol 177:3635–3643

Chang HD, Helbig C, Tykocinski L, Kreher S, Koeck J, Niesner U, Radbruch A (2007) Expression of IL-10 in Th memory lymphocytes is conditional on IL-12 or IL-4, unless the IL-10 gene is imprinted by GATA-3. Eur J Immunol 37:807–817

Chaudhry A, Samstein RM, Treuting P, Liang Y, Pils MC, Heinrich JM, Jack RS, Wunderlich FT, Bruning JC, Muller W, Rudensky AY (2011) Interleukin-10 signaling in regulatory T cells is required for suppression of Th17 cell-mediated inflammation. Immunity 34:566–578

Chihara N, Aranami T, Sato W, Miyazaki Y, Miyake S, Okamoto T, Ogawa M, Toda T, Yamamura T (2011) Interleukin 6 signaling promotes anti-aquaporin 4 autoantibody production from plasmablasts in neuromyelitis optica. Proc Natl Acad Sci U S A 108:3701–3706

Chu CQ, Wittmer S, Dalton DK (2000) Failure to suppress the expansion of the activated CD4 T cell population in interferon gamma-deficient mice leads to exacerbation of experimental autoimmune encephalomyelitis. J Exp Med 192:123–128

Codarri L, Gyulveszi G, Tosevski V, Hesske L, Fontana A, Magnenat L, Suter T, Becher B (2011) RORgammat drives production of the cytokine GM-CSF in helper T cells, which is essential for the effector phase of autoimmune neuroinflammation. Nat Immunol 12:560–567

Coombes JL, Powrie F (2008) Dendritic cells in intestinal immune regulation. Nat Rev Immunol 8:435–446

Coombes JL, Siddiqui KR, Arancibia-Carcamo CV, Hall J, Sun CM, Belkaid Y, Powrie F (2007) A functionally specialized population of mucosal CD103+ DCs induces Foxp+ regulatory T cells via a TGF-beta and retinoic acid-dependent mechanism. J Exp Med 204:1757–1764

Cosmi L, Palma R De, Santarlasci V, Maggi L, Capone M, Frosali F, Rodolico G, Querci V, Abbate G, Angeli R, Berrino L, Fambrini M, Caproni M, Tonelli F, Lazzeri E, Parronchi P, Liotta F, Maggi E, Romagnani S, Annunziato F (2008) Human interleukin 17-producing cells originate from a CD161+ CD4+ T cell precursor. J Exp Med 205:1903–1916

Cua DJ, Tato CM (2010) Innate IL-17-producing cells: the sentinels of the immune system. Nat Rev Immunol 10:479–489

Cua DJ, Sherlock J, Chen Y, Murphy CA, Joyce B, Seymour B, Lucian L, To W, Kwan S, Churakova T, Zurawski S, Wiekowski M, Lira SA, Gorman D, Kastelein RA, Sedgwick JD (2003) Interleukin-23 rather than interleukin-12 is the critical cytokine for autoimmune inflammation of the brain. Nature 421:744–748

DePaolo RW, Abadie V, Tang F, Fehlner-Peach H, Hall JA, Wang W, Marietta EV, Kasarda DD, Waldmann TA, Murray JA, Semrad C, Kupfer SS, Belkaid Y, Guandalini S, Jabri B (2011) Co-adjuvant effects of retinoic acid and IL-15 induce inflammatory immunity to dietary antigens. Nature 471:220–224

Devadas S, Das J, Liu C, Zhang L, Roberts AI, Pan Z, Moore PA, Das G, Shi Y (2006) Granzyme B is critical for T cell receptor-induced cell death of type 2 helper T cells. Immunity 25:237–247

Duerr RH, Taylor KD, Brant SR, Rioux JD, Silverberg MS, Daly MJ, Steinhart AH, Abraham C, Regueiro M, Griffiths A, Dassopoulos T, Bitton A, Yang H, Targan S, Datta LW, Kistner EO, Schumm LP, Lee AT, Gregersen PK, Barmada MM, Rotter JI, Nicolae DL, Cho JH (2006) A genome-wide association study identifies IL23R as an inflammatory bowel disease gene. Science 314:1461–1463

Durelli L, Conti L, Clerico M, Boselli D, Contessa G, Ripellino P, Ferrero B, Eid P, Novelli F (2009) T-helper 17 cells expand in multiple sclerosis and are inhibited by interferon-beta. Ann Neurol 65:499–509

Ferber IA, Brocke S, Taylor-Edwards C, Ridgway W, Dinisco C, Steinman L, Dalton D, Fathman CG (1996) Mice with a disrupted IFN-gamma gene are susceptible to the induction of experimental autoimmune encephalomyelitis (EAE). J Immunol 156:5–7

Gabrysova L, Nicolson KS, Streeter HB, Verhagen J, Sabatos-Peyton CA, Morgan DJ, Wraith DC (2009) Negative feedback control of the autoimmune response through antigen-induced differentiation of IL-10-secreting Th1 cells. J Exp Med 206:1755–1767

Ghoreschi K, Laurence A, Yang XP, Tato CM, McGeachy MJ, Konkel JE, Ramos HL, Wei L, Davidson TS, Bouladoux N, Grainger JR, Chen Q, Kanno Y, Watford WT, Sun HW, Eberl G, Shevach EM, Belkaid Y, Cua DJ, Chen W, O'Shea JJ (2010) Generation of pathogenic T(H)17 cells in the absence of TGF-beta signalling. Nature 467:967–971

Haak S, Croxford AL, Kreymborg K, Heppner FL, Pouly S, Becher B, Waisman A (2009) IL-17 A and IL-17 F do not contribute vitally to autoimmune neuro-inflammation in mice. J Clin Invest 119:61–69

Harrington LE, Hatton RD, Mangan PR, Turner H, Murphy TL, Murphy KM, Weaver CT (2005) Interleukin 17-producing CD4+ effector T cells develop via a lineage distinct from the T helper type 1 and 2 lineages. Nat Immunol 6:1123–1132

Hegazy AN, Peine M, Helmstetter C, Panse I, Frohlich A, Bergthaler A, Flatz L, Pinschewer DD, Radbruch A, Lohning M (2010) Interferons direct Th2 cell reprogramming to generate a stable GATA-3(+)T-bet(+) cell subset with combined Th2 and Th1 cell functions. Immunity 32:116–128

Hirota K, Duarte JH, Veldhoen M, Hornsby E, Li Y, Cua DJ, Ahlfors H, Wilhelm C, Tolaini M, Menzel U, Garefalaki A, Potocnik AJ, Stockinger B (2011) Fate mapping of IL-17-producing T cells in inflammatory responses. Nat Immunol 12:255–263

Honda K, Littman DR (2012) The microbiome in infectious disease and inflammation. Annu Rev Immunol 30:759–795

Howell OW, Reeves CA, Nicholas R, Carassiti D, Radotra B, Gentleman SM, Serafini B, Aloisi F, Roncaroli F, Magliozzi R, Reynolds R (2011) Meningeal inflammation is widespread and linked to cortical pathology in multiple sclerosis. Brain 134:2755–2771

Hsieh CS, Macatonia SE, Tripp CS, Wolf SF, O'Garra A, Murphy KM (1993) Development of TH1 CD4+ T cells through IL-12 produced by Listeria-induced macrophages. Science 260:547–549

Hu W, Troutman TD, Edukulla R, Pasare C. 2011. Priming microenvironments dictate cytokine requirements for T Helper 17 cell lineage commitment. Immunity 35(6):1010–1022

Huber S, Gagliani N, Esplugues E, O'Connor W Jr, Huber FJ, Chaudhry A, Kamanaka M, Kobayashi Y, Booth CJ, Rudensky AY, Roncarolo MG, Battaglia M, Flavell RA (2011) Th17 cells express interleukin-10 receptor and are controlled by Foxp3 and Foxp3+ regulatory CD4+ T cells in an interleukin-10-dependent manner. Immunity 34:554–565

Ishizu T, Osoegawa M, Mei FJ, Kikuchi H, Tanaka M, Takakura Y, Minohara M, Murai H, Mihara F, Taniwaki T, Kira J (2005) Intrathecal activation of the IL-17/IL-8 axis in opticospinal multiple sclerosis. Brain 128:988–1002

Ivanov II, McKenzie BS, Zhou L, Tadokoro CE, Lepelley A, Lafaille JJ, Cua DJ, Littman DR (2006) The orphan nuclear receptor RORgammat directs the differentiation program of proinflammatory IL-17(+) T helper cells. Cell 126:1121–1133

Ivanov II, Atarashi K, Manel N, Brodie EL, Shima T, Karaoz U, Wei D, Goldfarb KC, Santee CA, Lynch SV, Tanoue T, Imaoka A, Itoh K, Takeda K, Umesaki Y, Honda K, Littman DR (2009) Induction of intestinal Th17 cells by segmented filamentous bacteria. Cell 139:485–498

Iwakura Y, Ishigame H, Saijo S, Nakae S (2011) Functional specialization of interleukin-17 family members. Immunity 34:149–162

Jager A, Dardalhon V, Sobel RA, Bettelli E, Kuchroo VK (2009) Th1, Th17, and Th9 effector cells induce experimental autoimmune encephalomyelitis with different pathological phenotypes. J Immunol 183:7169–7177

Jankovic D, Kullberg MC, Feng CG, Goldszmid RS, Collazo CM, Wilson M, Wynn TA, Kamanaka M, Flavell RA, Sher A (2007) Conventional T-bet(+)Foxp3(-) Th1 cells are the major source of host-protective regulatory IL-10 during intracellular protozoan infection. J Exp Med 204:273–283

Janson PC, Linton LB, Bergman EA, Marits P, Eberhardson M, Piehl F, Malmstrom V, Winqvist O (2011) Profiling of CD4+ T cells with epigenetic immune lineage analysis. J Immunol 186:92–102

Kang Z, Altuntas CZ, Gulen MF, Liu C, Giltiay N, Qin H, Liu L, Qian W, Ransohoff RM, Bergmann C, Stohlman S, Tuohy VK, Li X (2010) Astrocyte-restricted ablation of interleukin-17-induced Act1-mediated signaling ameliorates autoimmune encephalomyelitis. Immunity 32:414–425

Kappos L, Radue EW, O'Connor P, Polman C, Hohlfeld R, Calabresi P, Selmaj K, Agoropoulou C, Leyk M, Zhang-Auberson L, Burtin P (2010) A placebo-controlled trial of oral fingolimod in relapsing multiple sclerosis. New Engl J Med 362:387–401

Kebir H, Kreymborg K, Ifergan I, Dodelet-Devillers A, Cayrol R, Bernard M, Giuliani F, Arbour N, Becher B, Prat A (2007) Human T(H)17 lymphocytes promote blood-brain barrier disruption and central nervous system inflammation. Nat Med 13:1173–1175

Kebir H, Ifergan I, Alvarez JI, Bernard M, Poirier J, Arbour N, Duquette P, Prat A (2009) Preferential recruitment of interferon-gamma-expressing TH17 cells in multiple sclerosis. Ann Neurol 66:390–402

Kemp KL, Levin SD, Stein PL (2010) Lck regulates IL-10 expression in memory-like Th1 cells. Eur J Immunol 40:3210–3219

Kim SH, Kim W, Li XF, Jung IJ, Kim HJ. (2012) Does interferon beta treatment exacerbate neuromyelitis optica spectrum disorder? Mult Scler 18(10):1480–1483

Kivisakk P, Imitola J, Rasmussen S, Elyaman W, Zhu B, Ransohoff RM, Khoury SJ (2009) Localizing central nervous system immune surveillance: meningeal antigen-presenting cells activate T cells during experimental autoimmune encephalomyelitis. Ann Neurol 65:457–469

Kolls JK, Linden A (2004) Interleukin-17 family members and inflammation. Immunity 21:467–476

Komiyama Y, Nakae S, Matsuki T, Nambu A, Ishigame H, Kakuta S, Sudo K, Iwakura Y (2006) IL-17 plays an important role in the development of experimental autoimmune encephalomyelitis. J Immunol 177:566–573

Korn T, Petermann F. (2012) Development and function of interleukin 17-producing gammadelta T cells. Ann N Y Acad Sci 1247:34–45

Korn T, Bettelli E, Gao W, Awasthi A, Jager A, Strom TB, Oukka M, Kuchroo VK (2007) IL-21 initiates an alternative pathway to induce proinflammatory T(H)17 cells. Nature 448:484–487

Korn T, Mitsdoerffer M, Croxford AL, Awasthi A, Dardalhon VA, Galileos G, Vollmar P, Stritesky GL, Kaplan MH, Waisman A, Kuchroo VK, Oukka M (2008) IL-6 controls Th17 immunity in vivo by inhibiting the conversion of conventional T cells into Foxp3+ regulatory T cells. Proc Natl Acad Sci U S A 105:18460–18465

Korn T, Bettelli E, Oukka M, Kuchroo VK (2009) IL-17 and Th17 Cells. Annu Rev Immunol 27:485–517

Korn T, Mitsdoerffer M, Kuchroo VK (2010) Immunological basis for the development of tissue inflammation and organ-specific autoimmunity in animal models of multiple sclerosis. Results Probl Cell Differ 51:43–74

Kreymborg K, Etzensperger R, Dumoutier L, Haak S, Rebollo A, Buch T, Heppner FL, Renauld JC, Becher B (2007) IL-22 is expressed by Th17 cells in an IL-23-dependent fashion, but not required for the development of autoimmune encephalomyelitis. J Immunol 179:8098–8104

Krishnamoorthy G, Saxena A, Mars LT, Domingues HS, Mentele R, Ben-Nun A, Lassmann H, Dornmair K, Kurschus FC, Liblau RS, Wekerle H (2009) Myelin-specific T cells also recognize neuronal autoantigen in a transgenic mouse model of multiple sclerosis. Nat Med 15:626–632

Kroenke MA, Carlson TJ, Andjelkovic AV, Segal BM (2008) IL-12- and IL-23-modulated T cells induce distinct types of EAE based on histology, CNS chemokine profile, and response to cytokine inhibition. J Exp Med 205:1535–1541

Lafaille JJ, Keere FV, Hsu AL, Baron JL, Haas W, Raine CS, Tonegawa S (1997) Myelin basic protein-specific T helper 2 (Th2) cells cause experimental autoimmune encephalomyelitis in immunodeficient hosts rather than protect them from the disease. J Exp Med 186:307–312

Langrish CL, Chen Y, Blumenschein WM, Mattson J, Basham B, Sedgwick JD, McClanahan T, Kastelein RA, Cua DJ (2005) IL-23 drives a pathogenic T cell population that induces autoimmune inflammation. J Exp Med 201:233–240

Lazarevic V, Chen X, Shim JH, Hwang ES, Jang E, Bolm AN, Oukka M, Kuchroo VK, Glimcher LH (2011) T-bet represses T(H)17 differentiation by preventing Runx1-mediated activation of the gene encoding RORgammat. Nat Immunol 12:96–104

Lee YK, Turner H, Maynard CL, Oliver JR, Chen D, Elson CO, Weaver CT (2009) Late developmental plasticity in the T helper 17 lineage. Immunity 30:92–107

Lee LF, Axtell R, Tu GH, Logronio K, Dilley J, Yu J, Rickert M, Han B, Evering W, Walker MG, Shi J, Jong BA de, Killestein J, Polman CH, Steinman L, Lin JC. (2011a) IL-7 promotes T(H)1 development and serum IL-7 predicts clinical response to interferon-beta in multiple sclerosis. Sci Transl Med 3:93ra68

Lee YK, Menezes JS, Umesaki Y, Mazmanian SK (2011b) Proinflammatory T-cell responses to gut microbiota promote experimental autoimmune encephalomyelitis. Proc Natl Acad Sci U S A 108(Suppl 1):4615–4622
Lee Y, Awasthi A, Yosef N, Quintana FJ, Xiao S, Peters A, Wu C, Kleinewietfeld M, Kunder S, Hafler D, Sobel RA, Regev A. (2012) Induction and molecular signature of pathogenic Th17 cells. Nat Immunol 13(10):991–999
Lees JR, Golumbek PT, Sim J, Dorsey D, Russell JH (2008) Regional CNS responses to IFN-gamma determine lesion localization patterns during EAE pathogenesis. J Exp Med 205:2633–2642
Leonardi C, Matheson R, Zachariae C, Cameron G, Li L, Edson-Heredia E, Braun D, Banerjee S (2012) Anti-interleukin-17 monoclonal antibody ixekizumab in chronic plaque psoriasis. New Engl J Med 366:1190–1199
Li MO, Wan YY, Flavell RA (2007) T Cell-Produced Transforming Growth Factor-beta1 Controls T Cell Tolerance and Regulates Th1- and Th17-Cell Differentiation. Immunity 26:579–591
Liu J, Marino MW, Wong G, Grail D, Dunn A, Bettadapura J, Slavin AJ, Old L, Bernard CC (1998) TNF is a potent anti-inflammatory cytokine in autoimmune-mediated demyelination. Nat Med 4:78–83
Lock C, Hermans G, Pedotti R, Brendolan A, Schadt E, Garren H, Langer-Gould A, Strober S, Cannella B, Allard J, Klonowski P, Austin A, Lad N, Kaminski N, Galli SJ, Oksenberg JR, Raine CS, Heller R, Steinman L (2002) Gene-microarray analysis of multiple sclerosis lesions yields new targets validated in autoimmune encephalomyelitis. Nat Med 8:500–508
Magliozzi R, Howell O, Vora A, Serafini B, Nicholas R, Puopolo M, Reynolds R, Aloisi F (2007) Meningeal B-cell follicles in secondary progressive multiple sclerosis associate with early onset of disease and severe cortical pathology. Brain 130:1089–1104
Magliozzi R, Howell OW, Reeves C, Roncaroli F, Nicholas R, Serafini B, Aloisi F, Reynolds R (2010) A gradient of neuronal loss and meningeal inflammation in multiple sclerosis. Ann Neurol 68:477–493
Manel N, Unutmaz D, Littman DR (2008) The differentiation of human T(H)-17 cells requires transforming growth factor-beta and induction of the nuclear receptor RORgammat. Nat Immunol 9:641–649
Mangan PR, Harrington LE, O'Quinn DB, Helms WS, Bullard DC, Elson CO, Hatton RD, Wahl SM, Schoeb TR, Weaver CT (2006) Transforming growth factor-beta induces development of the T(H)17 lineage. Nature 441:231–234
Matusevicius D, Kivisakk P, He B, Kostulas N, Ozenci V, Fredrikson S, Link H (1999) Interleukin-17 mRNA expression in blood and CSF mononuclear cells is augmented in multiple sclerosis. Mult Scler 5:101–104
McGeachy MJ, Bak-Jensen KS, Chen Y, Tato CM, Blumenschein W, McClanahan T, Cua DJ (2007) TGF-beta and IL-6 drive the production of IL-17 and IL-10 by T cells and restrain T(H)-17 cell-mediated pathology. Nat Immunol 8:1390–1397
McGeachy MJ, Chen Y, Tato CM, Laurence A, Joyce-Shaikh B, Blumenschein WM, McClanahan TK, O'Shea JJ, Cua DJ (2009) The interleukin 23 receptor is essential for the terminal differentiation of interleukin 17-producing effector T helper cells in vivo. Nat Immunol 10:314–324
McQualter JL, Darwiche R, Ewing C, Onuki M, Kay TW, Hamilton JA, Reid HH, Bernard CC (2001) Granulocyte macrophage colony-stimulating factor: a new putative therapeutic target in multiple sclerosis. J Exp Med 194:873–882
Meares GP, Ma X, Qin H, Benveniste EN (2012) Regulation of CCL20 expression in astrocytes by IL-6 and IL-17. Glia 60:771–781
Mehling M, Lindberg R, Raulf F, Kuhle J, Hess C, Kappos L, Brinkmann V (2010) Th17 central memory T cells are reduced by FTY720 in patients with multiple sclerosis. Neurology 75:403–410
Mitsdoerffer M, Lee Y, Jager A, Kim HJ, Korn T, Kolls JK, Cantor H, Bettelli E, Kuchroo VK (2010) Proinflammatory T helper type 17 cells are effective B-cell helpers. Proc Natl Acad Sci U S A 107:14292–14297

Montes M, Zhang X, Berthelot L, Laplaud DA, Brouard S, Jin J, Rogan S, Armao D, Jewells V, Soulillou JP, Markovic-Plese S (2009) Oligoclonal myelin-reactive T-cell infiltrates derived from multiple sclerosis lesions are enriched in Th17 cells. Clin Immunol 130:133–144
Mosmann TR, Cherwinski H, Bond MW, Giedlin MA, Coffman RL (1986) Two types of murine helper T cell clone. I. Definition according to profiles of lymphokine activities and secreted proteins. J Immunol 136:2348–2357
Muranski P, Borman ZA, Kerkar SP, Klebanoff CA, Ji Y, Sanchez-Perez L, Sukumar M, Reger RN, Yu Z, Kern SJ, Roychoudhuri R, Ferreyra GA, Shen W, Durum SK, Feigenbaum L, Palmer DC, Antony PA, Chan CC, Laurence A, Danner RL, Gattinoni L, Restifo NP (2011) Th17 cells are long lived and retain a stem cell-like molecular signature. Immunity 35:972–985
Murphy KM, Reiner SL (2002) The lineage decisions of helper T cells. Nat Rev Immunol 2:933–944
Murphy E, Shibuya K, Hosken N, Openshaw P, Maino V, Davis K, Murphy K, O'Garra A (1996) Reversibility of T helper 1 and 2 populations is lost after long-term stimulation. J Exp Med 183:901–913
Nair RP, Duffin KC, Helms C, Ding J, Stuart PE, Goldgar D, Gudjonsson JE, Li Y, Tejasvi T, Feng BJ, Ruether A, Schreiber S, Weichenthal M, Gladman D, Rahman P, Schrodi SJ, Prahalad S, Guthery SL, Fischer J, Liao W, Kwok PY, Menter A, Lathrop GM, Wise CA, Begovich AB, Voorhees JJ, Elder JT, Krueger GG, Bowcock AM, Abecasis GR (2009) Genome-wide scan reveals association of psoriasis with IL-23 and NF-kappaB pathways. Nat Genet 41:199–204
Niess JH, Adler G (2010) Enteric flora expands gut lamina propria CX3CR1+ dendritic cells supporting inflammatory immune responses under normal and inflammatory conditions. J Immunol 184:2026–2037
Palace J, Leite MI, Nairne A, Vincent A (2010) Interferon beta treatment in neuromyelitis optica: increase in relapses and aquaporin 4 antibody titers. Arch Neurol 67:1016–1017
Panitch HS, Hirsch RL, Schindler J, Johnson KP (1987) Treatment of multiple sclerosis with gamma interferon: exacerbations associated with activation of the immune system. Neurology 37:1097–1102
Pantelyushin S, Haak S, Ingold B, Kulig P, Heppner FL, Navarini AA, Becher B. (2012) Rorgammat+ innate lymphocytes and gammadelta T cells initiate psoriasiform plaque formation in mice. J Clin Invest 122(6):2252–2256
Papp KA, Leonardi C, Menter A, Ortonne JP, Krueger JG, Kricorian G, Aras G, Li J, Russell CB, Thompson EH, Baumgartner S (2012) Brodalumab, an anti-interleukin-17-receptor antibody for psoriasis. New Engl J Med 366:1181–1189
Park H, Li Z, Yang XO, Chang SH, Nurieva R, Wang YH, Wang Y, Hood L, Zhu Z, Tian Q, Dong C (2005) A distinct lineage of CD4 T cells regulates tissue inflammation by producing interleukin 17. Nat Immunol 6:1133–1141
Paulos CM, Carpenito C, Plesa G, Suhoski MM, Varela-Rohena A, Golovina TN, Carroll RG, Riley JL, June CH. (2010) The inducible costimulator (ICOS) is critical for the development of human T(H)17 cells. Sci Transl Med 2:55ra78
Pepper M, Linehan JL, Pagan AJ, Zell T, Dileepan T, Cleary PP, Jenkins MK (2010) Different routes of bacterial infection induce long-lived TH1 memory cells and short-lived TH17 cells. Nat Immunol 11:83–89
Peters A, Pitcher LA, Sullivan JM, Mitsdoerffer M, Acton SE, Franz B, Wucherpfennig K, Turley S, Carroll MC, Sobel RA, Bettelli E, Kuchroo VK (2011) Th17 cells induce ectopic lymphoid follicles in central nervous system tissue inflammation. Immunity 35:986–996
Reboldi A, Coisne C, Baumjohann D, Benvenuto F, Bottinelli D, Lira S, Uccelli A, Lanzavecchia A, Engelhardt B, Sallusto F (2009) C-C chemokine receptor 6-regulated entry of TH-17 cells into the CNS through the choroid plexus is required for the initiation of EAE. Nat Immunol 10:514–523
Rothhammer V, Heink S, Petermann F, Srivastava R, Claussen MC, Hemmer B, Korn T (2011) Th17 lymphocytes traffic to the central nervous system independently of alpha4 integrin expression during EAE. J Exp Med 208:2465–2476
Round JL, Mazmanian SK (2010) Inducible Foxp3+ regulatory T-cell development by a commensal bacterium of the intestinal microbiota. Proc Natl Acad Sci U S A 107:12204–12209

Rouvier E, Luciani MF, Mattei MG, Denizot F, Golstein P (1993) CTLA-8, cloned from an activated T cell, bearing AU-rich messenger RNA instability sequences, and homologous to a herpesvirus saimiri gene. J Immunol 150:5445–5456

Samoilova EB, Horton JL, Hilliard B, Liu TS, Chen Y (1998) IL-6-deficient mice are resistant to experimental autoimmune encephalomyelitis: roles of IL-6 in the activation and differentiation of autoreactive T cells. J Immunol 161:6480–6486

Sawcer S, Hellenthal G, Pirinen M, Spencer CC, Patsopoulos NA, Moutsianas L, Dilthey A, Su Z, Freeman C, Hunt SE, Edkins S, Gray E, Booth DR, Potter SC, Goris A, Band G, Oturai AB, Strange A, Saarela J, Bellenguez C, Fontaine B, Gillman M, Hemmer B, Gwilliam R, Zipp F, Jayakumar A, Martin R, Leslie S, Hawkins S, Giannoulatou E, D'Alfonso S, Blackburn H, Boneschi FM, Liddle J, Harbo HF, Perez ML, Spurkland A, Waller MJ, Mycko MP, Ricketts M, Comabella M, Hammond N, Kockum I, McCann OT, Ban M, Whittaker P, Kemppinen A, Weston P, Hawkins C, Widaa S, Zajicek J, Dronov S, Robertson N, Bumpstead SJ, Barcellos LF, Ravindrarajah R, Abraham R, Alfredsson L, Ardlie K, Aubin C, Baker A, Baker K, Baranzini SE, Bergamaschi L, Bergamaschi R, Bernstein A, Berthele A, Boggild M, Bradfield JP, Brassat D, Broadley SA, Buck D, Butzkueven H, Capra R, Carroll WM, Cavalla P, Celius EG, Cepok S, Chiavacci R, Clerget-Darpoux F, Clysters K, Comi G, Cossburn M, Cournu-Rebeix I, Cox MB, Cozen W, Cree BA, Cross AH, Cusi D, Daly MJ, Davis E, Bakker PI de, Debouverie M, D'Hooghe MB, Dixon K, Dobosi R, Dubois B, Ellinghaus D, Elovaara I, Esposito F, Fontenille C, Foote S, Franke A, Galimberti D, Ghezzi A, Glessner J, Gomez R, Gout O, Graham C, Grant SF, Guerini FR, Hakonarson H, Hall P, Hamsten A, Hartung HP, Heard RN, Heath S, Hobart J, Hoshi M, Infante-Duarte C, Ingram G, Ingram W, Islam T, Jagodic M, Kabesch M, Kermode AG, Kilpatrick TJ, Kim C, Klopp N, Koivisto K, Larsson M, Lathrop M, Lechner-Scott JS, Leone MA, Leppa V, Liljedahl U, Bomfim IL, Lincoln RR, Link J, Liu J, Lorentzen AR, Lupoli S, Macciardi F, Mack T, Marriott M, Martinelli V, Mason D, McCauley JL, Mentch F, Mero IL, Mihalova T, Montalban X, Mottershead J, Myhr KM, Naldi P, Ollier W, Page A, Palotie A, Pelletier J, Piccio L, Pickersgill T, Piehl F, Pobywajlo S, Quach HL, Ramsay PP, Reunanen M, Reynolds R, Rioux JD, Rodegher M, Roesner S, Rubio JP, Ruckert IM, Salvetti M, Salvi E, Santaniello A, Schaefer CA, Schreiber S, Schulze C, Scott RJ, Sellebjerg F, Selmaj KW, Sexton D, Shen L, Simms-Acuna B, Skidmore S, Sleiman PM, Smestad C, Sorensen PS, Sondergaard HB, Stankovich J, Strange RC, Sulonen AM, Sundqvist E, Syvanen AC, Taddeo F, Taylor B, Blackwell JM, Tienari P, Bramon E, Tourbah A, Brown MA, Tronczynska E, Casas JP, Tubridy N, Corvin A, Vickery J, Jankowski J, Villoslada P, Markus HS, Wang K, Mathew CG, Wason J, Palmer CN, Wichmann HE, Plomin R, Willoughby E, Rautanen A, Winkelmann J, Wittig M, Trembath RC, Yaouanq J, Viswanathan AC, Zhang H, Wood NW, Zuvich R, Deloukas P, Langford C, Duncanson A, Oksenberg JR, Pericak-Vance MA, Haines JL, Olsson T, Hillert J, Ivinson AJ,Jager PL De, Peltonen L, Stewart GJ, Hafler DA, Hauser SL, McVean G, Donnelly P, Compston A (2011) Genetic risk and a primary role for cell-mediated immune mechanisms in multiple sclerosis. Nature 476:214–219

Segal BM, Constantinescu CS, Raychaudhuri A, Kim L, Fidelus-Gort R, Kasper LH (2008) Repeated subcutaneous injections of IL12/23 p40 neutralising antibody, ustekinumab, in patients with relapsing-remitting multiple sclerosis: a phase II, double-blind, placebo-controlled, randomised, dose-ranging study. Lancet Neurol 7:796–804

Serafini B, Rosicarelli B, Magliozzi R, Stigliano E, Aloisi F (2004) Detection of ectopic B-cell follicles with germinal centers in the meninges of patients with secondary progressive multiple sclerosis. Brain Pathol 14:164–174

Sherlock JP, Joyce-Shaikh B, Turner SP, Chao CC, Sathe M, Grein J, Gorman DM, Bowman EP, McClanahan TK, Yearley JH, Eberl G, Buckley CD, Kastelein RA, Pierce RH, Laface DM, Cua DJ (2012) IL-23 induces spondyloarthropathy by acting on ROR-gammat(+) CD3(+)CD4(−)CD8(−) entheseal resident T cells. Nat Med 18:1069–1076

Sokol CL, Barton GM, Farr AG, Medzhitov R (2008) A mechanism for the initiation of allergen-induced T helper type 2 responses. Nat Immunol 9:310–318

Sokol CL, Chu NQ, Yu S, Nish SA, Laufer TM, Medzhitov R (2009) Basophils function as antigen-presenting cells for an allergen-induced T helper type 2 response. Nat Immunol 10:713–720

Sonderegger I, Kisielow J, Meier R, King C, Kopf M (2008) IL-21 and IL-21R are not required for development of Th17 cells and autoimmunity in vivo. Eur J Immunol 38:1833–1838
Stromnes IM, Cerretti LM, Liggitt D, Harris RA, Goverman JM (2008) Differential regulation of central nervous system autoimmunity by T(H)1 and T(H)17 cells. Nat Med 14:337–342
Stumhofer JS, Laurence A, Wilson EH, Huang E, Tato CM, Johnson LM, Villarino AV, Huang Q, Yoshimura A, Sehy D, Saris CJ, O'Shea JJ, Hennighausen L, Ernst M, Hunter CA (2006) Interleukin 27 negatively regulates the development of interleukin 17-producing T helper cells during chronic inflammation of the central nervous system. Nat Immunol 7:937–945
Stumhofer JS, Silver JS, Laurence A, Porrett PM, Harris TH, Turka LA, Ernst M, Saris CJ, O'Shea JJ, Hunter CA (2007) Interleukins 27 and 6 induce STAT3-mediated T cell production of interleukin 10. Nat Immunol 8:1363–1371
Sugimoto K, Ogawa A, Mizoguchi E, Shimomura Y, Andoh A, Bhan AK, Blumberg RS, Xavier RJ, Mizoguchi A (2008) IL-22 ameliorates intestinal inflammation in a mouse model of ulcerative colitis. J Clin Invest 118:534–544
Sun CM, Hall JA, Blank RB, Bouladoux N, Oukka M, Mora JR, Belkaid Y (2007) Small intestine lamina propria dendritic cells promote de novo generation of Foxp3 T reg cells via retinoic acid. J Exp Med 204:1775–1785
Sutton C, Brereton C, Keogh B, Mills KH, Lavelle EC (2006) A crucial role for interleukin (IL)-1 in the induction of IL-17-producing T cells that mediate autoimmune encephalomyelitis. J Exp Med 203:1685–1691
Traugott U, Lebon P (1988) Multiple sclerosis: involvement of interferons in lesion pathogenesis. Ann Neurol 24:243–251
Travis MA, Reizis B, Melton AC, Masteller E, Tang Q, Proctor JM, Wang Y, Bernstein X, Huang X, Reichardt LF, Bluestone JA, Sheppard D (2007) Loss of integrin alpha(v)beta8 on dendritic cells causes autoimmunity and colitis in mice. Nature 449:361–365
Tzartos JS, Friese MA, Craner MJ, Palace J, Newcombe J, Esiri MM, Fugger L (2008) Interleukin-17 production in central nervous system-infiltrating T cells and glial cells is associated with active disease in multiple sclerosis. Am J Pathol 172:146–155
Uzawa A, Mori M, Ito M, Uchida T, Hayakawa S, Masuda S, Kuwabara S (2009) Markedly increased CSF interleukin-6 levels in neuromyelitis optica, but not in multiple sclerosis. J Neurol 256:2082–2084
Veldhoen M, Hocking RJ, Atkins CJ, Locksley RM, Stockinger B (2006a) TGFbeta in the context of an inflammatory cytokine milieu supports de novo differentiation of IL-17-producing T cells. Immunity 24:179–189
Veldhoen M, Hocking RJ, Flavell RA, Stockinger B (2006b) Signals mediated by transforming growth factor-beta initiate autoimmune encephalomyelitis, but chronic inflammation is needed to sustain disease. Nat Immunol 7:1151–1156
Weaver CT, Hatton RD, Mangan PR, Harrington LE (2007) IL-17 Family Cytokines and the Expanding Diversity of Effector T Cell Lineages. Annu Rev Immunol 25:821–852
Wensky AK, Furtado GC, Marcondes MC, Chen S, Manfra D, Lira SA, Zagzag D, Lafaille JJ (2005) IFN-gamma determines distinct clinical outcomes in autoimmune encephalomyelitis. J Immunol 174:1416–1423
Willenborg DO, Fordham S, Bernard CC, Cowden WB, Ramshaw IA (1996) IFN-gamma plays a critical down-regulatory role in the induction and effector phase of myelin oligodendrocyte glycoprotein-induced autoimmune encephalomyelitis. J Immunol 157:3223–3227
Wilson NJ, Boniface K, Chan JR, McKenzie BS, Blumenschein WM, Mattson JD, Basham B, Smith K, Chen T, Morel F, Lecron JC, Kastelein RA, Cua DJ, McClanahan TK, Bowman EP, de Waal Malefyt R (2007) Development, cytokine profile and function of human interleukin 17-producing helper T cells. Nat Immunol 8:950–957
Wu HJ, Ivanov II, Darce J, Hattori K, Shima T, Umesaki Y, Littman DR, Benoist C, Mathis D (2010) Gut-residing segmented filamentous bacteria drive autoimmune arthritis via T helper 17 cells. Immunity 32:815–827

Yang XO, Panopoulos AD, Nurieva R, Chang SH, Wang D, Watowich SS, Dong C (2007) STAT3 regulates cytokine-mediated generation of inflammatory helper T cells. J Biol Chem 282:9358–9363
Yang L, Anderson DE, Baecher-Allan C, Hastings WD, Bettelli E, Oukka M, Kuchroo VK, Hafler DA (2008a) IL-21 and TGF-beta are required for differentiation of human T(H)17 cells. Nature 454:350–352
Yang XO, Chang SH, Park H, Nurieva R, Shah B, Acero L, Wang YH, Schluns KS, Broaddus RR, Zhu Z, Dong C (2008b) Regulation of inflammatory responses by IL-17 F. J Exp Med 205:1063–1075
Yang XO, Pappu BP, Nurieva R, Akimzhanov A, Kang HS, Chung Y, Ma L, Shah B, Panopoulos AD, Schluns KS, Watowich SS, Tian Q, Jetten AM, Dong C (2008c) T Helper 17 Lineage Differentiation Is Programmed by Orphan Nuclear Receptors RORalpha and RORgamma. Immunity 28:29–39
Yao Z, Painter SL, Fanslow WC, Ulrich D, Macduff BM, Spriggs MK, Armitage RJ (1995) Human IL-17: a novel cytokine derived from T cells. J Immunol 155:5483–5486
Zenewicz LA, Yancopoulos GD, Valenzuela DM, Murphy AJ, Karow M, Flavell RA (2007) Interleukin-22 but not interleukin-17 provides protection to hepatocytes during acute liver inflammation. Immunity 27:647–659
Zhang X, Brunner T, Carter L, Dutton RW, Rogers P, Bradley L, Sato T, Reed JC, Green D, Swain SL (1997) Unequal death in T helper cell (Th)1 and Th2 effectors: Th1, but not Th2, effectors undergo rapid Fas/FasL-mediated apoptosis. J Exp Med 185:1837–1849
Zhou L, Ivanov II, Spolski R, Min R, Shenderov K, Egawa T, Levy DE, Leonard WJ, Littman DR (2007) IL-6 programs T(H)-17 cell differentiation by promoting sequential engagement of the IL-21 and IL-23 pathways. Nat Immunol 8:967–974
Zielinski CE, Mele F, Aschenbrenner D, Jarrossay D, Ronchi F, Gattorno M, Monticelli S, Lanzavecchia A, Sallusto F (2012) Pathogen-induced human TH17 cells produce IFN-gamma or IL-10 and are regulated by IL-1beta. Nature 484:514–518

Chapter 2
Regulatory T Cells in MS

Barbara B. Gawlik and David A. Hafler

2.1 Introduction

Multiple sclerosis (MS) is a multifocal demyelinating disease of the central nervous system (CNS), caused by an autoimmune response to self-antigens in a genetically susceptible individual. It is characterized by progressive neurodegeneration and by CNS lesions containing a high number of infiltrating autoreactive B and T cells. In healthy individuals, regulatory T (Treg) cells can control potentially pathogenic autoreactive T cells, while Treg cells in MS patients show insufficient regulatory abilities. The fact that autoreactive T cells can be found in the peripheral blood of healthy individuals without causing any autoimmune diseases underlies the importance of an efficient control of immune responses. Treg cells are key regulators of immune homeostasis and self-tolerance.

Treg cells have been defined as $CD4^+CD25^+FoxP3^+$ Tcells that are capable of modulating the immune function of various effector cells. Other T cells have been described to also possess regulatory activity such as IL-10- secreting type 1 regulatory (T_R1) cells and transforming growth factor β (TGFβ)-secreting T helper 3 (T_H3) cells (Roncarolo et al. 2001; Weiner 2001). The population of $CD4^+CD25^+FoxP3^+$ Treg cells comprises two subpopulations: naturally occurring and induced Treg cells (Curotto de Lafaille and Lafaille 2009). Naturally occurring Treg cells differ from induced Treg cells in being a distinct Treg cell subpopulation specialized for suppressive function that has been determined during its development in the thymus. Studies investigating immunological dysfunctions in autoimmune diseases need to consider the complex composition of the human Treg cell repertoire.

B. B. Gawlik (✉) · D. A. Hafler
Departments of Neurology and Immunobiology, Yale School of Medicine,
New Haven, CT 06520, USA
e-mail: barbara.gawlik@ukb.uni-bonn.de

T. Yamamura, B. Gran (eds.), *Multiple Sclerosis Immunology*,
DOI 10.1007/978-1-4614-7953-6_2, © Springer Science+Business Media New York 2013

2.2 Treg Cells

2.2.1 Cell Surface Characterization and Plasticity of Treg Cells

Treg cells were initially defined as $CD4^+CD25^+$ cells in mice. Human Treg cells have been described as a population of $CD4^+CD25^{high}$ T cells in the peripheral blood and the thymus (Taams et al. 2002; Baecher-Allan et al. 2001; Dieckmann et al. 2001; Jonuleit et al. 2001; Levings et al. 2001; Ng et al. 2001; Sakaguchi et al. 1995). The characterization of human $CD4^+$ Treg cells is complex as the human Treg cell population is heterogeneous (Miyara et al. 2009; Ito et al. 2008). Only 1–2 % of the total $CD4^+$T cell population in the human peripheral blood consist of $CD25^{high}$ T cells (Baecher-Allan et al. 2001). Moreover, the isolation of Treg cells with high CD25 expression would lead to the exclusion of the naive, $CD4^+FoxP3^{low}CD25^{mid}$ Treg cell population.

2.2.1.1 Forkhead Box P3 (FoxP3) Is Essential for Immune Homeostasis

The transcription factor FoxP3 has been established as a specific marker for mouse Treg cells and as a cell surface marker for human Treg cells (Fontenot et al. 2003; Hori et al. 2003; Roncador et al. 2001). The importance of FoxP3 for immune homeostasis can be illustrated by the observation that scurfy mice, X-chromosome-linked mouse mutants, show a defect in the FoxP3 gene and a lack of scurfin, the protein that is encoded by FoxP3. This defective gene function results in a lethal disorder in mice similar to the Wiskott–Aldrich syndrome, involving scaly skin, gastrointestinal bleeding, hepatosplenomegaly, and severe anemia. The disorder is mediated by $CD4^+CD8^-$ T cells whose activity has been shown to be improperly regulated in scurfy mice (Brunkow et al. 2001; Kanangat et al. 1996; Lyon et al. 1990; Blair et al. 1994). Moreover, mutations in human FoxP3 have been identified to cause the rare, fatal immunodysregulation, polyendocrinopathy, enteropathy, X-linked syndrome (IPEX). Affected patients show, among other symptoms, a neonatal onset of type 1 diabetes mellitus, immune dysregulation, anemia, eczema, thrombocytopenia, and hypothyroidism (Bennett et al. 2001; Wildin et al. 2001, 2002).

2.2.1.2 Cell Surface Characterization of Treg Cells

In the search for an additional marker for Treg cells, it has been observed by several groups that $CD4^+FoxP3^+$ T cells with high suppressive ability downregulate CD127 (IL-7Rα) on the cell surface (Liu et al. 2006; Seddiki et al. 2006a). High CD25 and low CD127 expression can therefore be used to isolate human Treg cells from the peripheral blood. However, it has also been described that nonregulatory $CD4^+$ T cells downregulate the expression of CD127 after they have been activated, indicating that low expression of CD127 combined with the expression of CD25 cannot be used to sufficiently distinguish between activated $CD4^+$ T cells and Treg cells (Mazzucchelli and Durum 2007). Moreover, the fact that nonregulatory $CD4^+CD25^+$ T cells expressing low levels of FoxP3 and CD127 exist, impairs the significance of a staining with CD25 and CD127 in order to isolate Treg cells (Miyara et al. 2009). These nonregulatory Treg cells produce proinflammatory cytokines such as IL-2 and interferon-γ (IFN-γ), but do not show suppressive ability in vitro. Thus, the methylation status of the FoxP3 gene can be linked to the difference between regulatory and nonregulatory $FoxP3^+$ T cells, with $FoxP3^+$ Treg cells being completely and nonregulatory $FoxP3^+CD4^+$ T cells being incompletely demethylated (Miyara et al. 2009). Even though CD62L (L-Selectin) is not exclusively expressed on Treg cells, it is considered an effective marker to discriminate Treg cells ($CD62L^+$) from activated $CD4^+$ T cells ($CD62L^{low}$) utilizing the fact that CD62L expression is downregulated after activation (Hamann et al. 2000). Reflecting their suppressive role, $CD25^+FoxP3^+$ Treg cells also express cytotoxic T lymphocyte antigen 4 (CTLA4 and glucocorticoid-induced TNF-receptor-related protein (GITR)). The expression of these molecules correlates with the expression of FoxP3. Nevertheless, these markers are not solely expressed on Treg cells (Levings et al. 2001; Fontenot et al. 2003; Hori et al. 2003; Khattri et al. 2003).

2.2.1.3 Treg Cell Plasticity

The human Treg cell population is characterized by a significant heterogeneity that needs to be taken into account when performing and analyzing suppression assays. In addition to the markers noted above, the expression of CD45RA or CD45RO identifies functionally different Treg cell phenotypes, "naive" and "effector" Treg cells (Miyara et al. 2009; Seddiki et al. 2006b; Valmori et al. 2005; Fritzsching et al. 2006). $CD45RA^+CD45RO^-FoxP3^{low}$-naive Treg cells express CD31 (PECAM1), a surface marker for cells that have emigrated from the thymus recently, but only low levels of FoxP3 (Miyara et al. 2009; Valmori et al. 2005; Fritzsching et al. 2006; Kimmig et al. 2002). Reflecting the finding that naive Treg cells are more common in the human cord blood, their proportion among the $CD4^+$ T cells in the human peripheral blood declines with age. In contrast to this, the proportion of effector Treg cells increases, with effector Treg cells being more prevalent in adults and elderly people (Miyara et al. 2009). After TCR stimulation, Treg cells with a naive phenotype proliferate, upregulate their FoxP3 expression, and convert to $CD45RO^+FoxP3^{high}$ effector Treg cells (Miyara et al. 2009). These effector T cells exhibit a strong suppressive activity, but are also highly susceptible to apoptosis after activation and during suppression (Jonuleit et al. 2001; Vukmanovic-Stejic et al. 2006).

The population of $CD4^+CD25^+FoxP3^+$ Treg cells can be subdivided into two subpopulations: natural, thymus-derived Treg cells and adaptive Treg cells, conventional $CD4^+$ T cells that have been induced in the periphery (Sakaguchi et al. 2010; Kretschmer et al. 2005; Apostolou and Boehme 2004; Curotto de Lafaille et al. 2004). It has been shown that $CD4^+$ T cells require TCR stimulation as well as the presence of TGF-beta and IL-2 to convert to $CD25^+FoxP3^+$ Treg cells

(Chen et al. 2003; Zheng et al. 2007). In a recent publication, Helios, a member of the Ikaros transcription factor family, has been described as a potential new marker for thymus-derived Treg cells. After Helios has been shown to be expressed in FoxP3$^+$ Treg cells in microarray analyses (Sugimoto et al. 2006), Thornton et al. (2010) have observed that Helios is expressed early in the thymic development. Concurrent with the appearance of FoxP3 on the mRNA level, the expression of Helios is significantly increased in thymic CD4$^+$CD25$^+$cells. FoxP3$^+$ Treg cells that were induced in the periphery did not express Helios. Even though Helios does not seem to be involved in the regulation of either FoxP3 expression or Treg cell function, it may be regarded as an important Treg cell marker that allows distinguishing between induced and thymus-derived Treg cells (Thornton et al. 2010).

Moreover, distinct, terminally differentiated subpopulations of Treg cells can be identified based on the level of major histocompatibility complex (MHC) class II determinants (DR) expression. MHC-DR$^+$ Treg cells express high levels of FoxP3, and account for approximately 20–30 % of human Treg cells and approximately one-third of the circulating MHC II$^+$CD4$^+$cells. These MHC-DR$^+$ Treg cells exhibit a FoxP3-associated early contact-dependent suppression and cytokine production, but do not secrete IL-10. In contrast, MHC-DR$^-$ Treg cells execute their suppressive activity through a late FoxP3-associated cell contact-mediated mechanism as well as IL-10 secretion (Baecher-Allan et al. 2006).

2.2.2 *Suppressive Activity*

2.2.2.1 Mechanisms of Treg Cell Suppression

Although Treg cells have been shown to play a crucial role in the immune system by controlling immune responses, no single mechanism of suppression used by Treg cells has emerged, suggesting that Tregs are endowed with a number of pathways each contributing to the regulatory functionality of this population of T cells. One possible mechanism of action is cytokine secretion. In vivo, Treg cells secrete the suppressive cytokines TGF-β and IL-10 (Powrie et al. 1996; Asseman et al. 1999). TGF-β has been shown to be essential for Treg cell-mediated suppression of effector CD4$^+$ T cells in a murine model for colitis (Fahlen et al. 2005). In this model, Treg cells were not able to control CD4$^+$ T cells that were not sensitive to TGF- β. However, Kullberg et al. (2005) have shown that TGF-β production by Treg cells is not essential for in vivo Treg suppression. Other murine models of autoimmune inflammation have shown that IL-10 production contributes to Treg cell-mediated immune suppression (Asseman et al. 1999; Annacker et al. 2001). In vitro, both, TGF-β and IL-10, are not required for suppression (Shevach 2009).

Other models of Treg suppression require cell–cell contact as one possible mechanism of suppression used by Treg cells. Nakamura et al. (2001) have shown that membrane-bound TGF-β contributes to cell–cell contact-mediated suppression. Furthermore, the cell surface molecules Fas, Granzyme B, LAG3, and CTLA-4 have been implicated in suppression (Huang et al. 2004; Janssens et al. 2003; Cao et al. 2007; Read et al. 2000). Despite various reports suggesting that cell surface molecules contribute to Treg-mediated suppression, the role of cell–cell contact may vary depending upon the particular Treg subpopulation and the organ system where the function is being observed.

In vitro, Treg cells can deprive other T cells of IL-2, suggesting that competition for growth factors might contribute to the suppressive capacity of Treg cells (de la Rosa et al. 2004, Barthlott et al. 2005). However, the suppressive function of Treg cells cannot be entirely explained by IL-2 deprivation of effector T cells, as IL-2 receptor-deficient Treg cells are fully able to suppress T cell proliferation in vitro (Fontenot et al. 2005). Furthermore, Treg cells can suppress IL-2 receptor-deficient effector T cells (Fontenot et al. 2005). As no unique mechanism has been identified to be required for suppression, it is very likely that different mechanisms contribute to the suppressive ability of Treg cells.

2.2.2.2 Immune Functions Regulated by Treg Cells

Besides modulating the function of $CD4^+$ T cells, Treg cells also regulate a broad variety of immune cells such as $CD4^+$ and $CD8^+$ T cells, B cells, natural killer (NK) cells, natural killer T (NKT) cells, and antigen-presenting cells (APCs), through the suppression of activation, proliferation, and cytokine production (Zhao et al. 2006; Azuma et al. 2003; Ralainirina et al. 2007; Taams et al. 2005; Misra et al. 2004). As a basic prerequisite in order to execute their full suppressive potential, Treg cells must be activated through their T cell receptor (TCR; Baecher-Allan et al. 2001; Dieckman et al. 2001; Jonuleit et al. 2001). Interestingly, after being activated, they do not need to be viable in coculture to be capable to suppress the cell function of responder cells. In addition, the strength of T cell stimulation strongly influences whether suppression or proliferation occurs. It has been shown that effector T cells that have been activated in the presence of strong costimulatory signals seem to be refractory to Treg cell-induced suppression (Baecher-Allan et al. 2001, 2002). Moreover, the resistance of effector T cells to regulation through Treg cells-mediated mechanisms increases when the strength of TCR signals received by the effector T cells is increased (Baecher-Allan et al. 2001).

Moreover, various groups have described the occurrence of human Treg cells that secrete the proinflammatory cytokine IL-17 (Koenen et al. 2008; Beriou et al. 2009; Ayyoub et al. 2009). These cells have been shown to express RORγ t, a specific transcription factor for T_H17 cells (Koenen et al. 2008, Ayyoub et al. 2009). Beriou et al. (2009) have identified a subset of Treg cells within a $CD4^+CD45RA^-CD25^{high}CCRC6^+HLA\text{-}DR^-FoxP3^+$ population that is capable of producing IL-17. The presence of IL-1beta and IL-6 during activation of the cells was required for the production of IL-17. Interestingly, $IL\text{-}17^+/FoxP3^+$ clones from this subpopulation were able to alternately suppress Treg cells or secrete high levels of IL-17, depending on the stimuli.

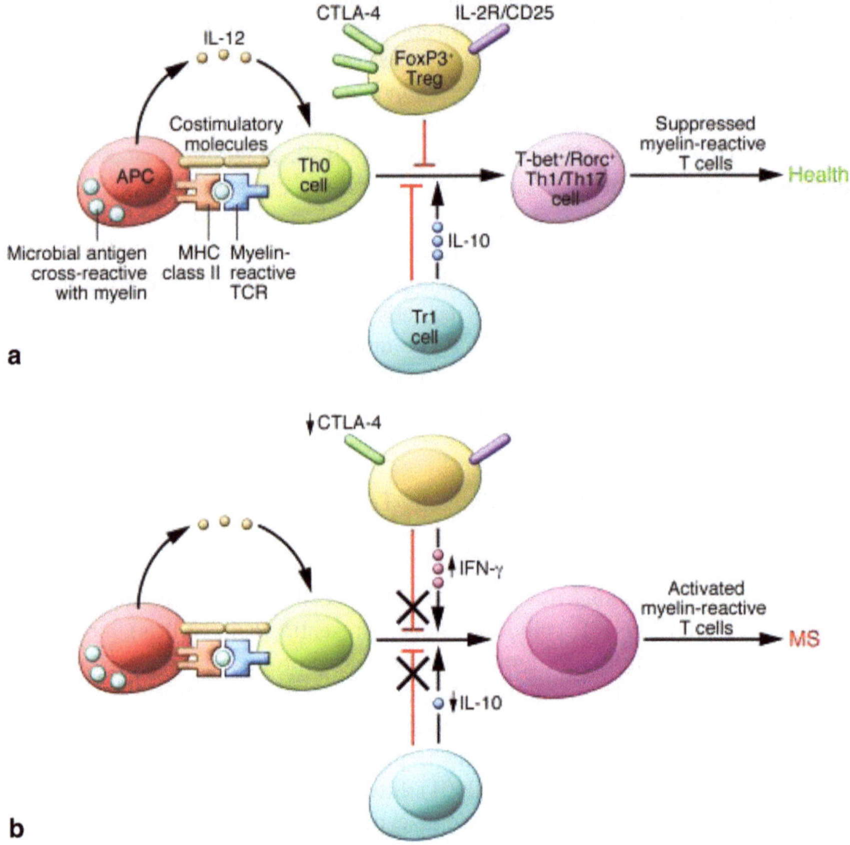

Fig. 2.1 Role of FoxP3+ Treg cells in immune regulation. **a** In healthy individuals, Treg cells modulate the immune function through the suppression of activation, proliferation and cytokine production, thereby interacting with various cell types. **b** In patients with MS, the immunoregulatory function of Treg cells is impaired. The frequency of IFN-γ producing T_H1-like cells is increased (Nylander and Hafler 2012)

In recent publications, Eos, a zinc-finger transcription factor of the Ikaros family, has been identified as an important element of FoxP3-mediated suppressive activity of Treg cells. Pan et al. (2009) have demonstrated that Eos induces gene silencing in Treg cells by directly interacting with FoxP3. Eos has been shown to coimmunoprecipitate with FoxP3. The secretion of IL-2 by transduced primary $CD4^+$ T cells was inhibited by the expression of full-length FoxP3. In contrast, the expression of ΔFoxP3 (a 51-amino acid fragment of FoxP3 that is necessary to bind to the C-terminal region of Eos) reversed this effect. After a knockdown of Eos in the same cells, the FoxP3-dependent suppression of IL-2 was abrogated. Moreover, the same group investigated the effect of an Eos-knockdown on a FoxP3-dependent gene set from Treg cells (Pan et al. 2009). Strikingly, more than 70 % of genes affected by a Eos-knockdown in Treg cells were FoxP3-dependent, and 90 % of the genes that are usually downregulated by FoxP3 expression were no longer inhibited after a knockdown of Eos.

Another cell type that executes regulatory effects is the T_R1 T cell. T_R1 cells are induced through activating signals such as CD3/CD46 cross-linking or IL-27 and TGFβ. They are characterized by the secretion of high levels of the highly immunosuppressive cytokine IL-10 as well as the lack of IL-4 expression and no or only low expression of IL-2. T_R1 cells modulate immune function through IL-10 secretion by inhibiting effector function and activation of various cell types (Roncarolo et al. 2001; Fig. 2.1).

2.3 Treg Cells in MS

The role of Treg cells in the development and in the course of MS has been in the focus of intensive clinical and basic research in the past years. These studies have investigated the frequency as well as the immune-modulating function of Treg cells, thereby considering disease activity and therapy status.

2.3.1 Frequency of Treg Cells in the Peripheral Blood of MS Patients

The frequency of $CD4^+CD25^{high}$ Treg cells in patients with MS has been investigated by various groups. Viglietta et al. (2004) first reported that while there were no significant differences in the frequency of $CD4^+CD25^{high}$ Treg cells in the peripheral blood of 15 untreated relapsing remitting MS (RRMS) patients and 21 healthy controls, there were differences in function that are discussed below. A similar result has been reported by a different group, which has analyzed $CD4^+CD25^{high}$ Treg cells from 73 RRMS patients and 73 healthy controls (Haas et al. 2005). Moreover, Feger et al. (2007) have observed no differences in the frequency of $CD4^+CD25^+$ Treg cells in the blood of 40 healthy controls and 36 untreated patients with different disease subtypes, including clinically isolated syndrome (CIS), RRMS, secondary progressive MS (SPMS), and primary progressive MS (PPMS).

2.3.2 Frequency of Treg Cells in the CSF of MS Patients

Treg cells have been identified in the cerebrospinal fluid (CSF) of MS patients. It has been observed by Haas et al. (2005) that the number of $CD4^+CD25^+$ Treg cells in the CSF and the peripheral blood of 15 untreated RRMS patients did not differ significantly. Nevertheless, in another study, the CSF of 14 untreated CIS and RRMS patients and 9 patients with other, nonautoimmune neurological diseases has been analyzed. The frequency of $CD4^+CD25^+FoxP3^+$ Treg cells in the CSF of the MS patients was significantly increased compared with peripheral blood of the MS patients. In contrast to this, patients with other neurological diseases did not show elevated Treg cell levels in the CSF compared with the blood. These data suggest that Treg cells are selectively enriched in the CSF of MS patients in order to fight autoimmune processes (Feger et al. 2007). In a recent report, Fritzsching et al. (2006) have compared the frequency of $CD4^+CD25^+FoxP3^+$ Treg cells in the CSF of 17 treatment-naive MS patients with the number of Treg cells in the peripheral blood. $CD45RO^{high}CD95^{high}$ Treg cells have been shown to be highly sensitive to CD95L-induced apoptosis. Strikingly, this subpopulation was increased in the CSF of MS patients compared with the peripheral blood. The Fritzsching group therefore hypothesizes that Treg cells may be eliminated in the CNS through CD95L-mediated apoptosis. Interestingly, the same group has also examined brain biopsies of 16 untreated RRMS patients. No Treg cells were detectable in 30 % of the biopsies; the number of $FoxP3^+$ Tcell was generally low in the analyzed brain tissue (Fritzsching et al. 2011).

2.3.3 *Function of Treg Cells in MS*

2.3.3.1 Function of $CD4^+CD25^+$ Treg Cells Is Impaired

Even though frequency of Treg cells in the peripheral blood of MS patients does not differ in comparison to healthy controls, the immunomodulatory function of Treg cells has been shown to be impaired in MS patients (Kumar et al. 2006, Baecher-Allan et al. 2004). Viglietta et al. (2004) have analyzed samples from untreated RRMS patients. When cocultured with $CD4^+CD25^-$ responder cells, $CD4^+CD25^{high}$ Treg cells from healthy subjects effectively suppressed the proliferation of the responder cells. In striking contrast to this, $CD4^+CD25^{high}$ Treg cells from MS patients showed an inadequate suppressive ability and inhibited proliferation only poorly. A similar observation has been made after coculturing $CD4^+CD25^{high}$ Treg cells from MS patients with $CD4^+CD25^-$ responder cells from either patients or healthy controls. The Treg cells were incapable of suppressing responder cell proliferation, while $CD4^+CD25^-$ responder cells from MS patients could be suppressed by $CD4^+CD25^{high}$ Treg cells from healthy controls, indicating that a defect in the regulatory function of the Treg cells themselves is responsible for the impaired suppressive ability. Moreover, single-cell cloning experiments were performed. Strikingly, the cloning frequency of $CD4^+CD25^{high}$ T cells was significantly decreased in MS patients compared with healthy controls. Furthermore, Huan et al. (2005) have shown that the levels of FoxP3 mRNA and protein expression are reduced in $CD4^+CD25^+$ Treg cells from untreated MS patients compared with healthy controls, indicating a correlation between the reduced FoxP3 expression and the impaired suppressive capacity of Treg cells in MS patients.

2.3.3.2 Frequency and Suppressive Function of $CD31^+$-Naive Treg Cells Are Altered

An altered Treg cell subpopulation has been described by Haas et al. (2007) $CD4^+CD25^+FoxP3^+$ Treg cells that enter the circulation and coexpress CD31 are defined as recent thymic emigrants (RTEs). The number of RTEs decreases with age and is significantly diminished in RRMS patients compared with healthy controls. The reduced de novo generation of $CD31^+$-naive Treg cells was compensated by an increase in the amount of memory Treg cells so that the total Treg cell number was stable. The differences in the functional capacity of Treg cells between MS patients and healthy controls were neutralized by depletion of $CD31^+$ T cells, indicating that RTEs contribute to the functional characteristics of the Treg cell population.

Although a defect in Treg cells function has been observed in patients with RRMS, the suppressive capacity of Treg cells from patients with SPMS does not seem to be impaired (Venken et al. 2006). The reduced suppressive ability of the Treg cells has been correlated with a decreased FoxP3 expression in RRMS patients (Venken et al. 2008a). Moreover, the Venken group has compared the frequency and function of naive ($CD4^+CD25^+CD127^{low}CD45RA^+$) and memory ($CD4^+CD25^+CD127^{low}CD45RO^+$) Treg cells from untreated RRMS and SPMS patients with short and long disease duration, respectively. The suppressive capacity of naive Treg cells was decreased in all groups compared with healthy controls; in contrast, the suppressive function of memory Treg cells was similar to healthy controls and was increased in SPMS patients and RRMS patients with a long disease duration ($\geq$ 10 years) compared with RRMS patients with a short disease duration ($<$ 10 years). When comparing the frequency of naive and memory Treg cells of early (disease duration $<$ 10 years) and chronic (disease duration $\geq$ 10 years) untreated MS patients, they observed that both groups showed decreased numbers of naive Treg cells. The frequency of memory Treg cells was increased in chronic patients. Interestingly, the proportion of $CD31^+$ memory Treg cells was diminished in early MS patients, suggesting a high cell turnover in early disease (Venken et al. 2008b).

2.3.3.3 IFN-γ-Secreting T_H1-Like T Cells Are More Prevalent in MS Patients

$CD4^+CD25^{high}FoxP3^+$ Treg cells isolated ex vivo from patients with untreated RRMS show a T helper type 1 (T_H1)-like phenotype after stimulation with PMA and ionomycin. The frequency of these IFN-γ- secreting T_H1-like T cells was higher in untreated RRMS patients compared with healthy controls (Fig. 2.2). Treg cells and responder T cells from patients with RRMS have been cultured with an IFN-γ-specific antibody showing that blocking IFN-γ leads to a significantly elevated suppressive capacity of the Treg cells, thereby confirming that the suppressive ability of Treg cells from RRMS patients is decreased by IFN-γ production. Moreover, a comparison of Treg cells from IFN-β-treated RRMS patients with Treg cells from healthy controls has shown a similar frequency of IFN-γ-secreting $FoxP3^+$ T cells in both groups. Comparable results have been reported for type 1 diabetes (Dominguez-Villar et al. 2011, McClymont et al. 2011).

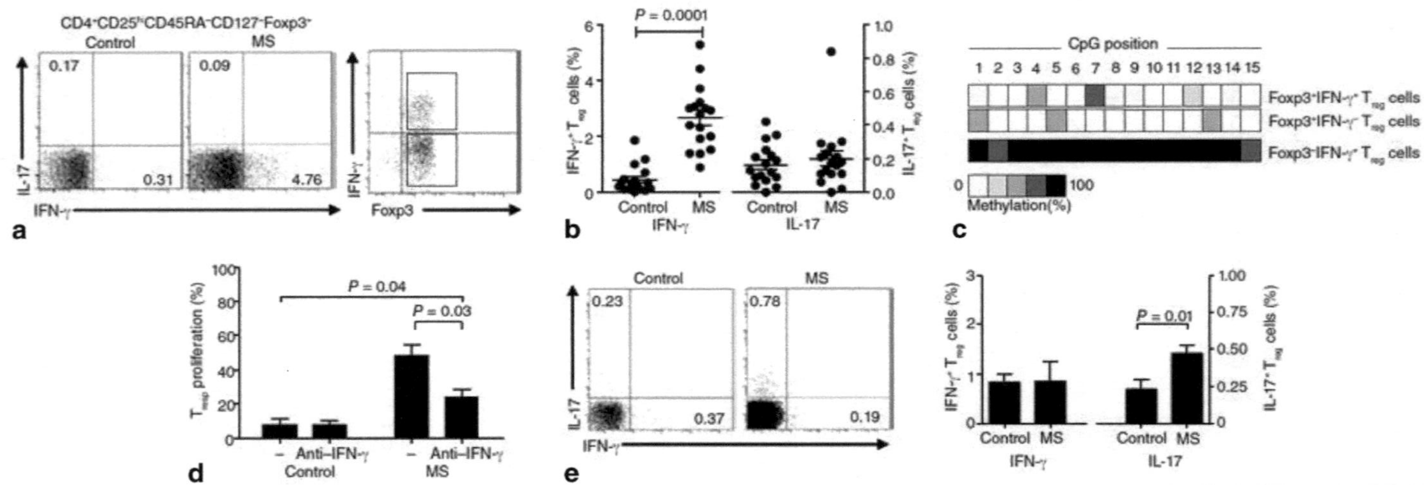

Fig. 2.2 Treg cells from individuals with RRMS secrete IFN-γ ex vivo. **a** The frequency of FACS-sorted IFN-γ^+ and IL-17^+ Treg cells in healthy control individuals (*left*) and untreated individuals with RRMS (*middle*, $n = 17$) gated on Foxp3^+ Treg cells. *Right*, purity analysis of the sorted IFN-γ^+Foxp3^+ and IFN-γ^-Foxp3^+ populations from subjects with RRMS used for methylation analysis in (c). **b** Percentage of IFN-γ^+Foxp3^+ and IL-17^+Foxp3^+ Treg cells ($n = 17$) as a proportion of total Foxp3^+ Treg cells. **c** Representative example of methylation analysis of the TSDR region of the FOXP3 locus in sorted IFN-γ^+Foxp3^+ and IFN-γ^-Foxp3^+ Treg cells from subjects with RRMS. An analysis of IFN-γ^+Foxp3^- memory T cells from subjects with RRMS is shown as a control. **d** Proliferation of Tresp cells cultured with ex vivo FACS-sorted Treg cells from healthy control subjects and untreated subjects with MS (Treg cell:Tresp cell ratio of 1:2) in the presence or absence of an IFN-γ-specific antibody ($n = 4$). **e** The frequency of IFN-γ^+ and IL-17^+ Treg cells in healthy control subjects (*left*) or IFN-β-treated patients with RRMS (*right*) as assessed by intracellular cytokine staining and FACS analysis. The bar diagram (*right*) shows the percentage of IFN-γ^+Foxp3^+ and IL-17^+Foxp3^+ cells as a proportion of total Foxp3^+ Treg cells in healthy controls or IFN-β-treated patients with RRMS ($n = 12$). (Dominguez-Villar et al. 2011, Copywright 2011)

2.3.3.4 CD46-Activated T Cells Have an Impaired Immunomodulatory Function

A defect of suppressive function has also been described for other regulatory cells, such as T_R1 cells. T_R1 cells are characterized by the secretion of high levels of IL-10 (Roncarolo et al. 2001; Groux et al. 1997). It has been observed that the immunoregulatory function of CD46-activated T cells is impaired in patients diagnosed with MS. CD46 is a costimulatory membrane molecule with two cytoplasmatic isoforms, Cyt1 (16 amino acids) and Cyt2 (23 amino acids). CD46-costimulated T cells acquire a T_R1-like phenotype in the presence of IL-2 with IL-10 and granzyme B production, but can also show a T_H1-like response, characterized by elevated levels of IL-2, IL-10, and IFN-γ and decreased secretion of IL-5. $CD4^+$ T cells from healthy controls and from untreated or IFN-β- treated patients with RRMS were stimulated with anti-CD3 and either anti-CD28 or anti-CD46 antibodies in the presence of IL-2. The IL-10 secretion of CD46-activated T cells from treated and untreated MS patients was significantly diminished compared with healthy controls, while INF-γ production did not significantly change in any of the groups. This effect could not be observed for CD28- stimulated T cells, and is therefore specific to CD46. Moreover, it has been detected that the CD46 isoform Cyt2 is significantly higher expressed in T cells from MS patients compared with healthy controls. In a murine model, Cyt2 is associated with an enhancement of inflammatory processes, while the other isoform, Cyt1, seems to inhibit inflammation (Astier et al. 2006; Marie et al. 2002).

2.3.3.5 Allele of CD58 Locus Has a Protective Effect

In the past years, genetic analyses such as genome-wide association studies (GWAS) have contributed greatly to the expansion of our knowledge of MS. In several GWAS, multiple susceptibility loci have been identified that are associated with the risk of developing the disease. Some of these loci, such as IL2RA (CD25), IL7RA, and CD58, are of particular interest as they have been shown to be linked to the function of Treg cells (Jager et al. 2009; Sawcer et al. 2005, 2011).

Recently, the protective effect of the $rs2300747^G$ allele of the CD58 locus has been described. CD58 (LFA-3) influences TCR signaling through the engagement of its receptor CD2. CD2 enhances the suppressive function of human Treg cells through costimulation and, moreover, by promoting FoxP3 expression. An enhanced CD58 mRNA expression has been observed in lymphoblastic cell lines and peripheral blood mononuclear cells (PBMCs) from patients with RRMS or CIS. Furthermore, it has been shown in a different set of patients that CD58 mRNA expression levels were higher in those patients who were in clinical remission, suggesting that elevated levels of CD58 RNA expression may play a role in minimizing inflammation in MS patients by enhancing the function of $CD4^+CD25^{high}$ Treg cells through CD2-mediated upregulation of FoxP3 expression (Jager et al. 2009).

2.3.4 Treg Cells in Experimental Autoimmune Encephalomyelitis (EAE)

In the investigation of immunological mechanisms, which contribute to the pathogenesis of MS, the use of EAE, and the mouse model of MS, has led to important observations. Many groups have described the complex role of Treg cells in the development and control of EAE. The CNS shows an increased proliferation of Treg cells during inflammation (O'Connor et al. 2007). It has been shown by several groups that murine $CD4^+CD25^+FoxP3^+$ T cells accumulate in the CNS, and that this accumulation correlates with recovery (Korn et al. 2007, McGeachy et al. 2005). Nevertheless, the accumulated cells do not have the functional capacity to effectively suppress effector T cells during the peak of EAE (Korn et al. 2007). As mentioned above, a subset of $CD4^+FoxP3^+$ Treg cells with the ability to produce IL-17 under certain inflammatory conditions has been identified in the human peripheral blood. Treg cells taken from the CNS of mice with EAE did not secrete IL-17 in the presence of IL-6. It has been observed that Treg cells from the CNS of these mice were lacking the IL-6 receptor chains, CD126 and gp130, suggesting a reduced responsiveness to IL-6 (O'Connor et al. 2012).

2.3.4.1 Adoptive Transfer of Treg Cells Has a Protective Effect

In 1994, Lafaille et al. (1994) have shown that the development of spontaneous EAE is increased in immunodeficient TCR myelin basic protein (MBP) transgenic mice. For these experiments, TCR transgenic mice were crossed with recombinant activating gene (RAG)-1 gene-deficient mice in order to generate mice with no lymphocytes but $CD4^+$ T cells expressing TCRs specific for MBP. All TCR transgenic RAG-1-deficient (T/R^-) mice developed spontaneous EAE, while only some mice with an intact RAG-1 gene (T/R^+) were affected, suggesting that nontransgenic lymphocytes have a protective effect. Moreover, it has been observed that an early transfer of total splenocytes or $CD4^+$ T cells from normal donor mice into T/R^- mice can prevent EAE in T/R^- mice. The same group has also described that $CD4^+$ T cells expressing endogenous α and β TCR chains are required to protect T/R^+ from developing spontaneous EAE. These observations have been interpreted in favor of the immunomodulatory effect of Treg cells on the development of EAE (Olivares-Villagomez et al. 1998).

These conclusions have been supported by a study of Hori et al. (2002) on the effect of $CD25^+CD4^+$ Treg cells on the development of EAE in TCR MBP RAG-1-deficient mice. In contrast to T/R^- mice, T/R^+ mice contain $CD25^+CD4^+$ T cells. The adoptive transfer of $CD25^+4^+$ T cells from either wild-type or T/R^+ mice into T/R^- mice prevented T/R^- mice from developing EAE. Moreover, Kohm et al. (2002) have observed that the adoptive transfer of $CD4^+CD25^+$ Treg cells results in a decreased CNS infiltration and in protection from myelin oligodendrocyte glycoprotein (MOG)- induced EAE in C57BL/6 mice, underlining the protective effect of Treg cells. In addition to this, Treg cells have been shown to have the potential to inhibit the cytokine production and proliferation of MOG_{35-55}-specific Th1 cells in vitro.

Passive transfer of $CD4^{+}CD25^{+}$ CNS-derived Treg cells in low numbers that were isolated from mice that were in the recovery phase of MOG- induced EAE has been shown to protect C57BL/6 mice from the development of EAE. In contrast, the same number of $CD4^{+}CD25^{+}$ Treg cells from naive lymph nodes did not have the same effect, indicating that antigen-specific Treg cells that have been isolated from the inflamed tissue seem to be more potent to suppress inflammation (McGeachy et al. 2005).

2.3.4.2 Differences in Disease Susceptibility

Not all mouse strains are equally or at all susceptible to the induction of EAE. Although B10.S mice are highly resistant, SJL mice show a high susceptibility to PLP139-151-induced EAE. Reddy et al. (2004, 2005) have demonstrated that after using PLP139-151 tetramers, both mouse strains do not show significant differences in the frequency of tetramer-positive T cells in the naive compartment. Interestingly, most tetramer-positive T cells in SJL mice were $CD4^{+}CD25^{-}$; while PLP139-151 tetramer-reactive T cells in B10.S mice have been shown to be $CD4^{+}CD25^{+}$. After depletion of $CD4^{+}CD25^{+}$ T cells through administration of anti-CD25 antibody, the susceptibility of B10.S to the induction of EAE has been shown to be increased. This observation indicates that B10 mice have strong Treg cell population and underlines the importance of $CD4^{+}CD25^{+}$ Treg cells in the regulation autoimmune diseases. Interestingly, the depletion of Treg cells before induction of PLP139-151-mediated EAE leads to a greater degree of susceptibility to EAE in male mice compared with nontransgenic controls and female mice.

2.3.4.3 Depletion of $CD25^{+}$ Increases Disease Severity

This observation is supported by another study, in which it has been demonstrated that the depletion of $CD25^{+}$ Treg cells in C57Bl/6 mice by anti-CD25 antibodies has been shown to inhibit the recovery from the MOG- induced EAE. Furthermore, the resistance to reinduction of EAE is removed when Treg cells are depleted (McGeachy et al. 2005). Another important study reports that SJL mice show an increased severity of PLP139-151-induced EAE after administration of anti-CD25 antibodies in order to reduce $CD25^{+}CD4^{+}$ T cells. Although cells from the lymph nodes of anti-CD25 antibody-treated mice produced more IFN-γ after stimulation with PLP139-151 in vitro, the IL-10 secretion of these cells was significantly reduced. The adoptive transfer of $CD25^{+}CD4^{+}$ T cells from naive SJL mice into mice before induction of EAE decreased disease severity, illustrating the suppressive *capacity* of Treg cells (Zhang et al. 2004).

2.3.5 *Treg Cells and MS Therapy*

A therapeutic strategy to recover immune function in MS patients could be the restoration of impaired Treg cell function. Some immunomodulatory MS treatments, such as glatiramer acetate (GA) and IFN-β, have been described to partially execute their therapeutic effect through Treg cells.

Treatment with GA has been shown to increase the FoxP3 expression of Treg cells from MS patients (Hong et al. 2005). In a recent study, the blood of 15 RRMS patients has been analyzed before and after long-term treatment with GA. Before treatment with GA (baseline) the proportions of naive and recent thymic emigrant Treg cells within the total Treg cell population were decreased compared with healthy controls. Interestingly, this effect was reversed after the patients had received treatment with GA for up to 6 months. Moreover, the impaired suppressive function of the total Treg cells was improved compared with the baseline results (Haas et al. 2009). In addition to this, it has been observed that treatment with GA leads to an upregulation of specific $CD8^+$ T cells responses (Karandikar et al. 2002). GA-reactive $CD8^+$ T cells have been shown to execute suppressive function. Although the suppressive ability of $CD8^+$ T cells was reduced in untreated MS patients compared with healthy controls, it was significantly enhanced in GA-treated MS patients, suggesting that treatment with GA has the potential to modulate immune responses directly during ongoing therapy (Tennakoon et al. 2006).

Another potent therapeutic agent is IFN-β. Blood samples of 22 untreated RRMS patients were analyzed before and after treatment with IFN-β-1a. The suppressive function of $CD4^+CD25^+$ Treg cells was impaired at baseline, but was restored after 6 months of treatment (Andres et al. 2007). Furthermore, Vandenbark et al. (2009) have reported elevated FoxP3 mRNA levels in RRMS patients that have been treated with IFN-β-1a for 12 months compared with their own baseline results and to untreated RRMS patients and healthy controls. Nevertheless, the FoxP3 protein levels did not differ significantly from those observed in untreated RRMS patients and healthy controls. Interestingly, one group has observed no differences in the frequency of $CD4^+CD25^{high}$ Treg cells in the blood patients treated with GA and/or IFN-β-1a compared with untreated MS patients and healthy controls (Putheti et al. 2004).

Natalizumab, a monoclonal antibody against the α-4 chain of very late activation antigen 4 (VLA-4), is an efficient drug in the treatment of MS. However, it does not seem to influence the suppressive capacity of $CD4^+CD25^+FoxP3^+$ Treg cells (Stenner et al. 2008, Ramos-Cejudo et al. 2011).

2.4 Conclusion

MS is an autoimmune disease caused by uncontrolled autoreactive T and B cells. The failure of Treg cells to suppress these immune cells in MS patients plays an important role in disease onset and progression. Although the frequency of $CD4^+CD25^{high}$ Treg cells is not altered in MS patients as compared with healthy controls, the suppressive capacity of Treg cells is impaired in MS patients. Recent studies have shown that Treg cells in MS patients can exhibit effector T cell functions, such as IFN-γ production. Modification of Treg cell activity is therefore a promising approach for the development of new experimental therapies for MS and other autoimmune diseases.

Treg cells are key regulators of the immune system. Imbalance of Treg cells and effector immune cells contributes to the development of various autoimmune diseases. Lessons learned from Treg studies in MS patients and EAE mouse models might therefore not only contribute to a better understanding of MS development and progression, but also provide insights into other autoimmune diseases.

References

Andres C de, Aristimuno C, Las HV de, Martinez-Gines ML, Bartolome M, Arroyo R et al (2007) Interferon beta-1a therapy enhances CD4+ regulatory T-cell function: an ex vivo and in vitro longitudinal study in relapsing-remitting multiple sclerosis. J Neuroimmunol 182(1–2):204–211. doi:10.1016/j.jneuroim.2006.09.012 (PubMed PMID: 17157927)

Annacker O, Pimenta-Araujo R, Burlen-Defranoux O, Barbosa TC, Cumano A, Bandeira A (2001) CD25+ CD4+ T cells regulate the expansion of peripheral CD4 T cells through the production of IL-10. J Immunol 166(5):3008–3018 (PubMed PMID: 11207250)

Apostolou I, Boehmer H von (2004) In vivo instruction of suppressor commitment in naive T cells. J Exp Med 199(10):1401–1408. doi:10.1084/jem.20040249 (PubMed PMID: 15148338; PubMed Central PMCID: PMC2211808)

Asseman C, Mauze S, Leach MW, Coffman RL, Powrie F (1999) An essential role for interleukin 10 in the function of regulatory T cells that inhibit intestinal inflammation. J Exp Med 190(7):995–1004 (PubMed PMID: 10510089; PubMed Central PMCID: PMC2195650)

Astier AL, Meiffren G, Freeman S, Hafler DA (2006) Alterations in CD46-mediated Tr1 regulatory T cells in patients with multiple sclerosis. J Clin Invest 116(12):3252–3257. doi:10.1172/JCI29251 (PubMed PMID: 17099776; PubMed Central PMCID: PMC1635165)

Ayyoub M, Deknuydt F, Raimbaud I, Dousset C, Leveque L, Bioley G et al (2009) Human memory FOXP3+ Tregs secrete IL-17 ex vivo and constitutively express the T(H)17 lineage-specific transcription factor RORgamma t. Proc Natl Acad Sci U S A 106(21):8635–8640. doi:10.1073/pnas.0900621106 (PubMed PMID: 19439651; PubMed Central PMCID: PMC2688993)

Azuma T, Takahashi T, Kunisato A, Kitamura T, Hirai H (2003) Human $CD4^{+}$ $CD25^{+}$ regulatory T cells suppress NKT cell functions. Cancer Res 63(15):4516–4520 (PubMed PMID: 12907625)

Baecher-Allan C, Brown JA, Freeman GJ, Hafler DA (2001) CD4+CD25high regulatory cells in human peripheral blood. J Immunol 167(3):1245–1253 (PubMed PMID: 11466340)

Baecher-Allan C, Viglietta V, Hafler DA (2002) Inhibition of human CD4(+)CD25(+ high) regulatory T cell function. J Immunol 169(11):6210–6217 (PubMed PMID: 12444126)

Baecher-Allan C, Hafler DA (2004) Suppressor T cells in human diseases. J Exp Med 200(3):273–276. doi:10.1084/jem.20040812 (PubMed PMID: 15280423; PubMed Central PMCID: PMC2211973)

Baecher-Allan C, Wolf E, Hafler DA (2006) MHC class II expression identifies functionally distinct human regulatory T cells. J Immunol 176(8):4622–4631 (PubMed PMID: 16585553)

Barthlott T, Moncrieffe H, Veldhoen M, Atkins CJ, Christensen J, O'Garra A et al (2005) CD25+CD4+ T cells compete with naive CD4+ T cells for IL-2 and exploit it for the induction of IL-10 production. Int Immunol 17(3):279–288. doi:dxh207[pii]10.1093/intimm/dxh207 (PubMed PMID: 15684039)

Bennett CL, Christie J, Ramsdell F, Brunkow ME, Ferguson PJ, Whitesell L et al (2001) The immune dysregulation, polyendocrinopathy, enteropathy, X-linked syndrome (IPEX) is caused by mutations of FOXP3. Nat Genet 27(1):20–21. doi:10.1038/83713 (PubMed PMID: 11137993)

Beriou G, Costantino CM, Ashley CW, Yang L, Kuchroo VK, Baecher-Allan C et al (2009) IL-17-producing human peripheral regulatory T cells retain suppressive function. Blood 113(18):4240–4249. doi:10.1182/blood-2008-10-183251 (PubMed PMID: 19171879; PubMed Central PMCID: PMC2676084)

Blair PJ, Bultman SJ, Haas JC, Rouse BT, Wilkinson JE, Godfrey VL (1994) CD4+CD8- T cells are the effector cells in disease pathogenesis in the scurfy (sf) mouse. J Immunol 153(8):3764–74 (PubMed PMID: 7930593)

Brunkow ME, Jeffery EW, Hjerrild KA, Paeper B, Clark LB, Yasayko SA et al (2001) Disruption of a new forkhead/winged-helix protein, scurfin, results in the fatal lymphoproliferative disorder of the scurfy mouse. Nat Genet 27(1):68–73. doi:10.1038/83784 (PubMed PMID: 11138001)

Cao X, Cai SF, Fehniger TA, Song J, Collins LI, Piwnica-Worms DR et al (2007) Granzyme B and perforin are important for regulatory T cell-mediated suppression of tumor clearance. Immunity 27(4):635–646. doi:S1074-7613(07)00444-X[pii]10.1016/j.immuni.2007.08.014 (PubMed PMID: 17919943)

Chen W, Jin W, Hardegen N, Lei KJ, Li L, Marinos N et al (2003) Conversion of peripheral CD4+CD25- naive T cells to CD4+CD25+ regulatory T cells by TGF-beta induction of transcription factor Foxp3. J Exp Med 198(12):1875–1886. doi:10.1084/jem.20030152 (PubMed PMID: 14676299; PubMed Central PMCID: PMC2194145)

Curotto de Lafaille MA, Lafaille JJ (2009) Natural and adaptive foxp3+ regulatory T cells: more of the same or a division of labor? Immunity 30(5):626–635. doi:10.1016/j.immuni.2009.05.002 (PubMed PMID: 19464985)

Curotto de Lafaille MA, Lino AC, Kutchukhidze N, Lafaille JJ. (2004) CD25- T cells generate CD25+ Foxp3+ regulatory T cells by peripheral expansion. J Immunol 173(12):7259–7268 (PubMed PMID: 15585848)

de la Rosa M, Rutz S, Dorninger H, Scheffold A (2004) Interleukin-2 is essential for CD4+CD25+ regulatory T cell function. Eur J Immunol 34(9):2480–2488. doi:10.1002/eji.200425274c (PubMed PMID: 15307180)

Dieckmann D, Plottner H, Berchtold S, Berger T, Schuler G (2001) Ex vivo isolation and characterization of CD4(+)CD25(+) T cells with regulatory properties from human blood. J Exp Med 193(11):1303–1310 (PubMed PMID: 11390437; PubMed Central PMCID: PMC2193384)

Dominguez-Villar M, Baecher-Allan CM, Hafler DA (2011) Identification of T helper type 1-like, Foxp3+ regulatory T cells in human autoimmune disease. Nature Med 17(6):673–675. doi:10.1038/nm.2389 (PubMed PMID: 21540856)

Fahlen L, Read S, Gorelik L, Hurst SD, Coffman RL, Flavell RA et al (2005) T cells that cannot respond to TGF-beta escape control by CD4(+)CD25(+) regulatory T cells. J Exp Med 201(5):737–746. doi:jem.20040685[pii]10.1084/jem.20040685 (PubMed PMID: 15753207; PubMed Central PMCID: PMC2212836)

Feger U, Luther C, Poeschel S, Melms A, Tolosa E, Wiendl H (2007) Increased frequency of CD4+ CD25+ regulatory T cells in the cerebrospinal fluid but not in the blood of multiple sclerosis patients. Clin Exp Immunol 147(3):412–418. doi:10.1111/j.1365-2249.2006.03271.x (PubMed PMID: 17302889; PubMed Central PMCID: PMC1810482)

Fontenot JD, Gavin MA, Rudensky AY (2003) Foxp3 programs the development and function of CD4+CD25+ regulatory T cells. Nat Immunol 4(4):330–336. doi:10.1038/ni904 (PubMed PMID: 12612578)

Fontenot JD, Rasmussen JP, Gavin MA, Rudensky AY (2005) A function for interleukin 2 in Foxp3-expressing regulatory T cells. Nat Immunol 6(11):1142–1151. doi:ni1263[pii]10.1038/ni1263 (PubMed PMID: 16227984)

Fritzsching B, Oberle N, Pauly E, Geffers R, Buer J, Poschl J et al (2006) Naive regulatory T cells: a novel subpopulation defined by resistance toward CD95 L-mediated cell death. Blood 108(10):3371–3378 doi:10.1182/blood-2006-02-005660 (PubMed PMID: 16868256)

Fritzsching B, Haas J, Konig F, Kunz P, Fritzsching E, Poschl J et al (2011) Intracerebral human regulatory T cells: analysis of CD4+ CD25+ FOXP3+ T cells in brain lesions and cerebrospinal fluid of multiple sclerosis patients. PloS one 6(3):e17988. doi:10.1371/journal.pone.0017988 (PubMed PMID: 21437244; PubMed Central PMCID: PMC3060879)

Groux H, O'Garra A, Bigler M, Rouleau M, Antonenko S, Vries JEdeetal (1997) A CD4+ T-cell subset inhibits antigen-specific T-cell responses and prevents colitis. Nature 389(6652):737–742 doi:10.1038/39614 (PubMed PMID: 9338786)

Haas J, Hug A, Viehover A, Fritzsching B, Falk CS, Filser A et al (2005) Reduced suppressive effect of CD4+CD25high regulatory T cells on the T cell immune response against myelin oligodendrocyte glycoprotein in patients with multiple sclerosis. Eur J Immunol 35(11):3343–3352. doi:10.1002/eji.200526065 (PubMed PMID: 16206232)

Haas J, Fritzsching B, Trubswetter P, Korporal M, Milkova L, Fritz B et al (2007) Prevalence of newly generated naive regulatory T cells (Treg) is critical for Treg suppressive function and determines Treg dysfunction in multiple sclerosis. J Immunol 179(2):1322–1330 (PubMed PMID: 17617625)

Haas J, Korporal M, Balint B, Fritzsching B, Schwarz A, Wildemann B (2009) Glatiramer acetate improves regulatory T-cell function by expansion of naive CD4(+)CD25(+)FOXP3(+)CD31(+) T-cells in patients with multiple sclerosis. J Neuroimmunol 16(1–2):113–117. doi:10.1016/j.jneuroim.2009.06.011 (PubMed PMID: 19646767)

Hamann A, Klugewitz K, Austrup F, Jablonski-Westrich D (2000) Activation induces rapid and profound alterations in the trafficking of T cells. Eur J Immunol 30(11):3207–3218. doi:10.1002/1521-4141(200011)30:11<3207::AID-IMMU3207>3.0.CO;2-L (PubMed PMID: 11093136)

Hong J, Li N, Zhang X, Zheng B, Zhang JZ (2005) Induction of CD4+CD25+ regulatory T cells by copolymer-I through activation of transcription factor Foxp3. Proc Natl Acad Sci U S A 102(18):6449–6454. doi:10.1073/pnas.0502187102 (PubMed PMID: 15851684; PubMed Central PMCID: PMC1088385)

Hori S, Haury M, Coutinho A, Demengeot J. (2002) Specificity requirements for selection and effector functions of CD25+4+ regulatory T cells in anti-myelin basic protein T cell receptor transgenic mice. Proc Natl Acad Sci U S A 99(12):8213–8218. doi:10.1073/pnas.122224799 (PubMed PMID: 12034883; PubMed Central PMCID: PMC123047)

Hori S, Nomura T, Sakaguchi S. (2003) Control of regulatory T cell development by the transcription factor Foxp3. Science 299(5609):1057–1061. doi:10.1126/science.1079490 (PubMed PMID: 12522256)

Huan J, Culbertson N, Spencer L, Bartholomew R, Burrows GG, Chou YK et al (2005) Decreased FOXP3 levels in multiple sclerosis patients. J Neurosci Res 81(1):45–52. doi:10.1002/jnr.20522 (PubMed PMID: 15952173)

Huang CT, Workman CJ, Flies D, Pan X, Marson AL, Zhou G et al (2004) Role of LAG-3 in regulatory T cells. Immunity 21(4):503–513. doi:S1074761304002468[pii]10.1016/j.immuni.2004.08.010 (PubMed PMID: 15485628)

Ito T, Hanabuchi S, Wang YH, Park WR, Arima K, Bover L et al (2008) Two functional subsets of FOXP3+ regulatory T cells in human thymus and periphery. Immunity 28(6):870–880. doi:10.1016/j.immuni.2008.03.018 (PubMed PMID: 18513999; PubMed Central PMCID: PMC2709453)

Jager PL De, Jia X, Wang J, de Bakker PI, Ottoboni L, Aggarwal NT, et al (2009) Meta-analysis of genome scans and replication identify CD6, IRF8 and TNFRSF1A as new multiple sclerosis susceptibility loci. Nat genet 41(7):776–82. doi:10.1038/ng.401 (PubMed PMID: 19525953; PubMed Central PMCID: PMC2757648)

Janssens W, Carlier V, Wu B, VanderElst L, Jacquemin MG, Saint-Remy JM (2003) CD4+CD25+ T cells lyse antigen-presenting B cells by Fas–Fas ligand interaction in an epitope-specific manner. J Immunol 171(9):4604–4612 (PubMed PMID: 14568934)

Jonuleit H, Schmitt E, Stassen M, Tuettenberg A, Knop J, Enk AH (2001) Identification and functional characterization of human CD4(+)CD25(+) T cells with regulatory properties isolated from peripheral blood. J Exp Med 193(11):1285–1294 (PubMed PMID: 11390435; PubMed Central PMCID: PMC2193380)

Kanangat S, Blair P, Reddy R, Daheshia M, Godfrey V, Rouse BT et al (1996) Disease in the scurfy (sf) mouse is associated with overexpression of cytokine genes. Eur J Immunol 26(1):161–165. doi:10.1002/eji.1830260125 (PubMed PMID: 8566060)

Karandikar NJ, Crawford MP, Yan X, Ratts RB, Brenchley JM, Ambrozak DR et al (2002) Glatiramer acetate (Copaxone) therapy induces CD8(+) T cell responses in patients with multiple sclerosis. J Clin Invest 109(5):641–649. doi:10.1172/JCI14380 (PubMed PMID: 11877472; PubMed Central PMCID: PMC150895)

Khattri R, Cox T, Yasayko SA, Ramsdell F. (2003) An essential role for Scurfin in CD4+CD25+ T regulatory cells. Nature Immunol 4(4):337–342. doi:10.1038/ni909 (PubMed PMID: 12612581)

Kimmig S, Przybylski GK, Schmidt CA, Laurisch K, Mowes B, Radbruch A et al (2002) Two subsets of naive T helper cells with distinct T cell receptor excision circle content in human adult peripheral blood. J Exp Med 195(6):789–794 (PubMed PMID: 11901204; PubMed Central PMCID: PMC2193736)

Koenen HJ, Smeets RL, Vink PM, Rijssen E van, Boots AM, Joosten I (2008) Human CD25highFoxp3pos regulatory T cells differentiate into IL-17-producing cells. Blood 112(6):2340–2352. doi:10.1182/blood-2008-01-133967 (PubMed PMID: 18617638)

Kohm AP, Carpentier PA, Anger HA, Miller SD. (2002) Cutting edge: CD4+CD25+ regulatory T cells suppress antigen-specific autoreactive immune responses and central nervous system inflammation during active experimental autoimmune encephalomyelitis. J Immunol 169(9):4712–6 (PubMed PMID: 12391178)

Korn T, Reddy J, Gao W, Bettelli E, Awasthi A, Petersen TR et al (2007) Myelin-specific regulatory T cells accumulate in the CNS but fail to control autoimmune inflammation. Nature Med 13(4):423–431. doi:10.1038/nm1564 (PubMed PMID: 17384649)

Kretschmer K, Apostolou I, Hawiger D, Khazaie K, Nussenzweig MC, Boehmer H von (2005) Inducing and expanding regulatory T cell populations by foreign antigen. Nature Immunol 6(12):1219–1227. doi:10.1038/ni1265 (PubMed PMID: 16244650)

Kullberg MC, Hay V, Cheever AW, Mamura M, Sher A, Letterio JJ et al (2005) TGF-beta1 production by CD4+CD25+ regulatory T cells is not essential for suppression of intestinal inflammation. Eur J Immunol;35(10):2886–2895. doi:10.1002/eji.200526106 (PubMed PMID: 16180248)

Kumar M, Putzki N, Limmroth V, Remus R, Lindemann M, Knop D et al (2006) CD4+CD25+FoxP3+ T lymphocytes fail to suppress myelin basic protein-induced proliferation in patients with multiple sclerosis. J Neuroimmunol 180(1–2):178–84. doi:10.1016/j.jneuroim.2006.08.003 (PubMed PMID: 17011048)

Lafaille JJ, Nagashima K, Katsuki M, Tonegawa S. (1994) High incidence of spontaneous autoimmune encephalomyelitis in immunodeficient anti-myelin basic protein T cell receptor transgenic mice. Cell 78(3):399–408 (PubMed PMID: 7520367)

Levings MK, Sangregorio R, Roncarolo MG (2001) Human CD25(+)CD4(+) T regulatory cells suppress naive and memory T cell proliferation and can be expanded in vitro without loss of function. J Exp Med 193(11):1295–302 (PubMed PMID: 11390436; PubMed Central PMCID: PMC2193376)

Liu W, Putnam AL, Xu-Yu Z, Szot GL, Lee MR, Zhu S et al (2006) CD127 expression inversely correlates with FoxP3 and suppressive function of human CD4+ T reg cells. J Exp Med 203(7):1701–1711. doi:10.1084/jem.20060772 (PubMed PMID: 16818678; PubMed Central PMCID: PMC2118339)

Lyon MF, Peters J, Glenister PH, Ball S, Wright E (1990) The scurfy mouse mutant has previously unrecognized hematological abnormalities and resembles Wiskott-Aldrich syndrome. Proc Natl Acad Sci U S A 87(7):2433–2437 (PubMed PMID: 2320565; PubMed Central PMCID: PMC53703)

Marie JC, Astier AL, Rivailler P, Rabourdin-Combe C, Wild TF, Horvat B (2002) Linking innate and acquired immunity: divergent role of CD46 cytoplasmic domains in T cell induced inflammation. Nat Immunol 3(7):659–666. doi:10.1038/ni810 (PubMed PMID: 12055630)

Mazzucchelli R, Durum SK (2007) Interleukin-7 receptor expression: intelligent design. Nat Rev Immunol 7(2):144–154. doi:10.1038/nri2023 (PubMed PMID: 17259970)

McClymont SA, Putnam AL, Lee MR, Esensten JH, Liu W, Hulme MA et al (2011) Plasticity of human regulatory T cells in healthy subjects and patients with type 1 diabetes. J Immunol 186(7):3918–3926. doi:10.4049/jimmunol.1003099 (PubMed PMID: 21368230; PubMed Central PMCID: PMC3091943)

McGeachy MJ, Stephens LA, Anderton SM (2005) Natural recovery and protection from autoimmune encephalomyelitis: contribution of CD4+CD25+ regulatory cells within the central nervous system. J Immunol 175(5):3025–3032 (PubMed PMID: 16116190)

Misra N, Bayry J, Lacroix-Desmazes S, Kazatchkine MD, Kaveri SV (2004) Cutting edge: human CD4+CD25+ T cells restrain the maturation and antigen-presenting function of dendritic cells. J Immunol 172(8):4676–4680 (PubMed PMID: 15067041)

Miyara M, Yoshioka Y, Kitoh A, Shima T, Wing K, Niwa A et al (2009) Functional delineation and differentiation dynamics of human CD4+ T cells expressing the FoxP3 transcription factor. Immunity 30(6):899–911. doi:10.1016/j.immuni.2009.03.019 (PubMed PMID: 19464196)

Nakamura K, Kitani A, Strober W (2001) Cell contact-dependent immunosuppression by CD4(+)CD25(+) regulatory T cells is mediated by cell surface-bound transforming growth factor beta. J Exp Med 194(5):629–644 (PubMed PMID: 11535631; PubMed Central PMCID: PMC2195935)

Ng WF, Duggan PJ, Ponchel F, Matarese G, Lombardi G, Edwards AD et al (2001) Human CD4(+)CD25(+) cells: a naturally occurring population of regulatory T cells. Blood 98(9):2736–2744 (PubMed PMID: 11675346)

Nylander A, Hafler DA (2012) Multiple sclerosis. J Clin Invest 122(4):1180–1188. doi:10.1172/JCI58649 (Reproduced with permission of the J Clin Invest)

O'Connor RA, Floess S, Huehn J, Jones SA, Anderton SM (2012) Foxp3(+) Treg cells in the inflamed CNS are insensitive to IL-6-driven IL-17 production. Eur J Immunol 42(5):1174–1179. doi:10.1002/eji.201142216 (PubMed PMID: 22539291)

O'Connor RA, Malpass KH, Anderton SM (2007) The inflamed central nervous system drives the activation and rapid proliferation of Foxp3+ regulatory T cells. J Immunol 179(2):958–966 (PubMed PMID: 17617587)

Olivares-Villagomez D, Wang Y, Lafaille JJ (1998) Regulatory CD4(+) T cells expressing endogenous T cell receptor chains protect myelin basic protein-specific transgenic mice from spontaneous autoimmune encephalomyelitis. J Exp Med 188(10):1883–1894 (PubMed PMID: 9815266; PubMed Central PMCID: PMC2212402)

Pan F, Yu H, Dang EV, Barbi J, Pan X, Grosso JF et al (2009) Eos mediates Foxp3-dependent gene silencing in CD4+ regulatory T cells. Science 325(5944):1142–1146. doi:10.1126/science.1176077 (PubMed PMID: 19696312; PubMed Central PMCID: PMC2859703)

Powrie F, Carlino J, Leach MW, Mauze S, Coffman RL (1996) A critical role for transforming growth factor-beta but not interleukin 4 in the suppression of T helper type 1-mediated colitis by CD45RB(low) CD4+ T cells. J Exp Med 83(6):2669–2674 (PubMed PMID: 8676088; PubMed Central PMCID: PMC2192626)

Putheti P, Pettersson A, Soderstrom M, Link H, Huang YM (2004) Circulating CD4+CD25+ T regulatory cells are not altered in multiple sclerosis and unaffected by disease-modulating drugs. J Clin Immunol 24(2):155–161. doi:10.1023/B:JOCI.0000019780.93817.82 (PubMed PMID: 15024182)

Ralainirina N, Poli A, Michel T, Poos L, Andres E, Hentges F et al (2007) Control of NK cell functions by CD4+CD25+ regulatory T cells. J Leukoc Biol 81(1):144–153. doi:10.1189/jlb.0606409 (PubMed PMID: 16959895)

Ramos-Cejudo J, Oreja-Guevara C, Stark Aroeira L, Rodriguez de Antonio L, Chamorro B, Diez-Tejedor E (2011) Treatment with natalizumab in relapsing-remitting multiple sclerosis patients induces changes in inflammatory mechanism. J Clin Immunol 31(4):623–631. doi:10.1007/s10875-011-9522-x (PubMed PMID: 21491095; PubMed Central PMCID: PMC3155864)

Read S, Malmstrom V, Powrie F (2000) Cytotoxic T lymphocyte-associated antigen 4 plays an essential role in the function of CD25(+)CD4(+) regulatory cells that control intestinal inflammation. J Exp Med 192(2):295–302 (PubMed PMID: 10899916; PubMed Central PMCID: PMC2193261)

Reddy J, Illes Z, Zhang X, Encinas J, Pyrdol J, Nicholson L et al (2004) Myelin proteolipid protein-specific CD4+CD25+ regulatory cells mediate genetic resistance to experimental autoimmune encephalomyelitis. Proc Natl Acad Sci U S A 101(43):15434–15439. doi:10.1073/pnas.0404444101 (PubMed PMID: 15492218; PubMed Central PMCID: PMC524444)

Reddy J, Waldner H, Zhang X, Illes Z, Wucherpfennig KW, Sobel RA et al (2005) Cutting edge: CD4+CD25+ regulatory T cells contribute to gender differences in susceptibility to experimental autoimmune encephalomyelitis. J Immunol 175(9):5591–5595 (PubMed PMID: 16237044)

Roncador G, Brown PJ, Maestre L, Hue S, Martinez-Torrecuadrada JL, Ling KL et al (2001) Analysis of FOXP3 protein expression in human CD4+CD25+ regulatory T cells at the single-cell level. Eur J Immunol 35(6):1681–91. doi:10.1002/eji.200526189 (PubMed PMID: 15902688)

Roncarolo MG, Bacchetta R, Bordignon C, Narula S Levings MK (2001) Type 1 T regulatory cells. Immunol Rev 182:68–79 (PubMed PMID: 11722624)

Sakaguchi S, Sakaguchi N, Asano M, Itoh M, Toda M (1995) Immunologic self-tolerance maintained by activated T cells expressing IL-2 receptor alpha-chains (CD25). Breakdown of a single mechanism of self-tolerance causes various autoimmune diseases. J Immunol 155(3):1151–1164 (PubMed PMID: 7636184)

Sakaguchi S, Miyara M, Costantino CM, Hafler DA (2010) FOXP3+ regulatory T cells in the human immune system. Nature Rev Immunol 10(7):490–500. doi:10.1038/nri2785 (PubMed PMID: 20559327)

Sawcer S, Ban M, Maranian M, Yeo TW, Compston A, Kirby A et al (2005) A high-density screen for linkage in multiple sclerosis. Am J Human Genet 77(3):454–467. doi:10.1086/444547 (PubMed PMID: 16080120; PubMed Central PMCID: PMC1226210)

Sawcer S, Hellenthal G, Pirinen M, Spencer CC, Patsopoulos NA, Moutsianas L et al (2011) Genetic risk and a primary role for cell-mediated immune mechanisms in multiple sclerosis. Nature 476(7359):214–219. doi:10.1038/nature10251 (PubMed PMID: 21833088; PubMed Central PMCID: PMC3182531)

Seddiki N, Santner-Nanan B, Martinson J, Zaunders J, Sasson S, Landay A et al (2006a) Expression of interleukin (IL)-2 and IL-7 receptors discriminates between human regulatory and activated T cells. J Exp Med 203(7):1693–1700. doi:10.1084/jem.20060468 (PubMed PMID: 16818676; PubMed Central PMCID: PMC2118333)

Seddiki N, Santner-Nanan B, Tangye SG, Alexander SI, Solomon M, Lee S et al (2006b) Persistence of naive CD45RA+ regulatory T cells in adult life. Blood 107(7):2830–2838. doi:10.1182/blood-2005-06-2403 (PubMed PMID: 16332974)

Shevach EM (2009) Mechanisms of foxp3+ T regulatory cell-mediated suppression. Immunity 30(5):636–45. doi:S1074-7613(09)00197-6[pii]10.1016/j.immuni.2009.04.010 (PubMed PMID: 19464986)

Stenner MP, Waschbisch A, Buck D, Doerck S, Einsele H, Toyka KV et al (2008) Effects of natalizumab treatment on Foxp3+ T regulatory cells. PloS one 3(10):e3319. doi:10.1371/journal.pone.0003319 (PubMed PMID: 18836525; PubMed Central PMCID: PMC2553177)

Sugimoto N, Oida T, Hirota K, Nakamura K, Nomura T, Uchiyama T et al (2006) Foxp3-dependent and -independent molecules specific for CD25+CD4+ natural regulatory T cells revealed by DNA microarray analysis. Int Immunol 18(8):1197–1209. doi:10.1093/intimm/dxl060 (PubMed PMID: 16772372)

Taams LS, Vukmanovic-Stejic M, Smith J, Dunne PJ, Fletcher JM, Plunkett FJ et al (2002) Antigen-specific T cell suppression by human CD4+ CD25+ regulatory T cells. European J Immunol 32(6):1621–1630. doi:10.1002/1521-4141(200206)32:6<1621::AID-IMMU1621>3.0.CO;2-Q (PubMed PMID: 12115645)

Taams LS, Amelsfort JM van, Tiemessen MM, Jacobs KM, Jong EC de, Akbar AN et al (2005) Modulation of monocyte/macrophage function by human CD4+CD25+ regulatory T cells. Human Immunol 66(3):222–230. doi:10.1016/j.humimm.2004.12.006 (PubMed PMID: 15784460)

Tennakoon DK, Mehta RS, Ortega SB, Bhoj V, Racke MK, Karandikar NJ (2006) Therapeutic induction of regulatory, cytotoxic CD8+ T cells in multiple sclerosis. J Immunol 176(11):7119–7129 (PubMed PMID: 16709875)

Thornton AM, Korty PE, Tran DQ, Wohlfert EA, Murray PE, Belkaid Y et al (2010) Expression of Helios, an Ikaros transcription factor family member, differentiates thymic-derived from peripherally induced Foxp3+ T regulatory cells. J Immunol;184(7):3433–3441. doi:10.4049/jimmunol.0904028 (PubMed PMID: 20181882)

Valmori D, Merlo A, Souleimanian NE, Hesdorffer CS, Ayyoub M (2005) A peripheral circulating compartment of natural naive CD4 Tregs. J Clin Invest 115(7):1953–1962. doi:10.1172/JCI23963 (PubMed PMID: 16007258; PubMed Central PMCID: PMC1159133)

Vandenbark AA, Huan J, Agotsch M, La Tocha D, Goelz S, Offner H et al (2009) Interferon-beta-1a treatment increases CD56bright natural killer cells and CD4+CD25+Foxp3 expression in subjects with multiple sclerosis. J Neuroimmunol 215(1–2):125–128. doi:10.1016/j.jneuroim.2009.08.007 (PubMed PMID: 19758707)

Venken K, Hellings N, Hensen K, Rummens JL, Medaer R, D'Hooghe MB et al (2006) Secondary progressive in contrast to relapsing-remitting multiple sclerosis patients show a normal CD4+CD25+ regulatory T-cell function and FOXP3 expression. J Neurosci Res 83(8):1432–1446. doi:10.1002/jnr.20852 (PubMed PMID: 16583400)

Venken K, Hellings N, Thewissen M, Somers V, Hensen K, Rummens JL et al (2008a) Compromised CD4+ CD25(high) regulatory T-cell function in patients with relapsing-remitting multiple sclerosis is correlated with a reduced frequency of FOXP3-positive cells and reduced FOXP3 expression at the single-cell level. Immunology 123(1):79–89. doi:10.1111/j.1365-2567.2007.02690.x (PubMed PMID: 17897326; PubMed Central PMCID: PMC2433271)

Venken K, Hellings N, Broekmans T, Hensen K, Rummens JL, Stinissen P (2008b) Natural naive CD4+CD25+CD127low regulatory T cell (Treg) development and function are disturbed in multiple sclerosis patients: recovery of memory Treg homeostasis during disease progression. J Immunol 180(9):6411–6420 (PubMed PMID: 18424765)

Viglietta V, Baecher-Allan C, Weiner HL, Hafler DA. (2004) Loss of functional suppression by CD4+CD25+ regulatory T cells in patients with multiple sclerosis. J Exp Med 199(7):971–979. doi:10.1084/jem.20031579 (PubMed PMID: 15067033; PubMed Central PMCID: PMC2211881)

Vukmanovic-Stejic M, Zhang Y, Cook JE, Fletcher JM, McQuaid A, Masters JE et al (2006) Human CD4+CD25hi Foxp3+ regulatory T cells are derived by rapid turnover of memory populations in vivo. J Clin Invest 116(9):2423–2433. doi:10.1172/JCI28941 (PubMed PMID: 16955142; PubMed Central PMCID: PMC1555646)

Weiner HL (2001) Induction and mechanism of action of transforming growth factor-beta-secreting Th3 regulatory cells. Immunol Rev 182:207–214 (PubMed PMID: 11722636)

Wildin RS, Ramsdell F, Peake J, Faravelli F, Casanova JL, Buist N et al (2001) X-linked neonatal diabetes mellitus, enteropathy and endocrinopathy syndrome is the human equivalent of mouse scurfy. Nature Genet 27(1):18–20 doi:10.1038/83707 (PubMed PMID: 11137992)

Wildin RS, Smyk-Pearson S, Filipovich AH (2002) Clinical and molecular features of the immunodysregulation, polyendocrinopathy, enteropathy, X linked (IPEX) syndrome. J Med Genet 39(8):537–545 (PubMed PMID: 12161590; PubMed Central PMCID: PMC1735203)

Zhang X, Koldzic DN, Izikson L, Reddy J, Nazareno RF, Sakaguchi S et al (2004) IL-10 is involved in the suppression of experimental autoimmune encephalomyelitis by CD25+CD4+ regulatory T cells. Int Immunol 16(2):249–256 (PubMed PMID: 14734610)

Zhao DM, Thornton AM, DiPaolo RJ, Shevach EM (2006) Activated CD4+CD25+ T cells selectively kill B lymphocytes. Blood 107(10):3925–3932. doi:10.1182/blood-2005-11-4502 (PubMed PMID: 16418326; PubMed Central PMCID: PMC1895290)

Zheng SG, Wang J, Wang P, Gray JD, Horwitz DA (2007) IL-2 is essential for TGF-beta to convert naive CD4+CD25- cells to CD25+ Foxp3+ regulatory T cells and for expansion of these cells. J Immunol 178(4):2018–2027 (PubMed PMID: 17277105)

Chapter 3
T-bet: A Critical Regulator of Encephalitogenic T Cells

Amy E. Lovett-Racke and Michael K. Racke

Abstract T-bet is a transcription factor that regulates CD4 Th1 cell differentiation and mice deficient in T-bet fail to develop experimental autoimmune encephalomyelitis, demonstrating its critical role in the generation of immune-mediated demyelinating disease. More importantly, silencing T-bet in a model for multiple sclerosis (MS) demonstrates that it is a viable therapeutic target. T-bet has been found to correlate with disease activity and therapeutic efficacy, suggesting that it may also be a biomarker for MS. Defining the role of T-bet in generating encephalitogenic T cells and their effector functions may provide insight into the mechanisms that underlie the pathology of MS lesions.

3.1 Introduction

T-bet was originally cloned and characterized in 2000 by Laurie Glimcher's laboratory in an effort to dissect the regulatory pathway that ultimately led to the development of Th1 cells (Szabo et al. 2000). Under the hypothesis that the *IL2, IFNg*, and *TNFb* genes would all be regulated by a common transcription factor, which would result in Th1 cells, since the expression of these cytokines defines Th1 cells, at least one hybrid system utilizing an IL-2 promoter–reporter construct was used to identify mRNA that was differentially expressed in Th1 cells relative to Th2 cells. Sequence homology to the T box family of transcription factors was the basis for the name T-bet, *T b*ox expressed in *T* cells. T-bet is a 530 amino acid protein encoded by the *Tbx21* gene on chromosome 17 in humans and chromosome 11 in mice, and it contains a 189 amino acid T box DNA-binding domain. T-bet was found to directly regulate the expression of IFNγ and repress the expression of Th2 cytokines (Szabo et al. 2000; Finotto et al. 2002; Lovett-Racke et al. 2004; Hwang et al. 2005; Jenner et al. 2009). Since myelin-specific Th1 cells were capable of

A. E. Lovett-Racke (✉)
Department of Microbial Infection and Immunity, The Ohio State University, Columbus, OH 43210, USA
e-mail: amy.lovett-racke@osumc.edu

M. K. Racke
Department of Neurology, The Ohio State University, Columbus, OH 43210, USA
e-mail: michael.racke@osumc.edu

T. Yamamura, B. Gran (eds.), *Multiple Sclerosis Immunology*,
DOI 10.1007/978-1-4614-7953-6_3, © Springer Science+Business Media New York 2013

inducing experimental autoimmune encephalomyelitis (EAE), a model of multiple sclerosis (MS), and Th1 cells were found in the central nervous system (CNS) of MS patients, a tremendous amount of research has focused on the role of Th1 cells and associated signaling pathways as a means to understand the pathophysiology of MS (McDonald and Swanborg 1988; Ando et al. 1989; Waldburger et al. 1996; Yura et al. 2001; Lovett-Racke et al. 2004; Gocke et al. 2007; Yang et al. 2009). T-bet, a Th1-associated transcription factor, has been found to be a critical factor in the development of encephalitogenic CD4 T cells in EAE, as well as an effective therapeutic target (Lovett-Racke et al. 2004; Bettelli et al. 2004; Gocke et al. 2007; Yang et al. 2009). Furthermore, T-bet has been identified as a potential biomarker for disease activity and therapeutic efficacy in MS patients (Nath et al. 2004; Frisullo et al. 2006; Peng et al. 2006; Frisullo et al. 2007; Drulovic et al. 2009; Iorio et al. 2009; Kleiter et al. 2010; Frisullo et al. 2011). Thus, T-bet provides insight into the mechanisms by which CD4 T cells mediate CNS lesion development, as well as a potential therapeutic target for the treatment of MS.

3.2 Characterization of the Immune Response in Multiple Sclerosis

MS is an old disease whose pathology was not formally articulated until the nineteenth century when Jean-Marie Charcot described CNS lesions associated with episodic neurological deficits.

> On histological sections, multiple sclerosis lesions contain perivascular inflammation and demyelination. Plaques occur anywhere within the white matter of the central nervous system. The most frequently affected sites are optic nerves, brainstem, cerebellum and spinal cord. Lesions in these areas often correlate with clinical systems. In the cerebral hemispheres, periventricular distribution of plaques is often seen. When plaques are adjacent to the cortex, subcortical myelinated nerves are often spared. Plaques located near the gray matter may spread into the gray matter, including deep nuclei and the cortex. Axons are spared within the initial lesions, but are later destroyed (Charcot 1968; translated from French).

Although tremendous research has been done to understand the pathophysiology of MS, Charcot's initial description is still as accurate a description of the MS lesions as any published since that time. In addition, the components of the lesions as delineated by Charcot, inflammation, demyelination, and axonal destruction, have been the basis of most research on MS. Since inflammation appears to be the predecessor of the demyelination and axonal damage, characterization of the inflammatory response has been a priority in MS research. As our understanding of immunology has evolved over the past decades, our understanding of the inflammatory response in the CNS of MS patients has also evolved, yet the cause of the disease remains unknown and our ability to modify the disease course limited.

3.3 CD4 T Cell Lineages

The hallmark observation that CD4 T cells can express distinct cytokine profiles and play different roles in protective immunity has shed light on the differential role of CD4 T cell lineages in health and disease. The original observation that effector CD4 T cells primarily expressed the signature cytokines IFNγ or IL-4, known as T-helper 1 (Th1) or T-helper 2 (Th2) cells, respectively, prompted interest in how these two lineages develop (Mosmann et al. 1986). T cell receptor (TCR) binding to MHC/peptide complexes (signal 1) and CD28 interaction with CD80/CD86 (signal 2) are the initial activation signals required for the activation of T cells via antigen-presenting cells (APCs; Fig. 3.1; June et al. 1990). However, cytokines produced in the microenvironment provide critical signals that determine the lineage commitment of CD4 T cells. If the environment is rich in IFNγ and IL-12, CD4 T cells differentiate into Th1 cells (Figs. 3.1 and 3.2). All CD4 T cells express the interferon receptor, which when engaged, results in the phosphorylation of the transcription factor STAT1 and translocation to the nucleus (Fig. 3.2a; Afkarian et al. 2002). STAT1 contributes to the expression of T-bet, the master regulator of Th1 cells (Fig. 3.2b–c; Lovett-Racke et al. 2004). There is a positive feedback loop between STAT1 and T-bet that promotes the Th1 phenotype and induces the expression of the IL-12 receptor β2 chain (IL12Rβ2). When the IL12Rβ2 chain pairs with the constitutively expressed IL12Rβ1 chain, this allows IL-12 signaling to occur. IL-12 receptor signaling causes phosphorylation of STAT4, translocation to the nucleus, and binding to the *Ifng* gene promoter (Fig. 3.2d; Jacobson et al. 1995). In conjunction with STAT1 and T-bet, STAT4 induces expression of IFNγ and lineage commitment to a Th1 phenotype (Fig. 3.2e). Since Th1 cells express IFNγ and IFNγ initiates the differentiation of Th1 cells, the microenvironment will continue to favor the differentiation of naive CD4 T cells into Th1 cells, and thus an immune response to a particular antigen is typically dominated by a specific CD4 T cell lineage. Similarly, CD4 Th2 cells are generated by IL-4 receptor signaling that causes phosphorylation of STAT6, translocation to the nucleus, and binding to the *gata3* gene promoter (Hsieh et al. 1992; Hou et al. 1994; Zheng and Flavell 1997). GATA3 is the master transcriptional regulator of Th2 cells that promotes the expression of IL-4 as well as other Th2-associated cytokines such as IL-5 and IL-13.

More recently, a unique population of CD4 T cells known as Th17 cells has been identified as another lineage defined by the expression of IL-17 (Yao et al. 1995). IL-6 appears to be the critical cytokine for the differentiation of naive CD4 T cells into Th17 cells (Veldhoen et al. 2006; Bettelli et al. 2006; Mangan et al. 2006; Acosta-Rodriguiz et al. 2007; Wilson et al. 2007; Yang et al. 2008a, 2008b; Yang et al. 2009; Ghoreschi et al. 2010). IL-6 receptor signaling causes the phosphorylation of STAT3, which in coordination with the transcription factor RORγt induce IL-17 expression (Fig. 3.2g–h). However, other cytokines have been implicated to enhance Th17 commitment in conjunction with IL-6, namely TGFβ in murine T cells (Figs. 3.1 and 3.2g) and TGFβ, IL-1β, and IL-21 in human T cells. Myelin-specific Th1 and Th17 cells are present in mice with EAE and MS patients, and both populations appear to mediate CNS pathology (Traugott and Lebon 1988; McDonald and

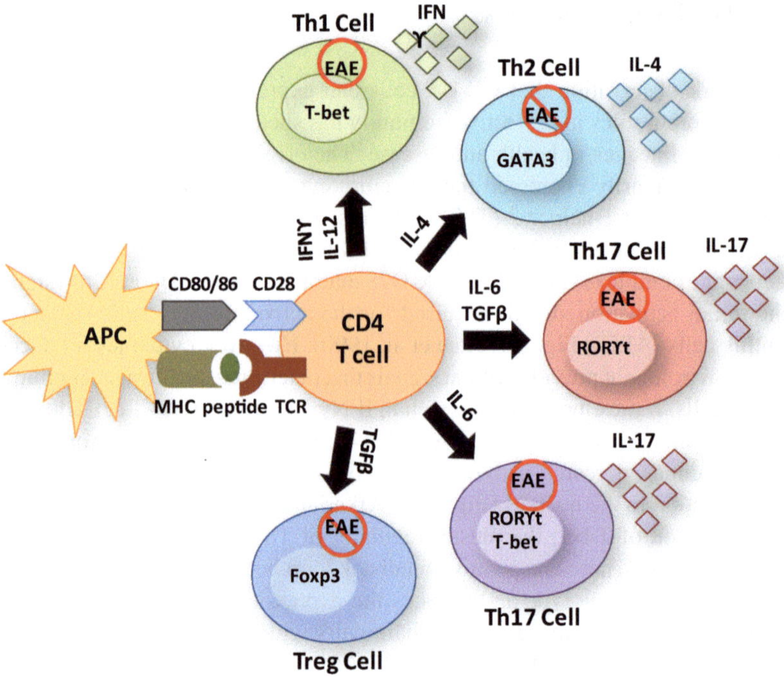

Fig. 3.1 Differentiation of CD4 T cells into effector T cells that mediate central nervous system (CNS) demyelination. Naive CD4 T cells engage antigen-presenting cells (APC) to become activated. Both MHC/peptide engagement with the T cell receptor (TCR) and costimulation mediated by CD80/86 (B7.1/B7.2) with CD28 is required to initiate T cells activation. These activated T cells have the capacity to differentiate into different T cell lineages depending on the cytokines in the local environment. IFNγ and IL-12 promote the differentiation of Th1 cells, which are primarily regulated by the transcription factor T-bet, express IFNγ, and can mediate experimental autoimmune encephalomyelitis (EAE). Th2 cells depend on IL-4 activation via the transcription GATA3 and typically are associated with EAE resistance. Th17 cells can be generated in the presence of IL-6 in the presence or absence of TGFβ; however, only Th17 generated in the absence of TGFβ are capable of causing EAE due to the negative regulation of T-bet by TGFβ. CD4 T cells can also develop into a regulatory population that limits the activation and effector functions of other CD4 T cells

Swanborg 1988; Ando et al. 1989; Waldburger et al. 1996; Yura et al. 2001; Lock et al. 2002; Lovett-Racke et al. 2004; Gocke et al. 2007; Kroenke and Segal 2007; Tzartos et al. 2008; Yang et al. 2009).

CD4-positive T cells may also develop into a regulatory population that plays a vital role in controlling and dampening of effector T cells to maintain the balance between protection and potential immune-mediated pathology (Kumar et al. 1996; Hori et al. 2003). CD4-regulatory T cells (Tregs) can develop in the thymus or in the periphery. TGFβ signaling is believed to be the critical cytokine signaling required for Treg development, which induces the expression of Foxp3, the transcription factor required for Treg development and function (Fig. 3.1; Marie et al. 2005). These four dominant populations of CD4 T cells provide molecular signals to other cells of the

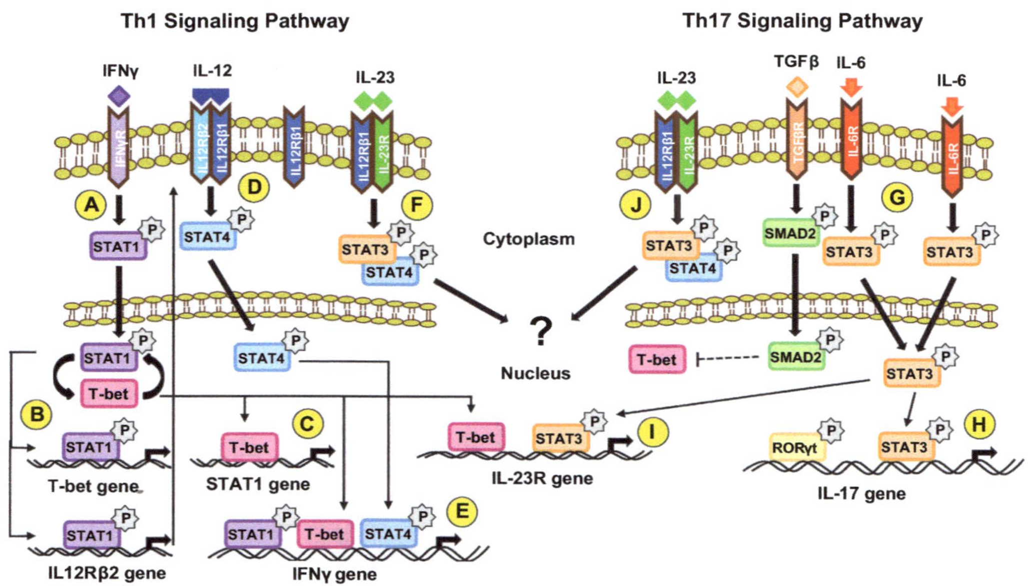

Fig. 3.2 Th1 and Th17 cells have the capacity to cause immune-mediated demyelinating disease via signaling pathways dependent on T-bet. Both Th1 and Th17 cells can cause experimental autoimmune encephalomyelitis (EAE) and both populations are present in multiple sclerosis (MS) lesions. (**a**) Th1 cells differentiate due to the initial signaling via the IFNγ receptor resulting in STAT1 phosphorylation and translocation to the nucleus whereby T-bet and STAT1 regulate each other's expression in a positive feedback loop and induce expression of the IL-12 receptor β2 chain (**b**). T-bet regulates STAT1 and IL-23 receptor expression (**c**). IL-12 receptor signaling can proceed (**d**), resulting in STAT4 phosphorylation and translocation to the nucleus, which ultimately leads to the activation of the IFNγ gene (**e**). The IL-23 receptor is upregulated during T cell differentiation (**f**), at least partially due to T-bet, and this is necessary for critical signals required for acquisition of an encephalitogenic phenotype. (**g**) IL-6 signaling during T cell activation favors Th17 development via phosphorylation of STAT3, a transcription factor that coordinates with RORγt to regulate IL-17 gene transcription (**h**). Phosphorylation STAT3 also contributes to the expression of the IL-23 receptor gene, making transcription factors commonly associated with both Th1 and Th17 cells necessary for induction of the IL-23 receptor (**i**). However, it is unknown what critical function is induced by IL-23 receptor signaling

immune system, which coordinate an immune response to protect us from pathogens and cancer. The effectiveness of our immune system is evident in that the vast majority of us live long and healthy lives. However, approximately 5 % of the population suffers from some form of autoimmunity and since autoimmunity is mediated by adaptive immune responses, a tremendous amount of research has focused on the role of CD4 T cells in the onset and progression of autoimmune diseases. Although the pathology of autoimmune diseases may be caused by auto-antibodies or cytotoxic CD8 T cells, CD4 T cells play vital roles in the development of antibodies and CD8 T cells, making CD4 T cells a potential common link among all autoimmune diseases.

3.4 Role of CD4 T Cells in Experimental Autoimmune Encephalomyelitis

EAE has been used as a model for MS research since the 1960s. The model originated from the observation that a small number of individuals who received the rabies virus vaccine, a live-attenuated vaccine grown in the CNS of rabbits, developed encephalomyelitis. Investigation into the cause of the postvaccine encephalomyelitis led to the discovery that the CNS material that contaminated the vaccine could induce a hypersensitivity reaction that resulted in an immune-mediated encephalomyelitis and the onset of symptoms reminiscent of MS (Rivers et al. 1933). EAE is typically induced in rodents by subcutaneous immunization of myelin proteins or peptides emulsified in Complete Freund's Adjuvant (CFA). However, adoptive transfer of myelin-specific CD4 Th1 cells into naive recipient mice will also result in EAE development (McDonald and Swanborg 1988; Ando et al. 1989; Waldburger et al. 1996; Yura et al. 2001; Lovett-Racke et al. 2004; Gocke et al. 2007; Yang et al. 2009), supporting the hypothesis that CD4 T cells are the primary mediator of this model autoimmune disease.

Since myelin-specific Th1 cells were sufficient to induce EAE in mice, research on the role of T cells in MS focused on Th1 cells. Several studies that reduced IFNγ in myelin-specific T cells prior to transfer to recipient mice found that changing the signaling pathways, which are necessary for Th1 cell differentiation, diminishes the encephalitogenic capacity of these myelin-specific CD4 T cells (Racke et al. 1994; Racke et al. 1995; Lovett-Racke et al. 2004). Furthermore, mice deficient in STAT4 and T-bet, two transcription factors that play vital roles in the Th1 differentiation pathway, were resistant to EAE induction, supporting the hypothesis that EAE is mediated by Th1 cells (Chitnis et al. 2001; Bettelli et al. 2004; Nath et al. 2006). To determine whether IFNγ was a potential therapeutic target, EAE experiments in mice deficient in IFNγ signaling were performed. Contrary to expectations, mice deficient in IFNγ were susceptible to EAE (Ferber et al. 1996). In addition, systemic treatment of mice with IFNγ-neutralizing antibodies did not suppress EAE (Lublin et al. 1993; Heremans et al. 1996; Willenborg et al. 1996). Together, these studies indicate that IFNγ is not essential for the development of encephalitogenic T cells in mice; however, molecules in the Th1 differentiation pathway are necessary.

The observation that CD4 Th1 cells were sufficient to cause EAE, yet IFNγ was dispensable, prompted the investigation of other cytokines in the development and function of encephalitogenic T cells. Since IL-12 was a key cytokine necessary for Th1 cell differentiation, the components of IL-12 and the IL-12 receptor were analyzed using mice genetically deficient in each subunit of the IL-12 cytokine and receptor. IL-12 is a heterodimer composed of a p40 and p35 subunit. Mice deficient in the IL-12p40 were resistant to EAE, yet mice deficient in IL-12p35 remained susceptible to EAE (Becher et al. 2002; Gran et al. 2002). Since IL-12p40 was also a component of IL-23 (Oppmann et al. 2000), EAE was evaluated in mice deficient in the IL-23-specific subunit, p19. IL-23p19-deficient mice were protected from EAE induction, similar to the IL-12p40-deficient mice, indicating that IL-23 signaling was necessary for EAE development (Cua et al. 2003). Culturing of myelin-specific T cells isolated from immunized mice with IL-23 promoted the expansion of myelin-specific IL-17-producing T cells (Langrish et al. 2005). In addition, transfer of these IL-23-expanded T cells into naive mice resulted in EAE, leading to speculation that Th17 cells were actually the primary encephalitogenic CD4 T cell population in EAE and perhaps MS. However, mice deficient in IL-17 remained susceptible to EAE, although the disease may be less severe, suggesting that IL-17 is also not necessary for the development of encephalitogenic T cells (Komiyama et al. 2006; Haak et al. 2009). These data indicate that IL-23, an APC-produced cytokine, is necessary for the development of encephalitogenic T cells. Yet, IFNγ and IL-17, the cytokines that define Th1 and Th17 cells, are not essential.

So what molecules expressed by myelin-specific CD4 effector T cells are required for encephalitogenicity? Use of genetic knock-out mice has shown that GM-CSF (Ponomarev et al. 2007; Codarri et al. 2011; El-Behi et al. 2011), STAT4 (Chitnis et al. 2001), and T-bet (Bettelli et al. 2004; Nath et al. 2006) are required for T cell encephalitogenicity. GM-CSF, a cytokine expressed by numerous cell types including macrophages, endothelial cells, and fibroblasts, is expressed by both Th1 and Th17 cells. However, STAT4 and T-bet are transcription factors that are typically associated with Th1 cells, making it unclear why deletion of these genes would result in EAE resistance if Th17 cells are sufficient to induce EAE. Suppression of T-bet with an siRNA in mice found that not only was EAE inhibited, but both Th1 and Th17 cells failed to differentiate indicating that T-bet was affecting both encephalitogenic T cell populations (Gocke et al. 2007; Yang et al. 2009). Thus, the contribution of T-bet in regulating genes in encephalitogenic T cells must extend beyond IFNγ and Th1-associated genes.

3.5 Role of T-bet in Regulating Gene Expression in CD4 T Cells

T-bet was originally described as the "master" regulator of Th1 cell differentiation because it directly regulates the expression of the IFNγ in CD4 T cells (Szabo et al. 2000). In naive CD4 T cells, the *Ifng* gene is epigenetically repressed by histone 3 lysine 4 trimethylation (H3K27me3; Fig. 3.3). Upon T cell activation and differentiation into a Th1 phenotype, T-bet physically associates with the *Ifng* promoter. This

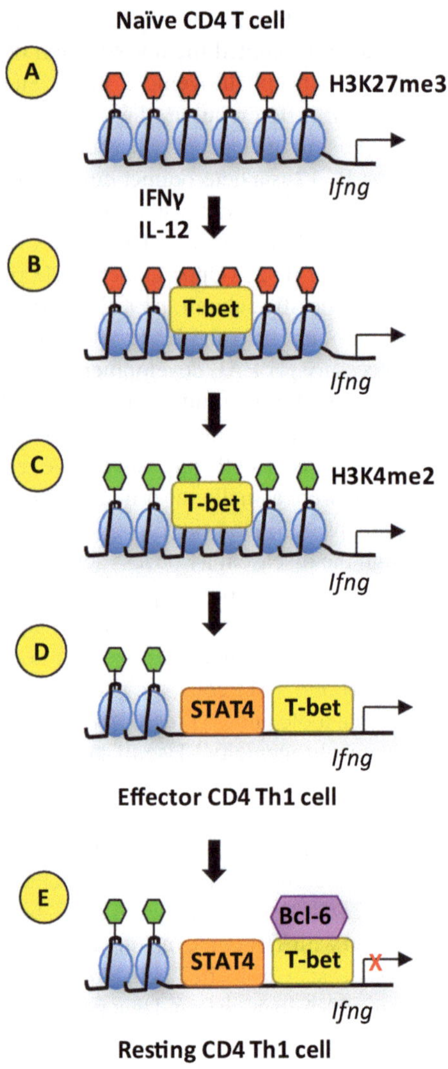

Fig. 3.3 T-bet is the critical transcription factor for the regulation of the IFNγ gene. **a** IFNγ gene is epigenetically repressed via H3K27me3 in naive CD4 T cells. **b** IFNγ and IL-12 receptor signaling induces T-bet, which recruits H3K27 demethylase complexes to the *Ifng* loci to reverse the epigenetically repressed state. **c** T-bet recruits a permissive H3K4 methyl transferase to establish a permissive epigenetic state via H3K4me2. **d** Chromatin remodeling allows Th1-associated transcription factors to bind and promote IFNγ production and the Th1 phenotype. **e** T-bet recruits the transcriptional repressor Bcl-6 to the *Ifng* loci late in Th1 cell differentiation to limit IFNγ production and return Th1 cells to a resting state

causes recruitment of H3K27 demethylase complexes to the *Ifng* loci to reverse the epigenetically repressed state (Lewis et al. 2007; Miller et al. 2008). T-bet subsequently recruits a permissive H3K4 methyl transferase to establish a permissive epigenetic state via H3K4me2, resulting in chromatin remodeling which allows T-bet and STAT4 to bind to the *Ifng* promoter. Typically within 3 days of activation, a naive CD4 T cell will express IFNγ and commit to a Th1 lineage. However, T-bet also plays a repressive role in Th1 cells by recruiting Bcl-6 to the *Ifng* loci late in Th1 cell differentiation (Oestreich et al. 2011). This results in reducing IFNγ production and return to a resting state of Th1 cells, probably to limit the effector function of Th1 cells, minimize tissue damage, and reduce the potential for autoimmunity.

T-bet-deficient mice are resistant to EAE development (Bettelli et al. 2004; Lovett-Racke et al. 2004; Nath et al. 2006), while IFNγ-deficient mice remain susceptible to EAE (Ferber et al. 1996). This suggests that T-bet must regulate genes other than *Ifng* that are necessary for EAE development. Since it had been shown that suppressing T-bet not only reduced Th1 cells but also Th17 cells in mice with EAE, T-bet may be regulating gene(s) common to both Th1 and Th17 cells (Gocke et al. 2007; Yang et al. 2009). Using chromatin immunoprecipitation assays, as well as overexpression of T-bet in cell lines, T-bet was found to positively regulate the expression of the *Il23r* gene (Gocke et al. 2007). It had previously been observed that IL-23 and IL-23 receptor-deficient mice were resistant to EAE suggesting that IL-23 receptor signaling is a vital component of EAE regardless of whether it is mediated by Th1 or Th17 cells (Zhang et al. 2003; Cua et al. 2003). Prior to the discovery of Th17 cells, it had been shown that IL-23 receptor was expressed on activated T cells that were largely of a Th1 phenotype (Oppmann et al. 2000; Parham et al. 2002), so it is feasible that IL-23 may affect both Th1 and Th17 cells. In addition, IL-23 had been shown to promote the expansion of encephalitogenic Th17 cells (Langrish et al. 2005), while neutralizing IL-23 can ameliorate EAE (Chen et al. 2006). It was also shown that IL-23 produced by microglia and CNS-infiltrating macrophages was necessary for the onset of EAE, indicating that myelin-specific T cells required IL-23 receptor expression to mediate demyelination in the CNS (Becher et al. 2003). Using primary microglia cultures, it was found that IFNγ enhanced IL-23 expression, supporting the hypothesis that CNS-infiltrating Th1 cells may contribute to expansion of Th17 cells in the CNS via their production of IFNγ. Similarly, Th17 cells are found in the CNS of mice with EAE induced by adoptive transfer of myelin-specific Th1 cells (Gocke et al. 2007; Lees et al. 2008). Thus, T-bet appears to be critical for EAE due to its role in upregulating the expression of the IL-23 receptor during T cell activation and differentiation.

It had been shown that CD4 T cell lineage commitment is determined by the interaction of T-bet and GATA-3. T-bet represses Th2 cell differentiation by a tyrosine kinase-mediated interaction with GATA-3 (Hwang et al. 2005). Since encephalitogenic CD4 T cells could be both Th1 and Th17, this led to the intriguing question as to what was the role of T-bet in encephalitogenic Th17 cells, beyond IL-23 receptor expression. As previously mentioned, silencing T-bet in wild-type mice with EAE results in fewer Th17 cells. However, induction of EAE in T-bet-deficient mice results in a significant population of myelin-specific Th17 cells, yet these T-bet- deficient mice fail to develop EAE (Yang et al. 2009). This suggests that T-bet is critical in the development of encephalitogenic Th17 cells, but not in the development of CD4 T cells that are capable of expressing IL-17. Several studies showed that naive murine T cells could be differentiated into Th17 cells with IL-6 and TGFβ (Fig. 3.1; Veldhoen et al. 2006; Bettelli et al. 2006; Mangan et al. 2006). However, these differentiation conditions failed to generate Th17 cells that could induce EAE when transferred into wild-type mice, suggesting that the in vivo conditions that generate encephalitogenic T cells must be different (Yang et al. 2009; Ghoreschi et al. 2010). It was subsequently shown that differentiation of naive T cells with IL-6, in the absence of TGFβ and cytokines that promote Th1 or Th2 cells, generates Th17 cells capable of transferring EAE (Fig. 3.1; Yang et al. 2009; Ghoreschi et al. 2010). This observation was consistent with a previous study that found that TGFβ is a negative regulator of T-bet (Gorelik et al. 2002; Park et al. 2005). Therefore, Th17-inducing conditions that included TGFβ-generated T cells failed to express T-bet. Although these T cells expressed significant amounts of IL-17, they were T-bet-negative and lacked a critical element of an encephalitogenic T cell. However, encephalitogenic T cells from wild-type mice had T-bet-positive Th17 cells, and Th17 cells differentiated in vivo with IL-6 in the absence of TGFβ also expressed T-bet, indicating that T-bet was a critical factor in encephalitogenic T cells regardless of whether they expressed a Th1 or Th17 phenotype (Yang et al. 2009).

T-bet has been implicated in the regulation of other molecules associated with the Th1 phenotype and encephalitogenicity. For example, T-bet has been shown to be required for optimal migration of Th1 cells into tissues. T-bet appears to regulate the binding of Th1 cells to P-selectin, an adhesion molecule expressed on inflamed endothelium (Lord et al. 2005). T-bet has also been found to regulate the chemokine receptor CXCR3, which is highly expressed on encephalitogenic Th1 cells (Qin et al. 1998; Sallusto et al. 1998; Beima et al. 2006). This led to speculation that CXCR3 may be vital to T cell trafficking to the CNS and thus, T-bet may be critical due to its role in upregulating CXCR3 expression on CD4 T cells. Although CXCR3 inhibitors have been shown to slightly diminish EAE severity (Kohler et al. 2008; Ni et al. 2009; Sporici and Issekutz 2010), CXCR3-deficient mice remain susceptible to EAE (Liu et al. 2006; Muller et al. 2007) indicating that CXCR3 is not critical to EAE development and, therefore, it is not an essential element regulated by T-bet. This indicates that the diminished trafficking capacity of T-bet-deficient CD4 T cells is probably mediated by a mechanism independent of CXCR3.

CD80/86 on APCs interaction with C28 on T cells is necessary to activate naive T cells in conjunction with TCR engagement (Fig. 3.1). However, memory and effector T cell populations do not require this costimulation signal via CD28, making it possible for memory and effector T cells to function in a rapid and precise manner (Dubey et al. 1996; Yi-qun et al. 1996; Lovett-Racke et al. 1998). More recently, it was discovered that there were other costimulatory molecules, such as inducible costimulator (ICOS) expressed on memory and effector T cells that contribute to their effector function. Inhibition of ICOS after the induction of EAE attenuated the disease (Rottman et al. 2001; Sporici et al. 2001). Ex vivo analysis of the CNS of these mice showed that the myelin-specific CD4 T cells became activated, produced IL-2, and trafficked to the CNS. However, IFNγ production was diminished and enhanced the apoptosis of memory T cells. T-bet was found to bind the ICOS promoter to regulate ICOS expression in conjunction with the transcription factor, NFATc2 (Tan et al. 2008). Since T-bet is not expressed in naive T cells and only expressed following T cell differentiation, the induction of ICOS in memory and effector T cells is temporally consistent with T-bet expression. In human T cells, ICOS was found to dramatically enhance the expansion of IFNγ + IL-17 + T cells, which have been found to have enhanced proinflammatory effector function in EAE and other diseases (Paulos et al. 2010). Interestingly, these cells also express high levels of T-bet, suggesting that T-bet may be enhancing the pathogenic potential of IFNγ + IL-17 + T cells via ICOS costimulation.

In 2001, a large-scale sequencing of cDNA libraries acquired from CNS lesions from MS patients found enhanced expression of osteopontin, a cytokine previously associated with bone formation (Chabas et al. 2001). Rats with EAE were also found to have enhanced osteopontin expression in their CNS. Although mice deficient in osteopontin develop EAE, the disease is less severe, had fewer relapses, and diminished proinflammatory cytokine expression (Chabas et al. 2001; Jansson et al. 2002). T-bet was found to at least partially regulate osteopontin expression, and T-bet-dependent osteopontin expression is necessary for optimal differentiation of Th1 cells (Shinohara et al. 2005). Osteopontin was subsequently found to initiate recurrent relapses and enhance neurological deficits in mice with EAE via enhanced survival of myelin-specific T cells (Hur et al. 2007). T-bet had originally been considered a transcription factor, critical in the initial differentiation of CD4 T cells, but this study indicates that T-bet function in effector and memory T cells via ICOS and osteopontin may be just as important in demyelinating autoimmunity. This was validated in treatment studies of EAE with an siRNA specific for T-bet in which disease was virtually halted in mice when T-bet was suppressed (Gocke et al. 2007). Furthermore, osteopontin levels are elevated in the CSF and serum of MS patients, and elevated osteopontin in the CSF appears to be correlated with relapses (Bornsen et al. 2011; Wen et al. 2012), reminiscent of elevated T-bet levels in MS patients (Frisullo et al. 2009; Kleiter et al. 2010).

T cell Ig- and mucin-domain-containing molecule 3 (Tim-3) was found to be expressed by Th1 cells and blockade of Tim-3 in EAE results in enhanced disease severity, suggesting that Tim-3 plays a role in limiting the effector function of Th1 cells (Monney et al. 2002; Khademi et al. 2004). Tim-3 was also found to be expressed on resident CNS cells in rats with EAE, suggesting that it may contribute CNS autoimmunity in the target organ as well as the infiltrating T cells (Gielen et al. 2005). T cell clones from the CSF of MS patients found that Tim-3 and T-bet were reduced compared to clones derived from control subjects, and that the MS patient T cells had enhanced production of IFNγ suggesting that Tim-3 inversely correlates with IFNγ expression (Koguchi et al. 2006). Using an siRNA specific for Tim-3, T cell proliferation and IFNγ production were reduced, demonstrating the Tim-3 expression plays a significant role in Th1 cell function. CSF T cell clones with low Tim-3 levels also demonstrated resistance to inhibitor signals via CTLA-4, suggesting that their enhanced effector functions may be partially due to diminished regulation (Koguchi et al. 2006). Blockade of Tim-3 ex vivo in MS patients' CD4 T cells did not alter IFNγ production as it did in control subjects, demonstrating a defect in Tim-3 immunoregulation (Yang et al. 2008a, 2008b). Interestingly, glatiramer acetate or IFNβ treatment reversed the functional defect. Thus, dysregulated expression of Tim-3 in MS patients may contribute to disease pathology, and current immunomodulatory drugs may be beneficial at normalizing immune dysregulation mediated by Tim-3. T-bet was found to contribute to the expression of Tim-3 in Th1 cells (Anderson et al. 2010). Since Tim-3 plays a role in dampening Th1 responses, it appears that T-bet-regulated expression of Tim-3 plays a role in not only inducing Th1 responses, but also regulating them in a manner that limits Th1 effector functions. Since MS patients appear to have diminished Tim-3 expression in effector/memory

T cells, the balance of protective adaptive immune responses may be tipped such that proinflammatory T cells go unregulated for extended periods of time resulting in autoimmune tissue damage.

Together, these studies demonstrate that T-bet regulates the expression of several genes that play different roles in T cells' differentiation and effector functions. T-bet may be an effective therapeutic target in EAE due to its ability to modulate different mechanisms in T cells that are required for development, trafficking, and pathogenesis in immune-mediated demyelinating disease.

3.6 Relevance of T-bet in Multiple Sclerosis

It is clear that T-bet is an essential factor in encephalitogenic T cells in mice. Yet, its role in MS is much more difficult to assess. However, changes in T-bet levels have become a common measure of therapeutic potential of drugs evaluated in EAE and MS patients. T-bet levels in peripheral T cells are enhanced in MS patients during relapses relative to remission and are elevated in MS patients compared to healthy controls (Frisullo et al. 2006; Kleiter et al. 2010). In addition, pSTAT1, the transcription factor that is initially activated during Th1 cell differentiation (Fig. 3.1a) is also upregulated. Since pSTAT1 contributes to the expression of T-bet (Afkarian et al. 2002; Lovett-Racke et al. 2004), it is not surprising that T-bet and pSTAT1 levels have a positive correlation. In addition, T-bet and pSTAT1 levels correlated with active lesions in the CNS as determined by MRI, suggesting that T-bet may be a marker of disease activity in MS. Glucocorticoids, which have anti-inflammatory properties, have been used successfully to treat MS exacerbations for decades. Ex vivo analysis of T cells from MS patients treated with glucocorticoids found that T-bet and pSTAT1 were reduced, as well as IFNγ production by peripheral lymphocytes (Frisullo et al. 2007), indicating that T-bet may be a potential biomarker of therapeutic efficacy.

During pregnancy, MS patients have a reduced exacerbation rate compared to pre- and postpregnancy (Korn-Lubetzki et al. 1984). The mechanisms that underlie this protection probably lie in the immune-tolerant state that is induced to protect the fetus. Interestingly, relapse rates in women postdelivery are often enhanced but typically return to prepregnancy levels within 1 year. In pregnant MS patients, T-bet levels are reduced, consistent with an anti-inflammatory or tolerant state (Iorio et al. 2009). However, in MS patients who have a relapse after delivery or have new active lesions, T-bet and pSTAT1 levels are enhanced, as well as IFNγ and IL-17 levels. In addition, there is an increase in CD4+ CD25+ Foxp3+- regulatory T cell population during pregnancy that may be suppressing the T-bet + T cells. Again, this study indicates that T-bet may be a marker of disease activity in MS.

For the past two decades, IFNβ has been used as a therapy for relapsing–remitting MS. In a study to determine whether Th1 or Th17 cells were altered due to IFNβ therapy, IFNγ and T-bet mRNA levels were reduced at 1-year postinitiation of IFNβ therapy, while IL-17 and RORγt (the Th17-associated transcription factor) were unchanged (Drulovic et al. 2009). Analysis of IFNβ responders versus nonresponders found that reduced T-bet levels correlated with a favorable clinical response to IFNβ treatment, further supporting the role of T-bet as a critical molecule in MS pathogenesis and as a potential indicator of therapeutic efficacy.

More recently, T-bet expression has been evaluated in clinical trials of new potential therapies for MS. Statins, 3-hydroxy-3-mehtylglutaryl coenzyme-A reductase inhibitors that have traditionally been used to reduce cholesterol, have been found to have immunomodulatory effects. Due to their widespread use and good safety record, they have been evaluated in MS as potential therapies. In clinical trials, ex vivo analysis revealed that MS patients on statins had reduced T cell proliferation, reduced proinflammatory cytokine expression and reduced T-bet expression, as well as significant clinical benefit to the patients (Peng et al. 2006).

Although there is evidence that T-bet levels correlate with disease activity and treatment efficacy in MS patients, it is still unclear whether T-bet is aberrantly expressed in MS patients, perhaps making them more susceptible to proinflammatory responses and the development of autoimmunity. MS patients have an increased incidence of other Th1-mediated autoimmune diseases such as diabetes, thyroiditis, and psoriasis, suggesting that they may possess a bias toward robust Th1 responses that may make them susceptible to Th1-mediated autoimmune diseases (Roquer et al. 1987; Karni and Abramsky 1999; Sloka 2002; Annunziata et al. 2003; Nielsen et al. 2006). A comprehensive analysis of miRNA expression in naive CD4 T cells of MS patients suggested that MS patients may have an inherent propensity to differentiate into Th1 cells due to loss of miRNA-mediated regulation of genes in the Th2 pathway (Guerau-de-Arellano et al. 2011). Since miRNAs negatively regulate gene expression, enhanced miRNA expression will result in decreased target gene expression. It was found that MS patients have enhanced expression of miR-27, miR-128, and miR-340 in CD4 T cells, resulting in decreased expression of Bmi1, GATA3, and IL-4. Since GATA3 and T-bet compete for lineage commitment during activation of naive T cells, reduced GATA3 leads to a dominant Th1 response. This study suggests that T-bet may be aberrantly expressed in CD4 T cells of MS patients due to miRNA-mediated suppression of Th2-associated molecules.

Several studies found that T-bet and IFNγ expression were also regulated by miRNA (Ma et al. 2011; Steiner et al. 2011; Smith et al. 2012). IFNγ induces the expression of miR-29, as well as T-bet, in CD4 T cells (Smith et al. 2012). T-bet directly regulates the expression of IFNγ, committing the CD4 T cell to the Th1 lineage. However, miR-29 subsequently binds to the mRNA of T-bet and IFNγ, demonstrating that a negative feedback loop exists as an additional mechanism to maintain a proper balance of IFNγ and to dampen effector Th1 responses appropriately following an inflammatory response. In resting memory, CD4 T cells of MS patients, T-bet, and miR-29 levels are increased, compared to control subjects (Smith et al. 2012). However, activation of MS patient memory CD4 T cells results in a significant decrease in miR-29 levels indicating that the feedback loop between miR-29 and T-bet/IFNγ is dysregulated in MS patients. The diminished capacity of miR-29 to regulate T-bet levels may be another mechanism that may promote chronic inflammation in MS patients.

3.7 Is T-bet a Valid Therapeutic Target for Multiple Sclerosis?

The T-bet-regulated gene that has been studied the most extensively is IFNγ. The contradictory data on the role of IFNγ in EAE and MS suggest that care must be taken on how therapies may systemically alter IFNγ levels. So is T-bet a valid therapeutic target in light of the data of EAE when IFNγ is suppressed? The observation that IFNγ-deficient mice remained susceptible to EAE (Ferber et al. 1996), and often had a more severe disease course than wild-type controls, led to caution about using drugs that may dramatically effect IFNγ levels. The EAE data in IFNγ-deficient mice and mice treated with antibodies to neutralize IFNγ suggested the IFNγ may play a positive regulatory role in the disease course (Lublin et al. 1993; Ferber et al. 1996; Heremans et al. 1996; Willenborg et al. 1996). However, there were two small clinical trials in MS patients that may suggest that inhibiting IFNγ in humans may be beneficial. In the 1980s, it was recognized that cytokines regulate immune responses and it was hypothesized that IFNγ may be beneficial in normalizing the aberrant immune responses observed in MS patients. IFNγ was administered to MS patients, resulting in an increased number of clinical exacerbations in the patients (Panitch et al. 1987). Subsequently, it was observed that IFNγ induces apoptosis of human oligodendrocytes, the cells that make myelin, and IFNγ expression in MS lesions colocalizes with apoptotic oligodendrocytes (Vartanian et al. 1995; Baerwald and Popko 1998), suggesting that IFNγ may play a role in the demyelination observed in the CNS of MS patients. These observations led to a clinical trial in which an IFNγ-neutralizing antibody was administered to MS patients, resulting in a clinical benefit (Skurkovich et al. 2001). Due to the contradictory data between mice and humans, systemic blockade of IFNγ has not continued in humans. However, the beneficial observations in humans suggest that the Th1 pathway is a viable therapeutic target.

When T-bet is genetically deleted or when T-bet is suppressed systemically with siRNA, mice are resistant to EAE induction, supporting T-bet as an effective therapeutic target (Bettelli et al. 2004; Lovett-Racke et al. 2004). Moreover, administration of a T-bet siRNA after the onset of EAE suggests that T-bet is a potential therapeutic target for established autoimmune demyelinating disease (Gocke et al. 2007). This is a critical point since we cannot predict who will develop MS and, therefore, must develop therapeutics that can prevent the development of autoreactive T cells, as well as suppress the effector/memory T cells that are already mediating lesion formation in MS patients. Furthermore, in MS patients treated with nonspecific immunomodulatory drugs, T-bet is reduced in patients who have clinical benefit (Drulovic et al. 2009).

Although T-bet is expressed in most immune cells, its role in EAE appears to be primarily mediated by CD4 T cells. In addition, T-bet regulates IFNγ in CD4 T cells, but does not appear to regulate IFNγ expression extensively in other immune cells (Szabo et al. 2000; Szabo et al. 2002). Therefore, suppression of T-bet does not result in systemic loss of IFNγ production and any positive effects of IFNγ that may be mediated by other immune cells would not be dramatically affected by suppression of T-bet. Thus, targeting T-bet may have far fewer potential side effects compared to global suppression of IFNγ.

T-bet and GATA3, the Th2- associated transcription factor, physically associate and compete to dominate lineage-specific genes in order to generate Th1 or Th2 cells (Hwang et al. 2005; Jenner et al. 2009). There is concern that suppression of T-bet may make individuals susceptible to Th2-mediated diseases, since GATA3 will not be as tightly regulated in the absence of T-bet. T-bet-deficient mice develop lung pathology consistent with allergic asthma (Finotto et al. 2002), a classic Th2-mediated disease. However, in mice treated with a T-bet siRNA, no lung pathology was observed, suggesting that diminishing T-bet expression, as opposed to complete abrogation of T-bet, may not have the same outcome (Lovett-Racke et al. 2004). The observation that MS patients have a decreased incidence of allergy and asthma is evidence that their immune responses may be biased away from Th2 responses (Bergamaschi et al. 2009; Pedotti et al. 2009). Thus, reducing T-bet expression in MS patients may simply normalize immune responses such that proinflammatory T cell effector functions are reduced, but not such that Th2- mediated diseases are a real threat.

3.8 Conclusion

MS is a complex disease that involves both inflammation and neurodegeneration. Since the inflammation appears to precede pathology and neurological deficits, a tremendous amount of research has been devoted to understanding the inflammatory process that is occurring at the site of lesion formation. In this quest, effector CD4 T cells have been found to be at the center of the immune response that results in demyelination and axonal damage. Why and how CD4 T cells become programmed to enter the apparently healthy CNS and mediate damage is unclear. However, T-bet is one molecule that appears to be associated with the capacity of CD4 T cells to cause CNS injury. Due to its relatively limited expression in humans, it may be a viable therapeutic target for MS. In addition, defining the role of T-bet in generating encephalitogenic T cells and their effector functions provides insight into the mechanisms that underlie the pathology of MS lesions.

References

Acosta-Rodriguez EV, Napolitani G, Lanzavecchia A, Salluston F (2007) Interleukins 1beta and 6 but not transforming growth factor-beta are essential for the differentiation of interleukin 17-producing human T helper cells. Nat Immunol 8:942–949

Afkarian M, Sedy JR, Yang J, Jacobson NG, Cereg N, Yang SY, Murphy TL, Murphy KM (2002) T-bet is a STAT1-induced regulator of IL-12R expression in naïve CD4+ T cells. Nat Immunol 3:549–557

Anderson AC, Lord GM, Dardalhon V, Lee DH, Sabatos-Peyton CA, Glimcher LH, Kuchroo VK (2010) T-bet, a Th1 transcription factor regulates the expression of Tim-3. Eur J Immunol 40:859–866

Ando DG, Clayton J, Dono D, Urban JL, Sercarz EE (1989) Encephalitogenic T cells in the B10.PL model of experimental allergic encephalomyelitis (EAE) are of the Th-1 lymphokine subtype. Cell Immunol 124:132–43

Annunziata P, Morana P, Giorgio A, Galeazzi M, Campanella V, Lore F et al (2003) High frequency of psoriasis in relatives is associated with early onset in an Italian multiple sclerosis cohort. Acta Neurol Scand 108:327–331

Baerwald KD, Popko B (1998) Developing and mature oliodendrocytes respond differently to the immune cytokine interferon-gamma. J Neurosci Res 52:230–239

Becher B, Durell BG, Noelle R (2002) Experimental autoimmune encephalitis and inflammation in the absence of interleukin-12. J Clin Invest 110:493–497

Becher B, Durell BG, Noelle RJ (2003) IL-23 produced by CNS-resident cells controls T cell encephalitogenicity during the effector phase of experimental autoimmune encephalomyelitis. J Clin Invest 112:1186–1191

Beima KM, Miazgowicz MM, Lewis MD, Yan PS, Huang TH, Weinmann AS (2006) T-bet binding to newly identified target gene promoters is cell type-independent but results in variable context-dependent functional effects. J Biol Chem 281:11992–12000

Bergamaschi R, Villani S, Crabbio M, Ponzio M, Romani A, Verri A et al (2009) Inverse relationship between multiple sclerosis and allergic respiratory diseases. Neurol Sci 30:115–118

Bettelli E, Sullivan B, Szabo SJ, Sobel RA, Glimcher LH, Kuchroo VK (2004) Loss of T-bet but not STAT1, prevents the development of experimental autoimmune encephalomyelitis. J Exp Med 200:79–87

Bettelli E, Carrier Y, Gao W, Kom T, Strom TB, Oukka M, Weiner HL, Kuchroo VK (2006) Reciprocal developmental pathways for the generation of pathogenic effector TH17 and regulatory T cells. Nature 441:235–238

Bornsen L, Khademi M, Olsson T, Sorensen PS, Sellebjerg F (2011) Osteopontin concentrations are increased in cerebrospinal fluid during attacks of multiple sclerosis. Mult Scler 17:32–42

Chabas D, Baranzini SE, Mitchell D, Bernard CC, Rittling SR, Denhardt DT, Sobel RA, Lock C, Karpuj M, Pedotti R, Heller R, Oksenberg JR, Steinman L (2001) The influence of the proinflammatory cytokine, osteopontin, on autoimmune demyelinating disease. Science 294:1731–1735

Charcot JM (1968) Histologie de la sclerose en plaques Gazette des hopitaux. Paris 41:554–555

Chen Y, Langrish CL, McKenzie B, Joyce-Shaikh B, Stumhofer JS, McClanahan T, Blumenschein W, Churakovsa T, Low J, Presta L, Hunter CA, Kastelein RA, Cua DJ (2006) Anti-IL-23 therapy inhibits multiple inflammatory pathways and ameliorates autoimmune encephalomyelitis. J Clin Invest 116:1317–26

Chitnis T, Najafian N, Benou C, Salama AD, Grusby MJ, Sayegh MH, Khoury SJ (2001) Effect of targeted disruption of STAT4 and STAT6 on the induction of experimental autoimmune encephalomyelitis. J Clin Invest 108:739–747

Codarri L, Gyulveszi G, Tosevski V, Hesske L, Fontana A, Magnenat L, Suter T, Becher B (2011) RORγt drives production of the cytokine GM-CSF in helper T cells, which is essential for the effector phase of autoimmune neuroinflammation. Nat Immunol 12:560–567

Cua DJ, Sherlock J, Chen Y, Murphy CA, Joyce B, Seymour B, Lucian L, To W, Kwan S, Churakova T, Zurawski S, Wiekowski M, Lira SA, Gorman D, Kastelein RA, Sedgwick JD (2003) Interleukin-23 rather than interleukin-12 is the critical cytokine for autoimmune inflammation of the brain. Nature 421:744–748

Drulovic J, Savic E, Pekmezovic T, Mesaros S, Stojavljevic N, Dujmovic-Basiroski I, Kostic J, Vasic V, Stojkovic MM, Popadic D (2009) Expression of Th1 and Th17 cytokines and transcription factors in multiple sclerosis patients: Does baseline T-bet mRNA predict the response to interferon-beta treatment? J Neuroimmunol 215:90–95

Dubey C, Croft M, Swain SL (1996) Naïve and effector CD4 T cells differ in their requirements for T cell receptor versus costimulatory signals. J Immunol 157:3280–3289

El-Behi M, Ciric B, Dai H, Yan Y, Cullimore M, Safavi F, Zhang GX, Dittel BN, Rostami A (2011) The encephalitogenicity of T(H)17 cells is dependent on IL-1- and IL-23-induced production of the cytokine GM-CSF. Nat Immunol 12:568–575

Ferber IA, Brock S, Taylor-Edwards C, Ridgway W, Dinisco C, Steinman L, Dalton D, Fathman CG (1996) Mice with a disrupted IFN-gamma gene are susceptible to the induction of experimental autoimmune encephalomyelitis (EAE). J Immunol 156:5–7

Finotto S, Neurath MF, Glickman JN, Qin S, Lehr HA, Green FH, Ackerman K, Haley K, Galle PR, Szabo SJ, Drazen JM, De Sanctis GT, Glimcher LH (2002) Development of spontaneous airway changes consistent with human asthma in mice lacking T-bet. Science 295:336–338

Frisullo G, Angelucci F, Caggiula M, Nociti V, Iorio R, Patanella AK, Sancricca C, Mirabella M, Tonali PA, Batocchi AP (2006) pSTAT1, pSTAT3, and T-bet expression in peripheral blood mononuclear cells from relapsing-remitting multiple sclerosis patients correlates with disease activity. J Neurosci Res 84:1027–1036

Frisullo G, Nociti V, Iorio R, Patanella KA, Bianco A, Caggiula M, Sancricca C, Tonali PA, Mirabella M, Batocchi AP (2007) Glucocorticoid treatment reduces T-bet and pSTAT1 expression in mononuclear cells from relapsing remitting multiple sclerosis patients. Clin Immunol 124:284–293

Frisullo G, Nociti V, Iorio R, Patanella AK, Caggiula M, Marti A, Sancricca C, Angelucci F, Mirabella M, Tonali PA, Batocchi AP (2009) Regulatory T cells fail to suppress CD4+ T-bet + T cells in relapsing multiple sclerosis patients. Immunology 127:418–428

Frisullo G, Iorio R, Plantone D, Marti A, Nociti V, Patanella AD, Batocchi AP (2011) CD4+ T-bet+, CD4+ pSTAT3+ and CD8+ T-bet+ T cells accumulate in peripheral blood during NZB treatment. Mult Scler 17:556–566

Ghoreschi K, Laurence A, Yang XP, Tato CM, McGeachy MJ, Konkel JE, Ramos HL, Wei L, Davidson TS, Bouladoux N, Grainger JR, Chen Q, Kanno Y, Watford WT, Sun HW, Eberl G, Shevach EM, Belkaid Y, Cua DJ, Chen W, O'Shea JJ (2010) Generation of pathogenic T(H)17 cells in the absence of TGF-β signalling. Nature 467(7318):967–971. doi: 10.1038/nature09447

Gielen AW, Lobell A, Lidman O, Khademi M, Olsson T, Piehl F (2005) Expression of T cell immunoglobulin- and mucin-domain-containing molecules-1 and -3 (TIM-1 and -3) in the rat nervous and immune systems. J Neuroimmunol 164:93–104

Gocke AR, Cravens PD, Ben LH, Hussain RZ, Northrop SC, Racke MK, Lovett-Racke AE (2007) T-bet regulates the fate of Th1 and Th17 lymphocytes in autoimmunity. J Immunol 178:1341–1348

Gorelik L, Constant S, Flavell RA (2002) Mechanism of transforming growth factor beta-induced inhibition of T helper type 1 differentiation. J Exp Med 195:1499–1505

Gran B, Zhang GX, Yu S, Li J, Chen XH, Ventura ES, Kamoun M, Rostami A (2002) IL-12p35-deficient mice are susceptible to experimental autoimmune encephalomyelitis: evidence for redundancy in the IL-12 system in the induction of central nervous system autoimmune demyelination. J Immunol 169:7104–7410

Guerau-de-Arellano M, Smith KM, Godlewski J, Liu Y, winger R, Lawler SE, Whitacre CC, Racke MK, Lovett-Racke AE (2011) Micro-RNA dysregulation in multiple sclerosis favours pro-inflammatory T-cell-mediated autoimmunity. Brain 134:3578–89

Haak S, Croxford AL, Dreymborg K, Heppner FL, Pouly S, Becher B, Waisman A (2009) IL-17 A and IL-17 F do not contribute vitally to autoimmune neuro-inflammation in mice. J Clin Invest 119:61–69

Heremans H, Dillen C, Groenen M, Martens E, Billiau A (1996) Chronic relapsing experimental autoimmune encephalomyelitis (CREAE) in mice: enhancement by monoclonal antibodies against interferon-gamma. Eur J Immunol 26:2393–2398

Hori S, Takahashi T, Sakaguchi S (2003) Control autoimmunity by naturally arising regulatory CD4+ T cells. Adv Immunol 81:331–371

Hou J, Schindler U, Henzel WJ, Ho TC, Brasseur M, McKnight SL (1994) An interleukin-4-induced transcription factor: IL-4 Stat. Science 265:1701–1706

Hsieh CS, Heimberger AB, Gold JS, O'Garra A, Murphy KM (1992) Differential regulation of T helper phenotype development by interleukin 4 and 10 in an alpha beta T-cell-receptor transgenic system. Proc Natl Acad Sci U S A 89:6065–6069

Hur EM, Youssef S, Haws ME, Zhang SY, Sobel RA, Steinman L (2007) Osteopontin-induced relapse and progression of autoimmune brain disease through enhanced survival of activated T cells. Nat Immunol 8:74–83

Hwang ES, Szabo SJ, Schwartzberg PL, Glimcher LH (2005) T helper cell fate specified by kinase-mediated interaction of T-bet with GATA-3. Science 307:430–343

Iorio R, Frisullo G, Nociti V, Patanella KA, Bianco A, Marti A, Mirabella M, Tonali PA, Batocchi AP (2009) T-bet pSTAT1 and pSTAT3 expression in peripheral blood mononuclear cells during pregnancy correlates with post-partum activation of multiple sclerosis. Clin Immunol 131:70–83

Jacobson NF, Szabo SJ, Weber-Nordt RM, Zhong Z, Schreiber RD, Darnell JE, Murphy KM (1995) Interleukin 12 signaling in T helper type 1 (Th1) cells involves tyrosine phosphorylation of signal transducer and activator of transcription (Stat) 3 and Stat4. J Exp Med 181:1755–1762

Jansson M, Panoutsakopoulou V, Baker J, Klein L, Cantor H (2002) Cutting edge: Attenuated experimental autoimmune encephalomyelitis in eta-1/osteopontin-deficient mice. J Immunol 168:2096–2099

Jenner RG, Townsend MJ, Jackson I, Sun K, Bouwman RD, Young RA, Glimcher LH, Lord GM (2009) The transcription factors T-bet and GATA-3 control alternative pathways of T-cell differentiation through a shared set of target genes. Proc Natl Acad Sci U S A 106:17876–17881

June CH, Ledbetter JA, Linsley PS, Thompson CB (1990) Role of the CD28 receptor in T-cell activation. Immunol Today 11:211–216

Karni A, Abramsky O (1999) Association of MS with thyroid disorders. Neurology 53:883–885

Khademi M, Illes Z, Gielen AW, Marta M, Takazawa N, Baecher-Allan C, Brundin L, Hannerz J, Martin C, Harris RA, Hafler DA, Kuchroo VK, Olsson T, Piehl F, Wallstrom E (2004) T cell Ig- and mucin-domain-containing molecule-3 (TIM-3) and TIM-1 molecules are differentially expressed on human Th1 and Th2 cells and in cerebrospinal fluid-derived mononuclear cells in multiple sclerosis. J Immunol 172:7169–7176

Kleiter I, Song J, Lukas D, hasan M, Neumann B, Croxford AL, Pedre X, Hovelmeyer N, Yogev N, Mildner A, Prinz M, Wiese e, Reifenberg K, Bittner S, Siendl H, Steinman L, Becker C, Bogdahn U, Neurath MF, Steinbrecher A, Waisman A (2010) Smad7 in T cells drives T helper 1 responses in multiple sclerosis and experimental autoimmune encephalomyelitis. Brain 133:1067–1081

Koguchi K, Anderson DE, Yang L, O'Connor KC, Kuchroo VK, Hafler DA (2006) Dysregulated T cell expression of TIM3 in multiple sclerosis. J Exp Med 203:1413–1418

Kohler RE, Comerford I, Townley S, Haylock-Jacobs S, Clark-Lewis I, McColl SR (2008) Antagonism of the chemokine receptors CXCR3 and CXCR4 reduces the pathology of experimental autoimmune encephalomyelitis. Brain Pathol 18:504–516

Komiyama Y, Nakae S, Matsuki T, Nambu A, Ishigame H, Kakuta S, Suko K, Iwakura Y (2006) IL-17 plays an important role in the development of experimental autoimmune encephalomyelitis. J Immunol 177:566–573

Korn-Lubetzki I, Kahana E, Cooper G, Abramsky O (1984) Activity of multiple sclerosis during pregnancy and puerperium. Ann Neurol 16:229–231

Kroenke MA, Segal BM (2007) Th17 and Th1 responses directed against the immunizing epitope, as opposed to secondary epitopes, dominate the autoimmune repertoire during relapses of experimental autoimmune encephalomyelitis. J Neurosci Res 85:1685–1693

Kumar V, Stellrecht K, Sercarz E (1996) Inactivation of T cell receptor peptide-specific CD4 regulatory T cells induces chronic experimental autoimmune encephalomyelitis (EAE). J Exp Med 184:1609–1617

Langrish CL, Chen Y, Blumenschein WM, Mattson J, Basham B, Sedgwick JD, McClanahan T, Kastelein RA, Cua DJ (2005) IL-23 drives a pathogenic T cell population that induces autoimmune inflammation. J Exp Med 201:233–40

Lees JR, Iwakura Y, Russell JH (2008) Host T cells are the main producers of IL-17 within the central nervous system during initiation of experimental autoimmune encephalomyelitis induced by adoptive transfer of Th1 cell lines. J Immunol 180:8066–72

Lewis MD, Miller SA, Miazgowicz MM, Beima KM, Weinmann AS (2007) T-bet's ability to regulate individual target genes requires the conserved T-box domain to recruit histone methyltransferase activity and a separate family member-specific transactivation domain. Mol Cell Biol 27:8510–8521

Liu L, Huang D, Matsui M, He TT, Hu T, Demartino J, Lu B, Gerard C, Ransohoff RM (2006) Severe disease, unaltered leukocyte migration, and reduced IFN-gamma production in CXCR3-/- mice with experimental autoimmune encephalomyelitis. J Immunol 176:4399–4409

Lock C, Hermans G, Pedotti R, Brendolan A, Schadt E, Garren H, Langer-Gould A, Strober S, Cannella B, Allard J, Klonowski P, Austin A, Lad N, Kaminski N, Galli SJ, Oksenberg JK, Raine CS, Heller R, Steinman L (2002) Gene-microarray analysis of multiple sclerosis lesions yields new targets validated in autoimmune encephalomyelitis. Nat Med 8:500–508

Lord GM, Rao RM, Choe H, Sullivan BM, Lichtman AH, Luscinskas FW, Glimcher LH (2005) T-bet is required for optimal proinflammatory CD4+ T-cell trafficking. Blood 106:3432–3439

Lovett-Racke AE, Trotter JL, Lauber J, Perrin PJ, June CH, Racke MK (1998) Decreased dependence of myelin basic protein-reactive T cells on CD28-mediated costimulation in multiple sclerosis patients. A marker of activated/memory T cells. J Clin Invest 101:725–730

Lovett-Racke AE, Rocchini AE, Choy J, Northrop SC, Hussain RZ, Ratts RB, Sikder D, Racke MK (2004) Silencing T-bet defines a critical role in the differentiation of autoreactive T lymphocytes. Immunity 21:719–731

Lublin FD, Knobler RL, Kalman B, Goldhaber M, Marini J, Perrault M, D'Imperio C, Joseph J, Alkan SS, Korngold R (1993) Monoclonal anti-gamma interferon antibodies enhance experimental allergic encephalomyelitis. Autoimmunity 16:267–274

Ma F, Xu S, Liu X, Zhang Q, Xu X, Liu M, Hua M, Li N, Yao H, Cao X (2011) The microRNA miR-29 controls innate and adaptive immune responses to intracellular bacterial infection by targeting interferon-γ. Nat Immunol 12:861–869

Mangan PR, Harrington LE, O'Quinn DB, Helms WS, Bullard DC, Elson CO, Hatton RD, Wahl SM, Schoeb TR, Weaver CT (2006) Transforming growth factor-β induces development of the Th17 lineage. Nature 441:231–234

Marie JC, Letterio JJ, Gavin M, Rudensky AY (2005) TGF-beta1 maintains suppressor function and Foxp3 expression in CD4+ CD25 + regulatory T cells. J Exp Med 201:1061–1067

McDonald AH, Swanborg RH (1988) Antigen-specific inhibition of immune interferon production by suppressor cells of autoimmune encephalomyelitis. J Immunol 140:1132–1138

Miller SA, Huang AC, Miazgowicz MM, Brassil MM, Weinmann AS (2008) Coordinated but physically separable interaction with H3K27-demethylase and H3K4-methyltransferase activities are required for T-box protein-mediated activation of developmental gene expression. Genes Dev 22:2980–2993

Monney L, Sabatos CA, Gaglia JL, Ryu A, Waldner H, Chernova T, Manning S, Greenfield EA, Coyle AJ, Sobel RA, Freeman GJ, Kuchroo VK (2002) Th1-specific cell surface protein Tim-3 regulates macrophage activation and severity of an autoimmune disease. Nature 415:536–541

Mosmann TR, Cherwinski H, Bond MS, Giedlin MA, Coffman RL (1986) Two types of murine helper T cell clones. I Definition according to profiles of lymphokine activities and secreted proteins. J Immunol 136:2348–2357

Muller M, Carter SL, Hofer MJ, Manders P, Getts DR, Getts MT, Dreykluft A, Lu B, Gerard C, King NJ, Campbell IL (2007) CXCR3 signaling reduces severity of experimental autoimmune encephalomyelitis by controlling the parenchymal distribution of effector and regulatory T cells in the central nervous system. J Immunol 179:2774–2786

Nath N, Giri S, Prasad R, Singh AK, Singh I (2004) Potential targets of 3-hydroxy-3-methylglutaryl coenzyme A reductase inhibitor for multiple sclerosis therapy. J Immunol 172:1273–1286

Nath N, Prasad R, Giri S, Singh AK, Singh I (2006) T-bet is essential for the progression of experimental autoimmune encephalomyelitis. Immunology 118:384–391

Ni J, Zhu YN, Zhong XG, Ding Y, Hou LF, Tong XK, Tang W, Ono S, Yang YF, Zuo JP (2009) The chemokine receptor antagonist, TAK-779, decreased experimental autoimmune encephalomyelitis by reducing inflammatory cell migration into the central nervous system, without affecting T cell function. Br J Pharmacol 158:2046–2056

Nielsen NM, Westergaard T, Frisch M, Rostgaard K, Wohlfahrt J, Koch-Henriksen N et al (2006) Type 1 diabetes and multiple sclerosis: A Danish population-based cohort study. Arch Neurol 63:1001–1004

Oestreich KJ, Huang AC, Weinmann AS (2011) The lineage-defining factors T-bet and Bcl-6 collaborate to regulate Th1 gene expression patterns. J Exp Med 208:1001–1013

Oppmann B, Lesley R, Blom B, Timans JC, Xu Y, Hunte B, Vega F, Yu N, Wang J, Singh K, Zonin F, Vaisberg E, Churakova T, Liu M, Gorman D, Wagner J, Zurawski S, Liu Y, Abrams JS, Moore KW, Rennick D, Waal-Malefyt R de, Hannum C, Bazan JF, Kastelein RA (2000) Novel p19 protein engages IL-12p40 to form a cytokine, IL-23, with biological activities similar as well as distinct from IL-12. Immunity 13:715–725

Panitch HS, Hirsch RL, Haley AS, Johnson KP (1987) Exacerbation of multiple sclerosis in patients treated with gamma interferon. Lancet 1:893–895

Parham C, Chirica M, Timans J, Vaisberg E, Travis M, Cheung J, Pflanz S, Zhang R, Singh KP, Vega F, To W, Wagner J, O'Farrell AM, McClanahan T, Zurawski S, Hannum C, Gorman D, Rennick DM, Kastelein RA, de Waal Malefyt R, Moore KW (2002) A receptor for the heterodimeric cytokine IL-23 is composed of IL- 12Rbeta1 and a novel cytokine receptor subunit IL-23R. J Immunol 168:5699–5708

Park IK, Shultz LD, Letterio JJ, Gorham JD (2005) TGF-beta1 inhibits T-bet induction by IFN-gamma in murine CD4+ T cells through the protein tyrosine phosphatase Src homology region 2 domain-containing phosphatase-1. J Immunol 175:5666–5674

Paulos CM, Carpenito C, Plesa G, Suhoski MM, Varela-Rohena A, Golovina TN, Carroll RG, Riley JL, June CH (2010) The inducible costimulator (ICOS) is critical for the development of human T(H)17 cells. Sci Transl Med 2:55ra78

Pedotti R, Farinotti M, Falcone C, Borgonovo L, Confalonieri P, Campanella A et al (2009) Allergy and multiple sclerosis: a population-based case-control study. Mult Scler 15:899–906

Peng X, Jin J, Montes M, Sujkowski D, Tang Y, Smrtka J, Vollmer T, Singh I, Markovic-Plese S (2006) Immunomodulatory effects of 3-hydroxy-3-methylglutaryl coenzyme-A reductase inhibitors, potential therapy for relapsing remitting multiple sclerosis. J Neuroimmunol 178:130–139

Ponomarev ED, Shriver LP, Maresz K, Pedras-Vasconcelos J, Verthelyi D, Dittel BN (2007) GM-CSF production by autoreactive T cells is required for the activation of microglial cells and the onset of experimental autoimmune encephalomyelitis. J Immunol 178:39–48

Qin S, Rottman JB, Myers P, Kasam N, Weinblatt M, Loetscher M, Koch AE, Moser B, Mackay CR (1998) The chemokine receptors CXCR3 and CCR5 mark subsets of T cells associated with certain inflammatory reactions. J Clin Invest 101:746–754

Racke MK, Bonomo A, Scott DE, Cannella B, Levine A, Raine CS, Shevach EM, Rocken M (1994) Cytokine-induced immune deviation as a therapy for inflammatory autoimmune disease. J Exp Med 180:1961–1966

Racke MK, Burnett D, Pak SH, Albert PS, Cannella B, Raine CS, McFarlin DE, Scott DE (1995) Retinoid treatment of experimental allergic encephalomyelitis. IL-4 production correlates with improved disease course. J Immunol 154:450–458

Rivers RM, Spunt DH, Berry GP (1933) Observations on attempts to produce acute disseminated encephalomyelitis in monkeys. J Exp Med 58:39–53

Roquer J, Escudero D, Herraiz J, Maso E, Cano F (1987) Multiple sclerosis and Hashimoto's thyroiditis. J Neurol 234:23–24

Rottman JB, Smith T, Tonra JR, Ganley K, Bloom T, Silva R, Pierce B, Gutierrez-Ramos JC, Ozkaynak E, Coyle AJ (2001) The costimulatory molecule ICOS plays an important role in the immunopathogenesis of EAE. Nat Immunol 2:605–611

Sallusto F, Lenig D, Mackay CR, Lanzavecchia A (1998) Flexible programs of chemokine receptor expression on human polarized T helper 1 and 2 lymphocytes. J Exp Med 187:875–883

Shinohara ML, Jansson M, Hwang ES, Werneck MK, Glimcher LH, Cantor H (2005) T-bet-dependent expression of osteopontin contributes to T cell polarization. Proc Natl Acad Sci U S A 102:17101–17106

Skurkovich S, Boilo A, Beliaeva I, Buglak A, Alekseeva T, Smirnova N, Kulakova O, Tchechonin V, Gurova O, Deomina T, Favorova OO, Skurkovic B, Gusev E (2001) Randomized study of antibodies to IFN-gamma and TNF-alpha in secondary progressive multiple sclerosis. Mult Scler 7:277–284

Sloka S (2002) Observations on recent studies showing increased co-occurrence of autoimmune diseases. J Autoimmun 18:251–257

Smith KM, Guerau-de-Arellano M, Costinean S, Williams JL, Bottoni A, Mavrikis Cox G, Satoskar AR, Croce CM, Racke MK, Lovett-Racke AE, Whitacre CC (2012) miR-29ab1 deficiency identifies a negative feedback loop controlling Th1 bias that is dysregulated inmultiple sclerosis. J Immunol 189(4):1567–1576. doi: 10.4049/jimmunol.1103171. (Epub 2012 Jul 6)

Sporici RA, Beswick RL, von Allmen C, Rumbley CA, Hayden-Ledbetter M, Ledbetter JA, Perrin PJ (2001) ICOS ligand costimulation is required for T-cell encephalitogenicity. Clin Immunol 100:277–288

Sporici R, Issekutz TB (2010) CXCR3 blockade inhibits T-cell migration into the CNS during EAE and prevents development of adoptively transferred, but not actively induced disease. Eur J Immunol 40:2751–2761

Steiner DF, Thomas MF, Hu JK, Yang Z, Babiarz JE, Allen CD, Matloubian M, Blelloch R, Ansel KM (2011) MicroRNA-29 regulates T-box transcription factors and interferon-γ production in helper T cells. Immunity 36:169–181

Szabo SJ, Kim ST, Costa GL, Zhang X, Fathman CG, Glimcher LH (2000) A novel transcription factor, T-bet directs th1 lineage commitment. Cell 100:655–669

Szabo SJ, Sullivan BM, Stemmann C, Satoskar AR, Sleckman BP, Glimcher LH (2002) Distinct effects of T-bet in Th1 lineage commitment and IFN-γ production in CD4 and CD8 T cells. Science 295:338–342

Tan AH, Goh SY, Wong SC, Lam KP (2008) T helper cell-specific regulation of inducible costimulator expression via distinct mechanisms mediated by T-bet and GATA-3. J Biol Chem 283:128–136

Traugott U, Lebon P (1988) Multiple sclerosis: involvement of interferons in lesion pathogenesis. Ann Neurol 24:243–251

Tzartos JS, Friese MA, Craner MJ, Palace J, Newcombe J, Esiri MM, Fugger L (2008) Interleukin-17 production in central nervous system-infiltrating T cells and glial cells is associated with active disease in multiple sclerosis. Am J Pathol 172:146–155

Vartanian T, Li Y, Zhao M, Stefansson K (1995) Interferon-gamma-induced oligodendrocyte cell death: implications for the pathogenesis of multiple sclerosis. Mol Med 1:732–743

Veldhoen M, Hocking RJ, Atkins CJ, Locksley RM, Stockinger B (2006) TGFbeta in the context of an inflammatory cytokine nilieu supports de novo differentiation of IL-17-producing T cells. Immunity 24:179–189

Waldburger KE, Hastings RC, Schaub RG, Goldman SL, Leonard JP (1996) Adoptive transfer of experimental allergic encephalomyelitis after in vitro treatment with recombinant murine interleukin-12. Preferential expansion of interferon-gamma-producing cells and increased expression of macrophage-associated inducible nitric oxide synthase as immunomodulatory mechanisms. Am J Pathol 148:375–382

Wen ST, Liu GJ, Feng RN, Gong FC, Zhong H, Duan SR, Bi S (2012) Increased levels of IL-23 and osteopontin in serum and cerebrospinal fluid of multiple sclerosis patients. J Neuroimmunol 244:94–96

Willenborg DO, Fordham S, Bernard CC, Cowden WB, Ramshaw IA (1996) IFN-gamma plays a critical down-regulatory role in the induction and effector phase of myelin oligodendrocyte glycoprotein-induced autoimmune encephalomyelitis. J Immunol 157:3223–3227

Wilson NJ, Boniface K, Chan JR, McKenzie BS, Blumenschein WM, Mattson JD, Basham B, Smith K, Chen T, Morel F, Lecron JC, Kastelein RA, Cua DJ, McClanahan TK, Bowman EP, de Waal Malefyt R (2007) Development, cytokine profile and function of human interleukin 17-producing helper T cells. Nat Immunol 8:950–957

Yang L, Anderson D, Baecher-Allan C, Hastings WD, Bettelli E, Oukka M, Kuchroo VK and H (2008a) Il-21 and TGF-beta are required for differentiation of human T(H)17 cells. Nature 454:350–352

Yang L, Anderson DE, Kuchroo VK, Hafler DA (2008b) Lack of TIM-3 immunoregulation in multiple sclerosis. J Immunol 180:4409–4414

Yang Y, Weiner J, Liu Y, Smith AJ, Huss DJ, Winger R, Peng H, Cravens PD, Racke MK, Lovett-Racke AE (2009) T-bet is essential for encephalitogenicity of both Th1 and Th17 cells. J Exp Med 206:1549–1564

Yao Z, Painter SL, Fanslow WC, Ulrich D, Macduff BM, Springs MK, Armitage RJ (1995) Human IL-17: a novel cytokine derived from T cells. J Immunol 155:5483–5486

Yi-qun Z, Joost van Neerven RJ, Kasran A, Boer M de, Ceuppens JL (1996) Differential requirements for co-stimulatory signals from B7 family members by resting versus recently activated memory T cells towards soluble recall antigens. Int Immunol 8:37–44

Yura M, Takahashi I, Serada M, Koshio T, Nakagami K, Yuki Y, Kiyono H (2001) Role of MOG-stimulated Th1 type "light up" (GFP+) CD4+ T cells for the development of experimental autoimmune encephalomyelitis (EAE). J Autoimmun 17:17–25

Zhang GX, Yu S, Gran B, Li J, Siglienti I, Chen X, Calida D, Ventura E, Kamoun M, Rostami A (2003) Role of IL-12 receptor beta 1 in regulation of T cell response by APC in experimental autoimmune encephalomyelitis. J Immunol 171:4485–4492

Zheng W, Flavell RA (1997) The transcription factor GATA-3 is necessary and sufficient for Th2 cytokine gene expression in CD4 T cells. Cell 89:587–596

Chapter 4
Antigen-Presenting Cells in the Central Nervous System

Nathalie Koning, Juan M. Ilarregui, Juan J. García-Vallejo and Yvette van Kooyk

The immune system employs a combination of innate and adaptive immune responses to detect and eliminate danger such as infiltrating pathogens or excessive tissue destruction. Antigen-presenting cells (APC), such as dendritic cells (DC) and Macrophages (MΦ), are crucial for initiating innate immune responses and processing of antigen to facilitate adaptive T cell-mediated immunity. DC and MΦ arise mostly from myeloid progenitors in that exit the bone marrow and populate the tissues where they finish their differentiation and, in some cases, still replicate. While both DC and MΦ function in antigen uptake, processing, and presentation, DC are the most efficient in priming naïve T cells and triggering antigen-specific effector T cells. APC are localized in all peripheral tissues and act as a first line of defense by sensing alterations in their microenvironment. In response to a pathogen or tissue injury, DC travel to the draining lymph node where they arrive with a mature phenotype characterized by, among others, the upregulation of costimulatory molecules, and the production of inflammatory cytokines. In the lymph nodes, DC are fully capable of presenting antigens to naïve T cells. Importantly, as they are delicate sensors of their microenvironment, APC also control immunological homeostasis in tissues, and can reduce excessive tissue destruction through an effective reduction of immune activation. APC are thus highly versatile innate immune cells, depending on the environmental signals, can either promote activation of inflammatory T cells or dampen immune responses, for example, via the induction of regulatory T cells. In this review, we focus on how APC in the central nervous system (CNS) exert this dual function of keeping both immunologic silence as well as activation with a specific focus on glycan-binding proteins.

Y. v. Kooyk (✉) · N. Koning · J. M. Ilarregui · J. J. García-Vallejo
Department of Molecular Cell Biology and Immunology,
VU University Medical Center, 7057, 1007 MB Amsterdam, The Netherlands
e-mail: y.vankooyk@vumc.nl

T. Yamamura, B. Gran (eds.), *Multiple Sclerosis Immunology*,
DOI 10.1007/978-1-4614-7953-6_4, © Springer Science+Business Media New York 2013

4.1 Antigen-Presenting Cells Modulate Adaptive Immunity

DC and MΦ have classically been classified as belonging to the innate immune system but are crucial to trigger the adaptive immune system (Steinman et al. 2003; Sica and Mantovani 2012). In adaptive immunity, T and B cell responses are generated toward specific antigens and are long-lasting, resulting in T cell-mediated responses, such as $CD4^+$ T helper (Th) cells or $CD8^+$ cytotoxic T cells, or antibody responses. Intracellular and extracellular antigen captured and processed by DC can thus be presented into MHC class I or II molecules, to prime $CD8^+$ or $CD4^+$ T cells, respectively (Steinman et al. 2003; Steinman and Banchereau 2007; Banchereau and Steinman 1998; Fig. 4.1).

Depending on the nature of the antigen they encounter, DC and MΦ respond secreting a panel of cytokines that allow the differentiation of several types of Th cell subsets that exhibit different effector functions (Fig. 4.1). Thus, secretion of IL-12 by DC has shown to induce IFNγ-producing Th1 cells, which are involved in the clearance of intracellular pathogens. Secretion of IL-4 by DC results in the differentiation of IL-4-producing and IL-5-producing Th2 cells, which are crucial in the removal of extracellular pathogens and parasites. The production of IL-23 by DC, on the other hand, results in the differentiation of IL-17-producing Th17, which are necessary in the immunity against extracellular bacteria and have been implicated in autoimmune diseases (Idoyaga et al. 2011; Galea et al. 2005; Stockinger and Veldhoen 2007; Jadidi-Niaragh and Mirshafiey 2011; Zygmunt and Veldhoen 2011). In contrast, the induction of regulatory T cells (T_{Regs}) by DC has been shown to lead to the inhibition of immune responses, and therefore is crucial to control the balance of autoreactive effector T cells and to dampen excessive immune responses (Bacchetta et al. 2005; Fig. 4.1).

The innate immune response lacks antigen specificity, diversity, and memory and is triggered in response to a wide variety of antigens. For the recognition of danger (Matzinger 2002)—pathogens or inflammatory mediators—APC are equipped with pathogen recognition receptors (PRR) that recognize specific structures expressed on pathogens, also known as danger signals, or pathogen-associated molecular patterns (PAMPs). So far, nine families of PRRs have been identified, and the most studied are Toll-like receptors (TLRs) (Medzhitov and Janeway 2000a; b), nucleotide-binding oligomerization domain (NOD)-like receptors (NLRs) (Fritz et al. 2007; Fritz et al. 2005), retinoic acid-inducible gene 1 (RIG-I)-like receptors (RLRs) (Stancic et al. 2011; Heine 2011; Loo and Gale 2011), and C-type lectin receptors (CLRs) (van Kooyk and Geijtenbeek 2003). Upon pathogen recognition, signaling is initiated through NF-κB, MAP kinase, and interferon regulatory factor (IRF) pathways that lead to the transcriptional and posttranslational upregulation of gene transcripts encoding inflammatory cytokines, including IL-6, TNFα, IL-12, and IL-23. Some TLRs, such as TLR1, TLR2, TLR4, TLR5, and TLR6, are exclusively located at the cell membrane and recognize PAMPs located on the exterior of the pathogen. In contrast, other TLRs (TLR3, TLR7, TLR8, and TLR9) are located in endocytic compartments, where they are able to recognize RNA and unmethylated CpG

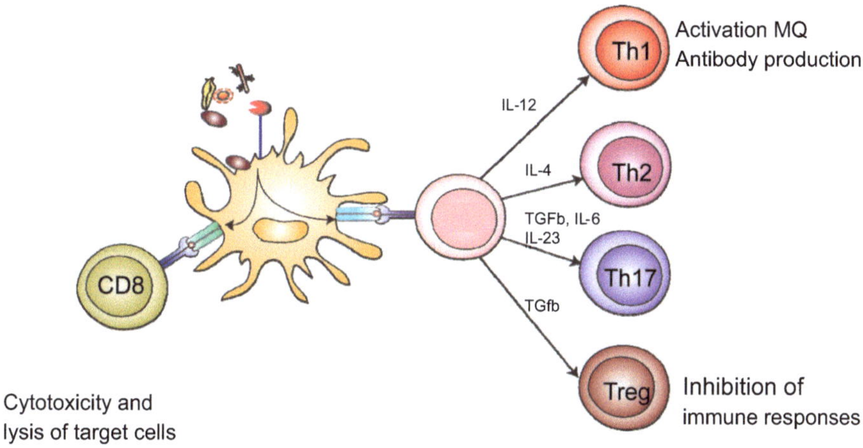

Fig. 4.1 Dendritic cells (DC) are crucial players in directing T cell responses. Innate recognition of pathogens and antigens by DC leads to processing and presentation of antigen to CD4 and/or CD8 T cells. The combination of innate receptors involved in the recognition of antigen determines the differentiation program of T cells that DC instruct. Depending on specific cytokines DC produce, CD4 T cells can differentiate into Th1, Th2, Th17, or Treg

DNA, for which internalization and partial degradation of the pathogen is required. Endogenous ligands, like heat shock proteins, have been described for TLRs as well (Ohashi et al. 2000). These proteins can be aberrantly expressed upon stress and/or released after necrosis. Also, NLRs are located in the cytosol and are involved in the recognition of microbial motifs as well as endogenous danger signals. Some NLRs participate in the induction and activation of the inflammasome, which is necessary for the production and secretion of mature IL-1β (Hanamsagar et al. 2012).

CLRs constitute a different group of PRRs that is characterized by a common feature, the presence of a C-type lectin domain (CTLD) in their amino acid sequence, a domain that mediates the recognition of glycans in a Ca^{2+}-dependent manner. Upon ligation, some receptors have the ability to, besides triggering ligand internalization, elicit an intracellular signaling cascade (Appelmelk et al. 2003; Figdor et al. 2002; Mitchell et al. 2001; Drickamer 1999; Gringhuis et al. 2007). An interesting aspect of CRL signaling is that it interferes with TLR signaling. This interference, or receptor cross-talk, often alters the cytokine secretion profile. In the case of dendritic cell-specific intercellular adhesion molecule-3-grabbing non-integrin (DC-SIGN) signaling, cross-talk results in an enhancement in IL-10 production with a simultaneous lowering of IL-12 production (Geijtenbeek et al. 2000a, b; Gringhuis et al. 2009).

Although CLRs are known as PRRs that respond to glycosylated antigens derived from pathogens, they also recognize glycosylated self-antigens and are also considered mediators of immune homeostasis (van Kooyk and Geijtenbeek 2003; Rabinovich and Toscano 2009; Geijtenbeek et al. 2004; van Kooyk and Rabinovich 2008; García-Vallejo and van Kooyk 2009). APC can express a large variety of CLR, of which DEC-205, DC-SIGN, macrophage galactose lectin (MGL), Mannose receptor (MR), and Clec9A are the best characterized. The glycan recognition and the exact ligand specificity of Dec205 (CD205) is not known, but those of DC-SIGN (CD209), MGL (CD301), CLEC9A, and MR (CD206) are described in detail (Steinman et al. 2003; Sica and Mantovani 2012; Steinman and Banchereau 2007; van Kooyk and Geijtenbeek 2002; Appelmelk et al. 2003; Zhang et al. 2012; Brown 2012; van Vliet et al. 2008; Chieppa et al. 2003; McKenzie et al. 2007). Different APC subsets may vary in the set of TLRs, NLRs, or CLRs they express. The net result in this receptor variability allows the recognition of distinct sets of pathogens and confers the ability to respond differently to pathogens and microenvironmental changes.

4.2 Glycan-Binding Receptors

Within the immune system, various classes of glycan-binding receptors (lectins) exist that recognize specific glycoconjugates (polysaccharides, glycolipids, proteoglycans, and glycoproteins). These receptors can either be secreted or found on the cell surface of immune cells. Where galectins are secreted, most C-type lectins are membrane-bound proteins. All these lectins contain one or more carbohydrate-recognition domains (CRDs) responsible for glycan binding (van Kooyk and Rabinovich 2008; Rabinovich et al. 2012).

Galectins, a highly conserved family of β-galactoside-binding lectins, recognize *N*-acetyllactosamine (LacNAc) on *N*-glycans and *O*-glycans on cell surface and matrix glycoproteins (van Gisbergen et al. 2005; Rabinovich and Croci 2012; Yang et al. 2008; Zhu et al. 2005). In addition, they regulate signal transduction and pre-mRNA splicing in a carbohydrate-independent fashion(McKenzie et al. 2007; Martinez-Pomares et al. 2006; Anderson et al. 2007; Liu et al. 2002). Through ligand binding, galectins induce the retention of their ligands at the cell surface, thereby increasing their responsiveness to extracellular inputs and prolonging intracellular signaling (Stancic et al. 2011; Rabinovich and Toscano 2009; Burgdorf et al. 2006; Singh et al. 2011). Some galectins, such as Gal-1 and Gal-3, are distributed in a wide variety of tissues (van Kooyk and Rabinovich 2008; van Vliet et al. 2007). In the immune system, galectins are mostly expressed by activated (but not resting) T and B cells, and they are significantly upregulated in activated MΦ, DC, and T_{Regs} cells.

CLRs are Ca^{2+}-dependent carbohydrate-binding proteins and consist of a large and diverse family of receptors. Several of these C-type lectins (the natural killer (NK) cell receptor-like family) do not have classical CRD and thus are not involved in protein–glycan interactions(Zelensky and Gready 2005). However, most CLRs are glycan-binding receptors as they carry one or more CRD regions. C-type lectins can be divided into two categories on the basis of an amino acid motif involved in glycan recognition and coordination of the Ca^{2+} ion. The mannose-specific CLRs (e.g., DC-SIGN and MR) contain an EPN (Glu-Pro-Asn) amino acid motif and have specificity for glycans bearing terminal mannose and/or fucose residues. In contrast, galactose-specific CLRs (e.g., MGL) contain a QPD (Gln-Pro-Asp) motif in the CRD and recognize glycans carrying terminal galactose or *N*-acetylgalactosamine

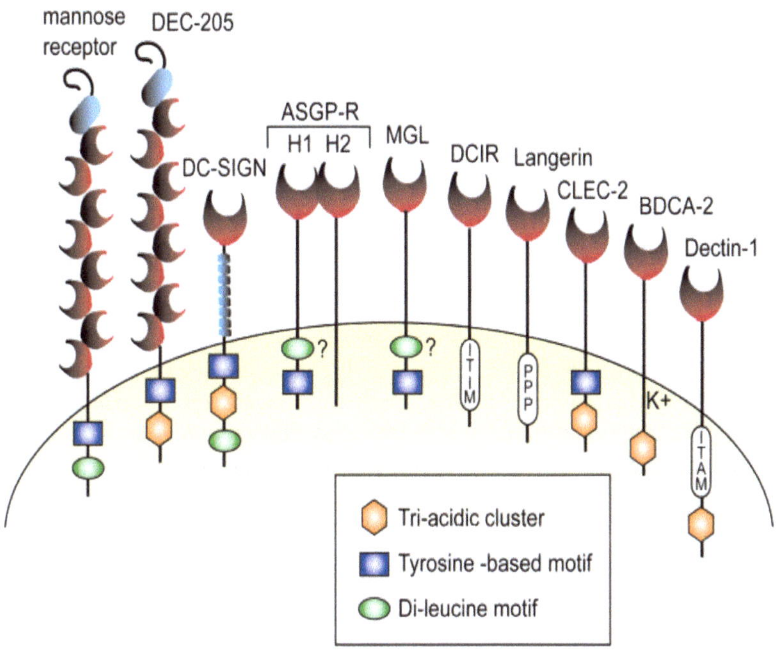

Fig. 4.2 Expression and variety of C-type lectins on antigen-presenting cells (APC)

(GalNAc). The type II subfamily of CLR, of which 17 members have been cloned in human, is mainly restricted APC, such as MΦ and DC.

Although a diverse range of CLRs is present on DC (Fig. 4.2), other cells of the immune system express CLRs as well. These include both the carbohydrate-binding, calcium-dependent CLRs as well as other receptors with a CTLD. On DC, both type I and type II CLRs are found. The type I CLRs have their N-terminus extracellular and contain multiple CRDs. In contrast, type II CLRs have only one CRD and their C-terminus extracellular (Figdor et al. 2002; van Vliet et al. 2006a, b).

On DC, CLRs have been shown to perform different function upon ligation of their glycan ligands. Besides recognition of glycan PAMPs on pathogens, CLRs can internalize glycan-carrying antigens and route them into MHC-I or MHC-II loading compartments (Idoyaga et al. 2011, Singh et al. 2011; van Vliet et al. 2006a, b; Bozzacco et al. 2007; Unger et al. 2007). Furthermore, some CLRs have been shown to mediate cell–cell interactions. For example, DC-SIGN is able to bind ICAM-3 on T cells (Geijtenbeek et al. 2004; Ginhoux et al. 2010) or ICAM-2 on endothelial cells (García-Vallejo et al. 2008) and thereby contribute to the interaction between DC and T cell, needed for efficient T cell activation, and DC migration. Lately, ligand-induced signaling has also been shown for CLRs (Gringhuis et al. 2009; Nimmerjahn et al. 2005). CLRs with signaling properties can be divided in four groups: the hemITAM group that is able to signal via an ITAM-like motif in the intracellular tail, an ITAM-coupled group that needs association to an ITAM-containing adaptor protein, which conducts the signal inside the cell, a group with an intracellular ITIM, and finally a group that lacks obvious signaling motifs (Schafer et al. 2012; Sancho and Reis e Sousa 2012). Even though most Ca^{2+}-dependent carbohydrate-binding CLRs belong to the latest group, they have been reported to modify TLR signaling.

4.3 Dendritic Cell-Specific Intercellular Adhesion Molecule-3-Grabbing Non-integrin, Mannose Receptor, and Macrophage Galactose Lectin

CLRs such as DC-SIGN, MR, and MGL are highly expressed on immature DC and on various MΦ. Maturation of DC often leads to a reduced expression of these lectins, indicating that their main function is in the innate recognition of antigen. Primarily, MGL is often upregulated on tolerogenic DC, illustrating a potential role for MGL to silence immune responses (van Vliet et al. 2006a, b; Koning et al. 2007; van Vliet et al. 2006a, b; Koning et al. 2009a, b; Mott et al. 2004).

One of the best characterized CLRs on DC is DC-SIGN. DC-SIGN is expressed mainly on DC and on a few types of MΦ(Geijtenbeek et al. 2000a, b; Davoust et al. 2008). There is no DC-SIGN expression found on other cells of the immune system. DC-SIGN has an EPN motif in the CRD and binds to both high mannose and fucose-containing glycans (e.g., Lewis-type glycans, a glycan structure consisting of one or two terminal fucoses on a (neo)lactosamine backbone) (Appelmelk et al. 2003; Mitchell et al. 2001). Several ligands for DC-SIGN have been described after the initial discovery of DC-SIGN binding to HIV and ICAM-3 (Geijtenbeek et al. 2000a, b). DC-SIGN ligands are present on various pathogens, such as viruses, bacteria, yeasts, and parasites (van Kooyk and Geijtenbeek 2003). However, DC-SIGN also interacts with different endogenous ligands. Adhesion molecules like ICAM-2, on vascular and lymphoid endothelium and Mac-1 and CEACAM-1 on neutrophils have been described to bind strongly to DC-SIGN (van Kooyk and Geijtenbeek 2008; García-Vallejo and van Kooyk 2009). Moreover, self-glycoproteins present in tumor-associated tissues, such as carcinoembryonic antigen (CEA) in colon cancer (van Gisbergen et al. 2005), or MOG in healthy brain tissues (Garcia-Vallejo et al. submitted), show binding activity to DC-SIGN. The diversity of DC-SIGN ligands is reflected in the different functional outcomes of ligand binding. Binding to cell-associated glycoproteins results in cell adhesion, while uptake of glycosylated antigen leads to presentation of antigen in MHC-I and MHC-II molecules, favoring $CD8^{+}$-mediated and $CD4^{+}$-mediated T cell responses (Singh et al. 2011; Burgdorf et al. 2008; Singh et al. 2009). Also, a signaling function has been described for DC-SIGN in relation to the specific carbohydrate it recognizes (Gringhuis and Geijtenbeek 2010). While mannose-type DC-SIGN-binding glycans induce more an inflammatory profile of cytokines IL12p70 and IL-6, the fucose-containing ligands like $Lewis^{X}$ established a reduced production of inflammatory cytokines, while promoting the production of the anti-inflammatory cytokine IL-10. Mannose-dependent

DC-SIGN signaling resulted in the activation of the kinase Raf-1, while signaling via fucose glycans was independent of Raf-1 (Gringhuis et al. 2009).

Although MR has a different glycan specificity than DC-SIGN, both CLRs also have an overlapping glycan recognition, mainly regarding mannosylated structures (McKenzie 2007; Martinez-Pomares et al. 2006). Similar to DC-SIGN, MR has been demonstrated to mediate antigen internalization and endocytic routing for presentation to $CD4^{+}$ and $CD8^{+}$ T cells (Burgdorf et al. 2006; Singh et al. 2011). Although self-glycoproteins have also been shown to interact with MR and anti-inflammatory cytokines are triggered, little is known on the exact signal transduction pathway triggered.

Distinct from DC-SIGN and MR, MGL recognizes glycans containing terminal GalNAc. MGL has been demonstrated to recognize several pathogens that expose these glycans, such as various bacteria and helminths (van Vliet et al. 2007). Also, MGL recognizes self-glycoproteins, such as MUC1, CD43, and CD45 (van Vliet et al. 2006a, b; Saeland et al. 2012). Triggering of MGL upon ligand binding has shown to induce an anti-inflammatory pathway by production of IL-10, whereas binding of MGL to the glycans on the phosphatase CD45 results in the inhibition of effector T cell function by reducing T cell proliferation, and inducing T cell death, implicating (van Vliet et al. 2006a, b) that MGL has an anti-inflammatory function (van Vliet et al. 2006a, b). Conclusively, CLRs are functionally diverse molecules but have in common that they modulate the outcome of the immune response.

4.4 Antigen-Presenting Cells in the Central Nervous System

The successful initiation of immune responses by the adaptive immune system is crucial for survival of the host. However, a sensitive organ like the CNS needs a shelter against inflammatory damage to protect its cells that generally have a low regenerative capacity. Several strategies have evolved, such as a lack of conventional lymphatic system and the presence of a blood–brain barrier that limits the infiltration of immune cells in the CNS. Although the CNS is considered to be "immune privileged," this does not mean that the CNS is immunologically unresponsive. In fact, the CNS contains many APC that are able to respond to danger stimuli, but yet they are equipped with molecules to control overt responses. Therefore, CNS APC are considered highly important in actively maintaining immune homeostasis. Different populations of myeloid cells in the CNS have been described: microglia, CNS-associated myeloid cells, and in some pathological conditions, CNS-infiltrating myeloid cells.

4.4.1 Microglia

Microglia are the brain-resident MΦ and are scattered throughout the CNS parenchyma, both in gray and white matter. The origin of microglia is widely debated, but recent murine studies suggest that microglia do not derive from precursors in the bone marrow, but rather from yolk sac MΦ that migrate into the CNS early in embryogenesis (Ginhoux et al. 2010). Also, turnover is not influenced by bone marrow-derived MΦ, but seems controlled by self-renewal within the CNS (Ajami et al. 2007). Microglia are small, ramified cells and have an immunologically quiescent phenotype. They closely resemble MΦ by sharing cell surface markers like CD11b and CD14 and have similar phagocytic capacity that allows them to take up material, such as myelin, from their environment. However, with low expression of MHC-II in the steady state, they do not exert substantial antigen-presenting properties. Despite their resting state, the fine cellular processes of microglia are highly motile and continually survey the microenvironment (Nimmerjahn et al. 2005). Microglia are essential in the development of the CNS by eliminating redundant synaptic connectivity through selective removal of developmental synapses via complement receptor 3 (Schafer et al. 2012). By further removal cellular debris, microglia can maintain CNS homeostasis. The CNS is extremely rich in expression of immune suppressive molecules such as CD200, CD47, and CD22 (Koning et al. 2007; Koning et al. 2009a, b; Mott et al. 2004) and soluble factors like TGFβ and prostaglandin, of which receptors are expressed on microglia. The strong interplay between microglia and other CNS cell types such as neurons, oligodendrocytes, and astrocytes via these molecules protects the CNS against disproportionate immune responses, by providing a high threshold for immune activation. Recently, it was shown that microglia express CLRs like MGL and DC-SIGN that stimulate anti-inflammatory cytokine production following interaction with its ligand expressed on myelin (Garcia-Vallejo et al. submitted), further supporting the function of microglia in immune homeostasis in the CNS.

Despite stringently controlled activation mechanisms, microglia are the first cells to rapidly respond to environmental changes caused by injury or inflammation (Davoust et al. 2008). Upon activation, they change to an amoeboid phenotype by retracting their protrusions, proliferate, and adopt a MΦ-like morphology and phenotype by an upregulation of MHC-II, and by the production of inflammatory cytokines and nitric oxide. However, TLR4-dependent activation of microglia reveals unique responses because they fail to upregulate molecules like TNFα and the chemokine receptor CCR7 (Clarkson et al. 2012; Melief et al. 2012), differentiating them from MΦ and stressing their homeostatic function.

Only in certain circumstances, immune activation can exacerbate, resulting in uncontrolled inflammation, such as seen in multiple sclerosis (MS). MS is a chronic demyelinating disease, characterized by activated and infiltrated leukocytes causing lesions throughout the brain. The etiology of MS remains unknown and it is debated whether it involves brain parenchymal factors or an initial peripheral event. However, in the MS brain, activated clusters of microglia are detected that may represent the earliest stage of lesion formation, they predominate in expanding MS lesions and may even have a higher capacity to phagocytose myelin compared to MΦ (Hatterer et al. 2008; Durafourt et al. 2012). With respect to T cell activation, it is not yet clear whether microglia are involved in the initial T cell activation or rather in the perpetuation of CNS inflammation. Although CNS antigens have been detected in the cervical lymph nodes, no studies have been reported that microglia can migrate to these lymph nodes. Despite upregulation of MHC-II upon microglia activation, the levels of costimulatory molecules remain low, making them poor activators of naïve T cells. It is therefore more likely that microglia aid in the reactivation of T cells after their infiltration into the CNS.

4.4.2 Central Nervous System-Associated Myeloid Cells

In contrast to microglia, CNS-associated APC are strategically located at the boundary between the CNS and the periphery, and are found in the meninges, the perivascular (Virchow-Robin) space of cerebral blood vessels between the endothelial vessel lining and the glia limitans, and in the choroid plexus. The highly vascularized choroid plexus is a structure in the cerebral ventricles that produces and secretes cerebrospinal fluid (CSF). CSF circulates from the ventricles through Virchow-Robin areas and the subarachnoid space, thereby bathing and buffering the CNS. Thus, CNS-associated APC are in close contact with CSF. Of note, we refer to this population as CNS-associated myeloid cells, but as this population has not yet been characterized in detail, it may very well represent different subsets of myeloid cells, including MΦ and perhaps DC, with separate specific immune functions (Fabriek et al. 2005; Ransohoff and Cardona 2010; de Vos et al. 2002; Ransohoff 2011). With eminent amounts of scavenger receptors, CLRs, MHC-II as well as costimulatory molecules expressed on their cell surface, CNS-associated APC scavenge substances derived from the CNS or from the circulation (Chamorro et al. 2009; Mato et al. 1996) and are capable of antigen presentation (Hickey and Kimura 1988). Their unique position bridges the CNS and the periphery, while assisting in the control of innate and adaptive immune responses. They generally express immune inhibitory and modulatory molecules, such as CD200R, MR, DC-SIGN, and CD163, by which they are ascribed to participate in immune surveillance and homeostasis (Gross et al. 2012; Koning et al. 2009a, b). Considered the gatekeepers of the brain, they monitor and respond to local changes in the microenvironment.

Interestingly, CNS MΦ are likely the first cells that leukocytes encounter when infiltrating the brain in MS and several lines of evidence point to an important role for these cells in facilitating inflammation, despite their homeostatic function in physiological conditions. Depriving the brain of MΦ by injecting clodronate-containing liposomes in the fourth ventricle of rat brains, ameliorated clinical signs of experimental autoimmune encephalomyelitis (EAE), the animal model for MS (Polfliet et al. 2002). Previously, Tran et al. showed that in the absence of MΦ, also by administration of clodronate-containing liposomes, leukocytes accumulated in the leptomeninges and perivascular spaces, but did not infiltrate the brain (Tran et al. 1998). The meninges of MS patients appeared to contain many T cells that are closely associated with meningeal APC (Androdias et al. 2010). Recent findings by Bartholomaus et al. extend these findings by imaging the initial event in EAE

(Bartholomäus et al. 2009). Following diapedesis of T cells into the meningeal abluminal vascular surface, mediated by adhesion molecules such as LFA-1 and VLA-4, T cells strongly interact with meningeal APC before invading the brain parenchyma. Indeed, it has been shown that $CD11c^{+}$ CNS myeloid cells, but neither microglia nor cells from the lymphoreticular system, are required for T cell invasion during EAE (Greter et al. 2005), thereby demonstrating that the contact between CNS-associated APC and T cell is, in fact, crucial in the development of neuroinflammation. The extensive interactions of infiltrating T cells with APC takes place in the subarachnoid space in the meninges, but also in the choroid plexus as recently published by Reboldi et al. (2009). They showed that the chemokine receptor CCR6 expressed on Th17 cells mediates the migration of T cells via its ligand CCL20 expressed on the choroid plexus epithelium. Mice lacking CCR6 were resistant to EAE because T cells accumulated in the choroid plexus, but failed to infiltrate the brain. These studies greatly enhance our understanding of the multifactorial processes of T cell diapedesis, CNS-associated APC–T cell interaction, and tissue invasion during brain inflammation. Although CNS-associated APC have a detrimental role in this process, the exact mechanism needs to be clarified, but likely involves presentation of foreign as well as self-antigens, such as myelin, and the production of mediators that trigger the inflammatory cascade. In addition, CNS-associated (subsets of) APC express DC-SIGN and MGL (unpublished data), and in contrast to microglia, also high levels of MR (Fig. 4.5). Given the immune modulatory properties of CLRs, depending on environmental antigens, it is highly interesting to understand their involvement in this process as well, as will be discussed later.

4.4.3 Inflammatory Central Nervous System-Infiltrating Myeloid Cells

During brain inflammation, infiltrating myeloid cells are found in the CNS. Within (chronic) active MS lesions, these cells are considered inflammatory monocytes that differentiate into MΦ, but are, in fact, indistinguishable from activated microglia. Also, the population of CNS-associated APC in the perivascular area, choroid plexus, and meninges expands with infiltrating myeloid cells, which, similar to CNS-associated cells, may contain multiple subsets. As such, nomenclature of this population varies in literature from infiltrating monocytes/MΦ and DC. Often, the distinction between MΦ and DC is based on the expression of CD11b/CD11c, but although these markers show higher expression on MΦ versus DC, they are not entirely MΦ- specific and DC-specific. However, while infiltrating MΦ in MS mainly phagocytose myelin, DC may primarily function in T cell (re)activation.

4.5 Central Nervous System Antigen-Presenting Cells in Priming and Reactivating T Cells in Autoimmune Disease

Given the fact that DC are the most effective APC, many studies have been performed to analyze whether in the brain DC derive from CNS precursors or rather infiltrate from the periphery. Within the context of CNS inflammation, it seems that DC in the brain are from bone marrow origin and therefore are derived from the periphery. Myeloid DC were found throughout the cerebellum and spinal cord (Kaunzner et al. 2012), as well as in meninges and parenchymal lesions in MS patients and in the CSF, where they express high levels of costimulatory molecules and CCR7, a chemokine receptor associated with DC maturation (Medzhitov and Janeway 2000a, b; Greter et al. 2005; Olson and Miller 2004). A well-established way of modeling aspects of MS is the induction of EAE by subcutaneous injection of fragments of myelin proteins (e.g., MOG or MBP), along with immunogenic boosters. Usually, around day 10 after immunization, motor weakness develops due to leukocyte accumulation in the spinal cord and inflammation, directed by myelin-specific T cells that are generated by myelin APC. Although the mechanisms to activate naïve T cell responses are well-studied, little is known about the APC requirements to reactivate fully primed T cells. A second way of inducing EAE is the adoptive transfer of myelin-specific $CD4^+$ Th cells. Using this model, it was demonstrated that microglia and peripheral APC have been excluded to play a role in T cell reactivation, but a population CNS-associated APC was postulated to present the cognate antigen to these activated T cells (Galea et al. 2005; Fritz et al. 2007; Stancic et al. 2011; Fabriek et al. 2005; Greter et al. 2005). Based on these studies, it is currently thought that DC can migrate as immature cells to the CNS, where they can further mature to reactivate infiltrating T cells. The question still remains whether maturated DC in neuroinflammation primarily reactivate infiltrating T cells, or whether they are also able to prime naïve T cells.

As part of its immune privileged status, the CNS lacks a conventional lymphatic system. Nevertheless, afferent immunity is intact as many studies suggest that antigens and cells from the CNS migrate to the cervical lymph nodes, although the mechanisms are as yet unclear. For example, antigens injected into the mouse CNS were taken up and processed by CNS-associated APC and resulted in specific immune responses in the cervical lymph nodes (Cserr and Knopf 1992; Cserr et al. 1992; Karman et al. 2004). Indeed, intracerebrally injected labeled mature DC as well as CSF-circulating DC were shown to migrate to cervical lymph nodes in mice (Hatterer et al. 2008; Karman et al. 2004). These processes are of utmost importance in brain inflammatory conditions such as MS. DC present in the meninges and perivascular space can efficiently present myelin (van Zwam et al. 2009, 2011; Kooi et al. 2009). This indicates that the afferent immunity is intact in the CNS and that antigens drain or traffic to the cervical lymph nodes. Mature DC injected i.c. have been shown to migrate to cervical lymph nodes in a CCR7-dependent and CXCR4-dependent manner. CNS-infiltrating DC are crucial for the local restimulation of encephalitogenic effector T cells (Clarkson et al. 2012; Hatterer et al. 2008) and may be further routed to the cervical lymph nodes. Here, APC have indeed been shown to contain CNS antigens although this was not only observed in MS patients but in healthy subjects as well (Boven et al. 2006). Interestingly, differences in inflammatory status of APC have been observed depending on whether the cells were loaded with neuronal or myelin antigens (van Zwam et al. 2009). Thus, it is likely that during neuroinflammation, CNS-associated APC and infiltrating DC are crucial for local restimulation of encephalitogenic effector T cells (Heine et al. 2011; Loo and Gale 2011; Clarkson et al. 2012; Leteux et al. 2000) directly in the CNS, as well as in the cervical lymph nodes (Hatterer et al. 2008) to prime naïve T cells. However, the mechanisms of migration as well as details on types of immune responses that are elicited in these lymph nodes need to be illuminated.

4.6 Immune Modulatory Effects of C-Type Lectins on Antigen-Presenting Cells in the Central Nervous System

Although the cause of MS is unknown, it is believed that once established, immune reactions against the CNS contribute to the significance of the disease progression. In particular, APC ingest debris from the damaged CNS tissue and process this material to antigenic fragments for presentation in MHC-I and MHC-II molecules in the context of costimulatory molecules and activate naïve T cells in the cervical lymph nodes (Ohashi et al. 2000; Fabriek et al. 2005; de Vos et al. 2002; Chavele et al. 2010), which differentiate in proinflammatory Th1 and Th17 cells or reactivate T cells upon CNS infiltration. Apart from priming naïve T cells, DC are also crucial in the control of homeostasis or the active inhibition of T cell-mediated immune responses by the induction of T_{Regs}. In this respect, DC have the capacity to vigorously eliminate activated T cells by the induction of apoptosis or anergy. The balance between effector T cells and T_{Regs} is driven by signals that DC receive from their environment to differentiate into an inflammatory or anti-inflammatory phenotype. In particular, exogenous factors, a reflection of the microenvironment, may play a crucial role in the DC differentiation program. In fact, there is ample evidence that DC can dampen inflammatory responses such as in EAE. IL-10, TGF-β, dexamethasone, and VitD3 have been shown to induce tolerogenic DC (Hanamsagar et al. 2012; Chamorro et al. 2009; Chavele et al. 2010) that in EAE models reduces the capacity to stimulate inflammatory T cells in spinal cords (Stancic et al. 2011; Ilarregui and Rabinovich 2010). Whereas injection of mature MOG- loaded DC prior to the induction of EAE decreases the frequency of T_{Regs} infiltrating the brain and increases the activation of CNS-infiltrating T cells, which is associated with the acceleration of clinical symptoms of EAE. Ex vivo-generated tolerogenic DC have been shown to reduce EAE symptoms by inducing a higher frequency of T_{Regs} and the production of IL-10 and TGF-β (Zhang et al. 2012; Brown 2012; Rabinovich and Croci 2012; Gross et al. 2012; Raïch-Regué et al. 2012). These studies indicate that peripheral injection of DC and the functional status of DC, being immunogenic or tolerogenic, is crucially affecting the type of DC that infiltrate the brain that can either increase CNS inflammation and cause damage or reduce brain CNS inflammation and allow tissue remodeling. In line with this, a schistosoma glycan, Lacto-*N*-fucopentaose III, was recently shown to reduce EAE severity and CNS inflammation by skewing the peripheral immune response to a Th2-dominant profile, increasing the population of IL-10-producing T cells, suppressing inflammation, while reducing the migration of DC to the CNS (Zhu et al. 2012). The schistosoma glycan, carrying Lewis^{X}-like structures, can be recognized by the CLR DC-SIGN and may negatively affect TLR signaling, leading to an anti-inflammatory phenotype of DC (Zhu et al. 2012).

Also, the recognition of the microenvironment, by CLRs in particular, is involved in the active suppression of DC activation upon recognition of ligands in their environment. Therefore, interactions of lectins with glycans are important in the homeostatic control by APC, a mechanism that is important in the healthy brain, but yet seems to fail in neuroinflammation.

4.6.1 Macrophage Galactose Lectin

MGL is a CLR mostly expressed by MΦ DC and mediates interactions with ligands on T cells via recognition of specific carbohydrate structures. Expression of the CLR MGL on tolerogenic APC provides a mechanism by which these cells control the inflammatory nature of effector T cells, by MGL dampening of the proinflammatory phenotype of T cells and the induction of T cell death. MGL thus provides an intrinsic mechanism that individually contributes to the resolution of inflammatory settings to dampen excessive immune responses. MGL is expressed on microglia in the brain as well as on DC in the cervical lymph nodes. Expression of MGL is increased during inflammatory condition within the brain. Moreover, the regulatory functions of MGL on APC are dictated by the presence of terminal GalNAc-exposing antigens that interact with MGL. MGL has shown to be a Th2-skewing receptor upon interaction with terminal GalNAc-containing pathogens. Binding of MGL has shown to lead to intracellular triggering events that lead to IL-10 induction and T cell anergy (van Vliet et al. 2008).

While MGL is both associated with a tolerogenic function in APC and has the capacity to generate a tolerogenic immune profile by altering the cytokine profile of DC to induce T_{Regs}, it is also involved in the recognition of glycan epitopes exposed on the phosphatase CD45 on effector T cells (van Kooyk and Rabinovich 2008; van Vliet et al. 2006a, b). Effector T cells present at the active phase of EAE or present in MS patients showed a higher frequency of MGL binding due to the glycosylation of CD45. MGL binding to this effector T cell population results in increased T cell death and a reduced T cell proliferation, illustrating an active role of MGL to dampen immune inflammation (Fig. 4.3).

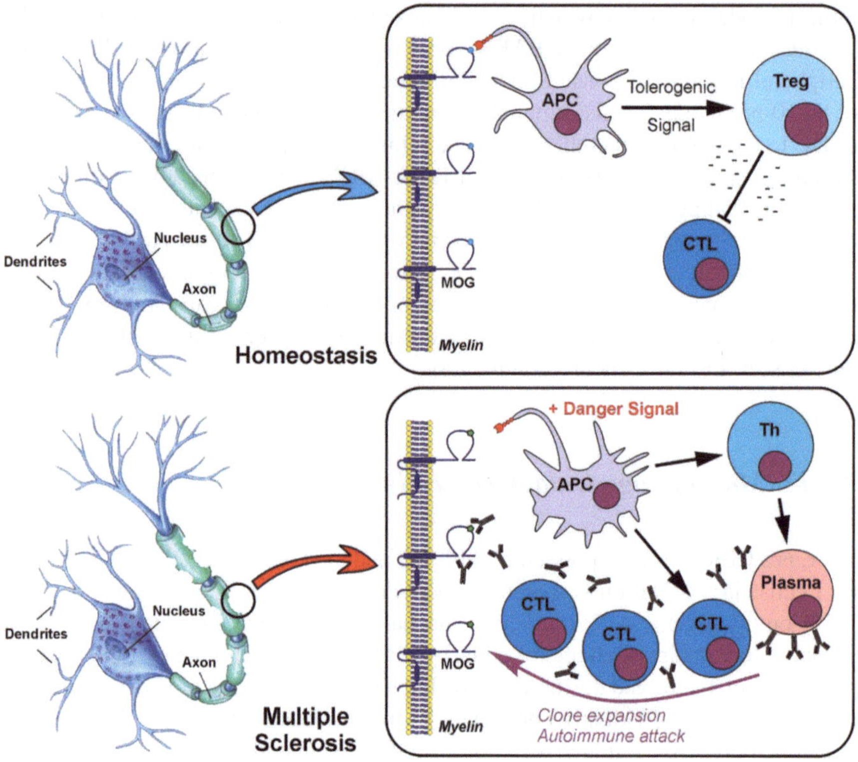

Fig. 4.3 Dual function of antigen-presenting cells (APC) on control of immune homeostasis in the central nervous system (CNS). By sampling glycosylated microenvironmental proteins such as myelin APC use C-type lectin receptors (CLR) to take up antigen for degradation. In healthy situation, these antigens induce homeostatic immune control by silencing effector T cells such as CD4 (Th) and CD8 T cells (CTLs) through enforcing the frequencies of Treg. In the situation of danger and the simultaneous reduction of inhibitory signals from the microenvironment due to altered glycosylation or loss of myelin uptake by APC, the frequency between Treg and effector T cells is out of balance, resulting in the clonal expansion of Th and CTLs to develop autoantibodies and CTLs to attack CNS tissues

4.7 Dendritic Cell-Specific Intercellular Adhesion Molecule-3-Grabbing Non-integrin

Other CLRs on APC, such as DC-SIGN, have shown to play a role in the control of immune homeostasis (Rabinovich and Toscano 2009; Geijtenbeek et al. 2004; van Kooyk and Rabinovich 2008; García-Vallejo and van Kooyk 2009). Although DC-SIGN recognizes many pathogens that expose carbohydrates, also self-glycoproteins have been described for this receptor. Interaction of these self-glycoproteins-carrying DC-SIGN ligands with DC-SIGN on DC results in antigen uptake (when the ligands are soluble), or contribute to adhesion interactions between cells (when the ligands are membrane-bound) (van Kooyk and Geijtenbeek 2002; Rabinovich and Toscano 2009). DC-SIGN has been shown to contribute to an anti-inflammatory signaling

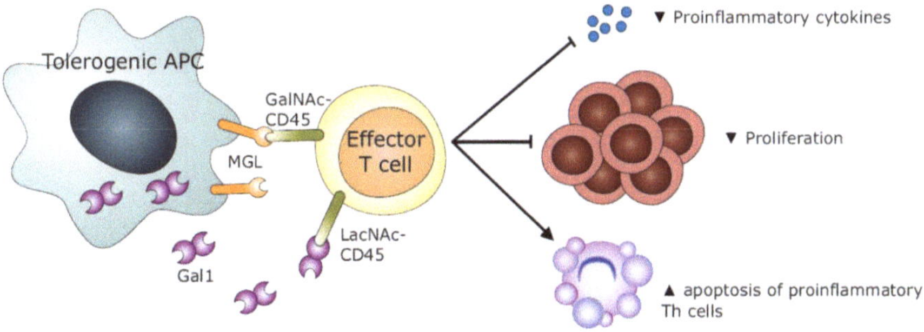

Fig. 4.4 Function of the C-type lectin receptors (CLR) MGL and Gal1 on tolerogenic antigen-presenting cells (APC) to suppress effector T cell function. MGL expressed on tolerogenic dendritic cells (DC) interact with unique glycosylated forms of CD45 expressed on effector T cells. Binding of MGL to the phosphatase CD45 reduces the proliferation of T cells, increases T cell death, and reduces the production of proinflammatory cytokines of effector T cells. Similar as MGL, secretion of Gal1 by tolerogenic DC binds CD45 on effector T cells and induces similar reduction of effector T cell function as MGL

circuit triggering IL-10 production depending on the type of glycan structure (mannose/fucose) that binds to the CRD.

CNS myelin is a highly glycosylated structure. Glycans can be found on several glycoproteins (e.g., MOG and MAG) and on glycolipids, such as cerebrosides. These glycan structures may potentially interact with CLR-expressing APC during the sampling of their microenvironment and contribute to the control of immune homeostasis. Thus, we can refer to the glycosylation status of myelin during homeostasis as a *healthy* glycosylation status. Glycosylation is very sensitive to extracellular cues and many stimuli have shown to affect the relative composition of the glycosylation machinery. Among the multiple stimuli known to affect glycosylation is inflammation (Delmotte et al. 2002; García-Vallejo et al. 2006), and thus, it is logical to postulate that the *healthy* glycosylation state of CNS myelin may become altered during local inflammation. The alteration of the glycosylation of glycoproteins and glycolipids in myelin may modify the recognition of myelin ligands by CLRs on CNS APC, which consequently could result in the loss of the strength of the immunoregulatory signaling controlling immune homeostasis in the CNS (Fig. 4.4). Microglia are CNS-based APC that continuously evaluate local changes in the CNS to activate the peripheral immune system during injury (Rabinovich and Toscano 2009; Olson and Miller 2004) or help maintain homeostasis in healthy conditions. On the other hand, also peripheral infiltrating APC present in the perivascular space, the meninges or the choroid plexus can sample CNS tissue in their microenvironment, and may induce inhibitory or stimulatory signals through interaction with incoming T cells.

4.7.1 Mannose Receptor

Also, MR is highly expressed on CNS-associated APC, MΦ, but not on microglia (Galea et al. 2005; Fabriek et al. 2005; Fig. 4.5). Similar to DC-SIGN,

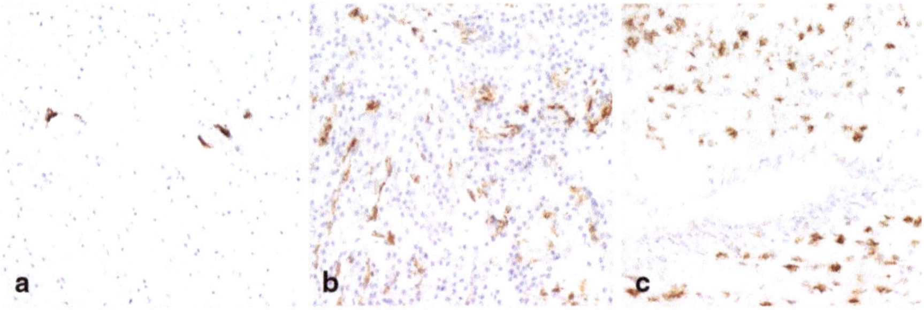

Fig. 4.5 Expression of the CLR MR on antigen-presenting cells (APC) in human central nervous system (CNS). Immunohistochemical staining shows MR expression on perivascular cell in the white matter (**a**), on irregular shaped cells within the choroid plexus (**b**), and in the meninges (**c**). Tissues are derived from human donors with nonneurological disease. Nuclei are stained in *blue*. Magnification × 20

MR recognizes carbohydrate structures for presentation to T cells. MR has two carbohydrate-binding domains. One of the CRD binds terminal mannose, fucose, and *N*-acetyl-glucosamine while the cystein-rich domain binds terminal sulfated *N*-acetyl-galactosamine, chondroitin sulfates A and B, and sulfated Lewis^{a} and Lewis^{X} (Leteux et al. 2000). Although little is known on the MR self-glycoprotein ligands, potential MR-binding structures may be present in the CNS. MR has been reported to be expressed primarily on alternative activated MΦ, and targeting of the MR with antibody-coupled antigen has been shown to result in IL-10 production, linking the expression of the MR on APC that are implicated in immune inhibition (Chieppa et al. 2003; Allavena et al. 2005, 2010). Also, MR-deficient mice have shown impaired clearance of inflammatory serum glycoproteins, corroborating its anti-inflammatory function (Chavele et al. 2010). On the other side, absence of MR in MΦ derived from $MR^{-/-}$ mice reduced LPS-mediated TNFα production compared to wild-type cells (Chavele et al. 2010). Similar to DC-SIGN, antigen targeting using MR-specific glycans can potentiate $CD8^{+}$ and $CD4^{+}$ responses. Thus, MR has a dual function, similar to DC-SIGN, in which anti-inflammatory and inflammatory functions depend on the signals the APC receives in combination with the CLR.

4.8 Galectins

To date, the best characterized galectins in CNS inflammation are Gal1, Gal3, and Gal9. These galectins are expressed in normal-appearing white matter (NAWM), microglia, astrocytes, and endothelial cell and are upregulated during MS (Stancic et al. 2011).

Gal1, a lectin associated with immune tolerance and T cell homeostasis (Rabinovich and Croci 2012), is upregulated in MS lesions and in activated microglia and downregulated in astrocytes, probably due to its release into the extracellular milieu (Stancic et al. 2011). Gal1 is also upregulated in the CNS during EAE, with the highest value at the peak of the disease. High Gal1 expression was observed on infiltrating $CD4^+$ T cells and $CD11b^+$ cells as well as on $GFAP^+$ astrocytes bordering the lesion area. Gal1 is similarly upregulated in DLNs and spleens in mice during the peak and resolution of EAE (Ilarregui et al. 2009). Gal1 is similarly upregulated in draining lymph nodes and spleens of mice during the peak and resolution phases of EAE (Ilarregui et al. 2009). The above mentioned results suggest the participation of Gal1 in limiting the inflammatory response in MS.

Gal1 binds to core 2 *O*-glycans decorating CD45 on microglial cells leading to microglia deactivation (Starossom et al. 2012). In line with these findings, therapeutic administration of 100 μg/day/mice of Gal1 ameliorates EAE, limiting microglia activation, axonal loss and demyelination, and promoting synaptic repair. (Starossom et al. 2012). Therefore, lack of endogenous Gal1 increases classical microglia activation promoting axonal damage during autoimmune neuroinflammation in mice. In the same manner, Gal1 binding to *N*-glycans and *O*-glycans on CD45 reduces the phosphatase activity of CD45 inducing T cell death (Rabinovich et al. 2012), similar to MGL (Fig. 4.3) leading to amelioration of autoimmune inflammation, as previously described for MGL (Rabinovich and Toscano 2009).

Due to its tolerogenic properties, recombinant Gal1 has been used as a treatment in several experimental models of autoimmune diseases to suppress chronic inflammation and to skew the balance of the immune responses toward a Th2-type cytokine profile (Rabinovich and Toscano 2009). Thus, administration of Gal1 reduces the severity of EAE by selective elimination of Th1 and Th17 pathogenic T cells (Rabinovich and Toscano 2009; Toscano et al. 2007; Offner et al. 1990). Moreover, $Gal1^{-/-}$ mice have an increased frequency of Th1 and Th17 cells and enhanced susceptibility to autoimmune neuroinflammation (Toscano et al. 2007). Taken together, these observations indicate an important role of Gal1 in "fine-tuning" the immunogenicity of DC in the context of EAE.

The tandem repeat galectin-type Gal9 is involved in central and peripheral tolerance by inducing apoptosis of thymocytes or effector T cells, respectively (Rabinovich and Croci 2012; Zhu et al. 2005; Zelensky and Gready 2005), and is upregulated in MS lesions (Anderson et al. 2007). In the microglia found in active MS lesions, Gal9 is located in the nuclei and cytosol, whereas it is only expressed in the cytosol in chronic inactive lesions (Stancic et al. 2011).

Gal9 can also bind the T cell immunoglobulin domain and mucin domain protein 3 (TIM-3), inducing apoptosis of thymocytes and effector Th1 cells. Gal9 also binds Th17 cells and induces their apoptosis, but in a TIM-3-independent manner (Zhu et al. 2005; Oomizu et al. 2012). In keeping with these findings, mice treated with recombinant Gal9 in the EAE model show reduced disease severity and mortality. TIM-3 is also expressed in DC but on the contrary, Gal9 induces a proinflammatory profile in these APC initiating a Th1-immune response. In accordance with these findings, mice treated with recombinant Gal9 during the induction of EAE show reduced disease severity and mortality (Zhu et al. 2005; Ilarregui et al. 2009). In addition, Gal9 knock-down or $Gal9^{-/-}$ mice suffer an exacerbated EAE in comparison to control mice (Oomizu et al. 2012). Moreover, monocytes and microglia from the active border regions of MS lesions express high levels of TIM-3 and astrocytes present in MS lesions express high levels of Gal9 relative to the quiescent center of MS lesions or to normal human CNS tissue (Stancic et al. 2011; Heine 2011; Loo and Gale 2011; Anderson et al. 2007). Collectively, these data may explain, at least in part, the sustained inflammation at the border region of MS lesions. As a member of the tandem repeat-type group, Gal9 posses two different CRDs, the one in the C-terminal domain is more potent in inducing T cell death than the N-terminal, while the CRD at the N-terminal domain is more effective in activating DC in a p38-dependent and AKT-dependent manner (Rabinovich and Croci 2012; Li et al. 2011). These data elucidate the contrasting effects observed between T cells and APC in the presence of Gal9.

On the other hand, Gal3, which has predominantly a proinflammatory role (Stancic et al. 2011; Ohashi et al. 2000; Rabinovich and Croci 2012; Yang et al. 2008), is upregulated in MS lesions and astrocytes. (Stancic et al. 2011; Hanamsagar et al. 2012). Similarly, in EAE experiments, Gal3 expression is upregulated in demyelinated areas, and in microglia and MΦ Gal3 appears to be involved in myelin phagocytosis (Reichert and Rotshenker 1999). Depending on whether it functions intracellularly or is added exogenously to T cells, Gal3 acts either protecting T cells from apoptosis or promoting cell death, respectively (Yang et al. 2008). However, in vivo studies support the notion that Gal3 promotes inflammatory response (Yang et al. 2008). Consequently, in EAE experiments, $Gal3^{-/-}$ mice develop lower clinical score accompanied by a decreased leukocyte infiltration, elevated frequency of $Foxp3^{+}$ T_{Regs} cells, and following antigen stimulation, draining lymph nodes T cells produce lower amounts of IL-6, IL-17, and IFNγ and higher levels of IL-10 and IL-5 compared to wild-type mice (Rabinovich and Toscano 2009; Jiang et al. 2009). In line with these results, Jeon et al. show that rat and mouse microglia and astrocytes treated with IFNγ induce Gal3 expression and secretion into the extracellular space (Jeon et al. 2010). Moreover, Gal3-treated primary microglia and astrocytes upregulate the expression of TNFα, IL-1β, and IL-12 (Jeon et al. 2010).

By contrast, infiltrating MΦ in relapsing–remitting EAE lesions as well as activated microglia in EAE and others models of CNS inflammation express high levels of Gal3 (Rabinovich et al. 2012; Toscano et al. 2007; Berard et al. 2010; Venkatesan et al. 2010). In these models, Gal3 plays a pivotal role in the phagocytosis of myelin since degenerated myelin inhibits remyelination by oligodendrocytes (Rabinovich and Croci 2012; Yang et al. 2008; Zhu et al. 2005; Kotter et al. 2006). These findings are particularly significant since Gal3 is present in microglia/MΦ that phagocytose myelin, and it has been shown in vitro that myelin phagocytosis induces a switch from a proinflammatory to an anti-inflammatory phenotype in MΦ (Anderson et al. 2007; Liu et al. 2002; Boven et al. 2006). Collectively, these data suggest a relevant role for galectins in MS pathophysiology.

4.9 Conclusion

CNS-resident APC of the CNS parenchyma, as well as of the perivascular, choroid plexus, and meningeal area are crucial for the control of immune homeostasis. They may sample their environment for antigens by means of their CLRs and scavenger receptors. Their strategic position has demonstrated their important function in the interaction with infiltrating T cells, in order to reactivate or inhibit these T cells, depending on the local signals they receive. Brain APC are, therefore, crucial in directing autoimmune diseases, either exacerbating or dampening inflammation, and their phenotype and functional status as a reflection of the CNS microenvironment may be more important than initially thought. A better understanding on how APC at different locations in the brain handle their microenvironmental changes is therefore essential in our understanding to design new therapies aimed at inhibiting both the initial and the chronic phase of autoimmune disease taking place in the CNS. Questions that need to be addressed in the future concern the inflammatory signals to recruit different APC populations into the brain, as well as the functional differences between infiltrating and resident APC and how they control their microenvironment at the molecular level. Furthermore, knowledge on how the cervical lymph nodes contribute to the onset and reactivation of autoimmune diseases is lacking, as well as on how CNS-associated APC subsets differentially contribute to T cell restimulation. Answers to these questions will help to design better therapies for CNS autoimmune and chronic inflammatory diseases that target subset-specific modulation of DC migration and activation status.

Acknowledgments Our work is financially supported by VENI NWO-ALW (grant 863.08.020) and VENI NWO-ZONMW ZonMw (grant 916.12.113), Dutch MS-Research Foundation (MS06–598 and MS05–560 567), and TIPharma TI-214.

References

Ajami B, Bennett JL, Krieger C, Tetzlaff W, Rossi FMV (2007) Local self-renewal can sustain CNS microglia maintenance and function throughout adult life. Nat Neurosci 10:1538–1543

Allavena P et al (2005) Anti-inflammatory properties of the novel antitumor agent yondelis (trabectedin): inhibition of macrophage differentiation and cytokine production. Cancer Res 65:2964–2971

Allavena P et al (2010) Engagement of the mannose receptor by tumoral mucins activates an immune suppressive phenotype in human tumor-associated macrophages. Clin Dev Immunol 2010:547179

Anderson AC et al (2007) Promotion of tissue inflammation by the immune receptor Tim-3 expressed on innate immune cells. Science 318:1141–1143

Androdias G et al (2010) Meningeal T cells associate with diffuse axonal loss in multiple sclerosis spinal cords. Ann Neurol 68:465–476

Appelmelk BJ et al (2003) Cutting edge: carbohydrate profiling identifies new pathogens that interact with dendritic cell-specific ICAM-3-grabbing nonintegrin on dendritic cells. J Immunol 170:1635–1639

Bacchetta R, Gregori S, Roncarolo M-G (2005) CD4+ regulatory T cells: mechanisms of induction and effector function. Autoimmun Rev 4:491–496
Banchereau J, Steinman RM (1998) Dendritic cells and the control of immunity. Nature 392:245–252
Bartholomäus I et al (2009) Effector T cell interactions with meningeal vascular structures in nascent autoimmune CNS lesions. Nature 462:94–98
Berard JL, Kerr BJ, Johnson HM, David S (2010) Differential expression of SOCS1 in macrophages in relapsing-remitting and chronic EAE and its role in disease severity. Glia 58:1816–1826
Boven LA et al (2006) Myelin-laden macrophages are anti-inflammatory, consistent with foam cells in multiple sclerosis. Brain 129:517–526
Bozzacco L et al (2007) DEC-205 receptor on dendritic cells mediates presentation of HIV gag protein to CD8+ T cells in a spectrum of human MHC I haplotypes. Proc Natl Acad Sci U S A 104:1289–1294
Brown GD (2012) Immunology: actin' dangerously. Nature 485:589–590
Burgdorf S, Lukacs-Kornek V, Kurts C (2006) The mannose receptor mediates uptake of soluble but not of cell-associated antigen for cross-presentation. J Immunol 176:6770–6776
Burgdorf S, Schölz C, Kautz A, Tampé R, Kurts C (2008) Spatial and mechanistic separation of cross-presentation and endogenous antigen presentation. Nat Immunol 9:558–566
Chamorro S et al (2009) TLR triggering on tolerogenic dendritic cells results in TLR2 up-regulation and a reduced proinflammatory immune program. J Immunol 183:2984–2994
Chavele K-M et al (2010) Mannose receptor interacts with Fc receptors and is critical for the development of crescentic glomerulonephritis in mice. J Clin Invest 120:1469–1478
Chieppa, M et al (2003) Cross-linking of the mannose receptor on monocyte-derived dendritic cells activates an anti-inflammatory immunosuppressive program. J Immunol 171:4552–4560
Clarkson BD et al (2012) Innate-adaptive crosstalk: how dendritic cells shape immune responses in the CNS. Adv Exp Med Biol 946:309–333
Cserr HF, Knopf PM (1992) Cervical lymphatics, the blood-brain barrier and the immunoreactivity of the brain: a new view. Immunol Today 13:507–512
Cserr HF, Harling-Berg CJ, Knopf PM (1992) Drainage of brain extracellular fluid into blood and deep cervical lymph and its immunological significance. Brain Pathol 2:269–276
Davoust N, Vuaillat C, Androdias G, Nataf S (2008) From bone marrow to microglia: barriers and avenues. Trends Immunol 29:227–234
de Vos AF et al (2002) Transfer of central nervous system autoantigens and presentation in secondary lymphoid organs. J Immunol 169:5415–5423
Delmotte P et al (2002) Tumor necrosis factor alpha increases the expression of glycosyltransferases and sulfotransferases responsible for the biosynthesis of sialylated and/or sulfated Lewis x epitopes in the human bronchial mucosa. J Biol Chem 277:424–431
Drickamer K (1999) C-type lectin-like domains. Curr Opin Struct Biol 9:585–590
Durafourt BA et al (2012) Comparison of polarization properties of human adult microglia and blood-derived macrophages. Glia 60:717–727
Fabriek BO et al (2005) CD163-positive perivascular macrophages in the human CNS express molecules for antigen recognition and presentation. Glia 51:297–305
Figdor CG, Kooyk Y van, Adema GJ (2002) C-type lectin receptors on dendritic cells and Langerhans cells. Nat Rev Immunol 2:77–84
Fritz JH, Girardin SE (2005) How Toll-like receptors and Nod-like receptors contribute to innate immunity in mammals. J Endotoxin Res 11:390–394
Fritz JH et al (2007) Nod1-mediated innate immune recognition of peptidoglycan contributes to the onset of adaptive immunity. Immunity 26:445–459
Galea I et al (2005) Mannose receptor expression specifically reveals perivascular macrophages in normal, injured, and diseased mouse brain. Glia 49:375–384
García-Vallejo JJ, Kooyk Y van (2009) Endogenous ligands for C-type lectin receptors: the true regulators of immune homeostasis. Immunol Rev 230:22–37

García-Vallejo JJ et al (2006) Activation of human endothelial cells by tumor necrosis factor-alpha results in profound changes in the expression of glycosylation-related genes. J Cell Physiol 206:203–210
García-Vallejo JJ et al (2008) DC-SIGN mediates adhesion and rolling of dendritic cells on primary human umbilical vein endothelial cells through LewisY antigen expressed on ICAM-2. Mol Immunol 45:2359–2369
García-Vallejo JJ et al Homeostatic interaction of CNS myelin with DC-SIGN-expressing APC prevents neuroinflammation, submitted
Geijtenbeek TB et al (2000a) DC-SIGN, a dendritic cell-specific HIV-1-binding protein that enhances trans-infection of T cells. Cell 100:587–597
Geijtenbeek TB et al (2000b) Identification of DC-SIGN, a novel dendritic cell-specific ICAM-3 receptor that supports primary immune responses. Cell 100:575–585
Geijtenbeek TBH, Vliet SJ van, Engering A, 't Hart BA, Kooyk Y van (2004) Self- and nonself-recognition by C-type lectins on dendritic cells. Annu Rev Immunol 22:33–54
Ginhoux F et al (2010) Fate mapping analysis reveals that adult microglia derive from primitive macrophages. Science 330:841–845
Greter M et al (2005) Dendritic cells permit immune invasion of the CNS in an animal model of multiple sclerosis. Nat Med 11:328–334
Gringhuis SI, Geijtenbeek TBH (2010) Carbohydrate signaling by C-type lectin DC-SIGN affects NF-kappaB activity. Meth Enzymol 480:151–164
Gringhuis SI et al (2007) C-type lectin DC-SIGN modulates Toll-like receptor signaling via Raf-1 kinase-dependent acetylation of transcription factor NF-kappaB. Immunity 26:605–616
Gringhuis SI, Dunnen denJ, Litjens M, Vlist M van der, Geijtenbeek TBH (2009) Carbohydrate-specific signaling through the DC-SIGN signalosome tailors immunity to Mycobacterium tuberculosis, HIV-1 and Helicobacter pylori. Nat Immunol 10:1081–1088
Gross CC, Jonuleit H, Wiendl H (2012) Fulfilling the dream: tolerogenic dendritic cells to treat multiple sclerosis. Eur J Immunol 42:569–572
Hanamsagar R, Hanke ML, Kielian T (2012) Toll-like receptor (TLR) and inflammasome actions in the central nervous system. Trends Immunol 33:333–342
Hatterer E, Touret M, Belin M-F, Honnorat J, Nataf S (2008) Cerebrospinal fluid dendritic cells infiltrate the brain parenchyma and target the cervical lymph nodes under neuroinflammatory conditions. PLoS ONE 3:e3321
Heine H (2011) TLRs, NLRs and RLRs: innate sensors and their impact on allergic diseases–a current view. Immunol Lett 139:14–24
Hickey WF, Kimura H (1988) Perivascular microglial cells of the CNS are bone marrow-derived and present antigen in vivo. Science 239:290–292
Idoyaga J et al (2011) Comparable T helper 1 (Th1) and CD8 T-cell immunity by targeting HIV gag p24 to CD8 dendritic cells within antibodies to Langerin, DEC205, and Clec9 A. Proc Natl Acad Sci U S A 108:2384–2389
Ilarregui JM, Rabinovich GA (2010) Tolerogenic dendritic cells in the control of autoimmune neuroinflammation: an emerging role of protein-glycan interactions. Neuroimmunomodulation 17:157–160
Ilarregui JM et al (2009) Tolerogenic signals delivered by dendritic cells to T cells through a galectin-1-driven immunoregulatory circuit involving interleukin 27 and interleukin 10. Nat Immunol 10:981–991
Jadidi-Niaragh F, Mirshafiey A (2011) Th17 cell, the new player of neuroinflammatory process in multiple sclerosis. Scand J Immunol 74:1–13
Jeon S-B et al (2010) Galectin-3 exerts cytokine-like regulatory actions through the JAK-STAT pathway. J Immunol 185:7037–7046
Jiang H-R et al (2009) Galectin-3 deficiency reduces the severity of experimental autoimmune encephalomyelitis. J Immunol 182:1167–1173
Karman J, Ling C, Sandor M, Fabry Z (2004) Initiation of immune responses in brain is promoted by local dendritic cells. J Immunol 173:2353–2361

Kaunzner UW et al (2012) Accumulation of resident and peripheral dendritic cells in the aging CNS. Neurobiol Aging 33:681–693.e1

Koning N, Bö L, Hoek RM, Huitinga I (2007) Downregulation of macrophage inhibitory molecules in multiple sclerosis lesions. Ann Neurol 62:504–514

Koning N, Swaab DF, Hoek RM, Huitinga I (2009a) Distribution of the immune inhibitory molecules CD200 and CD200R in the normal central nervous system and multiple sclerosis lesions suggests neuron-glia and glia-glia interactions. J Neuropathol Exp Neurol 68:159–167

Koning N, Uitdehaag BMJ, Huitinga I, Hoek RM (2009b) Restoring immune suppression in the multiple sclerosis brain. Prog Neurobiol 89:359–368

Kooi E-J et al (2009) Abundant extracellular myelin in the meninges of patients with multiple sclerosis. Neuropathol Appl Neurobiol 35:283–295

Kotter MR, Li W-W, Zhao C, Franklin RJM (2006) Myelin impairs CNS remyelination by inhibiting oligodendrocyte precursor cell differentiation. J Neurosci 26:328–332

Leteux C et al (2000) The cysteine-rich domain of the macrophage mannose receptor is a multispecific lectin that recognizes chondroitin sulfates A and B and sulfated oligosaccharides of blood group Lewis(a) and Lewis(x) types in addition to the sulfated N-glycans of lutropin. J Exp Med 191:1117–1126

Li Y et al (2011) The N- and C-terminal carbohydrate recognition domains of galectin-9 contribute differently to its multiple functions in innate immunity and adaptive immunity. Mol Immunol 48:670–677

Liu F-T, Patterson RJ, Wang JL (2002) Intracellular functions of galectins. Biochim Biophys Acta 1572:263–273

Loo Y-M, Gale M (2011) Immune signaling by RIG-I-like receptors. Immunity 34:680–692

Martinez-Pomares L et al (2006) Carbohydrate-independent recognition of collagens by the macrophage mannose receptor. Eur J Immunol 36:1074–1082

Mato M et al (1996) Involvement of specific macrophage-lineage cells surrounding arterioles in barrier and scavenger function in brain cortex. Proc Natl Acad Sci U S A 93:3269–3274

Matzinger P (2002) An innate sense of danger. Ann N Y Acad Sci 961:341–342

McKenzie EJ et al (2007) Mannose receptor expression and function define a new population of murine dendritic cells. J Immunol 178:4975–4983

Medzhitov R, Janeway C (2000a) The Toll receptor family and microbial recognition. Trends Microbiol 8:452–456

Medzhitov R, Janeway C (2000b) Innate immunity. N Engl J Med 343:338–344

Melief J et al (2012) Phenotyping primary human microglia: tight regulation of LPS responsiveness. Glia. doi:10.1002/glia.22370

Mitchell DA, Fadden AJ, Drickamer KA (2001) Novel mechanism of carbohydrate recognition by the C-type lectins DC-SIGN and DC-SIGNR. Subunit organization and binding to multivalent ligands. J Biol Chem 276:28939–28945

Mott RT et al (2004) Neuronal expression of CD22: novel mechanism for inhibiting microglial proinflammatory cytokine production. Glia 46:369–379

Nimmerjahn A, Kirchhoff F, Helmchen F (2005) Resting microglial cells are highly dynamic surveillants of brain parenchyma in vivo. Science 308:1314–1318

Offner H et al (1990) Recombinant human beta-galactoside binding lectin suppresses clinical and histological signs of experimental autoimmune encephalomyelitis. J Neuroimmunol 28:177–184

Ohashi K, Burkart V, Flohé S, Kolb H (2000) Cutting edge: heat shock protein 60 is a putative endogenous ligand of the toll-like receptor-4 complex. J Immunol 164:558–561

Olson JK, Miller SD (2004) Microglia initiate central nervous system innate and adaptive immune responses through multiple TLRs. J Immunol 173:3916–3924

Oomizu S et al (2012) Galectin-9 suppresses Th17 cell development in an IL-2-dependent but Tim-3-independent manner. Clin Immunol 143:51–58

Polfliet MMJ et al (2002) The role of perivascular and meningeal macrophages in experimental allergic encephalomyelitis. J Neuroimmunol 122:1–8

Rabinovich GA, Croci DO (2012) Regulatory circuits mediated by lectin-glycan interactions in autoimmunity and cancer. Immunity 36:322–335
Rabinovich GA, Toscano MA (2009) Turning 'sweet' on immunity: galectin-glycan interactions in immune tolerance and inflammation. Nat Rev Immunol 9:338–352
Rabinovich GA, Kooyk Y van, Cobb BA (2012) Glycobiology of immune responses. Ann N Y Acad Sci 1253:1–15
Raïch-Regué D et al (2012) Differential effects of monophosphoryl lipid A and cytokine cocktail as maturation stimuli of immunogenic and tolerogenic dendritic cells for immunotherapy. Vaccine 30:378–387
Ransohoff RM, Cardona AE (2010) The myeloid cells of the central nervous system parenchyma. Nature 468:253–262
Ransohoff RM (2011) Microglia and monocytes: 'tis plain the twain meet in the brain. Nat. Neurosci 14:1098–1100
Reboldi A et al (2009) C–C chemokine receptor 6-regulated entry of TH-17 cells into the CNS through the choroid plexus is required for the initiation of EAE. Nat Immunol 10:514–523
Reichert F, Rotshenker S (1999) Galectin-3/MAC-2 in experimental allergic encephalomyelitis. Exp Neurol 160:508–514
Saeland E et al (2012) Differential glycosylation of MUC1 and CEACAM5 between normal mucosa and tumour tissue of colon cancer patients. Int J Cancer 131:117–128
Sancho D, Reis e SousaC (2012) Signaling by myeloid C-type lectin receptors in immunity and homeostasis. Annu Rev Immunol 30:491–529
Schafer DP et al (2012) Microglia sculpt postnatal neural circuits in an activity and complement-dependent manner. Neuron 74:691–705
Sica A, Mantovani A (2012) Macrophage plasticity and polarization: in vivo veritas. J Clin Invest 122:787–795
Singh SK et al (2009) Targeting glycan modified OVA to murine DC-SIGN transgenic dendritic cells enhances MHC class I and II presentation. Mol Immunol 47:164–174
Singh SK et al (2011) Design of neo-glycoconjugates that target the mannose receptor and enhance TLR-independent cross-presentation and Th1 polarization. Eur J Immunol 41:916–925
Stancic M et al (2011) Increased expression of distinct galectins in multiple sclerosis lesions. Neuropathol Appl Neurobiol 37:654–671
Starossom SC, Mascanfroni ID, Imitola J, Cao L, Raddassi K, Hernandez SF, Bassil R, Croci DO, Cerliani JP, Wang Y et al (2012) Galectin-1 deactivates classically-activated microglia and protects from inflammation-induced neurodegeneration. (In Press)
Steinman RM, Banchereau J (2007) Taking dendritic cells into medicine. Nature 449:419–426
Steinman RM et al (2003) Dendritic cell function in vivo during the steady state: a role in peripheral tolerance. Ann N Y Acad Sci 987:15–25
Stockinger B, Veldhoen M (2007) Differentiation and function of Th17 T cells. Curr Opin Immunol 19:281–286
Toscano MA et al (2007) Differential glycosylation of TH1, TH2 and TH-17 effector cells selectively regulates susceptibility to cell death. Nat Immunol 8:825–834
Tran EH, Hoekstra K, Rooijen N van, Dijkstra CD, Owens T (1998) Immune invasion of the central nervous system parenchyma and experimental allergic encephalomyelitis, but not leukocyte extravasation from blood, are prevented in macrophage-depleted mice. J Immunol 161:3767–3775
Unger WWJ et al (2012) Glycan-modified liposomes boost CD4(+) and CD8(+) T-cell responses by targeting DC-SIGN on dendritic cells. J Control Release. doi:10.1016/j.jconrel.2012.02.007
van Gisbergen KPJM, Aarnoudse CA, Meijer GA, Geijtenbeek TBH, Kooyk Y van (2005) Dendritic cells recognize tumor-specific glycosylation of carcinoembryonic antigen on colorectal cancer cells through dendritic cell-specific intercellular adhesion molecule-3-grabbing nonintegrin. Cancer Res 65:5935–5944
van Kooyk Y, Geijtenbeek TBH (2002) A novel adhesion pathway that regulates dendritic cell trafficking and T cell interactions. Immunol Rev 186:47–56
van Kooyk Y, Geijtenbeek TBH (2003) DC-SIGN: escape mechanism for pathogens. Nat Rev Immunol 3:697–709

van Kooyk Y, Rabinovich GA (2008) Protein-glycan interactions in the control of innate and adaptive immune responses. Nat Immunol 9:593–601
van Vliet SJ, Gringhuis SI, Geijtenbeek TBH, Kooyk Y van (2006a) Regulation of effector T cells by antigen-presenting cells via interaction of the C-type lectin MGL with CD45. Nat Immunol 7:1200–1208
van Vliet SJ, Liempt E van, Geijtenbeek TBH, Kooyk Y van (2006b) Differential regulation of C-type lectin expression on tolerogenic dendritic cell subsets. Immunobiology 211:577–585
van Vliet SJ, Dunnen denJ, Gringhuis SI, Geijtenbeek TB, Kooyk Y van (2007) Innate signaling and regulation of dendritic cell immunity. Curr Opin Immunol 19:435–440
van Vliet SJ, Saeland E, Kooyk Y van (2008) Sweet preferences of MGL: carbohydrate specificity and function. Trends Immunol 29:83–90
van Zwam M et al (2009) Brain antigens in functionally distinct antigen-presenting cell populations in cervical lymph nodes in MS and EAE. J Mol Med 87:273–286
van Zwam M et al (2011) Myelin ingestion alters macrophage antigen-presenting function in vitro and in vivo. J Leukoc Biol 90:123–132
Venkatesan C, Chrzaszcz M, Choi N, Wainwright MS (2010) Chronic upregulation of activated microglia immunoreactive for galectin-3/Mac-2 and nerve growth factor following diffuse axonal injury. J Neuroinflammation 7:32
Yang R-Y, Rabinovich GAm, Liu F-T (2008) Galectins: structure, function and therapeutic potential. Expert Rev Mol Med 10:e17
Zelensky AN, Gready JE (2005) The C-type lectin-like domain superfamily. FEBS J 272:6179–6217
Zhang J-G et al (2012) The dendritic cell receptor Clec9 A binds damaged cells via exposed actin filaments. Immunity 36:646–657
Zhu C et al (2005) The Tim-3 ligand galectin-9 negatively regulates T helper type 1 immunity. Nat Immunol 6:1245–1252
Zhu B et al (2012) Immune modulation by Lacto-N-fucopentaose III in experimental autoimmune encephalomyelitis. Clin Immunol 142:351–361
Zygmunt B, Veldhoen MT (2011) Helper cell differentiation more than just cytokines. Adv Immunol 109:159–196

Chapter 5
The Role of B Cells in Multiple Sclerosis

Bernhard Hemmer, Markus C. Kowarik and Martin S. Weber

5.1 Introduction

B cells may have various roles in the pathogenesis of multiple sclerosis (MS), serving as a source of plasma cells that secrete autoreactive specific antibodies, but also as antigen-presenting cells for activation of encephalitogenic T cells. Data indicate that antibodies promote demyelination in MS and experimental autoimmune encephalomyelitis (EAE), the animal model of MS, while the role of B cells themselves in central nervous system (CNS) autoimmune disease is less clear. Like dendritic cells, B cells are professional antigen-presenting cells as defined by a constitutive expression of major histocompatibility complex (MHC) class II and an antigen-specific B cell receptor (BCR, membrane-associated Immunoglobulin (Ig)). Compared to other antigen-presenting cell populations, antigen-specific B cells are very competent in presentation of protein antigen when their BCR recognizes the same antigen as the responding T cells. As processing and presentation of CNS protein antigen is required for initiation of CNS autoimmune disease (Slavin et al. 2001), B cells and, in particular, B cells specific for CNS autoantigen may have an important role as antigen-presenting cells for the activation of myelin-specific T cells in MS.

B cells, plasma cells, and antibodies are commonly found in active CNS lesions in patients with MS. B cells isolated from CNS lesions as well as from the cerebrospinal fluid (CSF) show signs of clonal expansion and hypermutation suggesting their local activation. Plasma blasts maturating from these B cells were recently identified to contribute to the development of oligoclonal antibodies produced within the CSF, which remains a diagnostic hallmark finding in MS. Within the CNS, antibody deposition is associated with complement activation and demyelination, indicating antigen recognition-associated effector function. Although some studies indeed implied a disease-intrinsic and possibly pathogenic role of antibodies directed against

B. Hemmer (✉) · M. C. Kowarik · M. S. Weber
Department of Neurology, Technische Universität München, Klinikum rechts der Isar,
Department of Neurology, Ismaninger Strasse 22 Munich, Germany
e-mail: hemmer@tum.de

T. Yamamura, B. Gran (eds.), *Multiple Sclerosis Immunology*,
DOI 10.1007/978-1-4614-7953-6_5, © Springer Science+Business Media New York 2013

components of the myelin sheath, no unequivocal results on a decisive target antigen within the CNS persisted to date. In conclusion, various pathological, clinical, immunological, and experimental findings collectively indicate a pathogenic role of antibodies and B cells in MS, whereas several conceptual challenges, above all uncovering potential target antigens within the CNS, remain to be overcome.

5.2 Evidence for a Pathogenic Role of B cells and Autoantibodies Derived from Animal Models

The murine animal model of MS, EAE, is thought to be predominantly mediated by proinflammatory, self-reactive T cells (Zamvil and Steinman 1990). Strong evidence for this assumption derives from the fact that adoptive transfer of encephalitogenic T cells is sufficient to induce EAE in susceptible mice and that EAE can be actively induced in B cell-deficient mice (Zamvil et al. 1985; Lyons et al. 1999). In addition to infiltrating T cells and macrophages, B cells, plasma cells, and antibodies are, however, found in areas of myelin breakdown in EAE similar to active CNS lesions in patients with MS (Merkler et al. 2006; Prineas and Connell 1978). Although it is clear that B cells and antibodies by themselves are not capable of initiating inflammation in brain and spinal cord, certain EAE studies suggest that they might facilitate CNS damage and promote disease progression (Weber et al. 2010).

5.2.1 The Role of Antibodies in Experimental CNS Autoimmune Disease

Autoimmune T and B cell responses against CNS antigens remain a central component in the current view of MS pathogenesis. Myelin antigens are the prevalent putative targets studied in the field due to the often primarily demyelinating nature of inflammatory CNS lesions. Within candidate myelin antigens, myelin oligodendrocyte glycoprotein (MOG) is probably the most widely investigated due to its extracellular location on the outermost myelin lamellae. Such exposed location may make it an easily accessible target for an initial autoimmune attack against properly myelinated axons. The full-length MOG protein is constituted of 218 amino acids and is exclusively expressed within the CNS. Most importantly, MOG is highly encephalitogenic in the murine as well as in the marmoset EAE model.

Schluesener et al. (1987) reported more than 20 years ago that a monoclonal antibody directed against MOG exacerbated ongoing EAE in a rodent disease model. The authors demonstrated convincingly that the intravenous administration of this myelin-reactive antibody enhanced CNS demyelination and induced fatal relapses in recipient mice. Notwithstanding this seminal observation, it should be noted that the antibody was injected into already EAE-affected mice at a quantity that is unlikely to be produced endogenously. Experiments in B cell-deficient mice indeed indicate that B cells or antibodies are not required when the short encephalitogenic T cell-determinant peptide (p)35–55 is used to immunize mice in an active EAE induction protocol (Lyons et al. 2002). A crucial step in disease induction by active immunization is the presentation of the administered CNS autoantigen to naive encephalitogenic T cells by antigen-presenting cells in the context of MHC class II. Short peptides, such as MOG p35–55, are known to be most efficiently phagocytosed and presented by dendritic cells and macrophages (Constant et al. 1995a, b), so that B cell encounter with the peptide antigen rarely occurs. Moreover, B cells cannot process and present peptide antigens as efficiently as entire proteins even if they possess a BCR for the protein from which the peptide was derived. This results in two key features of this model of CNS autoimmune disease: B cell antigen presentation does not play a crucial role for EAE induction by MOG peptide and low anti-MOG antibody titers, if any, are generated.

In contrast, B cells and antibodies may be required for EAE induced by the recombinant (r) extracellular domain of MOG, as genetically B cell-deficient mice were found to be resistant to active immunization with human rMOG (Lyons et al. 1999). Reconstitution with the antigen-specific antibody was sufficient to restore EAE susceptibility, suggesting a crucial role for antibody-mediated antigen recognition in this model (Lyons et al. 2002). Unfortunately, the question as to whether B cells are required for MOG protein-induced EAE appears to be more complex and is still debated. Oliver et al. (2003) reported that immunization with either rat or human MOG leads to comparable titers of anti-MOG antibodies. However, only human (but not rat) MOG was reported to induce a B cell-dependent EAE model as evaluated by active immunization of B cell-deficient mice. The sequence of human MOG differs from rat MOG only at a few residues, including a proline for serine substitution at position 42, which encodes within the dominant T cell determinant of MOG p35–55. Substituting this amino acid with serine in human MOG p35–55 (resulting in the rat MOG sequence) substantially increased its encephalitogenicity (Oliver et al. 2003). Furthermore, exchanging the same residue within human MOG protein appears to be sufficient to restore EAE susceptibility in B cell-deficient mice, suggesting that B cells or B cell-derived products are specifically required to recognize human MOG protein due to the presence of proline at position 42 within the three-dimensional protein.

Furthermore, it is apparent that not all MOG-specific antibody responses are equally pathogenic. This can be determined by examining epitope recognition. In general, pathogenic MOG-specific antibodies recognize conformation-dependent MOG epitopes that are only available within the intact protein. Antibodies that are specific for linear determinants, although they may recognize antigens following tissue injury, are not thought to contribute to disease initiation or progression (Bourquin et al. 2003; von Budingen et al. 2002, 2004). Furthermore, immunization with either rat or human MOG leads to a considerable development of anti-MOG antibodies, whereas only immunization with human rMOG generates a pathogenic, EAE-enhancing MOG antibody response (Marta et al. 2005). Along the same lines, a transgenic mouse engineered to express the rearranged heavy chain of a pathogenic antibody recognizing a conformational determinant of MOG (8.18-C.5) developed more severe EAE with greater inflammation and demyelination compared with wild-type mice (Litzenburger et al. 1998). The fact that serum from these mice bound specifically to native, brain-derived MOG combined with the observed enhancement of CNS demyelination suggests a possible pathogenic role for plasma cell-secreted myelin-specific antibodies. Alternatively, although not mutually exclusive, accelerated EAE severity may reflect a pathogenic role for myelin-specific B cells in processing and presentation of myelin antigen to encephalitogenic T cells. Indeed, it has been shown that B cells carrying an antigen-specific BCR are highly efficient antigen-presenting cells when they encounter their specific antigen. Their efficacy may even exceed the efficacy of dendritic cells.

5.2.2 *The Role of B cells and Antibodies in Spontaneous EAE Models*

Recent efforts have been focused on developing EAE models, which do not require their active induction, as EAE induced by active immunization with self-antigen or passive transfer of encephalitogenic T cells is unlikely to fittingly reflect MS pathogenesis characterized by chronic inflammation and the lack of an apparent disease trigger. Generally, what these models have in common is that B cells, T cells, or both are genetically engineered to recognize CNS antigens at a higher frequency than mouse strains susceptible to induced EAE. Though it is debatable whether "spontaneously" occurring EAE in these transgenic mice reflects MS pathogenesis more closely, these models undoubtedly provide an excellent tool to study the interaction of self-reactive T cells, B cells, and antibodies.

The first of these spontaneous EAE models is produced by taking the already mentioned transgenic mice, in which a high frequency of B cells express a pathogenic antibody against MOG (MOG B cell-knocking), were crossed onto a line of transgenic mice in which a majority of T cells respond to MOG p35–55. Although it needs to be noted that approximately 40 % of these single-transgenic MOG T cell receptor transgenic mice were already affected by optic neuritis, they rarely revealed symptoms of spontaneous paralysis (Bettelli et al. 2006; Krishnamoorthy et al. 2006). However, in the double-transgenic mice, which also contain a high frequency of MOG recognizing B cells, approximately 60 % spontaneously developed a severe form of EAE with meningeal and parenchymal lesions (Bettelli et al. 2006; Krishnamoorthy et al. 2006). Interestingly, inflammatory lesions remained restricted to the spinal cord and optic nerves, not unlike in neuromyelitis optica (NMO) or Devic's disease, which selectively affects optic nerves and spinal cord, but spares the brain (Cree et al. 2002; Mandler et al. 1993). Intriguingly, this model suggests that myelin specificity of B cells and T cells is in principle sufficient to trigger spontaneous CNS autoimmune disease. It remains to be determined in further studies whether this spontaneous model primarily relates to the abundance of myelin-specific antibodies, or alternatively to the fact that MOG-specific B cells serve as efficient antigen-presenting cell for the activation of MOG p35–55-specific T cells in these mice.

Another more recently described spontaneous EAE model apparently also relies on the interaction of myelin-specific B cells and/or antibodies and T cells (Pollinger et al. 2009). In this model, T cells are genetically engineered to recognize MOG peptide 92–106 resulting in spontaneous relapsing-remitting EAE on the SJL/J background. Backcrossing these T cell transgenic mice to a line expressing the MOG-binding antibody 8.18-C.5 on B cells led to an earlier onset of an even more severe spontaneous EAE disease course. In single-T cell transgenic mice with later disease onset, myelin-specific B cells were shown to be recruited and expanded from the endogenous repertoire that results in development of pathogenic anti-MOG antibody titers comparable to those in wild-type mice actively immunized with rMOG. In both, single- and double-transgenic mice, anti-CD20-mediated B cell depletion could abrogate spontaneous EAE development, proving that endogenously recruited or transgenically engineered myelin-specific B cells or antibodies were indeed mandatory for initiation of spontaneous disease. Unexpectedly, myelin-specific B cells obtained from these mice were, however, unable to recognize the transgenic T cell determinant 92–106. Furthermore, spontaneous disease was not observed when MOG p92–106 T cell receptor transgenic mice were crossed onto a MOG-deficient background. Collectively, these findings indicate that in this model, activation of abundant MOG p92–106-specific T cells requires prior encounter of B cells with endogenous MOG. Similar to the spontaneous EAE model described in the previous paragraph, it remains yet unclear whether spontaneous CNS autoimmune disease in these mice relies primarily on cellular function of myelin-specific B cells or B cell-derived myelin-specific antibodies.

5.3 Evidence for a Pathogenic Role of B cells in Human Demyelinating Disorders

B cells are part of the adaptive immune system and are able to produce antibodies (Igs) against specific targets. B cells recognize antigens via their BCR and usually become activated through helper T cell stimulation. After the activation through different receptors and cytokines, B cells differentiate into mainly two subsets: plasma cells and memory cells. The B cell either becomes one of these cell types directly or may undergo a further differentiation step during a germinal center reaction. Thereby, the BCR specificity can be increased by mutations of the variable region Ig gene (somatic hypermutation) and eventually an Ig-class switch is induced. After these differentiation steps, B cells may turn into plasma blasts and plasma cells, which can persist in the bone marrow or tissue for long periods of time and release large amounts of antibodies. Alternatively, B cells may develop to B cell memory cells and turn into antibody-secreting cells at another point of time. Through this antibody secretion of plasma blasts/plasma cells against specific targets, B cells are essential to control microbial infections. On the other hand, a misguided immune reaction against self-inherent structures can lead to autoantibodies and may predispose to autoimmune disease.

Although the pathophysiological mechanism is still unclear, MS is often considered to be an autoimmune disorder in which T and B cells cause and maintain demyelination and axonal damage in the CNS. It has been known since the 1940s that more than 90 % of MS patients show an increased intrathecal production of Igs (Kabat et al. 1942), for which reason early MS research mainly focused on the humoral immune system. In the last decades, greater emphasis was placed on the pathogenic role of T cells. This was due to the fact that activated T cells are present in MS plaques, that certain MHC-II molecules (HLA-DR15, critical for antigen presentation to T cells) convey a risk for MS, and experimental allergic encephalomyelitis (EAE) can be solely initiated by myelin-reactive T cells. Nevertheless, a number of findings suggest that B cells may play an important role in MS:

1. B cells are present in active and inactive MS lesions.
2. Formation of B cell follicle-like structures can be observed in the brain meninges.
3. CSF changes in MS are characterized by increased B cell populations and show a persistence of intrathecal oligoclonal Ig bands.
4. B cells in CSF and brain lesions of MS patients show clonal expansion.
5. B cell targeting therapies have been shown to be effective in MS.

Although a number of studies have investigated the phenotype of B cells in MS lesions and in the CSF, there is little information about the exact mechanism of B cell trafficking across the blood–brain barrier and the blood–CSF barrier. Furthermore, the nature and the site of the antigenic stimuli that initiate and perpetuate the abnormal immune reactivity are still unknown.

5.3.1 Histopathologic Evidence for Involvement of B cells and Antibodies in MS and NMO

The pathologic hallmark of MS is the plaque, an area of white matter demyelination often accompanied by inflammation. Although a relative axonal sparing can be observed in lesions, axonal damage is present in active and chronic MS plaques and it is thought to be an essential cause for disease progression and nonremitting progress of clinical disability. Historically, MS plaques have been considered to primarily affect the white matter but recent pathological studies have found more extensive cortical demyelination than previously expected (Lucchinetti et al. 2011; Ozawa et al. 1994).

It has been proposed that MS is an autoimmune disease in which autoreactive lymphocytes drive an inflammatory process leading to macrophage recruitment and subsequent myelin/oligodendrocyte destruction. In general, the inflammatory infiltrates are composed of macrophages, T lymphocytes, B cells, and plasma blasts as well as activated microglial cells. The pathologic findings are similar to those found in some of the EAE models.

B cells and plasma blasts are found in active- and late-stage MS lesions. Molecular analysis of B cells in brain lesions shows an accumulation of clonotypic B cells with preferential use of particular variable (V) heavy (H) chain (VH) genes indicating a restricted local immune response (Baranzini et al. 1999; Owens et al. 1998). Furthermore, the consequence of several Ig-mediated effector functions can be found in MS plaques: capping of surface IgG on macrophages, which is involved in myelin breakdown, codeposition of IgG and complement proteins at plaque borders, and the presence of Igs and complement in areas of active myelin breakdown (Prineas and Graham 1981; Prineas et al. 1984). The proportion of T cells-/Ig-containing cells is lower in chronic MS lesions compared to early-MS lesions. In addition, B cell supporting factors like the cytokines APRIL and BAFF and the chemokines CXCL12 and CXL13 have been found to be upregulated in MS lesions (Krumbholz et al. 2006).

Both $CD4^+$ and $CD8^+$ T cells are found in MS lesions. $CD4^+$ T cells dominate the perivascular cuff, whereas $CD8^+$ T cells outnumber $CD4^+$ T cells in the parenchyma. It was furthermore, axonal destruction in MS lesions seems to be associated with the presence of $CD8^+$ T cells and macrophages. MS lesions are associated with an upregulation of proinflammatory cytokines and chemokines, e.g., interferon gamma and tumor necrosis factor alpha (TNF-α; Ozawa et al. 1994).

However, the exact pathogenic role of the inflammatory response in MS plaques is not clear. Inflammatory cells are not always present in areas of active demyelination and persistent inflammation is typically found in chronic active MS lesions. Besides the inflammatory functions of leukocytes, they also secrete growth factors, which might be of relevance for repair- and remyelination (Lassmann 2001; Ozawa et al. 1994).

Several studies have been aiming to identify correlations between immunopathological patterns and different clinical disease courses in MS patients. In general, four different immunopathological patterns of myelin destruction have been proposed (Lucchinetti et al. 2000). One of these patterns (pattern II) has been characterized as a mainly antibody- and complement (C9neo)-mediated myelin destruction (Storch et al. 1998). The other patterns suggest T cell-mediated demyelination (pattern I), oligodendrocyte dystrophy (pattern III), and primary oligodendrocyte degeneration (pattern IV; Ozawa et al. 1994). Although a high heterogeneity of lesion patterns has been described in the early phases of MS, homogeneity of pathological patterns can be found in active lesion of patients with established MS. In these patients, primarily an antibody- and complement-mediated demyelination could be found (Breij et al. 2008; Lassmann et al. 2001).

More recently, it has been shown that infiltrating B cells are not limited to the brain parenchyma, CSF, or perivascular space. Approximately, 30–40 % of MS patients with secondary progressive MS or long-standing disease display lymphoid-like follicles in the meninges (Magliozzi et al. 2007; Serafini et al. 2004). Furthermore, it can also be shown that in early MS there is meningeal inflammation with a strong topographic relation to cortical demyelination (Lucchinetti et al. 2011). B cell clones derived from meningeal aggregates of patients with long-lasting disease are also present in the CSF and brain parenchyma. This indicates that equilibrium exists between the various CNS B cell populations in MS patients (Lovato et al. 2011; Magliozzi et al. 2004).

5.3.2 *Evidence from the CSF*

Since brain interstitial fluid extravasates into the subarachnoid and ventricular spaces, the cellular and protein composition of human CSF can be a useful surrogate to monitor the microenvironment of the brain.

The assessment of CSF, especially the analysis of CSF cells and intrathecal Ig production, is an important tool in the diagnosis of MS (Farrell et al. 1985). Intrathecal Ig production in the CSF compartment with the formation of oligoclonal bands is a key feature and a relatively sensitive finding in MS. About 50–60 % of all diagnosed MS patients exhibit an intrathecal production of IgG. After separation of CSF Ig by electrophoresis, the IgG fraction is described as oligoclonal IgG bands (OCBs). This is true only in CSF IgG but not in serum where IgG appears polyclonal. OCBs extracted from the CNS have a similar pattern as from CSF of the same individuals strengthening the view that the CSF compartment reflects—at least partially—the milieu within the CNS itself. Furthermore, the oligoclonal IgG pattern shows local accumulation of restricted IgG specificities and is concomitant with a restricted Ig receptor repertoire in CSF (Baranzini et al. 1999; Owens et al. 2001, 1998). The relevance of CSF B cells in the production of OCBs, had been for a long time an open question. In a recent study, Obermeier et al. (2008) compared the IgG proteome in CSF and the IgG transcriptome from the B cellular compartment in CSF and found an overlap between both compartments. This strongly suggests that CSF B cells are indeed the source of OCB.

The occurrence of such OCBs in CSF is still the most reliable immunological test supporting clinical and MRI findings in establishing the diagnosis of MS. Hence, researchers have investigated the relevance of OCBs as potential biomarkers for the clinical outcome of patients with MS (Avasarala et al. 2001; Koch et al. 2007; Walsh and Tourtellotte 1986). OCB-negative MS patients seem to have a more benign disease course. The number of OCBs and the intrathecal IgG synthesis correlated with a more progressive outcome in a retrospective study (Izquierdo et al. 2002). However, this finding was not confirmed by another study. One study suggested that the presence of IgM OCBs predicts a higher probability for conversion to secondary progressive MS (SP-MS) and intrathecal IgM production predicts a higher progression rate, but this was also not confirmed by an independent study (Villar et al. 2002, 2003). However, OCBs are not unique to MS and can also be found in chronic infectious diseases of the CNS such as subacute sclerosing panencephalitis (Villar et al. 2002), neurosyphilis, mumps meningitis, progressive rubella panencephalitis, Borrelia burgdorferi meningoencephalitis (Martin et al. 1988), and cryptococcal meningitis (Owens et al. 2007). In each of these conditions, the oligoclonal IgG is directed against the causative agent whereas in MS the antigen against which the oligoclonal IgG is directed has yet to be identified.

In MS patient, CSF cell counts appear normal to slightly elevated and for the most part do not exceed 50 cells/μl. By means of fluorescence-activated cell sorting (FACS), it is possible to further quantify and differentially examine CSF cells according to their surface markers. Within the CSF compartment, $CD3^+$ T cells constituted the vast majority of CSF lymphocytes while B cells can hardly be detected under normal conditions (< 1 % of all mononuclear cells in the CSF; Cepok et al. 2001).

During neuroinflammation, a significant increase in CSF B cells can be observed (Cepok et al. 2003). In MS, $CD19^+$ CD138− B cells average 5 % of all mononuclear cells, $CD19^+CD138^+$ plasma blasts show values around 0.9 %. Interestingly, the percentage of B cells in the CSF does not correlate with the percentage of B cells in the blood. Also, the disruption of the blood–CSF barrier has no major impact on the distribution of B cells in the CSF (Kowarik et al. 2012).

Analysis of B cells present in the CSF of MS and other inflammatory neurological disorders identified B cell populations representing all stages of differentiation observed in secondary lymphoid follicles, indicating that the CNS can maintain a persistent B cell response. Detailed analyses of CSF B cells revealed that the majority of B cells display a phenotype of memory B cells and plasma blasts during neuroinflammation. These memory B cells outnumber naive B cells in the CSF, whereas naive B cells are more prevalent in the peripheral blood. This accumulation of memory B cells in the CSF is largely due to the recruitment of IgM−IgD− class switched memory B cells (Cepok et al. 2006). Also, a high proportion of plasma blasts can consistently be found in the CSF of patients with inflammatory CNS diseases, whereas plasma cells are only found at very low levels in the CSF compartment (Cepok et al. 2001, 2005a). This finding might be associated with the role of the chemokine CXCL13, a major B cell chemoattractant in the CSF. CXCL13 binds to the receptor CXCR5, is upregulated during neuroinflammation and correlates with CSF B cells, plasma blasts, and intrathecal Ig production (Kowarik et al. 2012). During maturation in the periphery, B cells undergo different modifications and a change of surface receptors to become plasma cells. This involves downregulation of the chemokine receptor CXCR5 and upregulation of the CXCR4 receptor and alpha4 beta1 integrins under the control of B-lymphocyte-induced maturation protein 1 (BLIMP-1). Consequently, the CXCL5 receptor is downregulated on B cells during the maturation to plasma cells, whereas other B cells, e.g., plasma blasts still express CXCR5. After CXCL13 is upregulated during neuroinflammation, mainly plasma blasts or B cells that express CXCR5 might be recruited to the CSF.

The role of plasma blasts as the main CSF effector B cells during neuroinflammation is further supported by the correlation with the intrathecal Ig synthesis (Winges et al. 2007). Furthermore, MS patients show clonally expanded plasma blast populations with extensive somatic hypermutation of their rearranged Ig genes. This indicates that CSF plasma blasts have not only encountered an antigen but were also expanded in a germinal center reaction (Owens et al. 2007). It is, however, still unclear whether this germinal center reaction takes place in the periphery or within the CNS. Also, the trafficking of B cells into the CNS and CSF is still unknown. While plasma blasts disappeared rapidly from the CSF after resolution of a CNS infection (Cepok et al. 2005a), these cells are continuously found throughout the disease course in MS patients. This suggests that plasma blasts can either persist or are continuously recruited to the CNS compartment in MS patients.

Concerning the clinical implication, plasma blasts correlate with the inflammatory parenchymal disease activity in MS patients as disclosed by MRI (Cepok et al. 2001). Also, the chemokine CXCL13, which at least partially reflects the humoral immune response in the CSF, has recently been suggested as a prognostic marker for MS and clinically isolated syndrome (CIS; Brettschneider et al. 2010).

5.3.3 Evidence for Pathogenic B Cell Function Within the CNS: B Cell Receptor (BCR) Rearrangement

During early maturation, B cells initiate gene rearrangement in order to express a unique receptor on their surface. Once this "naive" B cell binds it's antigen, it becomes activated and undergoes further differentiation into an antibody-secreting plasma cell. The clonal expansion of these B cells can be observed during neuroinflammation. Therefore, the assessment of these B cell clones helps to further understand the humoral immune response in MS.

In order to create a unique BCR in a single diploid cell, only one of the alleles is rearranged and expressed. The total number of antibody specificities available to an individual is known as the antibody/Ig repertoire, and in humans is at least 10^{11}. The human antibody repertoire uses 51 functional germline genes, which are divided into families based on sequence homology. Of the seven V_H families, the largest are V_H3 and V_H4 with 11 gene segments each. These gene segments are located relatively far away from each other and then brought together by DNA-modifying recombinases. The Ig gene segments are organized into three clusters of genetic loci, the kappa, lambda, and heavy chain loci, each of which can assemble a complete V-region sequence. The heavy chain V region is encoded in three gene segments: the V–segment (variable), D-segment (diversity), and J-segment (joining). The light chain V region is only encoded by V-segment and J-segment. The different gene segments are brought together by somatic recombination process (V(D)J recombination) to produce a complete V-region exon. The constant region of the heavy chain contains a series of gene segments arranged one after the other. Additional changes in the V-region of one clone are introduced by hypermutation during further maturation in the germinal center reaction. Thus, an intraclonal sequence diversification has repeatedly been observed within B and plasma cell clones.

Analyses of Ig oligoclonal heavy (H)- and light (L)-chain variable (V)-sequences recovered from MS plaques and CSF reveals clonal expansion, intraclonal sequence diversity, somatic hypermutation, and VH-gene segment bias; features consistent with a specific and targeted antigen response (Colombo et al. 2003, 2000; Haubold et al. 2004; Owens et al. 2003; Zhang et al. 2005).

It can be shown that the V_H usage in peripheral blood B cells of MS patients is similar to those of healthy individuals. The V_H usage approximates the germline prevalence or is slightly biased towards excess of V_H3 family sequences. However, in the CSF of MS patients, clonal expansion of B cells and a bias towards certain V_H has been observed (Owens et al. 2001). Also, patients with CIS showed clonal expansion and V_H bias, suggesting that B cell responses are established early in the disease course. Among $CD138^+$ plasma blasts, which are the primary inflammatory B cells in the CSF, around 64 % can be found in clonal populations in MS patients. Clonal expansion is not as prominent in the repertoire of CD19+CD138- B cell populations in the CSF. A striking feature of the plasma blast repertoire in MS CSF is the accumulation of cells expressing V_H4 family gene segments. On average, around 70 % of $CD138^+$ B cells use a functional V_H4 heavy chain sequence and most were V(D)J rearrangements of three specific gene segments. V_H4 bias in $CD19^+$ B cells was not as pronounced as in $CD138^+$ plasma blasts. As noted before, this V_H4 bias is not found in the peripheral blood but is restricted to the CSF compartment. An explanation might be that the CDR regions of these specific families form a favorable conformation for binding an unknown antigenic target in early MS (Owens et al. 2007).

The restricted V_H repertoires have been observed in response to both infectious and autoimmune disease. In subacute sclerosing panencephalitis, which is caused by measles virus, V_H1 was the predominant germline family used by $CD138^+$ plasma blasts. Concerning autoimmune diseases, VH family-biased B cell populations can be found in different compartments and different diseases. Splenic germinal center B cells from patients with systemic lupus erythematosus (SLE) demonstrate a bias towards the VH5 gene family and show an underrepresentation of VH1 family segments. In patients with rheumatoid arthritis (RA), synovial tissues contain memory B cells with a high proportion of VH4 family segments. In patients with ankylosing spondylitis (AS), VH4 usage is underrepresented while VH5 family usage is overrepresented. This VH repertoire bias may reflect the ongoing inflammatory activity and/or immunopathogenesis of the diseases (Owens et al. 2007).

In summary, CSF B cells, and especially the plasma blasts, in MS patients are extensively clonally expanded and display mutational patterns, which suggests that these cells underwent a maturation and selection during germinal center reaction. It is still unknown if this germinal center reaction takes place in the periphery or within the CNS itself. According to the latest pathological studies, the meninges might constitute a place for B cell maturation but whether this maturation indeed occurs in the meninges has remained uncertain (Lovato et al. 2011). The VH repertoire bias suggests a chronic B cell stimulation by a common mechanism or antigen target and thus may reflect the ongoing inflammatory activity and/or immunopathogenesis of the diseases.

Concerning the clinical implication of these findings, patients with CIS were analyzed according to their VH family preference and then correlated with clinical activity (Bennett et al. 2008; Cameron et al. 2009). Again, an overrepresentation of VH4 family germline segments could be found but also a bias towards VH2 was present in these patients. Overrepresented VH4 family germline sequences were found in 60 % of the repertoires. One-third of the VH4-biased repertoires exhibited coincident VH2 family sequence bias. CIS patients with a VH4 or VH2 bias converted to MS within the subsequent 6 months. In contrast, CIS subjects without a repertoire bias did not develop MS in a minimum follow-up period of 2 years. The presence of VH4 or VH2 repertoire bias correlated with subsequent clinical activity. Interestingly, the two germlines that are overrepresented in CIS, VH4, and VH2 are closely related based on nucleotide sequence homology in the framework1 and framework3 intervals. Since VH4 repertoire bias is evident in established demyelinating diseases, the early presence of VH4 bias at the time of CIS might indicate that the target of the humoral immune response does not change significantly over time. The V_H4 was independent of disease duration suggesting that the driving force for B cell clonal expansion might persist.

5.4 Evidence for a Pathogenic Role of Autoantibodies in MS and NMO

5.4.1 *Targets of Antibodies in MS*

Although a huge effort has been taken to search for the targets of the local immune response in MS, the antigens of the humoral immune response in the CNS are still largely unknown. MS lesions are focused on CNS white matter for which reason possible antigenic structures were suspected to be within this region (Rand et al. 1998). Initially, the main body of research provided evidence that the relevant components may be proteins of the myelin sheath, such as myelin basic protein (MBP), MOG, and proteolipid protein (PLP; Genain et al. 1999). Other data suggested that lipids or carbohydrates might constitute the targets of the humoral response. The immune response against myelin proteins has been extensively investigated (Berger et al. 2003). However, to date, controversial results have been obtained (Owens et al. 2009). In MS lesions, antibodies to myelin, especially MOG, were found by immunohistochemical analysis and IgGs extracted from inflamed CNS also recognized MOG (O'Connor et al. 2005; Reindl et al. 1999). Elevated antibody titers against MBP and/or MOG were also reported in serum and CSF of MS patients (Schmidt et al. 2001; Vogt et al. 2009). However, the difference between patients and controls is small (Karni et al. 1999; Kuhle et al. 2007; Lampasona et al. 2004; O'Connor et al. 2007; Rauer et al. 2006). Measuring antibody responses to CNS proteins is not trivial, especially in case of membrane proteins, which are highly folded, and the conformational epitopes represent targets of autoantibodies. The conformational epitopes are, however, not preserved in conventional assays such as ELISA or Western blot. This problem has recently been overcome by the development of cell-based antibody detection assays. Concerning MOG, the gold standard to prove potential antibody pathogenicity has become such a cell-based assay in which MOG is expressed by a transfected cell line (Lalive et al. 2006; Zhou et al. 2006). Through measurement of cell lysis, these assays allow determining whether antibodies are capable to target conformationally folded, cell membrane-embedded MOG. Using this technique, one study was able to demonstrate higher IgG antibody titers to native MOG in the serum of MS patients compared with non-MS control groups (Zhou et al. 2006). Several other groups have recently reported elevated titers of anti-MOG antibodies in young children with demyelinating CNS diseases such as MS or ADEM (Brilot et al. 2009; McLaughlin et al. 2009), using cell-based assays. Interestingly, high MOG antibody titers were primarily found in children below the age of 10 suggesting that in these children MOG might be a relevant autoantigen (Selter et al. 2010).

Given the presence of B cells, plasma blasts, and antibodies in MS lesions, antibody-dependent activation of complement in MS lesions and the favorable response of MS relapses to plasma exchange, it is conceivable that autoantibodies contribute to MS pathogenesis at least in a subset of MS patients. Identification of the target of the autoantibody response is highly challenging but may eventually lead to a better understanding of the disease pathogenesis. Many laboratories have been searching for such targets using a broad array of methodological approaches.

Since CNS-resident proteins might be the target of the antibody response, complementary DNA (cDNA) expression libraries generated from MS brain lesions were developed and probed with CSF antibodies with little success. Phage display libraries containing random short peptides or peptides derived from MS brain plaques were constructed and displayed on phage surface-enabled large-scale screening of CSF antibodies for identification of binding epitopes or mimotopes (Cortese et al. 1996). However, none of the identified targets has been confirmed to be strictly MS-associated.

Using a novel proteomic approach, some of us recently identified the potassium channel KIR4.1 as a possible target of serum antibodies in MS. KIR4.1, the major inward-rectifying potassium channel in the brain, is expressed on oligodendrocytes and a subset of astrocytes. Specific ELISA testing for serum IgG against KIR4.1 indicated the presence of serum antibodies in almost 50 % of MS patients whereas these antibodies are rarely found in patients with other neurological diseases and healthy subjects. The pathogenic role of Anti-KIR4.1 antibodies and its potential role as a clinical biomarker have to be further addressed in future studies (Srivastava et al. 2012).

Besides the autoimmune hypothesis, it is assumed that infectious agents may play a significant role in the pathogenesis of MS. The antibody reactivities against various pathogens have been investigated in CSF and serum of MS patients. Most discussed are Epstein–Barr virus (EBV), human herpes virus-6 (HHV-6), varicella zoster virus (VZV; Burgoon et al. 2009), and *Chlamydia pneumoniae*. The hypothesis is still attractive in view of other infectious diseases of the CNS, which cause inflammation and demyelination in humans such as SSPE- or HTLV-I-associated myelopathy (Vandvik et al. 1976). In these disorders, a comparable chronic immune response is observed in the CNS, including the occurrence of OCBs. Interestingly, the intrathecal Ig response and the OCBs contain antibodies specific for the causative agent. Similar to autoantibody studies, many researchers have reported on elevated antibody titers to a broad range of pathogens in MS patients, although most findings were not confirmed by independent studies. It is only in EBV that conclusive data on an increased antibody response are reported (Ascherio and Munger 2010; Cepok et al. 2005b). Using a phage display library technology, one group identified a 5-amino acid consensus sequence present in EBV nuclear antigen and a heat shock protein, alpha-B crystalline. Recently, another group identified antibodies to eight novel antigenic targets present in a subgroup of MS patients but not in controls (Somers et al. 2008). Using a human brain cDNA expression library combined with epitope mapping, Cepok et al. identified two different EBV proteins, the well-known EBNA-1 and a novel protein BRRF-2, as putative targets of the oligoclonal immune response in MS. While antibody titers to EBV proteins are elevated in serum and CSF of MS patients, it seems rather unlikey that EBV infects and persists in the brain of MS patients (Lassmann et al. 2011).

Recently, monoclonal recombinant antibodies (rAbs) were generated from clonally expanded and therefore most likely disease-relevant CSF IgG-secreting plasma cells and B cells of MS patients (Owens et al. 2009). This strategy allows to produce an unlimited amount of relevant Igs for large-scale screening of antibody binding using various antigens and tissues. Immunofluorescent staining of MS lesions tissue with rAb revealed reactivity to areas of myelin degradation or axons. However, specific reactivity of rAb to myelin epitopes could not be confirmed by immunostaining of MOG-, MBP-, and PLP-transfected cell lines or immunostaining of brain tissue sections. Screening of rAb reactivities to a larger number of different antigens, cells, and tissues will be the next step to determine the specificity of these rAbs.

5.4.2 *Targets of Antibodies in NMO*

NMO is a severe demyelinating disorder with predilection for the optic nerves and spinal cord. There is accumulating evidence that NMO is pathologically different from MS and represents a distinct disease entity. In 2004, Lennon and colleagues made the groundbreaking observation that the majority of NMO patients are seropositive for autoantibodies (NMO-IgG) against the aquaporin 4 (AQP4) water channel (Lennon et al. 2005). Subsequently, multiple researchers have used a variety of assays to document the sensitivity and specificity of AQP4 autoantibodies for NMO. In these studies, NMO IgG demonstrates approximately 70 % sensitivity and 85–100 % specificity for the disease (Jarius et al. 2008). NMO-IgG could also be detected in the serum of patients with NMO spectrum diseases such as longitudinally extensive transverse myelitis, recurrent optic neuritis, and Asian optic–spinal MS. Except in some individual studies, AQP4 antibodies are generally undetected in clinically defined MS (Paul et al. 2007).

Multiple lines of evidence support a pathogenic role of AQP4 antibodies in NMO. First, NMO IgG demonstrates high specificity for NMO and NMO spectrum diseases. Second, B cell- depleting therapies as well as plasma exchange have shown to be effective in the treatment of NMO. Third, in cultured cells and spinal cord explants, NMO-IgG binding to AQP4 causes complement activation and cytotoxicity. And, finally, administration of human NMO-IgG or cloned AQP4 rAbs to naive mice or to rats with preexisting neuroinflammation produces NMO-like pathology. Mechanistically, NMO-IgG binding to AQP4 on CNS astrocytes is thought to initiate several inflammatory events such as antibody-dependent complement activation and cell-mediated cytotoxicity, leukocyte recruitment, and cytokine release. All these events might lead to myelin damage but it still remains under debate, whether NMO-IgG causes astrocyte injury independent of antibody effector function (Bennett et al. 2009; Bradl et al. 2009).

AQP4 has been shown to be the target of a pathologic NMO-IgG in the majority of NMO patients, but the target of the immune response in about 30 % of seronegative patients remains unclear. Since there is no significant difference in the treatment response or CNS pathology between seronegative and seropositive patients, there might be additional target antigens, which have not been identified yet. Different antigens related to the same pathology can be found in other diseases such as myasthenia gravis, where muscle-specific tyrosine kinase and low-density lipoprotein receptor-related protein 4 have been identified as pathologic antigens.

Although AQP4 antibodies are highly sensitive and specific for NMO, the anti-AQP4 titer in affected individuals has not been proven to be an accurate indicator of disease severity or acute relapse. Nevertheless, a detailed understanding of the relationship between antibody titers and disease activity would have a considerable clinical impact. This would allow physicians to identify high-risk and low-risk patients and adopt immunosuppressive therapies accordingly. Further studies are needed to investigate the exact binding pattern of NMO antibodies to AQP4 and the pathological mechanisms, which lead to cell damage. Possibly, not all anti-AQP4-binding antibodies cause cell-mediated astrocyte injury and secondary myelin damage. A detailed understanding of the immune targets and immunopathogenesis of NMO will advance efforts to diagnose, monitor, and treat the spectrum of patients with demyelinating disorders.

5.5 B cells as a Therapeutic Target in MS

The greatest indirect evidence for a pathogenic role of B cells in MS and NMO is derived from recent clinical trials testing B cell-depleting anti-CD20 in these disorders. CD20 is a surface molecule, which is expressed on a broad range of cells of the B lineage throughout their maturation, starting from pre-B cells all the way up to mature and memory B cells. It is lost upon terminal B cell differentiation into plasma cells. Rituximab and its further humanized successor ocrelizumab and ofatumumab are monoclonal antibodies against CD20, which efficiently deplete circulating B cells through antibody effector mechanisms such as complement-dependent cytotoxicity, cellular cytotoxicity, as well as induction of apoptosis. Rituximab was originally developed for treatment of non-Hodgkin's B cell lymphoma and approved for this indication in 1997. Following several clinical trials, it was also approved for treatment of patients with RA not responding to TNF-α- blocking agents in 2006. Based on an ongoing shift in the field of MS research towards the understanding that besides T cells, B cells and B cell-related immune products may substantially contribute to MS pathogenesis, growing interest has developed for testing this therapeutic approach furthermore in MS. In a double-blind placebo-controlled phase II trial with patients with RR-MS, treatment with rituximab led to a rapid decline in newly developing (gadolinium-enhancing) inflammatory CNS lesions (Hauser et al. 2008). The trial included a total of 104 patients, 69 of whom received rituximab at a single course (administered intravenously 1,000 mg on days 1 and 15), while 35 patients received placebo. Despite the short trial period of 48 weeks, therapeutic B cell depletion was associated with a significant reduction in the number of experienced relapses. In treatment of primary progressive (PP)-MS, a double-blind, placebo-controlled phase II/III trial of rituximab was conducted, which included 439 patients who received rituximab (two infusions of 1,000 mg each, 2 weeks apart) or placebo every 24 weeks through week 96. Although the primary endpoint, time to confirmed disease progression, was not reached, rituximab significantly reduced lesion formation in a subgroup of younger patients with active CNS inflammation (Hawker et al. 2009).

In a recently reported 24-week, placebo-controlled and active comparator Phase II study of ocrelizumab, a further humanized anti-CD20 antibody, a total of 220 RR-MS patients were randomized to one of four arms: 600 mg of ocrelizumab, 2,000 mg of ocrelizumab (2 infusions at days 1 and 15), placebo or interferon beta-1a 30 μg i.m. weekly as an open-label arm. This trial demonstrated that ocrelizumab, similar to rituximab, significantly reduced development of new inflammatory CNS lesions as well as the annualized relapse rate compared to placebo or to interferon beta-1a (Kappos et al. 2010). Regarding both drugs' mechanism of action, abolishment of cellular B cell functions rather than a secondary decline in potentially pathogenic antibodies is believed to account for this rapid halt on lesion development. Immunological analysis of PBMC from patients with RR-MS revealed that anti-CD20 B cell depletion was associated with a diminished proliferation and proinflammatory differentiation of T cells, suggesting that abrogation of B cell antigen presentation may be an important mechanism for the prompt effect of anti-CD20 in treatment of MS (Bar-Or et al. 2010).

References

Ascherio A, Munger KL (2010) Epstein-barr virus infection and multiple sclerosis: a review. J Neuroimmune Pharmacol 5(3):271–277

Avasarala JR, Cross AH, Trotter JL (2001) Oligoclonal band number as a marker for prognosis in multiple sclerosis. Arch Neurol 58(12):2044–2045

Bar-Or A et al (2010) Abnormal B-cell cytokine responses a trigger of T-cell-mediated disease in MS? Ann Neurol 67(4):452–461

Baranzini SE et al (1999) B cell repertoire diversity and clonal expansion in multiple sclerosis brain lesions. J Immunol 163(9):5133–5144

Bennett JL et al (2008) CSF IgG heavy-chain bias in patients at the time of a clinically isolated syndrome. J Neuroimmunol 199(1–2):126–132

Bennett JL et al (2009) Intrathecal pathogenic anti-aquaporin-4 antibodies in early neuromyelitis optica. Ann Neurol 66(5):617–629

Berger T et al (2003) Antimyelin antibodies as a predictor of clinically definite multiple sclerosis after a first demyelinating event. N Engl J Med 349(2):139–145

Bettelli E et al (2006) Myelin oligodendrocyte glycoprotein-specific T and B cells cooperate to induce a Devic-like disease in mice. J Clin Invest 116(9):2393–2402

Bourquin C et al (2003) Selective unresponsiveness to conformational B cell epitopes of the myelin oligodendrocyte glycoprotein in H-2b mice. J Immunol 171(1):455–461

Bradl M et al (2009) Neuromyelitis optica: pathogenicity of patient immunoglobulin in vivo. Ann Neurol 66(5):630–643

Breij EC et al (2008) Homogeneity of active demyelinating lesions in established multiple sclerosis. Ann Neurol 63(1):16–25

Brilot F et al (2009) Antibodies to native myelin oligodendrocyte glycoprotein in children with inflammatory demyelinating central nervous system disease. Ann Neurol 66(6):833–842

Burgoon MP et al (2009) Varicella zoster virus is not a disease-relevant antigen in multiple sclerosis. Ann Neurol 65(4):474–479

Brettschneider J, Czerwoniak A, Senel M, Fang L, Kassubek J, Pinkhardt E, Lauda F, Kapfer T, Jesse S, Lehmensiek V, Ludolph AC, Otto M, Tumani H (2010) The chemokine CXCL13 is a prognostic marker in clinically isolated syndrome (CIS). PLoS One 5(8):e11986. doi:10.1371/journal.pone.0011986

Cameron EM et al (2009) Potential of a unique antibody gene signature to predict conversion to clinically definite multiple sclerosis. J Neuroimmunol 213(1–2):123–130
Cepok S et al (2001) Patterns of cerebrospinal fluid pathology correlate with disease progression in multiple sclerosis. Brain 124(Pt 11):2169–2176
Cepok S et al (2003) The immune response at onset and during recovery from Borrelia burgdorferi meningoradiculitis. Arch Neurol 60(6):849–855
Cepok S et al (2005a) Short-lived plasma blasts are the main B cell effector subset during the course of multiple sclerosis. Brain 128(Pt 7):1667–1676
Cepok S et al (2005b) Identification of Epstein-Barr virus proteins as putative targets of the immune response in multiple sclerosis. J Clin Invest 115(5):1352–1360
Cepok S et al (2006) Accumulation of class switched IgD-IgM- memory B cells in the cerebrospinal fluid during neuro-inflammation. J Neuroimmunol 180(1–2):33–39
Colombo M et al (2000) Accumulation of clonally related B lymphocytes in the cerebrospinal fluid of multiple sclerosis patients. J Immunol 164(5):2782–2789
Colombo M et al (2003) Maintenance of B lymphocyte-related clones in the cerebrospinal fluid of multiple sclerosis patients. Eur J Immunol 33(12):3433–3438
Constant S et al (1995a) Peptide and protein antigens require distinct antigen-presenting cell subsets for the priming of CD4+ T cells. J Immunol 154(10):4915–4923
Constant S et al (1995b) B lymphocytes can be competent antigen-presenting cells for priming CD4+ T cells to protein antigens in vivo. J Immunol 155(8):3734–3741
Cortese I et al (1996) Identification of peptides specific for cerebrospinal fluid antibodies in multiple sclerosis by using phage libraries. Proc Natl Acad Sci U S A 93(20):11063–11067
Cree BA, Goodin DS, Hauser SL (2002) Neuromyelitis optica. Semin Neurol 22(2):105–122
Farrell MA et al (1985) Oligoclonal bands in multiple sclerosis: clinical-pathologic correlation. Neurology 35(2):212–218
Genain CP et al (1999) Identification of autoantibodies associated with myelin damage in multiple sclerosis. Nat Med 5(2):170–175
Haubold K et al (2004) B-lymphocyte and plasma cell clonal expansion in monosymptomatic optic neuritis cerebrospinal fluid. Ann Neurol 56(1):97–107
Hauser SL et al (2008) B-cell depletion with rituximab in relapsing-remitting multiple sclerosis. N Engl J Med 358(7):676–688
Hawker K et al (2009) Rituximab in patients with primary progressive multiple sclerosis: results of a randomized double-blind placebo-controlled multicenter trial. Ann Neurol 66(4):460–471
Izquierdo G et al (2002) Intrathecal IgG synthesis: marker of progression in multiple sclerosis patients. Acta Neurol Scand 105(3):158–163
Jarius S et al (2008) Antibody to aquaporin-4 in the long-term course of neuromyelitis optica. Brain 131(Pt 11):3072–3080
Kabat EA, Moore DH, Landow H (1942) An electrophoretic study of the protein components in cerebrospinal fluid and their relationship to the serum proteins. J Clin Invest 21(5):571–577
Kappos L, O'Connor P, Bar-Or A, Li D, Barkhof F, Yin M, Glanzman R, Tinbergen J, Hauser S (2010) Efficacy and safety of ocrelizumab in patients with relapsing-remitting multiple sclerosis: results of a phase II randomised placebo-controlled multicentre trial. Presented at the Congress of the European Committee for Treatment and Research in Multiple Sclerosis
Karni A et al (1999) Elevated levels of antibody to myelin oligodendrocyte glycoprotein is not specific for patients with multiple sclerosis. Arch Neurol 56(3):311–315
Koch M et al (2007) Cerebrospinal fluid oligoclonal bands and progression of disability in multiple sclerosis. Eur J Neurol 14(7):797–800
Kowarik MC et al (2012) CXCL13 is the major determinant for B cell recruitment to the CSF during neuro-inflammation. J Neuroinflammation 16(9):93
Krishnamoorthy G et al (2006) Spontaneous opticospinal encephalomyelitis in a double-transgenic mouse model of autoimmune T cell/B cell cooperation. J Clin Invest 116(9):2385–2392
Krumbholz M et al (2006) Chemokines in multiple sclerosis: CXCL12 and CXCL13 up-regulation is differentially linked to CNS immune cell recruitment. Brain 129(Pt 1):200–211

Kuhle J et al (2007) Lack of association between antimyelin antibodies and progression to multiple sclerosis. N Engl J Med 356(4):371–378

Lalive PH et al (2006) Antibodies to native myelin oligodendrocyte glycoprotein are serologic markers of early inflammation in multiple sclerosis. Proc Natl Acad Sci U S A 103(7):2280–2285

Lampasona V et al (2004) Similar low frequency of anti-MOG IgG and IgM in MS patients and healthy subjects. Neurology 62(11):2092–2094

Lassmann H, Bruck W, Lucchinetti C (2001) Heterogeneity of multiple sclerosis pathogenesis: implications for diagnosis and therapy. Trends Mol Med 7(3):115–121

Lassmann H, Niedobitek G, Aloisi F, Middeldorp JM, NeuroproMiSe EBV Working Group (2011) Epstein-Barr virus in the multiple sclerosis brain: a controversial issue-report on a focused workshop held in the Centre for Brain Research of the Medical University of Vienna, Austria. Brain 134(Pt 9):2772-2286

Lennon VA et al (2005) IgG marker of optic-spinal multiple sclerosis binds to the aquaporin-4 water channel. J Exp Med 202(4):473–477

Litzenburger T et al (1998) B lymphocytes producing demyelinating autoantibodies: development and function in gene-targeted transgenic mice. J Exp Med 188(1):169–180

Lovato L et al (2011) Related B cell clones populate the meninges and parenchyma of patients with multiple sclerosis. Brain 134(Pt 2):534–541

Lucchinetti C, Brück W, Parisi J, Scheithauer B, Rodriguez M, Lassmann H (2000) Heterogeneity of multiple sclerosis lesions: implications for the pathogenesis of demyelination. Ann Neurol 47(6):707-717

Lucchinetti C et al (2011) Inflammatory cortical Demyelination in early multiple sclerosis. N Engl J Med 365(23):2188–2197

Lyons JA et al (1999) B cells are critical to induction of experimental allergic encephalomyelitis by protein but not by a short encephalitogenic peptide. Eur J Immunol 29(11):3432–3439

Lyons JA, Ramsbottom MJ, Cross AH (2002) Critical role of antigen-specific antibody in experimental autoimmune encephalomyelitis induced by recombinant myelin oligodendrocyte glycoprotein. Eur J Immunol 32(7):1905–1913

Magliozzi R et al (2004) Intracerebral expression of CXCL13 and BAFF is accompanied by formation of lymphoid follicle-like structures in the meninges of mice with relapsing experimental autoimmune encephalomyelitis. J Neuroimmunol 148(1–2):11–23

Magliozzi R et al (2007) Meningeal B-cell follicles in secondary progressive multiple sclerosis associate with early onset of disease and severe cortical pathology. Brain 130(Pt 4):1089–1104

Mandler RN et al (1993) Devic's neuromyelitis optica: a clinicopathological study of 8 patients. Ann Neurol 34(2):162–168

Marta CB et al (2005) Pathogenic myelin oligodendrocyte glycoprotein antibodies recognize glycosylated epitopes and perturb oligodendrocyte physiology. Proc Natl Acad Sci U S A 102(39):13992–13997

Martin R et al (1988) Persistent intrathecal secretion of oligoclonal, Borrelia burgdorferi-specific IgG in chronic meningoradiculomyelitis. J Neurol 235(4):229–233

McLaughlin KA et al (2009) Age-dependent B cell autoimmunity to a myelin surface antigen in pediatric multiple sclerosis. J Immunol 183(6):4067–4076

Merkler D et al (2006) Myelin oligodendrocyte glycoprotein-induced experimental autoimmune encephalomyelitis in the common marmoset reflects the immunopathology of pattern II multiple sclerosis lesions. Mult Scler 12(4):369–374

O'Connor KC et al (2005) Antibodies from inflamed central nervous system tissue recognize myelin oligodendrocyte glycoprotein. J Immunol 175(3):1974–1982

O'Connor KC et al (2007) Self-antigen tetramers discriminate between myelin autoantibodies to native or denatured protein. Nat Med 13(2):211–217

Obermeier B et al (2008) Matching of oligoclonal immunoglobulin transcriptomes and proteomes of cerebrospinal fluid in multiple sclerosis. Nat Med 14(6):688–693

Oliver AR, Lyon GM, Ruddle NH (2003) Rat and human myelin oligodendrocyte glycoproteins induce experimental autoimmune encephalomyelitis by different mechanisms in C57BL/6 mice. J Immunol 171(1):462–468

Owens GP et al (1998) Restricted use of VH4 germline segments in an acute multiple sclerosis brain. Ann Neurol 43(2):236–243
Owens GP et al (2001) The immunoglobulin G heavy chain repertoire in multiple sclerosis plaques is distinct from the heavy chain repertoire in peripheral blood lymphocytes. Clin Immunol 98(2):258–263
Owens GP et al (2003) Single-cell repertoire analysis demonstrates that clonal expansion is a prominent feature of the B cell response in multiple sclerosis cerebrospinal fluid. J Immunol 171(5):2725–2733
Owens GP et al (2007) VH4 gene segments dominate the intrathecal humoral immune response in multiple sclerosis. J Immunol 179(9):6343–6351
Owens GP et al (2009) Antibodies produced by clonally expanded plasma cells in multiple sclerosis cerebrospinal fluid. Ann Neurol 65(6):639–649
Ozawa K et al (1994) Patterns of oligodendroglia pathology in multiple sclerosis. Brain 117 (Pt 6):1311–1322
Paul F et al (2007) Antibody to aquaporin 4 in the diagnosis of neuromyelitis optica. PLoS Med 4(4):e133
Pollinger B et al (2009) Spontaneous relapsing-remitting EAE in the SJL/J mouse: MOG-reactive transgenic T cells recruit endogenous MOG-specific B cells. J Exp Med 206(6):1303–1316
Prineas JW, Connell F (1978) The fine structure of chronically active multiple sclerosis plaques. Neurology 28(9 Pt 2):68–75
Prineas JW, Graham JS (1981) Multiple sclerosis: capping of surface immunoglobulin G on macrophages engaged in myelin breakdown. Ann Neurol 10(2):149–158
Prineas JW et al (1984) Continual breakdown and regeneration of myelin in progressive multiple sclerosis plaques. Ann N Y Acad Sci 436:11–32
Rand KH et al (1998) Molecular approach to find target(s) for oligoclonal bands in multiple sclerosis. J Neurol Neurosurg Psychiatry 65(1):48–55
Rauer S et al (2006) Antimyelin antibodies and the risk of relapse in patients with a primary demyelinating event. J Neurol Neurosurg Psychiatry 77(6):739–742
Reindl M et al (1999) Antibodies against the myelin oligodendrocyte glycoprotein and the myelin basic protein in multiple sclerosis and other neurological diseases: a comparative study. Brain 122(Pt 11):2047–2056
Schluesener HJ et al (1987) A monoclonal antibody against a myelin oligodendrocyte glycoprotein induces relapses and demyelination in central nervous system autoimmune disease. J Immunol 139(12):4016–4021
Schmidt S et al (2001) Serum autoantibody responses to myelin oligodendrocyte glycoprotein and myelin basic protein in X-linked adrenoleukodystrophy and multiple sclerosis. J Neuroimmunol 119(1):88–94
Selter RC et al (2010) Antibody responses to EBV and native MOG in pediatric inflammatory demyelinating CNS diseases. Neurology 74(21):1711–1715
Serafini B et al (2004) Detection of ectopic B-cell follicles with germinal centers in the meninges of patients with secondary progressive multiple sclerosis. Brain Pathol 14(2):164–174
Slavin AJ et al (2001) Requirement for endocytic antigen processing and influence of invariant chain and H-2M deficiencies in CNS autoimmunity. J Clin Invest 108(8):1133–1139
Somers V et al (2008) Autoantibody profiling in multiple sclerosis reveals novel antigenic candidates. J Immunol 180(6):3957–3963
Srivastava R et al (2012) Potassium channel KIR4.1 as an immune target in multiple sclerosis. N Engl J Med 267(2):115–123
Storch MK et al (1998) Multiple sclerosis: in situ evidence for antibody- and complement-mediated demyelination. Ann Neurol 43(4):465–471
Vandvik B et al (1976) Oligoclonal measles virus-specific IgG antibodies isolated from cerebrospinal fluids, brain extracts, and sera from patients with subacute sclerosing panencephalitis and multiple sclerosis. Scand J Immunol 5(8):979–992
Villar LM et al (2002) Intrathecal IgM synthesis predicts the onset of new relapses and a worse disease course in MS. Neurology 59(4):555–559

Villar LM et al (2003) Intrathecal IgM synthesis is a prognostic factor in multiple sclerosis. Ann Neurol 53(2):222–226

Vogt MH et al (2009) Cerebrospinal fluid anti-myelin antibodies are related to magnetic resonance measures of disease activity in multiple sclerosis. J Neurol Neurosurg Psychiatry 80(10):1110–1115

von Budingen HC et al (2002) Molecular characterization of antibody specificities against myelin/oligodendrocyte glycoprotein in autoimmune demyelination. Proc Natl Acad Sci U S A 99(12):8207–8212

von Budingen HC et al (2004) Frontline: epitope recognition on the myelin/oligodendrocyte glycoprotein differentially influences disease phenotype and antibody effector functions in autoimmune demyelination. Eur J Immunol 34(8):2072–2083

Walsh MJ, Tourtellotte WW (1986) Temporal invariance and clonal uniformity of brain and cerebrospinal IgG, IgA, and IgM in multiple sclerosis. J Exp Med 163(1):41–53

Weber MS, Prod'homme T, Patarroyo JC, Molnarfi N, Karnezis T, Lehmann-Horn K, Danilenko DM, Eastham-Anderson J, Slavin AJ, Linington C, Bernard CC, Martin F, Zamvil SS (2010) B-cell activation influences T-cell polarization and outcome of anti-CD20 B-cell depletion in central nervous system autoimmunity. Ann Neurol 68(3):369-383. doi:10.1002/ana.22081

Winges KM et al (2007) Analysis of multiple sclerosis cerebrospinal fluid reveals a continuum of clonally related antibody-secreting cells that are predominantly plasma blasts. J Neuroimmunol 192(1–2):226–234

Zamvil S et al (1985) T cell clones specific for myelin basic protein induce relapsing EAE and demyelination. Nature 317:355–358

Zamvil SS, Steinman L (1990) The T lymphocyte in experimental allergic encephalomyelitis. Ann Rev Immunol 8:579–621

Zhang Y et al (2005) Axon reactive B cells clonally expanded in the cerebrospinal fluid of patients with multiple sclerosis. J Clin Immunol 25(3):254–264

Zhou D et al (2006) Identification of a pathogenic antibody response to native myelin oligodendrocyte glycoprotein in multiple sclerosis. Proc Natl Acad Sci U S A 103(50):19057–19062

Chapter 6
Diet, Gut Flora, and Multiple Sclerosis: Current Research and Future Perspectives

Takashi Yamamura and Sachiko Miyake

6.1 Introduction

Multiple sclerosis (MS) is an autoimmune disease, which is continuously increasing in developed countries over the last decades (Bach 2002). Efforts to analyze epidemiological data sometimes lead to a breakthrough, such as identifying a preventive strategy for a disease. In fact, long-standing efforts to understand the correlation between a greater risk of MS and higher latitude have identified lower serum levels of vitamin D3 resulting from a reduced exposure to sunlight as a manageable risk factor for MS (Mahon et al. 2003; Munger et al. 2006). As such, research into elucidating the causes of the increased prevalence and incidence of MS is very important and could be rewarding.

It is worthwhile to mention that the increase in the number of patients with MS is particularly remarkable in Japan, where the number of officially registered patients increased more than 15-fold between 1980 and 2010 (Fig. 6.1a). It was argued that the increase in the number of Japanese patients with MS might be due to a better awareness of the disease, or improvement in health care system and medical technology, including availability of magnetic resonance imaging (MRI) scans across the country. However, this is obviously not the case as has been discussed by Houzen et al. (2008, 2012) in interpreting their epidemiological data in Hokkaido. Generally speaking, an increase in such a short time period should be attributed to environmental changes and not to genetic factors.

In addition to vitamin D3 deficiency, Epstein–Barr (EB) virus infection and cigarette smoking are known risk factors for MS in developed countries (Ascherio and Munger 2007). However, it is unlikely that the Japanese people born in the last half century have been exposed more heavily to these risk factors than before. In fact, the number of people who smoke is decreasing in Japan like in other developed countries. The latest research has indicated that a higher concentration of salt in diet

T. Yamamura (✉) · S. Miyake
Department of Immunology, National Institute of Neuroscience,
National Center of Neurology and Psychiatry, Tokyo, Japan
e-mail: yamamura@ncnp.go.jp

T. Yamamura, B. Gran (eds.), *Multiple Sclerosis Immunology*,
DOI 10.1007/978-1-4614-7953-6_6, © Springer Science+Business Media New York 2013

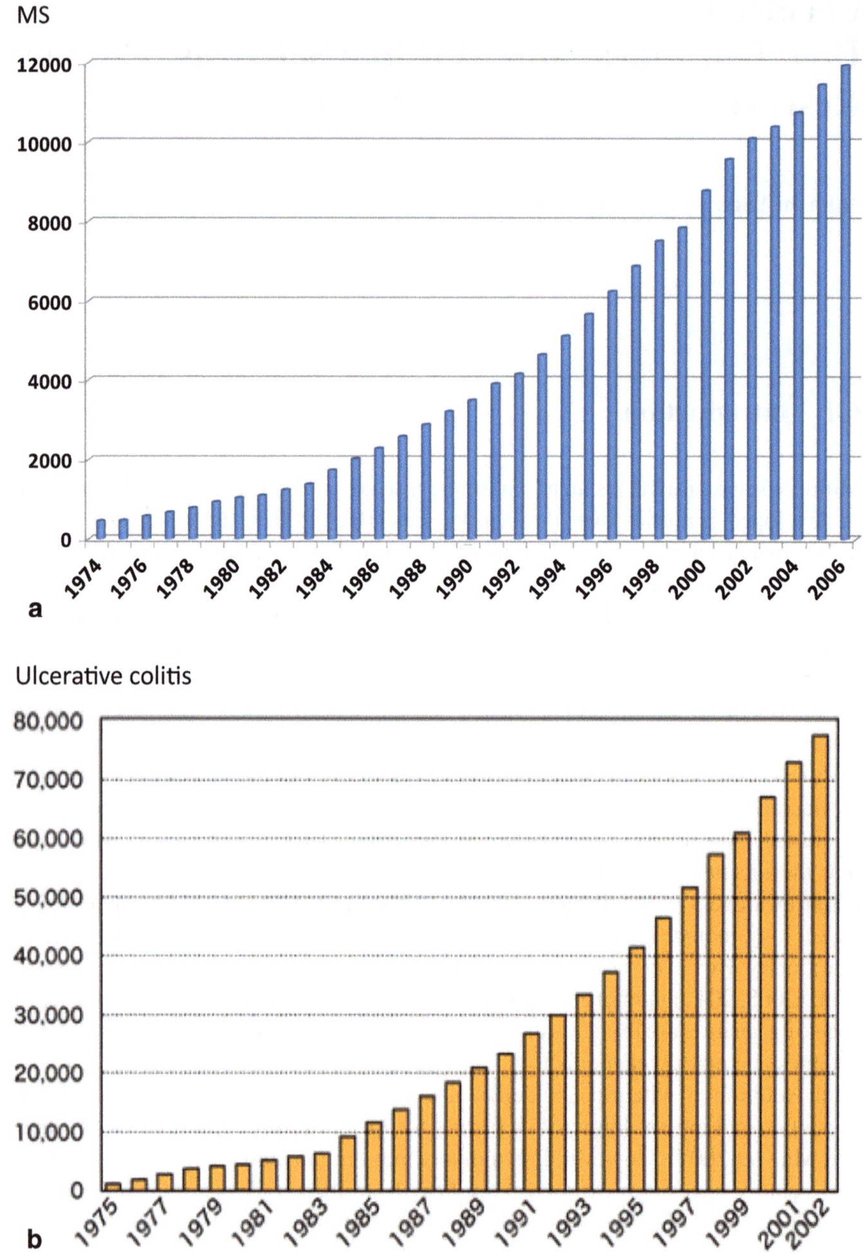

Fig. 6.1 Increased numbers of patients with **(a)** multiple sclerosis (MS) and **(b)** ulcerative colitis (inflammatory bowel diseases) in Japan

may be a risk factor for MS (Wu et al. 2013; Kleinewietfeld et al. 2013). However, according to the health report released by the Ministry of Health and Welfare of Japan, salt consumption is not increasing but rather decreasing in Japan.

It is broadly recognized that westernized lifestyle, including more intake of high-fat Western diet, has been prevailing all over Japan, which accounts for an increased prevalence of diabetes and obesity in Japan. As high-fat diet is thought to be a risk factor of MS (Ascherio and Munger 2007), we assume that westernization of our eating habits could have greatly altered the immune system of our body, leading to the increase of MS in Japan.

In this chapter, entitled "Diet, gut flora, and multiple sclerosis," we overview the past research and recent progress in this field and discuss how Western diet influences gut flora (diet–microbiota interaction) and what products from gut bacteria alter the immune balance (microbiota–immune interaction) towards developing autoimmune diseases like MS. We also discuss which products of gut bacteria or which components within the diet would interact with Th17 (T helper 17) cells or regulatory cells, including Foxp3^{+} regulatory T cells (Tregs), invariant natural killer T (iNKT) cells (Bendelac et al. 2007; Yamamura et al. 2007), and mucosal-associated invariant T (MAIT) cells (Treiner et al. 2003, 2005).

6.2 Is There a Problem with the Gut Flora in Multiple Sclerosis?

We started asking this question around 2004 when some immunologists emphasized the importance of intestinal lymphocytes and their dependence on commensal gut flora (Macpherson and Harris 2004). In 2006, we reported that commensal flora-dependent lymphocytes called MAIT cells play a regulatory role in experimental autoimmune encephalomyelitis (EAE; Croxford et al. 2006). We then raised a possibility that an alteration of gut flora may modulate the immunoregulatory system, involving MAIT cells, and thereby influence the development of MS. However, this idea was not readily accepted because very little was known about the mechanism by which commensal flora influences the immune system. In addition, only few people paid attention to the fact that the bowel dysfunction is a common symptom of MS, but cannot be ascribed to neural dysfunction (Chia et al. 1995).

We were encouraged to pursue the research after noticing that the cases of ulcerative colitis (UC) and Crohn's disease (CD) are also greatly increasing in Japan (Fig. 6.1b). Unlike MS, an etiological role of intestinal microbes was already recognized in the inflammatory bowel diseases (IBD; Sartor 2004; O'Hara and Shanahan 2006). Notably, patients having both MS and IBD have been sporadically reported (Rang et al. 1982; Kimura et al. 2000). With relevance to this, a recent genome-wide association study demonstrated single-nucleotide polymorphisms (SNPs) shared by MS and IBD (International Multiple Sclerosis Genetics Consortium et al. 2011). However, the concurrence of MS and IBD had not been correlated to a common environmental factor that increases the risk of developing these inflammatory diseases. We then hypothesized that more intake of Western diet, high in fat and sugar but low in fiber (plant polysaccharide), might have altered the intestinal commensal flora not only in IBD but also in MS, and increased a risk of Japanese people developing MS. Subsequently, we verified this postulate in EAE by altering gut flora with oral antibiotics treatment. By altering the gut commensal flora of the mice, we were able to suppress clinical and pathological signs of EAE and inhibit T cell production of proinflammatory cytokines (Yokote et al. 2008). Subsequently, we found that independent works from the USA and Germany reported on the role of commensal intestinal bacteria in the development of EAE (Ochoa-Reparaz et al. 2009; Lee et al. 2011; Berer et al. 2011).

6.3 Diet and the Gut Microbiota

Diet has a considerable impact on shaping the repertoire of gut intestinal microbiota (Maslowski and Mackay 2011; De Filippo et al. 2010; Turnbaugh et al. 2009; Nagy-Szakal 2013). Recent analysis of human fecal microbiome actually demonstrated that gut bacteria from African children are highly enriched in *Bacteroides* bacteria having genes encoding enzymes that catalyze plant polysaccharides (De Filippo et al. 2010). As African children take more dietary fibers than European children, this result can be interpreted as intake of high-fiber diet induces enrichment for commensal bacteria that can deal with it. Interestingly, it is also of note that an enzyme to digest carbohydrates present only in marine products was specifically found in the intestinal microbiota of Japanese people (Hehemann et al. 2010). The gene encoding the same enzyme was not present in the gut microbiota of French people. The authors speculated that this gene could have been transferred from marine bacteria to the intestinal bacteria of the Japanese people, as a result of long tradition of eating fish, shellfish, and seaweeds. In addition to these association studies, interventional works in rodent and human showed that changing diet composition would alter the composition of intestinal flora (Berer et al. 2011; Maslowski and Mackay 2011). For example, by switching a high-fiber, low-fat diet to a low-fiber, high-fat diet, microbial compositions of humanized gnotobiotic mice change very rapidly (Turnbaugh et al. 2009). In another study, cellulose supplementation to the diet during the early life stage of mice altered the composition of intestinal flora and prevented development of colitis induced in adult (Nagy-Szakal 2013).

Gut commensal microbiota are not harmful but rather accomplish a variety of beneficial functions for promoting and maintaining health, such as synthesizing vitamins and producing short-chain fatty acids (SCFAs) with anti-inflammatory activity. SCFA, including acetate, propionate, and butyrate, is synthesized through fermenting digestion of dietary fiber by commensal bacteria in the gut. Butyrate is known to exert anti-inflammatory functions via inhibition of NFκB activation and IκBα degradation (Segain et al. 2000). Recent works have shown that fecal bacterium capable of synthesizing butyrate is reduced in the intestinal lumen of patients with active CD (Sokol et al. 2008), indicating the protective role of such bacteria in the pathogenesis of IBD.

6.4 Roles of Gut Commensal Flora in Animal Models of Multiple Sclerosis

Roles of commensal bacteria in the pathogenesis of IBD are broadly supported by results of rodent and human studies. By contrast, it remained obscure for years whether the gut microbiota could affect systemic immune responses beyond the gut and alter the inflammatory pathology in extraintestinal organs. As mentioned previously, the research of EAE has proven that the role of commensal flora is not restricted to the pathogenesis of intestinal inflammation but to the autoimmune disease in the organ distant from the gut. Yokote et al. (2008) induced EAE with myelin oligodendrocyte glycoprotein (MOG) 35–55 peptide in B6 mice that were orally given antibiotics, and showed that antibiotics treatment alters the composition of intestinal microbiota and reduces the clinical and pathological grades of EAE. The suppressed signs of EAE were associated with reduced Th1 and Th17 responses to the sensitized peptide MOG 35–55 in the draining lymph nodes. T cells isolated from the gut-associated lymph nodes showed a selectively suppressed IL-17 production. Interestingly, the effect of antibiotics treatment was not reproduced in mice that were deficient for iNKT cells, indicating the possible involvement of iNKT cells in the suppression of EAE.

In 2009, Ivanov et al. (2009) described that Th17 cell abundance in the lamina propria of the intestine differs very much between B6 mice obtained from different sources. Intensive analysis showed that intestinal Th17 cells are heavily influenced by a bacterium called segmented filamentous bacterium (SFB), which is differentially colonized in independent colonies. In 2011, Lee et al. (2011) have reported that although germ-free mice are very resistant against induction of EAE, colonizing the mice with SFB would restore the susceptibility to EAE, which coincides with the Th17 cell dependence on SFB. In contrast, Berer et al. (2011) described that germ-free mice are susceptible to induction of EAE. Instead, they showed that the commensal flora greatly affects the development of disease in their spontaneous EAE model created by genetic engineering (Berer et al. 2011). Although details have not been published yet, bacterium other than SFB may be critical in the development of the spontaneous EAE.

6.5 Gut Microbiota and Regulatory Cells

Whereas autoaggressive T cells, including Th17 and Th1 cells, trigger the inflammation in organ-specific autoimmune diseases, regulatory cells play a counteracting role in downmodulating the activity of pathogenic T cells. Accumulating evidences now indicate that regulatory cells are also influenced by gut commensal microbiota. Although MAIT cells are widely known to depend on the commensal intestinal flora (Treiner et al. 2003, 2005), recent works have revealed that Foxp3^{+} Tregs (Round and Mazmanian 2010; Ochoa-Reparaz et al. 2010; Atarashi et al. 2011) as well as iNKT cells (Wei et al. 2010; Wingender et al. 2012; Olszak et al. 2012) are influenced by compositions of gut commensal flora. Reduced numbers or altered functions of these regulatory cells have been linked with the pathogenesis of MS (Venken et al. 2008; Illes et al. 2000; Araki et al. 2003; Miyazaki et al. 2011). An interesting question that remains to be answered is whether an alteration of commensal flora would account for the dysfunction of these regulatory cells in MS.

6.5.1 Foxp3$^+$ Tregs

CD4$^+$ T cells expressing the transcription factor Foxp3 and known as Foxp3$^+$ Tregs play a critical role in the control of autoimmune diseases such as MS (Venken et al. 2008). Recent works have indicated that a zwitterionic capsular polysaccharide A (PSA) of human *Bacteroides fragilis* (*B. fragilis*) could induce the Foxp3$^+$ Tregs in mice. Round and Mazmanian (2010) demonstrated that monocolonization of germ-free mice with *B. fragilis* increased the suppressive functions of Tregs in the gut, and further revealed that PSA from *B. fragilis* would mediate the conversion of CD4$^+$ T cells into Foxp3$^+$ Tregs. Kasper and colleagues showed that oral PSA treatment is protective against EAE. They suggested that PSA-induced CD103$^+$ dendritic cells would contribute to the EAE suppression by inducing IL-10- producing Tregs (Ochoa-Reparaz et al. 2010).

After showing that Foxp3$^+$ Tregs are particularly enriched in colon, Atarashi et al. (2011) revealed that spore-forming colon bacteria, particularly clusters IV and XIVa of *Clostridium* species, are essential for promoting accumulation of Foxp3$^+$ Tregs in the colonic mucosa. They also showed that oral inoculation of the *Clostridium* species during early life of conventionally reared mice would protect against colitis development and systemic IgE responses in adult. Although the precise mechanism of inducing Tregs remains unclear, these works indicate that inoculation of bacterium or their component capable of inducing Tregs may be considered as a therapeutic option for immune-mediated diseases in the future.

6.5.2 iNKT Cells

iNKT cells are unique T lymphocytes that express invariant T cell antigen receptor (TCR), which comprises an invariant α-chain and a noninvariant β-chain biased for usage of particular Vβ gene segments (Fig. 6.2; Bendelac et al. 2007; Yamamura et al. 2007). Unlike conventional T cells, the invariant T cells express NK cell markers such as NK1.1 in mice and recognize glycolipid antigen bound to CD1d, a non-classical major histocompatibility complex (MHC) class I-like molecule. Functional uniqueness of the cells is its ability to produce excessive amounts of proinflammatory cytokines (interferon-γ) and anti-inflammatory cytokines (IL-4, IL-13) within hours after TCR ligation. iNKT cells play either protective or augmenting effects in models of autoimmunity, depending on the context of how they are stimulated. Full stimulation of the cells with α-galactosylceramide, a strong agonist for iNKT cells,

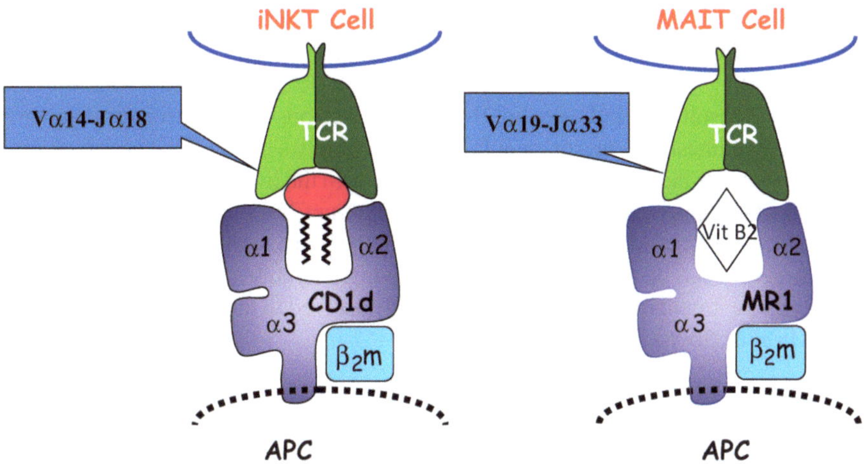

Fig. 6.2 Mice invariant natural killer T (iNKT) cells and mucosal-associated invariant T (MAIT) cells. *TCR* T cell antigen receptor, *APC* antigen-presenting cell

leads to production of both pro- and anti-inflammatory cytokines; whereas a partial agonist such as OCH (Miyamoto et al. 2001), an analogue of α-galactosylceramide with shorter lipid tail, would selectively induce production of anti-inflammatory cytokines (Bendelac et al. 2007; Yamamura et al. 2007; Miyamoto et al. 2001; Oki et al. 2004). iNKT cells are reduced in number in the peripheral blood of MS (Illes et al. 2000; Araki et al. 2003), but can be detected in brain lesions of MS (Illes et al. 2000). The cells can be identified by flow cytometry as cells stained with CD1d tetramer loaded with α-galactosylceramide. iNKT cells react to various lipid ligands derived from bacteria (Yamamura et al. 2007; Kinjo et al. 2005; Chang et al. 2011). For example, lipid ligands derived from *Sphingomonas* bacterium (Kinjo et al. 2005) would stimulate iNKT cells in a CD1d-restricted manner.

It has recently been demonstrated in germ-free mice or restricted flora (RF) mice that iNKT cells are also under control of gut commensal microbiota (Wei et al. 2010; Wingender et al. 2012; Olszak et al. 2012). Whereas Braun and Kronenberg observed a moderate reduction of iNKT cells in germ-free mice, they also noted a more remarkable iNKT cell reduction in RF mice (Wei et al. 2010). The NKT cell reduction in RF mice was mediated by cytolytic killing of iNKT cells by $CD8^+$ T cells. In another study, they also showed the functional immaturity of iNKT cells in germ-free mice. The NKT cell functions were restored after inoculating the mice with *Sphingomonas* bacteria that carry lipid ligands for iNKT cells (Wingender et al. 2012). Blumberg et al. described that in germ-free mice iNKT cells are accumulated in the lamina propria of colon and lung. The abnormal accumulation of iNKT cells was then interpreted as accounting for an increased morbidity of the mice following induction of IBD or allergic asthmas in adulthood (Olszak et al. 2012). Colonization with conventional flora during early life prevented the accumulation of iNKT cells and reduced the morbidity of accompanying pathology in the colon or lung.

We have previously described that preventive antibiotics treatment for EAE in B6 mice did not show any effect in mice deficient for iNKT cells, including β2-microglobulin$^{-/-}$ mice, CD1d$^{-/-}$ mice, and TCR Jα281$^{-/-}$ mice (Yokote et al. 2008). This result may indicate that iNKT cells may possess a sensor for detecting the change of intestinal environment following antibiotics treatment. It is also of note that high-fat diet induces a reduction of iNKT cells in the liver (Miyazaki et al. 2008; Ma et al. 2008) and reduces the ability of mice to mount Th1 responses after exposure to α-galactosylceramide. It remains unclear whether the alterations of iNKT cells by a high-fat diet can be explained by accompanying alterations of gut flora, although probiotics treatment restores iNKT cell defects observed in the mice given a high-fat diet (Ma et al. 2008).

6.5.3 Mucosal Associated Invariant T Cells

MAIT cells are invariant T cells with an invariant TCR α-chain and semi-invariant β-chain, reminiscent of iNKT cells (Fig. 6.2; Treiner et al. 2003, 2005). MAIT cells are abundantly present in the peripheral blood of healthy subjects, but are significantly reduced in number in MS (Miyazaki et al. 2011). Possibly, reflecting their abundance in human, MAIT cells can be readily detected in the cerebrospinal fluid and brain lesions of MS (Illes et al. 2004). MAIT cells could inhibit development of EAE (Croxford et al. 2006), but would augment the autoimmune pathology in arthritis models (Chiba et al. 2012). Previous works showed that MAIT cells are restricted by MR1, a nonclassical MHC class I-like molecule (Treiner et al. 2003, 2005). Although TCR ligands for MAIT cells are present in numerous bacteria and yeast, its identity remains unclear. A recent study showed that crystal structure of MR1 molecule is best suited for binding a ligand originating from vitamin metabolites (Kjer-Nielsen et al. 2013). They demonstrated that a metabolite of folic acid (Vit B9) is a potential ligand for MAIT cells, as it was present as making a complex with MR1. However, since the pterin ring of the metabolite, potentially recognized by MAIT-TCR, was sequestered within MR1, the Vit B9 metabolite was not licensed as an MAIT ligand. Further study has revealed that a metabolite of riboflavin (Vit B2) would bind to MR1 and stimulate MAIT cells in an MR1-restricted manner. This striking work indicates that microbial synthesis of Vit B2 may be critical for producing MAIT cell ligands and maintaining MAIT cells in the gut mucosa. Its implications in biology and medicine remain to be further explored.

6.6 Perspectives

Results of experimental works as well as epidemiological studies allow us to support the importance of intestinal environment in maintaining health, which is greatly affected by microbiota–immune as well as diet–microbiota interactions. Of particular interest, nutritional factors previously reported to show protective effects on MS include vegetable protein, dietary fiber, cereal fiber, vitamin C, thiamin, riboflavin, calcium, and potassium (Ghadirian et al. 1998). As discussed earlier, dietary fibers promote bacterial production of butyrate capable of maintaining intestinal homeostasis, whereas riboflavin metabolites may be able to stimulate MAIT cells. It is also of note that green vegetables contain ligands for aryl hydrocarbon receptor expressed by Th17 cells (Veldhoen et al. 2008). Along with rapid progress in basic research, anecdotal or fragmental works, supporting diet therapy of MS, could be now reevaluated based on more solid scientific background.

Opposed to traditional views, we now know that changing diet compositions could very rapidly alter gut flora and the immune system. In rodent, antibiotics treatment during the induction phase of EAE just for 1 week was found to significantly downmodulate clinical and pathological signs of EAE (unpublished data). Lately, we have more chances to see Japanese patients with MS in our clinic in Tokyo, who have developed the disease in Western countries during their transient stay for study or business, or patients with MS who lived abroad before diagnosis. Similarly, a twin study for IBD in Germany indicated that living abroad before diagnosis is among the risk factors for IBD, in addition to westernization, cigarette smoking, and dietary habit (Spehlman et al. 2012). As such, epidemiological analysis regarding MS should be extended to people who were only transiently exposed to certain environmental risks. Applying modern techniques for analyzing lymphocytes, intestinal content, and microbiome, research into "Diet, gut microbiota, and MS" will possibly reveal a role of particular gut bacterium in the pathogenesis of MS or lead to a preventive strategy for MS, including science-based diet therapy.

References

Araki M, Kondo T, Gumperz JE, Brenner MB, Miyake S, Yamamura T (2003) Th2 bias of $CD4^+$ NKT cells derived from multiple sclerosis in remission. Int Immunol 15:279–288

Ascherio A, Munger KL (2007) Environmental risk factors for multiple sclerosis. Part II: noninfectious factors. Ann Neurol 61:504–513

Atarashi K, Tanoue T, Shima T, Imaoka A, Kuwahara T, Momose Y, Cheng G, Yamasaki S, Saito T, Ohba Y, Taniguchi T, Takeda K, Hori S, Ivanov II, Umesaki Y, Itoh K, Honda K (2011) Induction of colonic regulatory T cells by indigenous Clostridium species. Science 331:337–341

Bach J-F (2002) The effect of infections on susceptibility to autoimmune and allergic diseases. N Eng J Med 347:911–920

Bendelac A, Savage PB, Teyton L (2007) The biology of NKT cells. Ann Rev Immunol 25:297–336

Berer K, Mues M, Koutrolos M, Rasbi ZA, Boziki M, Johner C, Wekerle H, Krishnamoorthy G (2011) Commensal microbiota and myelin autoantigen cooperate to trigger autoimmune demyelination. Nature 479:538–541

Chang Y-J, Kim HY, Albacker LA, Lee H-H, Baumgarth N, Akira S, Savage P, Endo S, Yamamura T, Maaskant J, Kitano N, Singh A, Bhatt A, Besra G, van den Elzen P, Appelmelk B, Franck RW, Chen G, DeKruyff R, Shimamura M, Illarionov P, Umetsu D (2011) Influenza A infection in suckling mice expands a population of NKT cells that protects mice as adults from airway hyperreactivity. J Clin Invest 121:57–69

Chia Y-W, Fowler CJ, Kamm MA, Henry MM, Lemieux M-C, Swash M (1995) Prevalence of bowel dysfunction in patients with multiple sclerosis and bladder dysfunction. J Neurol 242:105–108

Chiba A, Tajima R, Tomi C, Miyazaki Y, Yamamura T, Miyake S (2012) Mucosal-associated invariant T cells promote inflammation and exacerbate disease in murine models of arthritis. Arthritis Rheum 64:153–161

Croxford JL, Miyake S, Huang Y-Y, Shimamura M, Yamamura T (2006) Invariant V(alpha)19iαT cells regulate autoimmune inflammation. Nat Immunol 7:987–994

De Filippo C, Cavalieri D, Paola M, Ramazzotti M, Poullet JB, Massart S, Collini S, Pieraccini G, Lionettei P (2010) Impact of diet in shaping gut microbiota revealed by a comparative study in children from Europe and rural Africa. PNAS 107:14691–14696

Ghadirian P, Jain M, Ducic S, Shatenstein B, Morisset R (1998) Nutritional factors in the aetiology of multiple sclerosis: a case-control study in Montreal, Canada. Int J Epidemiol 27:845–852

Hehemann J-H, Correc G, Barbeyron T, Helbert W, Czjzek M, Michel G (2010) Transfer of carbohydrate-active enzyme from marine bacteria to Japanese gut microbiota. Nature 464:908–912

Houzen H, Niino M, Hata D, Nakano F, Kikuchi S, Fukazawa T, Sasaki H (2008) Increasing prevalence and incidence of multiple sclerosis in northern Japan. Mult Scler 14:887–892

Houzen H, Niino M, Hirotani M, Fukazawa T, Kikuchi S, Tanaka K, Sasaki H (2012) Increased prevalence, incidence and female predominance in multiple sclerosis in northern Japan. J Neurol Sci 323:117–122

Illes Z, Kondo T, Newcombe J, Oka N, Tabira T, Yamamura T (2000) Differential expression of natural killer T cell Vα24JαQ invariant TCR chain in the lesions of multiple sclerosis and chronic inflammatory demyelinating polyneuropathy. J Immunol 164:4375–4381

Illes Z, Shimamura M, Newcombe J, Oka N, Yamamura T (2004) Accumulation of Vα7.2-Jα33 invariant T cells in autoimmune inflammatory lesions of the nervous system. Int Immunol 16:223–230

International Multiple Sclerosis Genetics Consortium et al (2011) Genetic risk and a primary role for cell-mediated immune mechanisms in multiple sclerosis. Nature 476:214–219

Ivanov II, Atarashi K, Manel N, Brodie EL, Shima T, Karaoz U, Wei D, Goldfarb KC, Santee CA, Lynch SV, Tanoue T, Imaoka A, Itoh K, Takeda K, Umesaki Y, Honda K, Littman DR (2009) Induction of intestinal Th17 cells by segmented filamentous bacteria. Cell 139:485–498

Kimura K, Hunter SF, Thollander MS, Loftus EV, Melton LJ, O'Brien PC, Rodriguez M, Phillips SF (2000) Concurrence of inflammatory bowel disease and multiple sclerosis. Mayo Clin Proc 75:802–806

Kinjo Y, Wu D, Kim G, Xing GW, Poles MA, Ho DD, Tsuji M, Kawahara K, Wong CH, Kronenberg M (2005) Recognition of bacterial glycosphingolipids by natural killer T cells. Nature 434:520–525

Kjer-Nielsen L et al (2013) MR1 presents microbial vitamin B metabolites to MAIT cells. Nature 491:717–723

Kleinewietfeld M, Manzel A, Titze J, Kvakan H, Yosef N, Linker RA, Muller DN, Hafler DA (2013) Sodium chloride drives autoimmune disease by the induction of pathogenic TH17 cells. Nature 496:518–522. doi:10.1038

Lee YK, Menezes JS, Umesaki Y, Mazmanian SK (2011) Proinflammatory T-cell responses to gut microbiota promote experimental autoimmune encephalomyelitis. PNAS 108:4615–4622

Ma X, Hua J, Li Z (2008) Probiotics improve high fat diet-induced hepatic steatosis and insulin resistance by increasing hepatic NKT cells. J Hepatol 49:821–830

Macpherson AJ, Harris NL (2004) Interactions between commensal intestinal bacteria and the immune system. Nat Rev Immunol 4:478–485

Mahon BD, Gordon SA, Cruz J, Cosman F, Cantorna MT (2003) Cytokine profile in patients with multiple sclerosis following vitamin D supplementation. J Neuroimmunol 134:128–132

Maslowski K, Mackay CR (2011) Diet, gut microbiota and immune responses. Nat Immunol 12:5–9

Miyamoto K, Miyake S, Yamamura T (2001) A synthetic glycolipid prevents autoimmune encephalomyelitis by inducing TH2 bias of natural killer T cells. Nature 413:531–534

Miyazaki Y, Iwabuchi K, Iwata D, Miyazaki A, Kon Y, Niino M, Kikuchi S, Yanagawa Y, Kaer LV, Sasaki H, Onoe K (2008) Effect of high fat diet on NKT cell function and NKT cell-mediated regulation of Th1 responses. Scand J Immunol 67:230–237

Miyazaki Y, Miyake S, Chiba A, Lantz O, Yamamura T (2011) Mucosal-associated invariant T cells regulate T helper type 1 response in multiple sclerosis. Int Immunol 23:332–337

Munger KL, Levin LI, Hollis BW, Howard NS, Ascherio A (2006) Serum 25-hydroxyvitamine D levels and risk of multiple sclerosis. JAMA 296:2832–2838

Nagy-Szakal D, Hollister EB, Luna RA, Szigeti R, Tatevian N, Smith CW, Versalovic J, Kellermayer R (2013) Cellulose supplementation early in life ameliorates colitis in adult mice. PLoS One 8:e56685

O'Hara AM, Shanahan F (2006) The gut flora as a forgotten organ. EMBO Rep 7:688–693

Ochoa-Reparaz J, Mielcarz DW, Ditrio LE, Burroughs AR, Fourean DM, Haque-Begum S, Kasper LH (2009) Role of gut commensal microflora in the development of experimental autoimmune encephalomyelitis. J Immunol 183:6041–6050

Ochoa-Reparaz J, Mielcarz DW, Wang Y, Begum-Haque S, Sasgupta S, Kasper DL, Kasper LH (2010) A polysaccharide from the human commensal *Bacteroides fragilis* protects against CNS demyelinating disease. Mucosal Immunol 3:487–495

Oki S, Chiba A, Yamamura T, Miyake S (2004) The clinical implication and molecular mechanism of preferential Il-4 production by modified glycolipid-stimulated NKT cells. J Clin Invest 113:1631–1640

Olszak T, An D, Zeissig S, Vera MP, Richter J, Franke A, Glickman JN, Siebert R, Baron R, Kasper DL, Blumberg RS (2012) Microbial exposure during early life has persistent effects on natural killer T cell function. Science 336:489–493

Rang EH, Brooke BN, Taylor JH (1982) Association of ulcerative colitis with multiple sclerosis. Lancet 2:555

Round JL, Mazmanian SK (2010) Inducible Foxp3^{+} regulatory T-cell development by a commensal bacterium of the intestinal microbiota. PNAS 107:12204–12209

Sartor RB (2004) Therapeutic manipulation of the enteric microflora in inflammatory bowel diseases: antibiotics, probiotics, and prebiotics. Gastroenterology 126:1620–1633

Segain J-P, de la Bletiere DR, Bourreille A, Leray V, Gervois N, Rosales C, Ferrier L, Bonnet C, Blottiere HM, Galmiche J-P (2000) Butyrate inhibits inflammatory responses through NFkB inhibition: implications for Crohn's disease. Gut 47:397–403

Sokol H et al (2008) *Faecalibacterium prausnitzii* is an anti-inflammatory commensal bacterium identified by gut microbiota analysis of Crohn disease patients. PNAS 105:16731–16736

Spehlman ME, Begun AZ, Saroglou E, Hinrichs F, Tiemann U, Raedler A, Schreiber S (2012) Risk factors in German twins with inflammatory bowel diseases: results of a questionnaire-based survey. J Crohns Colitis 6:29–42

Treiner E et al (2003) Selection of evolutionarily conserved mucosal-associated invariant T cells by MR1. Nature 422:164–169

Treiner E, Duban L, Mour IC, Hansen T, Gilfillan S, Lantz O (2005) Mucosal-associated invariant T (MAIT) cells: an evolutionarily conserved T cell subset. Microbes Infect 7:552–559

Turnbaugh PJ, Ridaura VK, Faith JJ, Rey FE, Knight R, Gordon JI (2009) The effect of diet on the human gut microbiome: a metagenomic analysis in humanized gnotobiotic mice. Sci Transl Med 1:6ra14

Veldhoen M, Hirota K, Westendorf AM, Buer J, Dumoutier L, Renauld J-C, Stockinger B (2008) The arylhydrocarbon receptor links TH17-cell-mediated autoimmunity to environmental toxins. Nature 453:106–110

Venken K, Hellings N, Thewissen M, Somers V, Hensen K, Rummens J-L, Medaer R, Hupperts R, Stinissen P (2008) Compromised CD4^{+} CD25^{high} regulatory T-cell function in patients with relapsing-remitting multiple sclerosis is correlated with a reduced frequency of FOXP3-positive cells and reduced FOXP3 expression at the single cell level. Immunology 123:79–89

Wei B, Wingender G, Fujiwara D, Chen DY, McPherson M, Brewer S, Borneman J, Kronenberg M, Braun J (2010) Commensal microbiota and CD8^{+} T cells shape the formation of invariant NKT cells. J Immunol 184:1218–1226

Wingender G, Stepniak D, Krebs P, Lin L, McBride S, Wei B, Braun J, Mazmanian SK, Kronenberg M (2012) Intestinal microbes affect phenotypes and functions of invariant natural killer T cells in mice. Gastroenterology 143:418–428

Wu C, Yosef N, Thalhamer T, Zhu C, Xiao S, Kishi Y, Regev A, Kuchroo VK (2013) Induction of pathogenic TH17 cells by inducible salt-sensing kinase SGK1. Nature 496:513–517. doi:10.1038

Yamamura T, Sakuishi K, Illes Z, Miyake S (2007) Understanding the behavior of invariant NKT cells in autoimmune diseases. J Neuroimmunol 191:8–15

Yokote H, Miyake S, Croxford JL, Oki S, Mizusawa H, Yamamura T (2008) NKT cell-dependent amelioration of a mouse model of multiple sclerosis by altering gut flora. Am J Pathol 173:1714–1723

Chapter 7
GM-CSF in Autoimmune Inflammation of the Central Nervous System

Mohamed El-Behi, Bogoljub Ciric and Abdolmohamad Rostami

7.1 Introduction

Multiple sclerosis (MS) is an autoimmune demyelinating disease of the central nervous system (CNS). MS was first described over a century ago, and despite advances in therapy, it remains the major disabling neurological disease in young adults (Noseworthy et al. 2000). It is believed that MS, like its animal model, experimental autoimmune encephalomyelitis (EAE), is mediated by myelin-specific $CD4^+$ T cells that infiltrate the CNS (Kuchroo et al. 2002). In the CNS, these autoreactive $CD4^+$ T cells are activated by local and invading antigen-presenting cells (APCs), and then initiate inflammation by secreting various proinflammatory mediators that attract and activate other immune cells, including monocytes, B cells, $CD8^+$ T cells, and granulocytes (Williams et al. 1994). Accumulation of immune cells in localized CNS areas leads to injury and remodeling of local CNS tissue and formation of MS lesions or plaques, resulting in loss of neurologic function and disability (Williams et al. 1994). $CD4^+$ T cells are viewed as pivotal in initiation and evolution of these processes of autoimmune CNS inflammation.

It was thought that the Th1 subset of $CD4^+$ T cells that produce IFN-γ, and are driven by IL-12 were the only pathogenic Th lineage in MS and EAE (Kuchroo et al. 2002). Several observations supported an important role of Th1 cells and IFN-γ in pathogenesis of EAE and MS. In CNS lesions, IFN-γ is abundant in both EAE and MS and administration of IFN-γ to MS patients worsened disease severity (Ando et al. 1989; Panitch et al. 1987; Traugott and Lebon 1988). T-bet is the master transcription factor in Th1 lineage differentiation and T-bet$^{-/-}$ mice are resistant to EAE (Bettelli et al. 2004). Similarly, mice lacking STAT4$^{-/-}$, a transcription factor involved in IL-12 signaling, have impaired IFN-γ production in response to IL-12 and

M. El-Behi (✉)
Institut du Cerveau et de la Moelle Epinière, INSERM U975, Paris, France
e-mail: mohamed.elbehi@icm-institute.org

B. Ciric · A. Rostami
Department of Neurology, Thomas Jefferson University, Philadelphia, PA 19107, USA

T. Yamamura, B. Gran (eds.), *Multiple Sclerosis Immunology*,
DOI 10.1007/978-1-4614-7953-6_7, © Springer Science+Business Media New York 2013

are resistant to the induction of EAE (Chitnis et al. 2001). However, it has now been shown that neither IFN-γ nor IL-12 is necessary for EAE development and that both of them actually suppress disease. These surprising findings contradicted the Th1 paradigm (Gran et al. 2002; Krakowski and Owens 1996; Tran et al. 2000; Zhang et al. 2003). The identification of the cytokine IL-23 as pivotal in EAE pathogenesis and its fundamental role in the biology of IL-17A- producing CD4^{+} T (Th17) cell lineage led to a new model of autoimmune CNS inflammation, with Th17 cells as its principal cellular mediators (Cua et al. 2003; Harrington et al. 2005; Ivanov et al. 2006; Langrish et al. 2005; Park et al. 2005). Support for this view came from data showing that IL-23$^{-/-}$ mice do not develop Th17 cells after immunization and are resistant to EAE induction (Cua et al. 2003; Langrish et al. 2005). Furthermore, IL-17A-deficient animals developed less severe EAE and administration of IL-17 neutralizing antibodies (Abs) ameliorated disease (Hofstetter et al. 2005; Ishigame et al. 2009; Nakae et al. 2003). Elevated amounts of IL-17A have been found in brain lesions and cerebrospinal fluid of MS patients (Lock et al. 2002; Matusevicius et al. 1999), and IL-17A facilitated migration of human Th17 cells through the blood–brain barrier (BBB) by disrupting endothelial cell tight junctions (Kebir et al. 2007). However, other studies showed that neither IL-17A nor IL-17F plays a significant role in EAE development (Haak et al. 2009). Although the majority of available data show that IL-17A is a contributing factor, its relevance in EAE pathogenesis requires further elucidation. One possibility is that IL-17A directs the localization of CNS inflammation. Indeed, both myelin-specific Th1 and Th17 cells can transfer EAE to naive recipients, inducing similar clinical impairment but with a distinct type and localization of lesions (Kroenke et al. 2008; Stromnes et al. 2008). Th17 cells mainly induced brain inflammation, whereas mice that received Th1 cells developed spinal cord lesions (Kroenke et al. 2008; Stromnes et al. 2008). Furthermore, Th1 and Th17 cells, perhaps due to effects of their respective hallmark cytokines, IFN-γ and IL-17A, attract distinct types of myeloid cells into the CNS. In Th1-mediated EAE, inflammatory CNS infiltrate is dominated by monocytes, whereas large proportions of granulocytes and, in particular, neutrophils are present in the infiltrate when Th17 cells are the principal mediators of CNS inflammation (Kroenke et al. 2008). Collectively, these data demonstrate that, while contributing to disease, neither IFN-γ nor IL-17 is crucial for EAE susceptibility and that other product(s), some of them possibly yet unknown, secreted by Th1 and Th17 cells play a major role in disease development.

Although Th17 cells require exposure to IL-23 to become encephalitogenic (McGeachy et al. 2009), the initial commitment of murine naive T cells toward Th17 lineage is directed by TGF-β and IL-6 (Bettelli et al. 2006; Veldhoen et al. 2006) or IL-21 (Korn et al. 2007). IL-23 itself cannot drive the initial development of Th17 cells, but it is required for maturation of Th17 cells into fully functional effector cells (McGeachy et al. 2009). The mechanisms underlying functional dependency of Th17 cells on IL-23 are not fully understood.

A recent article presents the finding that, among different TGF-β isoforms, TGF-β3 in combination with IL-6 induces highly pathogenic Th17 cells (Lee et al. 2012). Furthermore, TGF-β3 production by developing Th17 cells is dependent on IL-23

(Lee et al. 2012). Th17 cells secrete a range of mediators, including IL-17A, IL-17F, IL-22, and granulocyte–macrophage colony-stimulating factor (GM-CSF). Although IL-17A contributes to the inflammatory capacity of Th17 cells in EAE, the studies mentioned earlier show that IL-17A$^{-/-}$ mice are still susceptible to disease, albeit less than wild-type (WT) mice (Haak et al. 2009; Hofstetter et al. 2005; Ishigame et al. 2009; Nakae et al. 2003). Similarly, IL-22 is not required for the development of EAE, which raises the question which factor(s) mediate(s) Th17 cell pathogenicity (Kreymborg et al. 2007). Among T cell cytokines, TGF-β production by T cells seems to be necessary for EAE development; however, TGF-β acts primarily in an autocrine manner, by stabilizing the Th17 lineage, but does not directly contribute to the disease process (Gutcher et al. 2011). Interest in GM-CSF has been invigorated by recent findings showing that GM-CSF production by Th17 cells is driven by IL-23, revealing a link between IL-23-dependent disease development and GM-CSF as a downstream effector that promotes disease processes (Codarri et al. 2011; El-Behi et al. 2011; Figs. 7.1 and 7.2). Thus, GM-CSF produced by Th17 cells plays a fundamental and nonredundant role in pathogenesis of EAE, making this cytokine an important candidate for designing future therapeutic strategies (Becher and Segal 2011; Codarri et al. 2011; El-Behi et al. 2011; King et al. 2010; Kroenke et al. 2010; McGeachy 2011; Ponomarev et al. 2007; Sonderegger et al. 2008; Figs. 7.1 and 7.2).

In this chapter, we describe recent advances in our knowledge of GM-CSF biology, such as its cellular sources and targets, and possible mechanisms of its action in EAE and MS. Regulation of GM-CSF expression in Th cells by cytokines such as TGF-β, IL-23, IL-12, IL-27, and IL-1β and transcription factors T-bet and RORγt are also discussed.

7.2 Biology of GM-CSF

Colony-stimulating factors (CSFs), such as GM-CSF, granulocyte colony-stimulating factor (G-CSF), and macrophage colony-stimulating factor (M-CSF) regulate the homeostasis of several hematopoietic cell types that originate from bone marrow multipotent progenitors. G-CSF and M-CSF stimulate production of either granulocytes or monocytes/macrophages, respectively, whereas GM-CSF stimulates development of both cell types (Burgess and Metcalf 1980).

In addition to its roles in the growth and maturation of bone marrow precursor cells, GM-CSF regulates the functional activities of several myeloid effector cells, including macrophages, neutrophils, basophils, and eosinophils, as well as dendritic cell (DC) maturation (Burgess and Metcalf 1980). Systemic administration of GM-CSF, or increase in its levels due to inflammation or infection, leads to the mobilization of monocytes and other myeloid populations from bone marrow to blood (Hart et al. 1988). GM-CSF primes monocytes for an increased in vitro response to other stimuli such as LPS or IFN-γ (Fleetwood et al. 2005; Hamilton and Anderson 2004; Stanley and Burgess 1983). GM-CSF can also mobilize precursors of non-hematopoietic lineages, such as endothelial cells (Takahashi et al. 1999). GM-CSF

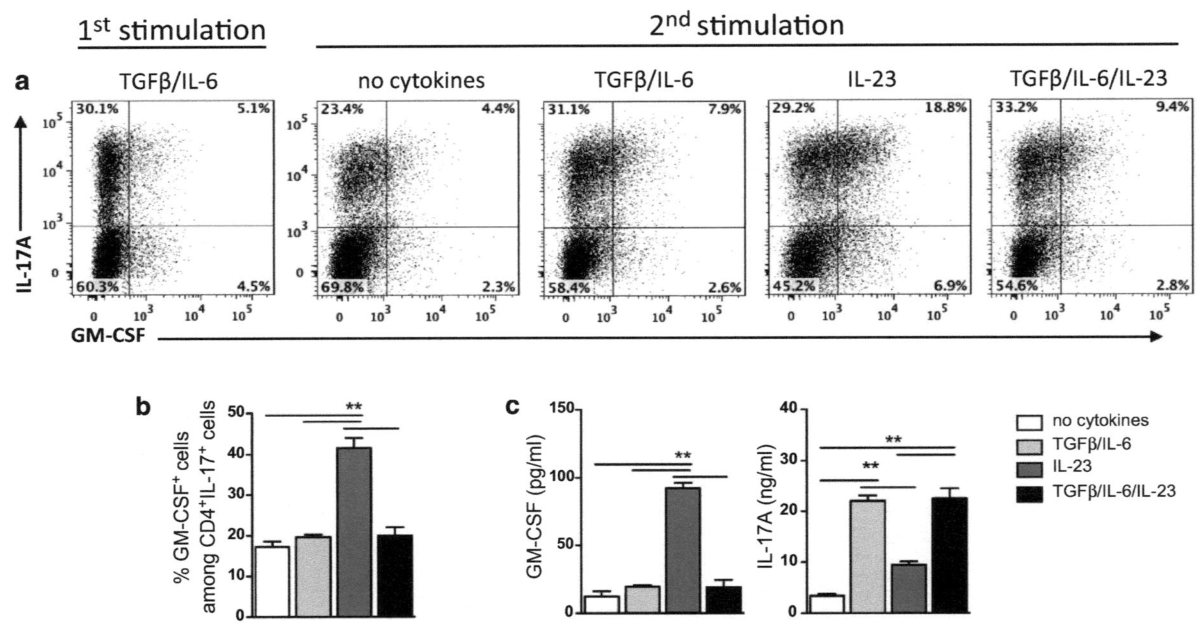

Fig. 7.1 IL-23 upregulates GM-CSF expression in Th17 cells. **a** Flow cytometry of $CD4^+$ cells among $CD4^+CD25^-CD62L^{hi}CD44^{lo}$ T cells sorted by flow cytometry from the spleens of C57BL/6 mice, then activated for 72 h with anti-CD3 and anti-CD28 in the presence of TGF-β plus IL-6, anti-IFN-γ, and anti-IL-4 (1st stimulation), allowed to "rest" for 2 days in the presence of IL-2, then reactivated for 72 h with anti-CD3 and anti-CD28 (2nd stimulation) in the presence of no cytokines, TGF-β plus IL-6, IL-23 alone, or TGF-β, IL-6, and IL-23, and then stimulated with the phorbol ester PMA and ionomycin in the presence of GolgiPlug for the final 4 h and stained. **b** Frequency of $GM\text{-}CSF^+$ cells among $CD4^+IL\text{-}17A^+$ cells after the second stimulation in **a**. **c** Enzyme-linked immunosorbent assay (ELISA) of GM-CSF and IL-17A in culture supernatants after the second stimulation in **a**. *GM-CSF* granulocyte–macrophage colony-stimulating factor, *TGF* transforming growth factor, *IL* interleukin. (Figure first published in *Nature Immunology*, El-Behi et al. 2011)

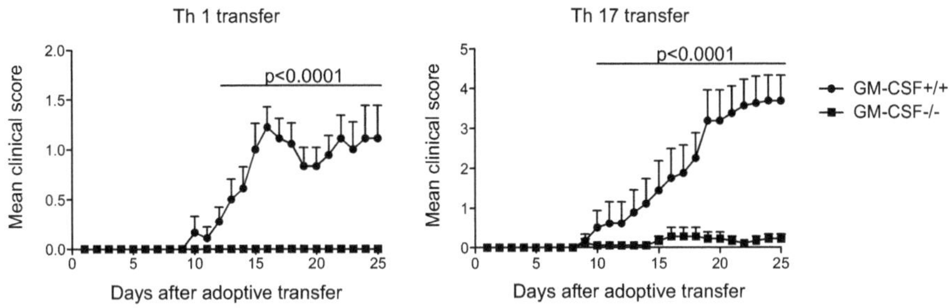

Fig. 7.2 GM-CSF production by Th1 and Th17 cells is required for their encephalitogenicity. Wild-type or Csf2$^{-/-}$ MBP$_{(Ac1-11)}$ TCR–transgenic splenocytes were activated for 72 h with MBP$_{(Ac1-11)}$ in the presence of IL-12 (Th1 conditions) or TGF-β plus IL-6, anti-IFN-γ, and anti-IL-4 (Th17 conditions), then allowed to "rest" for 2 days in the presence of IL-2 and then reactivated for 72 h with MBP$_{(Ac1-11)}$ in the presence of IL-12 (Th1 conditions) or IL-23 (Th17 conditions). Clinical scores of mice that received 5×10^6 MBP$_{(Ac1-11)}$-specific wild-type or Csf2$^{-/-}$ Th1 or Th17 cells enriched by magnetic beads after the second stimulation in the presence of IL-23, followed by intraperitoneal injection of pertussis toxin on days 0 and 2 after transfer are shown. Data are representative of two independent experiments. *Error bars* standard error of the mean, *GM-CSF* granulocyte–macrophage colony-stimulating factor, *Th* T helper cell. (Figure first published in *Nature Immunology*, El-Behi et al. 2011)

is widely used as an adjuvant (Armitage 1998), and inflammatory DCs, in particular, appear to depend on GM-CSF for their in vivo generation (Shortman and Naik 2007). Overall, GM-CSF can be viewed as a major regulator in the control of granulocyte and macrophage lineage populations at all stages of maturation.

GM-CSF is a secreted single-chain glycosylated protein of 23 kDa (Whetton and Dexter 1989), which can be produced by either bone marrow-derived cells, such as activated T cells (Codarri et al. 2011; El-Behi et al. 2011; Ponomarev et al. 2007) and monocytes/macrophages (Hamilton 1994), or by resident tissue cells, including renal parenchymal cells (Timoshanko et al. 2005), fibroblasts (Zucali et al. 1986), endothelial cells (Bagby et al. 1986), chondrocytes (Campbell et al. 1991; Leizer et al. 1990), and smooth muscle cells (Filonzi et al. 1993). GM-CSF acts through binding to its heterodimeric receptor. The GM-CSF receptor (CSF2R) is composed of a specific ligand-binding subunit (CSF2Rα) that binds GM-CSF with low affinity, and a common signal-transduction subunit (CSF2Rβ; Gearing et al. 1989; Metcalf 1993; Whetton and Dexter 1989), which is shared with the receptors for IL-3 and IL-5 (Hercus et al. 2009; Kitamura et al. 1991; Tavernier et al. 1991). In addition to leukocytes, nonhematopoietic cell types (i.e., keratinocytes, smooth muscle cells, endothelial cells, epithelial cells, and neurons) can also express CSF2R and respond to GM-CSF stimulation (Baldwin et al. 1989; Bussolino et al. 1989; Bussolino et al. 1991; Choi et al. 2007; Dedhar et al. 1988; Hancock et al. 1988; Rivas et al. 1998; Soldi et al. 1997). The binding of GM-CSF to its receptor initiates signal transduction involving JAK2, STAT5, and MAPK (Dijkers et al. 1999; Jenkins et al. 1998).

Mice deficient in GM-CSF or CSF2R develop normally and without significant alterations in myeloid cell numbers or their phenotype in steady state conditions (Robb et al. 1995; Stanley et al. 1994). However, these mice have a defect in alveolar macrophage maturation, resulting in alveolar proteinosis (Stanley et al. 1994). Some findings suggest that GM-CSF plays a major role in local tissue myelopoiesis at the site of injury and/or infection rather than participating only in the central production of myeloid cells in bone marrow (Fleetwood et al. 2005; Shibasaki et al. 2007). After infectious challenge, GM-CSF$^{-/-}$ mice develop altered immune responses to several types of pathogens, but not all, indicating an important role for GM-CSF in host response to microbes (Bender et al. 1993; LeVine et al. 1999; Riopel et al. 2001; Zhan et al. 1998). In addition, mice overexpressing GM-CSF develop a multiorgan tissue damage syndrome characterized by large infiltration of activated macrophages (Lang et al. 1987). Furthermore, several inflammatory mediators were augmented in these mice, suggesting that GM-CSF may regulate expression of other cytokines (Lang et al. 1987).

Consistent with its proinflammatory functions, GM-CSF blocking resulted in suppression of disease in virtually all animal models of inflammation and autoimmunity that have been tested. GM-CSF has well-established roles in the following diseases: arthritis (Campbell et al. 1998; Cook et al. 2001), autoimmune CNS inflammation (McQualter et al. 2001), nephritis (Kitching et al. 2002; Timoshanko et al. 2005), lung diseases (Bozinovski et al. 2004; Bozinovski et al. 2002; Cates et al. 2004; Vlahos et al. 2006; Yamashita et al. 2002), atherosclerosis and vascular injury (Ditiatkovski et al. 2006; Shindo et al. 1999), cancer (reviewed in Armitage 1998), obesity (Reed et al. 2005), and type 1 diabetes mellitus (Gaudreau et al. 2007). In summary, GM-CSF can be viewed as a major inflammatory mediator and thus represents a potential therapeutic target in a number of inflammatory diseases.

7.3 GM-CSF as a T Cell Cytokine

GM-CSF impacts the biology of several cell types in steady state and/or in inflammatory conditions as well. The fact that GM-CSF deficiency or blockade ameliorates disease in most CD4$^+$ T cell-driven experimental models of autoimmunity and inflammation suggests that CD4$^+$ T lymphocytes are important producers of GM-CSF. Indeed, both human and mouse GM-CSF have been cloned using cDNA from activated T cells (Cantrell et al. 1985; Gough et al. 1985). Several types of T lymphocytes, including CD4$^+$ and CD8$^+$ T cells, secrete GM-CSF (Min et al. 2010). Interestingly, when naive or effector populations were compared for their GM-CSF secretion profile, naive CD4$^+$ T cells did not produce GM-CSF whereas naive CD8$^+$ T cells did, suggesting that GM-CSF is regulated differently in these two cell types (Min et al. 2010). In addition to CD4$^+$ and CD8$^+$ T cells, natural killer T (NKT) cells and epidermal T lymphocytes produced the largest amounts of GM-CSF while GM-CSF was barely detectable in CD4$^+$CD25$^+$ regulatory T cells (Tregs) or $\gamma\delta$ T cells cultures (Min et al. 2010). However, during EAE, CNS-infiltrating $\gamma\delta$ T cells expressed GM-CSF, which suggests that an inflammatory environment can induce GM-CSF in these cells (Lukens et al. 2012).

Among various CD4$^+$ T cell subsets, GM-CSF is secreted by Th1, Th2, and Th17 cells (Infante-Duarte et al. 2000; Quill et al. 1989). Depending on experimental conditions, several investigators have shown that CD4$^+$ T cells secrete variable amounts of GM-CSF after stimulation with anti-CD3 Ab (Horwood et al. 1998; Leppkes et al. 2009; Marti et al. 1996). Early studies concluded that GM-CSF promotes T cell proliferation because of its ability to augment immune responses to tumor antigens (Disis et al. 1996; Dranoff et al. 1993). However, GM-CSF cannot directly influence T cell biology given that T cells do not express the GM-CSF receptor (Miyamoto et al. 2002; Park et al. 1986). Thus, when isolated T cells of naive GM-CSF$^{-/-}$ mice were stimulated with anti-CD3 Ab, their proliferation was similar to T cells of WT mice, indicating that the proliferative potential of T cells is independent of GM-CSF (Wada et al. 1997). In contrast, splenocytes from immunized GM-CSF$^{-/-}$ mice showed impaired proliferative response in comparison with splenocytes from WT mice (Wada et al. 1997). When GM-CSF$^{-/-}$ T cells were stimulated in the presence of GM-CSF$^{+/+}$ APCs, proliferation was still reduced, demonstrating that GM-CSF produced by T cells plays an important role in immune response (Sonderegger et al. 2008; Wada et al. 1997). Sonderegger et al. (2008) have identified a possible mechanism of action of T cell-derived GM-CSF in development of T cell response. The authors have demonstrated that GM-CSF produced by CD4$^+$ T cells stimulates IL-6 and IL-23 secretion by APCs, which in turn promotes T cell proliferation and survival (Fig. 7.3). Although these data demonstrate that GM-CSF production by T cells contributes indirectly to their proliferation in vitro, it cannot be excluded that non-T cell sources of GM-CSF are also important for T cell functions in vivo.

7.4 GM-CSF in Autoimmune CNS Inflammation

GM-CSF is detectable in healthy human and mouse CNS and is produced mainly by astrocytes (Dame et al. 1999; Malipiero et al. 1990). It has been proposed that GM-CSF, together with other cytokines produced by astrocytes, may contribute to local regulation of microglia function (Franzen et al. 2004; Malipiero et al. 1990). Indeed, GM-CSF can stimulate the antigen-presenting capacity of quiescent microglia cells (Re et al. 2002; Fig. 7.3). GM-CSFR is expressed in neurons and several glial cells, including astrocytes and oligodendrocytes, suggesting that GM-CSF can regulate the physiology of these cells as well (Sawada et al. 1993). Whether GM-CSF signaling in these glial cells has an effect on CNS inflammation has not been investigated.

GM-CSF is essential for the development and progression of EAE. Mice deficient in GM-CSF are resistant to EAE induction and blockade of GM-CSF in WT mice suppresses established disease (McQualter et al. 2001). Treatment of GM-CSF$^{-/-}$ mice with recombinant GM-CSF restored their susceptibility to EAE (McQualter et al. 2001). Overexpression of GM-CSF by encephalitogenic T cells resulted in more severe clinical disease (Marusic et al. 2002). In this model, GM-CSF-overexpressing T cells led to an increase in numbers of CNS-infiltrating cells and mice failed to recover from EAE (Marusic et al. 2002). In humans, as with most other cytokines,

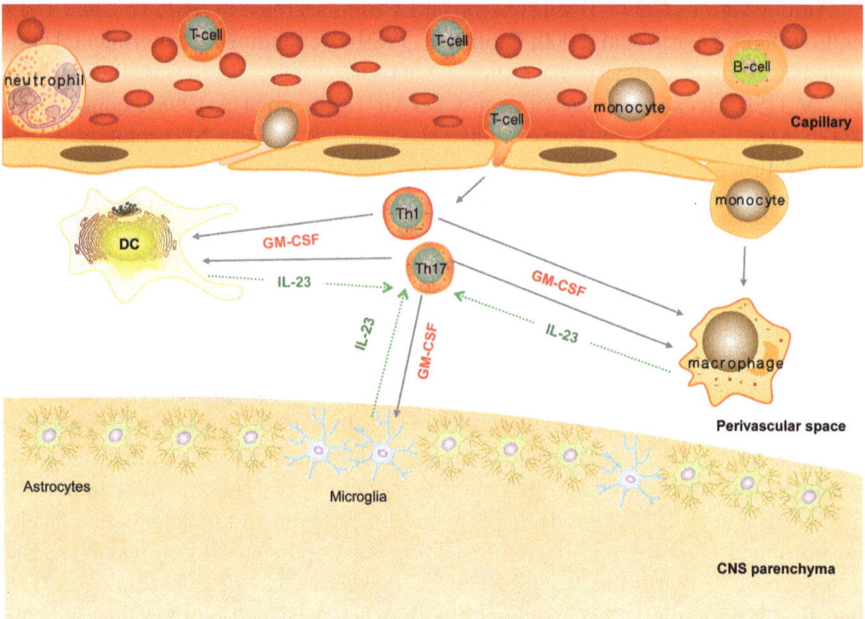

Fig. 7.3 Central role of GM-CSF in autoimmune CNS inflammation. Encephalitogenic Th1 and Th17 cells that have been activated in the periphery enter the circulation, cross the blood–brain barrier (BBB) to reach the perivascular space. GM-CSF produced by Th1 and Th17 cells triggers the recruitment of inflammatory macrophages and DCs to the CNS to initiate experimental autoimmune encephalomyelitis (EAE). In response to T cell-derived GM-CSF-infiltrating macrophages, DCs and resident microglia secrete IL-23, which in turn participates in Th17 cell reactivation and perpetuation of inflammation. *GM-CSF* granulocyte–macrophage colony-stimulating factor, *CNS* central nervous system, *DC* dendritic cell, *IL* interleukin, *Th* T helper cell

there is no direct evidence of the role played by GM-CSF in MS, but elevated GM-CSF in cerebrospinal fluid has been shown to correlate with the active phase of MS (Carrieri et al. 1998). These cumulative observations indicate that GM-CSF has a critical role in CNS autoimmunity.

Based on these data, subsequent studies have focused on defining the mechanism of action of GM-CSF in CNS inflammation. While various cells can produce it, GM-CSF from myelin-specific $CD4^+$ T cells is essential to EAE development (Codarri et al. 2011; El-Behi et al. 2011; Kroenke et al. 2010; Ponomarev et al. 2007), as other cellular sources of GM-CSF do not substantially contribute to disease induction. Initially, resistance of GM-$CSF^{-/-}$ mice to EAE was attributed solely to inefficient T cell priming in the periphery (McQualter et al. 2001). In subsequent studies using the adoptive EAE model, GM-$CSF^{-/-}$ MBP-specific T cells activated in vitro failed to induce EAE, even when activated in the presence of the GM-CSF source, indicating that a defect in T cell priming does not explain resistance to EAE of GM-$CSF^{-/-}$ mice (Ponomarev et al. 2007). These findings demonstrate that GM-CSF plays a crucial role in EAE during the effector and not the priming phase. The same authors have demonstrated that GM-CSF produced by T cells activates microglia and concluded that T cell-derived GM-CSF mediates EAE through a mechanism that likely relies on activation of microglia (Ponomarev et al. 2007; Fig. 7.3). These data were in agreement with previous studies showing that GM-CSF potently activates microglia (Aloisi et al. 2000; Re et al. 2002). However, the following observations demonstrated that CNS-invading myeloid cells rather than resident microglia are relevant targets of GM-CSF produced by encephalitogenic T cells (Codarri et al. 2011; Fig. 7.3). Chimeric mice generated by reconstitution of WT mice with bone marrow cells deficient in the GM-CSFR were resistant to EAE, whereas GM-CSFR$^{-/-}$ mice reconstituted with WT stem cells developed disease, demonstrating that GM-CSF responsiveness of radio-resistant microglia (or other CNS cell types) is not crucial to EAE development (Codarri et al. 2011; Fig. 7.3). Consistent with these findings, administration of recombinant GM-CSF to immunized GM-CSF$^{-/-}$ mice triggered Ly6C^{+} monocyte infiltration into the CNS, where they differentiated into inflammatory DCs and restored susceptibility to EAE (King et al. 2009). Additional data indicate that GM-CSF$^{-/-}$ mice are selectively deficient in a subset of dermal DCs expressing langerin and CD103, and depletion of this subset in WT mice conferred resistance to EAE (King et al. 2010). The authors concluded that CD103^{+} DCs play a crucial role in EAE development by acquiring the antigen after immunization and transporting it to draining lymph nodes, where an encephalitogenic immune response is then initiated. It is now clear that GM-CSF plays a crucial role in EAE during the effector phase of EAE and that peripheral myeloid cells are relevant cellular targets of its bioactivity. The action of GM-CSF on Ly6C^{+} inflammatory monocytic lineage (M1 monocytes) is likely responsible for crucial disease-promoting effects of GM-CSF in EAE. However, other myeloid cell types, especially CX3CR1^{+} resident (M2) monocytes and neutrophils, can be relevant targets of GM-CSF as well. Although GM-CSF responsiveness of microglia seems not to be important in EAE, in contrast with previous findings (Ponomarev et al. 2007), microglia have been shown to be important for CNS antigen presentation and additionally as mediators of epitope spreading in EAE (McMahon et al. 2005; McRae et al. 1995). Furthermore, activated microglia secrete IL-23 during disease progression, which can in turn sustain local inflammation and T cell activation (Becher et al. 2003; Li et al. 2008; Fig. 7.3). Given that GM-CSF plays a crucial role during the effector phase of EAE development, it is likely that the CNS represents the most important site of its action. Nonetheless, the importance of its systemic effects, such as mobilization of inflammatory monocytes from bone marrow, cannot be excluded at this point.

Both Th1 and Th17 cells can be encephalitogenic, and both lineages can produce GM-CSF, which raises the questions whether Th1 or Th17 cells are the major source of GM-CSF in EAE, and whether encephalitogenicity of both Th lineages depends on their GM-CSF production. Kroenke et al. (2008) have shown in an adoptive EAE model in SJL mice that administration of anti-GM-CSF mAb inhibited disease in mice that had received IL-23-stimulated myelin-specific CD4^{+} T cells (enriched Th17 cells) but not disease induced by transferring CD4^{+} T cells treated with IL-12 (enriched Th1 cells). These data indicate that Th17 cells could be the major producer of GM-CSF in EAE. Importantly, the data also suggest that, contrary to Th17 cells, encephalitogenicity of Th1 cells does not depend on their GM-CSF production, implying that other proinflammatory mediators produced by Th1 cells can substitute for GM-CSF. Given that in active EAE GM-CSF is necessary for disease to develop, the aforementioned findings suggest that active EAE is for the most part mediated by Th17 cells, with perhaps only marginal contribution of Th1 cells. This conclusion is in agreement with other lines of evidence (i.e., the crucial role of IL-23), demonstrating that Th17 cells play an essential role in EAE, whereas the role of Th1 cells can be considered negligible. However, the same group later reported that anti-GM-CSF treatment inhibits adoptive EAE mediated by IL-12-stimulated $CD4^+$ T cells (enriched Th1 cells) in C57Bl/6 mice (Kroenke et al. 2010), contradicting their earlier findings. The reason for this discrepancy is unclear but might be due to different strains of mice used. Nonetheless, these results preclude definitive conclusions on the most important Th source of GM-CSF in EAE, and on the role of GM-CSF in their encephalitogenicity. We have recently shown that encephalitogenicity of both Th1 and Th17 cells is equally dependent on their GM-CSF expression (El-Behi et al. 2011; Fig. 7.2). In support of our findings is the fact that encephalitogenic $CD4^+$ T cells deficient in both IFN-γ and IL-17A, but not GM-CSF, can transfer EAE (Codarri et al. 2011; Kroenke et al. 2010), demonstrating that this cytokine plays a crucial role in encephalitogenicity irrespective of the Th lineage that produces it. Furthermore, these findings have been reproduced using different strains of mice, which clearly emphasizes a central function of GM-CSF in autoimmune inflammation (Codarri et al. 2011).

It should be noted that the aforementioned conclusions on the role of GM-CSF in the encephalitogenicity of Th1 and Th17 cells come from adoptive EAE models. Even though these conclusions are likely to be fully applicable to active EAE, they do not answer whether Th1 or Th17 cells are the most important source of GM-CSF in active EAE. Alternatively, GM-CSF production by both Th lineages might be required for full EAE susceptibility. The question about the most important GM-CSF source mirrors one that has been raised ever since the Th17 lineage was discovered: what is the relative importance of Th1 and Th17 cells in EAE? This topic is still a matter of debate, given that available approaches do not enable its unambiguous experimental testing. The current prevailing view, based on substantial indirect evidence showing a strong correlation between anti-myelin Th17 responses and EAE, is that Th17 cells are necessary for EAE to develop, at least initially; whereas Th1 cells contribute to disease severity, but in a nonessential manner, and possibly more substantially later in disease. It is likely that the relative importance of Th1 and Th17 cells as the source of GM-CSF reflects their overall contribution to EAE development, with Th17 cells being initially the major producers of encephalitogenic GM-CSF, whereas later on the contribution of Th1 cell-derived GM-CSF becomes more significant, or even predominant. To test the relative importance of Th1 and Th17 cells as GM-CSF sources, we would need a model where one of these lineages does not produce GM-CSF, while the other retains its normal production. Another layer of complexity is added with the lineage plasticity between Th1 and Th17 cells

(Lee et al. 2009; Nurieva et al. 2009; Zhou et al. 2009). Th17 cells can progressively acquire expression of T-bet and IFN-γ, while losing expression of RORγt and IL-17A, blurring the distinction between Th1 and Th17 cells (Bending et al. 2009; Martin-Orozco et al. 2009). Of great importance are findings demonstrating that the vast majority of Th1 cells in the CNS of EAE mice arise from Th17 cells (Hirota et al. 2011). This study used a fate-reporter mouse in which cells that express IL-17A are permanently marked with enhanced yellow fluorescence protein (eYFP). During the course of EAE, $eYFP^+$ Th17 cells progressively extinguished IL-17A expression and began producing IFN-γ (Hirota et al. 2011). Most of the $IFN\text{-}\gamma^+IL\text{-}17A^-$ T cells found in the CNS were also $eYFP^+$ indicating that the majority of Th1 cells found in the CNS originated from Th17 cells (Hirota et al. 2011). Together with IFN-γ, these $eYFP^+$ Th1 cells also coexpressed several inflammatory cytokines, including GM-CSF. These data demonstrate that the major sources of GM-CSF in EAE are Th17 and ex-Th17 cells and not "conventional" Th1 cells.

7.5 Regulation of GM-CSF Production by T Cells

T cell production of GM-CSF can be influenced by multiple cytokines. Its expression is inhibited in the presence of TGF-β and by Th1 and Th2 cytokines IFN-γ and IL-4, respectively (Codarri et al. 2011; El-Behi et al. 2011; Sagawa et al. 1996; Fig. 7.1). The inhibition of GM-CSF production by TGF-β can explain why Th17 cells treated with TGF-β plus IL-6 are not pathogenic despite their abundant production of IL-17A (El-Behi et al. 2011; McGeachy et al. 2007). The anti-inflammatory cytokine IL-10 decreased production of GM-CSF in human peripheral blood mononuclear cells (PBMCs) stimulated with anti-CD3 Abs, whereas it did not have an effect of GM-CSF production by isolated $CD4^+$ T cells (El-Behi et al. 2011; Sagawa et al. 1996). These results suggest that IL-10 has an indirect effect on GM-CSF production by T cells, probably through an effect on APCs (Fiorentino et al. 1991). In contrast to the inhibitory effect of the aforementioned cytokines, IL-1β is a potent inducer of GM-CSF secretion by $CD4^+$ T cells (El-Behi et al. 2011; Lukens et al. 2012; Fig. 7.4). Furthermore, heterodimeric cytokines of the IL-12 family, including IL-12, IL-23, and IL-27, also regulate and have distinct effects on GM-CSF production by $CD4^+$ T cells (Fig. 7.5). IL-35, a recently identified member of the IL-12 cytokine family, is produced by activated Treg cells and is required for their suppressive activity (Collison et al. 2010). Although IL-35 is a potent inhibitor of cytokine production by T cells, its effects on GM-CSF production by T cells have not been investigated.

IL-12 and IL-27 are potent inhibitors of GM-CSF in Th1 cells whereas IL-23 drives production of GM-CSF by Th17 cells (Codarri et al. 2011; El-Behi et al. 2011; Young et al. 2012; Figs. 7.1 and 7.5). Interestingly, in contrast to its suppressive effect on Th17 differentiation, IL-27 did not suppress GM-CSF production by committed Th17 cells but inhibited GM-CSF expression in committed Th1 cells (Young et al. 2012). These results are consistent with findings showing that IL-27 does not suppress effector functions of committed Th17 cells during EAE (Diveu et al. 2009; El-behi

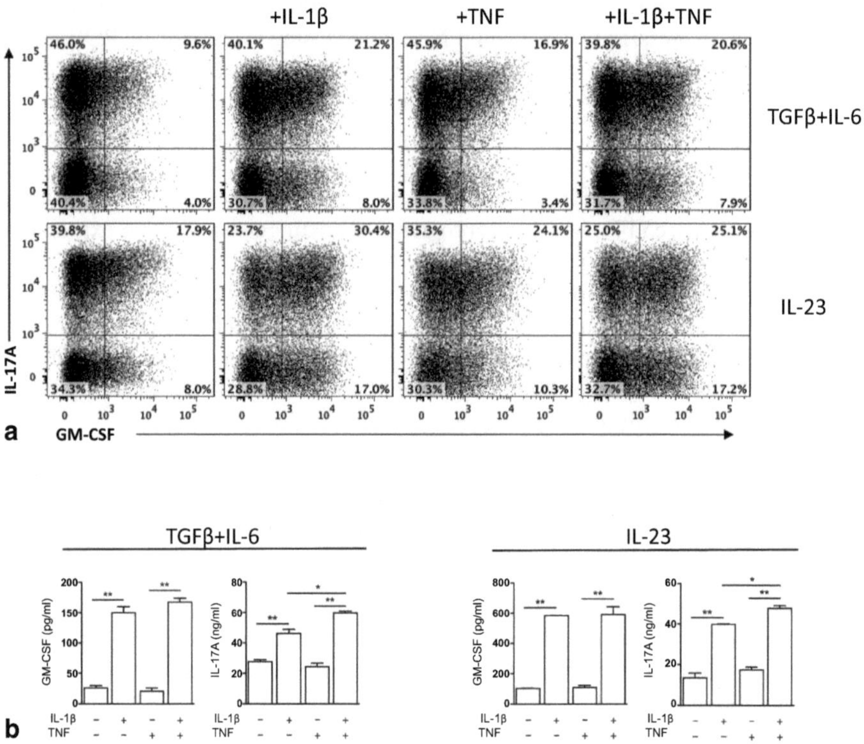

Fig. 7.4 IL-1β upregulates GM-CSF expression in Th17 cells. **a** Flow cytometry of $CD4^+$ cells among $CD4^+CD25^-CD62L^{hi}CD44^{lo}$ T cells sorted by flow cytometry from the spleens of C57BL/6 mice and differentiated into Th17 cells during the first stimulation, then reactivated for 72 h with anti-CD3 and anti-CD28 in the presence of either TGF-β plus IL-6 (*top row*) or IL-23 (*bottom row*) in the presence of no cytokines, IL-1β (10 ng/ml) or TNF (10 ng/ml), or both. **b** Enzyme-linked immunosorbent assay (ELISA) of GM-CSF and IL-17A in culture supernatants after the second stimulation in **a**. *GM-CSF* granulocyte–macrophage colony-stimulating factor, *TNF* tumor necrosis factor, *TGF* transforming growth factor, *IL* interleukin. (Figure first published in *Nature Immunology*, El-Behi et al. 2011)

et al. 2009). These data indicate that GM-CSF is differentially regulated in subsets of Th cells and identification of the molecular pathways that influence IL-23-mediated regulation of GM-CSF may provide potential therapeutic targets in CNS autoimmune diseases.

Th cell development is controlled by transcription factors that drive their commitment toward different lineages. Indeed, transcription factors T-bet, GATA-3, and RORγt drive Th1, Th2, and Th17 developmental programs, respectively. Given that all three Th lineages produce GM-CSF, it is likely that none of the aforementioned transcription factors solely controls GM-CSF expression in Th cells. Even though a positive correlation was found between GATA-3^+ cells and GM-CSF^+ cells in the nasal mucosa of patients with allergic rhinitis (Nakamura et al. 2000), suggesting

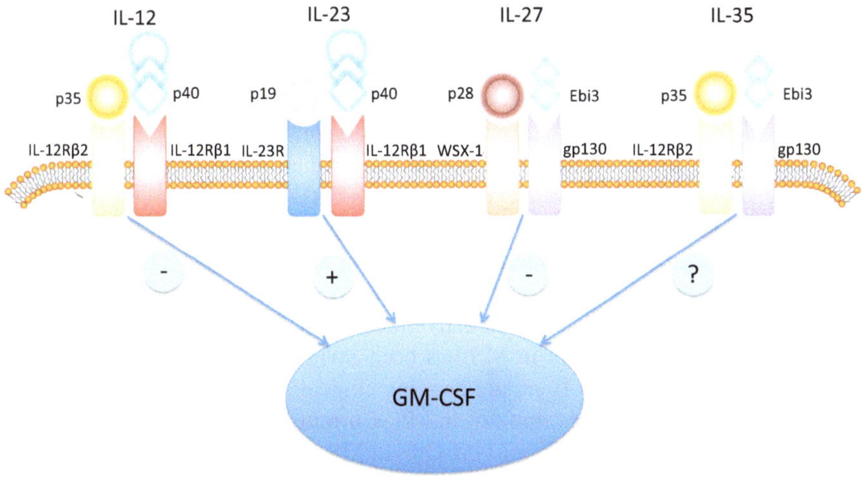

Fig. 7.5 Effect of cytokines from IL-12 family on GM-CSF production by T cells. The four members of the IL-12 cytokine family (IL-12, IL-23, IL-27, and IL-35) are represented together with their respective receptors. IL-12 and IL-27 inhibit GM-CSF production by Th cells, while IL-23 potentiates it. However, these effects can vary with Th lineage, as, for example, IL-27 inhibits GM-CSF production by Th1 cells, but not by Th17 cells. The effect of IL-35 on GM-CSF production is not known. *GM-CSF* granulocyte–macrophage colony-stimulating factor, *IL* interleukin

that GATA-3 is involved in GM-CSF expression, to the best of our knowledge there is no study directly analyzing the role of GATA-3 in GM-CSF production. In contrast to GATA-3, the roles of T-bet and RORγt in GM-CSF secretion have been studied. T-bet is clearly not involved in regulation of GM-CSF expression as T-bet-deficient Th1 and Th17 cells produce normal quantities of GM-CSF (El-Behi et al. 2011). Studies on the role of RORγt in GM-CSF expression gave conflicting results. In our study, purified Rorc$^{-/-}$ CD4^{+} T cells produced similar quantities of GM-CSF as WT when cultivated in vitro (El-Behi et al. 2011), whereas Codarri et al. found that Rorc$^{-/-}$ T cells are deficient in GM-CSF production (Codarri et al. 2011). In contrast, splenocytes of Rorc$^{-/-}$ mice immunized with MOG_{35-55} did not produce GM-CSF after ex vivo restimulation with MOG_{35-55} (El-Behi et al. 2011). We observed that splenocytes from Rorc$^{-/-}$ immunized mice have a reduced proportion of CD4^{+} T cells when compared to WT immunized mice, which may explain the reduced amount of GM-CSF produced by Rorc$^{-/-}$ splenocytes. These inconsistent findings warrant additional investigation to conclusively define the role of RORγt in GM-CSF production by T cells.

7.6 Conclusion and Perspectives

GM-CSF is essential for the development and progression of EAE. Mice deficient in GM-CSF are resistant to EAE induction, and blockade of GM-CSF in WT mice suppresses ongoing disease. While produced by several hematopoietic cell types,

GM-CSF from CD4$^+$ T cells is essential to EAE development, as other cellular sources of GM-CSF do not substantially contribute to disease induction. These insights were obtained from EAE models that rely on encephalitogenicity of CD4$^+$ T cells, whereas in MS, or certain types of MS, other cell types (i.e., CD8$^+$ T cells) might be pivotal in initiating and perpetuating CNS inflammation. CD8$^+$ T cells can produce large quantities of GM-CSF, suggesting that their pathogenicity in MS might also depend on GM-CSF. Given its crucial role in EAE, it is expected that GM-CSF also plays an important role in MS, making it a highly attractive therapeutic target. A compelling argument for targeting GM-CSF in MS is that its cellular source is likely to be irrelevant, as irrespective of whether MS is primarily mediated by Th1, Th17, Tc1, or Tc17 cells, its role in activation of myeloid cells remains the same. Interest in targeting GM-CSF in MS has been invigorated by the recent findings summarized in this review. There are ongoing clinical trials using anti-GM-CSF in several autoimmune diseases, but not in MS. Current knowledge provides a basic rationale for clinical testing of anti-GM-CSF in MS.

Acknowledgments We thank K. Regan for editorial assistance. This work was supported in part by the grants from National Institutes of Health (5R01NS046782 and 1U19A1082726), and the M.E. Groff Foundation.

References

Aloisi F, De Simone R, Columba-Cabezas S, Penna G, Adorini L (2000) Functional maturation of adult mouse resting microglia into an APC is promoted by granulocyte-macrophage colony-stimulating factor and interaction with Th1 cells. J Immunol 164:1705–1712

Ando DG, Clayton J, Kono D, Urban JL, Sercarz EE (1989) Encephalitogenic T cells in the B10.PL model of experimental allergic encephalomyelitis (EAE) are of the Th-1 lymphokine subtype. Cell Immunol 124:132–143

Armitage JO (1998) Emerging applications of recombinant human granulocyte-macrophage colony-stimulating factor. Blood 92:4491–4508

Bagby GC Jr, Dinarello CA, Wallace P, Wagner C, Hefeneider S, McCall E (1986) Interleukin 1 stimulates granulocyte macrophage colony-stimulating activity release by vascular endothelial cells. J Clin Invest 78:1316–1323

Baldwin GC, Gasson JC, Kaufman SE, Quan SG, Williams RE, Avalos BR, Gazdar AF, Golde DW, DiPersio JF (1989) Nonhematopoietic tumor cells express functional GM-CSF receptors. Blood 73:1033–1037

Becher B, Segal BM (2011) T(H)17 cytokines in autoimmune neuro-inflammation. Curr Opin Immunol 23:707–712

Becher B, Durell BG, Noelle RJ (2003) IL-23 produced by CNS-resident cells controls T cell encephalitogenicity during the effector phase of experimental autoimmune encephalomyelitis. J Clin Invest 112:1186–1191

Bender A, Amann U, Jager R, Nain M, Gemsa D (1993) Effect of granulocyte/macrophage colony-stimulating factor on human monocytes infected with influenza A virus. Enhancement of virus replication, cytokine release, and cytotoxicity. J Immunol 151:5416–5424

Bending D, De la Pena H, Veldhoen M, Phillips JM, Uyttenhove C, Stockinger B, Cooke A (2009) Highly purified Th17 cells from BDC2.5NOD mice convert into Th1-like cells in NOD/SCID recipient mice. J Clin Invest 119:565–572

Bettelli E, Sullivan B, Szabo SJ, Sobel RA, Glimcher LH, Kuchroo VK (2004) Loss of T-bet, but not STAT1, prevents the development of experimental autoimmune encephalomyelitis. J Exp Med 200:79–87
Bettelli E, Carrier Y, Gao W, Korn T, Strom TB, Oukka M, Weiner HL, Kuchroo VK (2006) Reciprocal developmental pathways for the generation of pathogenic effector TH17 and regulatory T cells. Nature 441:235–238
Bozinovski S, Jones JE, Vlahos R, Hamilton JA, Anderson GP (2002) Granulocyte/macrophage-colony-stimulating factor (GM-CSF) regulates lung innate immunity to lipopolysaccharide through Akt/Erk activation of NFkappa B and AP-1 in vivo. Journal Biol Chem 277:42808–42814
Bozinovski S, Jones J, Beavitt SJ, Cook AD, Hamilton JA, Anderson GP (2004) Innate immune responses to LPS in mouse lung are suppressed and reversed by neutralization of GM-CSF via repression of TLR-4. Am J Physiol Lung Cell Mol Physiol 286:L877–885
Burgess AW, Metcalf D (1980) The nature and action of granulocyte-macrophage colony stimulating factors. Blood 56:947–958
Bussolino F, Wang JM, Defilippi P, Turrini F, Sanavio F, Edgell CJ, Aglietta M, Arese P, Mantovani A (1989) Granulocyte- and granulocyte-macrophage-colony stimulating factors induce human endothelial cells to migrate and proliferate. Nature 337:471–473
Bussolino F, Ziche M, Wang JM, Alessi D, Morbidelli L, Cremona O, Bosia A, Marchisio PC, Mantovani A (1991) In vitro and in vivo activation of endothelial cells by colony-stimulating factors. J Clin Invest 87:986–995
Campbell IK, Novak U, Cebon J, Layton JE, Hamilton JA (1991) Human articular cartilage and chondrocytes produce hemopoietic colony-stimulating factors in culture in response to IL-1. J Immunol 147:1238–1246
Campbell IK, Rich MJ, Bischof RJ, Dunn AR, Grail D, Hamilton JA (1998) Protection from collagen-induced arthritis in granulocyte-macrophage colony-stimulating factor-deficient mice. J Immunol 161:3639–3644
Cantrell MA, Anderson D, Cerretti DP, Price V, McKereghan K, Tushinski RJ, Mochizuki DY, Larsen A, Grabstein K, Gillis S et al (1985) Cloning, sequence, and expression of a human granulocyte/macrophage colony-stimulating factor. Proc Natl Acad Sci U S A 82:6250–6254
Carrieri PB, Provitera V, De Rosa T, Tartaglia G, Gorga F, Perrella O (1998) Profile of cerebrospinal fluid and serum cytokines in patients with relapsing-remitting multiple sclerosis: a correlation with clinical activity. Immunopharmacol Immunotoxicol 20:373–382
Cates EC, Fattouh R, Wattie J, Inman MD, Goncharova S, Coyle AJ, Gutierrez-Ramos JC, Jordana M (2004) Intranasal exposure of mice to house dust mite elicits allergic airway inflammation via a GM-CSF-mediated mechanism. J Immunol 173:6384–6392
Chitnis T, Najafian N, Benou C, Salama AD, Grusby MJ, Sayegh MH, Khoury SJ (2001) Effect of targeted disruption of STAT4 and STAT6 on the induction of experimental autoimmune encephalomyelitis. J Clin Invest 108:739–747
Choi JK, Choi BH, Ha Y, Park H, Yoon SH, Park HC, Park SR (2007) Signal transduction pathways of GM-CSF in neural cell lines. Neurosci Lett 420:217–222
Codarri L, Gyulveszi G, Tosevski V, Hesske L, Fontana A, Magnenat L, Suter T, Becher B (2011) RORgammat drives production of the cytokine GM-CSF in helper T cells, which is essential for the effector phase of autoimmune neuroinflammation. Nat Immunol 12:560–567
Collison LW, Chaturvedi V, Henderson AL, Giacomin PR, Guy C, Bankoti J, Finkelstein D, Forbes K, Workman CJ, Brown SA et al (2010) IL-35-mediated induction of a potent regulatory T cell population. Nat Immunol 11:1093–1101
Cook AD, Braine EL, Campbell IK, Rich MJ, Hamilton JA (2001) Blockade of collagen-induced arthritis post-onset by antibody to granulocyte-macrophage colony-stimulating factor (GM-CSF): requirement for GM-CSF in the effector phase of disease. Arthritis Res 3:293–298
Cua DJ, Sherlock J, Chen Y, Murphy CA, Joyce B, Seymour B, Lucian L, To W, Kwan S, Churakova T et al (2003) Interleukin-23 rather than interleukin-12 is the critical cytokine for autoimmune inflammation of the brain. Nature 421:744–748

Dame JB, Christensen RD, Juul SE (1999) The distribution of granulocyte-macrophage colony-stimulating factor and its receptor in the developing human fetus. Pediatr Res 46:358–366

Dedhar S, Gaboury L, Galloway P, Eaves C (1988) Human granulocyte-macrophage colony-stimulating factor is a growth factor active on a variety of cell types of nonhemopoietic origin. Proc Natl Acad Sci U S A 85:9253–9257

Dijkers PF, van Dijk TB, de Groot RP, Raaijmakers JA, Lammers JW, Koenderman L, Coffer PJ (1999) Regulation and function of protein kinase B and MAP kinase activation by the IL-5/GM-CSF/IL-3 receptor. Oncogene 18:3334–3342

Disis ML, Bernhard H, Shiota FM, Hand SL, Gralow JR, Huseby ES, Gillis S, Cheever MA (1996) Granulocyte-macrophage colony-stimulating factor: an effective adjuvant for protein and peptide-based vaccines. Blood 88:202–210

Ditiatkovski M, Toh BH, Bobik A (2006) GM-CSF deficiency reduces macrophage PPAR-gamma expression and aggravates atherosclerosis in ApoE-deficient mice. Arterioscler Thromb Vasc Biol 26:2337–2344

Diveu C, McGeachy MJ, Boniface K, Stumhofer JS, Sathe M, Joyce-Shaikh B, Chen Y, Tato CM, McClanahan TK, de Waal MR et al (2009) IL-27 blocks RORc expression to inhibit lineage commitment of Th17 cells. J Immunol 182:5748–5756

Dranoff G, Jaffee E, Lazenby A, Golumbek P, Levitsky H, Brose K, Jackson V, Hamada H, Pardoll D, Mulligan RC (1993) Vaccination with irradiated tumor cells engineered to secrete murine granulocyte-macrophage colony-stimulating factor stimulates potent, specific, and long-lasting anti-tumor immunity. Proc Natl Acad Sci U S A 90:3539–3543

El-Behi M, Ciric B, Yu S, Zhang GX, Fitzgerald DC, Rostami A (2009) Differential effect of IL-27 on developing versus committed Th17 cells. J Immunol 183:4957–4967

El-Behi M, Ciric B, Dai H, Yan Y, Cullimore M, Safavi F, Zhang GX, Dittel BN, Rostami A (2011) The encephalitogenicity of T(H)17 cells is dependent on IL-1- and IL-23-induced production of the cytokine GM-CSF. Nat Immunol 12:568–575

Filonzi EL, Zoellner H, Stanton H, Hamilton JA (1993) Cytokine regulation of granulocyte-macrophage colony stimulating factor and macrophage colony-stimulating factor production in human arterial smooth muscle cells. Atherosclerosis 99:241–252

Fiorentino DF, Zlotnik A, Vieira P, Mosmann TR, Howard M, Moore KW, O'Garra A (1991) IL-10 acts on the antigen-presenting cell to inhibit cytokine production by Th1 cells. J Immunol 146:3444–3451

Fleetwood AJ, Cook AD, Hamilton JA (2005) Functions of granulocyte-macrophage colony-stimulating factor. Crit Rev Immunol 25:405–428

Franzen R, Bouhy D, Schoenen J (2004) Nervous system injury: focus on the inflammatory cytokine 'granulocyte-macrophage colony stimulating factor'. Neurosci Lett 361:76–78

Gaudreau S, Guindi C, Menard M, Besin G, Dupuis G, Amrani A (2007) Granulocyte-macrophage colony-stimulating factor prevents diabetes development in NOD mice by inducing tolerogenic dendritic cells that sustain the suppressive function of CD4 + CD25 + regulatory T cells. J Immunol 179:3638–3647

Gearing DP, King JA, Gough NM, Nicola NA (1989) Expression cloning of a receptor for human granulocyte-macrophage colony-stimulating factor. EMBO J 8:3667–3676

Gough NM, Metcalf D, Gough J, Grail D, Dunn AR (1985) Structure and expression of the mRNA for murine granulocyte-macrophage colony stimulating factor. EMBO J 4:645–653

Gran B, Zhang GX, Yu S, Li J, Chen XH, Ventura ES, Kamoun M, Rostami A (2002) IL-12p35-deficient mice are susceptible to experimental autoimmune encephalomyelitis: evidence for redundancy in the IL-12 system in the induction of central nervous system autoimmune demyelination. J Immunol 169:7104–7110

Gutcher I, Donkor MK, Ma Q, Rudensky AY, Flavell RA, Li MO (2011) Autocrine transforming growth factor-beta1 promotes in vivo Th17 cell differentiation. Immunity 34:396–408

Haak S, Croxford AL, Kreymborg K, Heppner FL, Pouly S, Becher B, Waisman A (2009) IL-17 A and IL-17 F do not contribute vitally to autoimmune neuro-inflammation in mice. J Clin Invest 119:61–69

Hamilton JA (1994) Coordinate and noncoordinate colony stimulating factor formation by human monocytes. J Leukoc Biol 55:355–361
Hamilton JA, Anderson GP (2004) GM-CSF Biology. Growth Factors 22:225–231
Hancock GE, Kaplan G, Cohn ZA (1988) Keratinocyte growth regulation by the products of immune cells. J Exp Med 168:1395–1402
Harrington LE, Hatton RD, Mangan PR, Turner H, Murphy TL, Murphy KM, Weaver CT (2005) Interleukin 17-producing CD4 + effector T cells develop via a lineage distinct from the T helper type 1 and 2 lineages. Nat Immunol 6:1123–1132
Hart PH, Whitty GA, Piccoli DS, Hamilton JA (1988) Synergistic activation of human monocytes by granulocyte-macrophage colony-stimulating factor and IFN-gamma. Increased TNF-alpha but not IL-1 activity. J Immunol 141:1516–1521
Hercus TR, Thomas D, Guthridge MA, Ekert PG, King-Scott J, Parker MW, Lopez AF (2009) The granulocyte-macrophage colony-stimulating factor receptor: linking its structure to cell signaling and its role in disease. Blood 114:1289–1298
Hirota K, Duarte JH, Veldhoen M, Hornsby E, Li Y, Cua DJ, Ahlfors H, Wilhelm C, Tolaini M, Menzel U et al (2011) Fate mapping of IL-17-producing T cells in inflammatory responses. Nat Immunol 12:255–263
Hofstetter HH, Ibrahim SM, Koczan D, Kruse N, Weishaupt A, Toyka KV, Gold R (2005) Therapeutic efficacy of IL-17 neutralization in murine experimental autoimmune encephalomyelitis. Cell Immunol 237:123–130
Horwood NJ, Udagawa N, Elliott J, Grail D, Okamura H, Kurimoto M, Dunn AR, Martin T, Gillespie MT (1998) Interleukin 18 inhibits osteoclast formation via T cell production of granulocyte macrophage colony-stimulating factor. J Clin Invest 101:595–603
Infante-Duarte C, Horton HF, Byrne MC, Kamradt T (2000) Microbial lipopeptides induce the production of IL-17 in Th cells. J Immunol 165:6107–6115
Ishigame H, Kakuta S, Nagai T, Kadoki M, Nambu A, Komiyama Y, Fujikado N, Tanahashi Y, Akitsu A, Kotaki H et al (2009) Differential roles of interleukin-17 A and -17 F in host defense against mucoepithelial bacterial infection and allergic responses. Immunity 30:108–119
Ivanov II, McKenzie BS, Zhou L, Tadokoro CE, Lepelley A, Lafaille JJ, Cua DJ, Littman DR (2006) The orphan nuclear receptor RORgammat directs the differentiation program of proinflammatory IL-17 + T helper cells. Cell 126:1121–1133
Jenkins BJ, Blake TJ, Gonda TJ (1998) Saturation mutagenesis of the beta subunit of the human granulocyte-macrophage colony-stimulating factor receptor shows clustering of constitutive mutations, activation of ERK MAP kinase and STAT pathways, and differential beta subunit tyrosine phosphorylation. Blood 92:1989–2002
Kebir H, Kreymborg K, Ifergan I, Dodelet-Devillers A, Cayrol R, Bernard M, Giuliani F, Arbour N, Becher B, Prat A (2007) Human TH17 lymphocytes promote blood-brain barrier disruption and central nervous system inflammation. Nat Med 13:1173–1175
King IL, Dickendesher TL, Segal BM (2009) Circulating Ly-6 C + myeloid precursors migrate to the CNS and play a pathogenic role during autoimmune demyelinating disease. Blood 113:3190–3197
King IL, Kroenke MA, Segal BM (2010) GM-CSF-dependent, CD103+ dermal dendritic cells play a critical role in Th effector cell differentiation after subcutaneous immunization. J Exp Med 207:953–961
Kitamura T, Sato N, Arai K, Miyajima A (1991) Expression cloning of the human IL-3 receptor cDNA reveals a shared beta subunit for the human IL-3 and GM-CSF receptors. Cell 66:1165–1174
Kitching AR, Ru Huang X, Turner AL, Tipping PG, Dunn AR, Holdsworth SR (2002) The requirement for granulocyte-macrophage colony-stimulating factor and granulocyte colony-stimulating factor in leukocyte-mediated immune glomerular injury. J Am Soc Nephrol 13:350–358
Korn T, Bettelli E, Gao W, Awasthi A, Jager A, Strom TB, Oukka M, Kuchroo VK (2007) IL-21 initiates an alternative pathway to induce proinflammatory T(H)17 cells. Nature 448:484–487

Krakowski M, Owens T (1996) Interferon-gamma confers resistance to experimental allergic encephalomyelitis. Eur J Immunol 26:1641–1646

Kreymborg K, Etzensperger R, Dumoutier L, Haak S, Rebollo A, Buch T, Heppner FL, Renauld JC, Becher B (2007) IL-22 is expressed by Th17 cells in an IL-23-dependent fashion, but not required for the development of autoimmune encephalomyelitis. J Immunol 179:8098–8104

Kroenke MA, Carlson TJ, Andjelkovic AV, Segal BM (2008) IL-12- and IL-23-modulated T cells induce distinct types of EAE based on histology, CNS chemokine profile, and response to cytokine inhibition. J Exp Med 205:1535–1541

Kroenke MA, Chensue SW, Segal BM (2010) EAE mediated by a non-IFN-gamma/non-IL-17 pathway. Eur J Immunol 40:2340–2348

Kuchroo VK, Anderson AC, Waldner H, Munder M, Bettelli E, Nicholson LB (2002) T cell response in experimental autoimmune encephalomyelitis (EAE): role of self and cross-reactive antigens in shaping, tuning, and regulating the autopathogenic T cell repertoire. Annu Rev Immunol 20:101–123

Lang RA, Metcalf D, Cuthbertson RA, Lyons I, Stanley E, Kelso A, Kannourakis G, Williamson DJ, Klintworth GK, Gonda TJ et al (1987) Transgenic mice expressing a hemopoietic growth factor gene (GM-CSF) develop accumulations of macrophages, blindness, and a fatal syndrome of tissue damage. Cell 51:675–686

Langrish CL, Chen Y, Blumenschein WM, Mattson J, Basham B, Sedgwick JD, McClanahan T, Kastelein RA, Cua DJ (2005) IL-23 drives a pathogenic T cell population that induces autoimmune inflammation. J Exp Med 201:233–240

Lee YK, Turner H, Maynard CL, Oliver JR, Chen D, Elson CO, Weaver CT (2009) Late developmental plasticity in the T helper 17 lineage. Immunity 30:92–107

Lee Y, Awasthi A, Yosef N, Quintana FJ, Xiao S, Peters A, Wu C, Kleinewietfeld M, Kunder S, Hafler DA et al (2012) Induction and molecular signature of pathogenic T(H)17 cells. Nat Immunol 13:991–999

Leizer T, Cebon J, Layton JE, Hamilton JA (1990) Cytokine regulation of colony-stimulating factor production in cultured human synovial fibroblasts: I. Induction of GM-CSF and G-CSF production by interleukin-1 and tumor necrosis factor. Blood 76:1989–1996

Leppkes M, Becker C, Ivanov II, Hirth S, Wirtz S, Neufert C, Pouly S, Murphy AJ, Valenzuela DM, Yancopoulos GD et al (2009) RORgamma-expressing Th17 cells induce murine chronic intestinal inflammation via redundant effects of IL-17 A and IL-17 F. Gastroenterology 136:257–267

LeVine AM, Reed JA, Kurak KE, Cianciolo E, Whitsett JA (1999) GM-CSF-deficient mice are susceptible to pulmonary group B streptococcal infection. J Clin Invest 103:563–569

Li Y, Chu N, Hu A, Gran B, Rostami A, Zhang GX (2008) Inducible IL-23p19 expression in human microglia via p38 MAPK and NF-kappaB signal pathways. Exp Mol Pathol 84:1–8

Lock C, Hermans G, Pedotti R, Brendolan A, Schadt E, Garren H, Langer-Gould A, Strober S, Cannella B, Allard J et al (2002) Gene-microarray analysis of multiple sclerosis lesions yields new targets validated in autoimmune encephalomyelitis. Nat Med 8:500–508

Lukens JR, Barr MJ, Chaplin DD, Chi H, Kanneganti TD (2012) Inflammasome-derived IL-1beta regulates the production of GM-CSF by CD4+ T cells and gammadelta T Cells. J Immunol 188:3107–3115

Malipiero UV, Frei K, Fontana A (1990) Production of hemopoietic colony-stimulating factors by astrocytes. J Immunol 144:3816–3821

Marti RM, Wasik MA, Kadin ME (1996) Constitutive secretion of GM-CSF by three different cell lines derived from a single patient with a progressive cutaneous lymphoproliferative disorder. Cytokine 8:323–329

Martin-Orozco N, Chung Y, Chang SH, Wang YH, Dong C (2009) Th17 cells promote pancreatic inflammation but only induce diabetes efficiently in lymphopenic hosts after conversion into Th1 cells. Eur J Immunol 39:216–224

Marusic S, Miyashiro JS, Douhan J 3rd, Konz RF, Xuan D, Pelker JW, Ling V, Leonard JP, Jacobs KA (2002) Local delivery of granulocyte macrophage colony-stimulating factor by retrovirally transduced antigen-specific T cells leads to severe, chronic experimental autoimmune encephalomyelitis in mice. Neurosci Lett 332:185–189

Matusevicius D, Kivisakk P, He B, Kostulas N, Ozenci V, Fredrikson S, Link H (1999) Interleukin-17 mRNA expression in blood and CSF mononuclear cells is augmented in multiple sclerosis. Mult Scler 5:101–104

McGeachy MJ (2011) GM-CSF: the secret weapon in the T(H)17 arsenal. Nat Immunol 12:521–522

McGeachy MJ, Bak-Jensen KS, Chen Y, Tato CM, Blumenschein W, McClanahan T, Cua DJ (2007) TGF-beta and IL-6 drive the production of IL-17 and IL-10 by T cells and restrain T(H)-17 cell-mediated pathology. Nat Immunol 8:1390–1397

McGeachy MJ, Chen Y, Tato CM, Laurence A, Joyce-Shaikh B, Blumenschein WM, McClanahan TK, O'Shea JJ, Cua DJ (2009) The interleukin 23 receptor is essential for the terminal differentiation of interleukin 17-producing effector T helper cells in vivo. Nat Immunol 10:314–324

McMahon EJ, Bailey SL, Castenada CV, Waldner H, Miller SD (2005) Epitope spreading initiates in the CNS in two mouse models of multiple sclerosis. Nat Med 11:335–339

McQualter JL, Darwiche R, Ewing C, Onuki M, Kay TW, Hamilton JA, Reid HH, Bernard CC (2001) Granulocyte macrophage colony-stimulating factor: a new putative therapeutic target in multiple sclerosis. J Exp Med 194:873–882

McRae BL, Vanderlugt CL, Dal Canto MC, Miller SD (1995) Functional evidence for epitope spreading in the relapsing pathology of experimental autoimmune encephalomyelitis. J Exp Med 182:75–85

Metcalf D (1993) The cellular basis for enhancement interactions between stem cell factor and the colony stimulating factors. Stem Cells 11(Suppl 2):1–11

Min L, Mohammad Isa SA, Shuai W, Piang CB, Nih FW, Kotaka M, Ruedl C (2010) Cutting edge: granulocyte-macrophage colony-stimulating factor is the major CD8 + T cell-derived licensing factor for dendritic cell activation. J Immunol 184:4625–4629

Miyamoto T, Iwasaki H, Reizis B, Ye M, Graf T, Weissman IL, Akashi K (2002) Myeloid or lymphoid promiscuity as a critical step in hematopoietic lineage commitment. Dev Cell 3:137–147

Nakae S, Nambu A, Sudo K, Iwakura Y (2003) Suppression of immune induction of collagen-induced arthritis in IL-17-deficient mice. J Immunol 171:6173–6177

Nakamura Y, Christodoulopoulos P, Cameron L, Wright E, Lavigne F, Toda M, Muro S, Ray A, Eidelman DH, Minshall E et al (2000) Upregulation of the transcription factor GATA-3 in upper airway mucosa after in vivo and in vitro allergen challenge. J Allergy Clin Immunol 105:1146–1152

Noseworthy JH, Lucchinetti C, Rodriguez M, Weinshenker BG (2000) Multiple sclerosis. N Engl J Med 343:938–952

Nurieva R, Yang XO, Chung Y, Dong C (2009) Cutting edge: in vitro generated Th17 cells maintain their cytokine expression program in normal but not lymphopenic hosts. J Immunol 182:2565–2568

Panitch HS, Hirsch RL, Schindler J, Johnson KP (1987) Treatment of multiple sclerosis with gamma interferon: exacerbations associated with activation of the immune system. Neurology 37:1097–1102

Park LS, Friend D, Gillis S, Urdal DL (1986) Characterization of the cell surface receptor for human granulocyte/macrophage colony-stimulating factor. J Exp Med 164:251–262

Park H, Li Z, Yang XO, Chang SH, Nurieva R, Wang YH, Wang Y, Hood L, Zhu Z, Tian Q et al (2005) A distinct lineage of CD4 T cells regulates tissue inflammation by producing interleukin 17. Nat Immunol 6:1133–1141

Ponomarev ED, Shriver LP, Maresz K, Pedras-Vasconcelos J, Verthelyi D, Dittel BN (2007) GM-CSF production by autoreactive T cells is required for the activation of microglial cells and the onset of experimental autoimmune encephalomyelitis. J Immunol 178:39–48

Quill H, Gaur A, Phipps RP (1989) Prostaglandin E2-dependent induction of granulocyte-macrophage colony-stimulating factor secretion by cloned murine helper T cells. J Immunol 142:813–818

Re F, Belyanskaya SL, Riese RJ, Cipriani B, Fischer FR, Granucci F, Ricciardi-Castagnoli P, Brosnan C, Stern LJ, Strominger JL et al (2002) Granulocyte-macrophage colony-stimulating factor induces an expression program in neonatal microglia that primes them for antigen presentation. J Immunol 169:2264–2273

Reed JA, Clegg DJ, Smith KB, Tolod-Richer EG, Matter EK, Picard LS, Seeley RJ (2005) GM-CSF action in the CNS decreases food intake and body weight. J Clin Invest 115:3035–3044

Riopel J, Tam M, Mohan K, Marino MW, Stevenson MM (2001) Granulocyte-macrophage colony-stimulating factor-deficient mice have impaired resistance to blood-stage malaria. Infect Immun 69:129–136

Rivas CI, Vera JC, Delgado-Lopez F, Heaney ML, Guaiquil VH, Zhang RH, Scher HI, Concha II, Nualart F, Cordon-Cardo C et al (1998) Expression of granulocyte-macrophage colony-stimulating factor receptors in human prostate cancer. Blood 91:1037–1043

Robb L, Drinkwater CC, Metcalf D, Li R, Kontgen F, Nicola NA, Begley CG (1995) Hematopoietic and lung abnormalities in mice with a null mutation of the common beta subunit of the receptors for granulocyte-macrophage colony-stimulating factor and interleukins 3 and 5. Proc Natl Acad Sci U S A 92:9565–9569

Sagawa K, Mochizuki M, Sugita S, Nagai K, Sudo T, Itoh K (1996) Suppression by IL-10 and IL-4 of cytokine production induced by two-way autologous mixed lymphocyte reaction. Cytokine 8:501–506

Sawada M, Itoh Y, Suzumura A, Marunouchi T (1993) Expression of cytokine receptors in cultured neuronal and glial cells. Neurosci Lett 160:131–134

Shibasaki T, Katayama N, Ohishi K, Fujieda A, Monma F, Nishi K, Masuya M, Shiku H (2007) IL-3 cannot replace GM-CSF in inducing human monocytes to differentiate into Langerhans cells. Int J Oncol 30:549–555

Shindo J, Ishibashi T, Yokoyama K, Nakazato K, Ohwada T, Shiomi M, Maruyama Y (1999) Granulocyte-macrophage colony-stimulating factor prevents the progression of atherosclerosis via changes in the cellular and extracellular composition of atherosclerotic lesions in watanabe heritable hyperlipidemic rabbits. Circulation 99:2150–2156

Shortman K, Naik SH (2007) Steady-state and inflammatory dendritic-cell development. Nature reviews. Immunology 7:19–30

Soldi R, Primo L, Brizzi MF, Sanavio F, Aglietta M, Polentarutti N, Pegoraro L, Mantovani A, Bussolino F (1997) Activation of JAK2 in human vascular endothelial cells by granulocyte-macrophage colony-stimulating factor. Blood 89:863–872

Sonderegger I, Iezzi G, Maier R, Schmitz N, Kurrer M, Kopf M (2008) GM-CSF mediates autoimmunity by enhancing IL-6-dependent Th17 cell development and survival. J Exp Med 205:2281–2294

Stanley IJ, Burgess AW (1983) Granulocyte macrophage-colony stimulating factor stimulates the synthesis of membrane and nuclear proteins in murine neutrophils. J Cell Biochem 23:241–258

Stanley E, Lieschke GJ, Grail D, Metcalf D, Hodgson G, Gall JA, Maher DW, Cebon J, Sinickas V, Dunn AR (1994) Granulocyte/macrophage colony-stimulating factor-deficient mice show no major perturbation of hematopoiesis but develop a characteristic pulmonary pathology. Proc Natl Acad Sci U S A 91:5592–5596

Stromnes IM, Cerretti LM, Liggitt D, Harris RA, Goverman JM (2008) Differential regulation of central nervous system autoimmunity by T(H)1 and T(H)17 cells. Nat Med 14:337–342

Takahashi T, Kalka C, Masuda H, Chen D, Silver M, Kearney M, Magner M, Isner JM, Asahara T (1999) Ischemia- and cytokine-induced mobilization of bone marrow-derived endothelial progenitor cells for neovascularization. Nat Med 5:434–438

Tavernier J, Devos R, Cornelis S, Tuypens T, Van der Heyden J, Fiers W, Plaetinck G (1991) A human high affinity interleukin-5 receptor (IL5R) is composed of an IL5-specific alpha chain and a beta chain shared with the receptor for GM-CSF. Cell 66:1175–1184

Timoshanko JR, Kitching AR, Semple TJ, Holdsworth SR, Tipping PG (2005) Granulocyte macrophage colony-stimulating factor expression by both renal parenchymal and immune cells mediates murine crescentic glomerulonephritis. J Am Soc Nephrol 16:2646–2656

Tran EH, Prince EN, Owens T (2000) IFN-gamma shapes immune invasion of the central nervous system via regulation of chemokines. J Immunol 164:2759–2768

Traugott U, Lebon P (1988) Multiple sclerosis: involvement of interferons in lesion pathogenesis. Ann Neurol 24:243–251

Veldhoen M, Hocking RJ, Atkins CJ, Locksley RM, Stockinger B (2006) TGFbeta in the context of an inflammatory cytokine milieu supports de novo differentiation of IL-17-producing T cells. Immunity 24:179–189

Vlahos R, Bozinovski S, Hamilton JA, Anderson GP (2006) Therapeutic potential of treating chronic obstructive pulmonary disease (COPD) by neutralising granulocyte macrophage-colony stimulating factor (GM-CSF). Pharmacol Ther 112:106–115

Wada H, Noguchi Y, Marino MW, Dunn AR, Old LJ (1997) T cell functions in granulocyte/macrophage colony-stimulating factor deficient mice. Proc Natl Acad Sci U S A 94:12557–12561

Whetton AD, Dexter TM (1989) Myeloid haemopoietic growth factors. Biochim Biophys Acta 989:111–132

Williams KC, Ulvestad E, Hickey WF (1994) Immunology of multiple sclerosis. Clin Neurosci 2:229–245

Yamashita N, Tashimo H, Ishida H, Kaneko F, Nakano J, Kato H, Hirai K, Horiuchi T, Ohta K (2002) Attenuation of airway hyperresponsiveness in a murine asthma model by neutralization of granulocyte-macrophage colony-stimulating factor (GM-CSF). Cell Immunol 219:92–97

Young A, Linehan E, Hams E, O'Hara Hall AC, McClurg A, Johnston JA, Hunter CA, Fallon PG, Fitzgerald DC (2012) Cutting edge: suppression of GM-CSF expression in murine and human T Cells by IL-27. J Immunol 189:2079–2083

Zhan Y, Lieschke GJ, Grail D, Dunn AR, Cheers C (1998) Essential roles for granulocyte-macrophage colony-stimulating factor (GM-CSF) and G-CSF in the sustained hematopoietic response of Listeria monocytogenes-infected mice. Blood 91:863–869

Zhang GX, Gran B, Yu S, Li J, Siglienti I, Chen X, Kamoun M, Rostami A (2003) Induction of experimental autoimmune encephalomyelitis in IL-12 receptor-beta 2-deficient mice: IL-12 responsiveness is not required in the pathogenesis of inflammatory demyelination in the central nervous system. J Immunol 170:2153–2160

Zhou L, Chong MM, Littman DR (2009) Plasticity of CD4 + T cell lineage differentiation. Immunity 30:646–655

Zucali JR, Dinarello CA, Oblon DJ, Gross MA, Anderson L, Weiner RS (1986) Interleukin 1 stimulates fibroblasts to produce granulocyte-macrophage colony-stimulating activity and prostaglandin E2. J Clin Invest 77:1857–1863

Chapter 8
The Role of Toll-Like Receptors in Multiple Sclerosis and Experimental Autoimmune Encephalomyelitis

Mukanthu H. Nyirenda, James Crooks and Bruno Gran

8.1 Introduction

Multiple sclerosis (MS) is a chronic disease of the central nervous system (CNS) characterized by inflammation, demyelination and axonal degeneration. The exact cause is unknown; however, both genetic and environmental factors are thought to be involved (Fischer and Ehlers 2008). MS may be mediated by $CD4^+$ T cells that are reactive against myelin antigens (Frohman et al. 2006). These cells are activated in the periphery and express adhesion molecules, which facilitate interactions with ligands present on vascular endothelial cells, resulting in extravasation from the circulation to the CNS compartment (Compston and Coles 2008). Once in the CNS, myelin-reactive $CD4^+$ T cells may be reactivated and lead to the characteristic demyelination and progressive axonal pathology (Frohman et al. 2005). $CD8^+$ T cells and B cells may also contribute to MS pathogenesis (Johnson et al. 2007; Hauser et al. 2008; Racke and Drew 2009).

Experimental autoimmune encephalomyelitis (EAE), an animal model for MS, has been a helpful tool for the study of human disease. EAE develops similar clinical and pathological features to MS. To induce EAE, laboratory animals are immunised with myelin-derived peptides in complete Freund's adjuvant (CFA). CFA contains killed *Mycobacterium tuberculosis* and pathogen-associated molecular patterns (PAMPs) from these bacteria that activate innate immune responses, which in turn promote pathogenic autoreactive T cell responses (Mills 2011). Immunisation usually also requires Pertussis toxin (PT) injection to promote CNS inflammatory infiltration. Many variations of EAE have been developed including acute monophasic, relapsing–remitting and chronic progressive models as well as models for optic neuritis. Importantly, different EAE models mimic different aspects of MS (Steinman and Zamvil 2006) and can be useful tools to address specific aspects of MS pathogenesis (O'Brien et al. 2008). So far, studies on EAE have led to significant breakthroughs

B. Gran (✉) · M. H. Nyirenda · J. Crooks
Division of Clinical Neurosciences, University of Nottingham, C Floor South Block, Queen's Medical Centre, Nottingham NG7 2UH, UK
e-mail: bruno.gran@nottingham.ac.uk

T. Yamamura, B. Gran (eds.), *Multiple Sclerosis Immunology*,
DOI 10.1007/978-1-4614-7953-6_8, © Springer Science+Business Media New York 2013

in understanding the biology of MS and have contributed to the development and approval of at least three MS therapies, glatiramer acetate (GA), mitoxantrone and natalizumab (Steinman and Zamvil 2006; O'Brien et al. 2008; Farooqi et al. 2010; Constantinescu et al. 2011; t Hart et al. 2011).

In addition to lymphocytes that control adaptive immune responses, innate immune cells such as dendritic cells (DCs) and tissue macrophages also play a role in controlling the pathogenesis of MS and EAE. These cells express pattern recognition receptors (PRRs) including Toll-like receptors (TLRs) that recognise PAMPs. Following ligand binding to TLRs, innate immune cells produce pro-inflammatory cytokines and can serve as antigen-presenting cells (APCs) to prime naïve T cells to recognise antigens in the presence of T cell stimuli and co-stimulatory molecules (Takeda and Akira 2005). Thus, TLRs play an important role in linking the innate to the adaptive immune response. In addition, glial cells including astrocytes and microglia play an important role in protecting the CNS against pathogenic insults. However, when chronically activated, such glial cells may contribute to the pathogenesis of MS. This may occur partly through PAMP binding to TLRs present on these cells, which can contribute to the reactivation of myelin-specific autoreactive T cells in the CNS (Sanders and De Keyser 2007; Nair et al. 2008). Interestingly, a variety of resident cells of the CNS express TLRs (Bsibsi et al. 2002). Depending on the TLR evaluated, TLR expression on CNS cells has been demonstrated to contribute to oligodendrocyte and neuron cell death (Lehnardt et al. 2003) or alternatively to be neuroprotective (Bsibsi et al. 2006). It is also interesting that some TLRs are expressed on B cell and T cell populations and that TLR signalling can directly alter adaptive immune responses (Kabelitz 2007; Lampropoulou et al. 2008; Nyirenda et al. 2011).

8.2 Toll-Like Receptors and Their Signalling Pathways

TLRs were the first PRRs to be identified. They are also the best characterized and recognise a wide range of PAMPs. TLRs were first discovered in the fruit fly *Drosophila melanogaster*. Their discovery was based on homology to the Drosophila ortholog protein, Toll (Lemaitre et al. 1996). Toll was found to be required in the fruit fly for proper embryonic development (Anderson et al. 1985). In addition, it was found that flies that lacked Toll were more susceptible to *Aspergillus fumigatus* infection (Lemaitre et al. 1996). This hinted to the possibility that Toll and related proteins may be important in innate immunity to pathogens and was subsequently found in mammals and was named Toll-like receptor (Rock et al. 1998). At least 13 TLRs are known so far in humans and mice (Akira 2003; Akira and Hemmi 2003; Pasare and Medzhitov 2004; Liu and Zhao 2007). Both humans and mice express TLR1–TLR9, in addition, humans, but not mice, express TLR10 and mice exclusively express TLR11–TLR13 (Chaturvedi and Pierce 2009). TLR1, TLR2, TLR4, TLR5 and TLR6 are localised on the cell surface and largely recognise microbial membrane components whereas TLR3, TLR7, TLR8 and TLR9 are expressed within endosomes and recognise nucleic acids (Blasius and Beutler 2010). Recently, it was shown that TLR11, a relative of TLR5 expressed on the cell surface, is also expressed in intracellular compartments (Pifer et al. 2011). TLR13 is also expressed in intracellular vesicles although its cognate PAMP has not yet been identified (Blasius and Beutler 2010).

In addition to TLRs, other PRRs exist that are also involved in PAMP recognition and the control of innate immunity. These include membrane-bound C-type lectin receptors (CLRs), cytosolic proteins such as nucleotide-binding oligomerization domain (NOD)-like receptors (NLRs), retinoic acid-inducible gene 1 (RIG-I)-like receptors (RLRs), unidentified proteins that mediate sensing of cytosolic DNA or retrovirus infection (Elinav et al. 2011; Kawai and Akira 2011). CLRs are a large superfamily of membrane proteins comprised of one or more C-type lectin-like domains, which largely elicit inflammatory responses by recognising fungal and bacterial PAMPs. RLRs, which include RIG-I, MDA5 and LGP2 are RNA helicases that recognise RNA species released into the cytoplasm in a variety of cell types and coordinate antiviral programmes via type I IFN induction (Kawai and Akira 2011). More than 20 members of the NLR family exist (Barbalat et al. 2011).

TLRs are type 1 membrane-spanning receptors that consist of extracellular leucine-rich repeats (LRRs), a transmembrane domain and a cytoplasmic Toll/interleukin-1 receptor (TIR) domain, the presence of which defines membership of the family. Downstream signalling is achieved by the presence of cytoplasmic TIR-containing adaptor proteins (Akira et al. 2006). There are five TIR domain-containing adaptors including MyD88, TIR domain-containing adaptor inducing IFN-β (TRIF; also known as TICAM −1), TIRAP/Mal, TRIF-related adaptor molecule (TRAM) and sterile-alpha and armadillo motif-containing protein (SARM) (Takeuchi and Akira 2010). TLR signalling can be divided into two distinct pathways depending on the usage of the distinct adaptor molecules, MyD88 and TRIF (Fig. 8.1).

MyD88 is essential for the downstream signalling of all known TLRs, except TLR3. Both TLR2 and TLR4 require TIRAP/Mal for bridging between TLR and MyD88. In contrast, TLR4 signalling following lipopolysaccharide (LPS) stimulation requires Mal, MyD88 and TRAM as a bridging adapter to TRIF to mediate MyD88-independent signalling (O'Neill and Bowie 2007). MyD88 interacts with IL-1R-associated kinase (IRAK)-4, a serine/threonine kinase with an N-terminal death domain. IRAK-4 activates other IRAK family members, IRAK-1 and IRAK-2 (Kawagoe et al. 2008). The IRAKs then dissociate from MyD88 and interact with TNFR-associated factor 6 (TRAF6). TRAF6 acts as an ubiquitin E3 ligases and with its E2 counterparts, Uev1A and Ubc13, catalyses the formation of a lysine 63 (K63)-linked polyubiquitin chain on TRAF6 as well as the generation of an unconjugated free polyubiquitin chain (Xia et al. 2009; Takeuchi and Akira 2010).

A complex of TGF-β-activated kinase 1 (TAK1), TAK1-binding protein 1 (TAB1), TAB2 and TAB3 is activated by the unconjugated free K63 polyubiquitin chain and phosphorylates Ikβ kinase (IKK)-β and MAP kinase kinase 6. Consequently, the IKK complex composed of IKK-α, IKK-β and NF-κβ essential modulator (NEMO), phosphorylates IκB, an NF-κB inhibitory protein (Takeuchi and Akira 2010). Phosphorylated IκB undergoes degradation by the ubiquitin-proteasome system, enabling

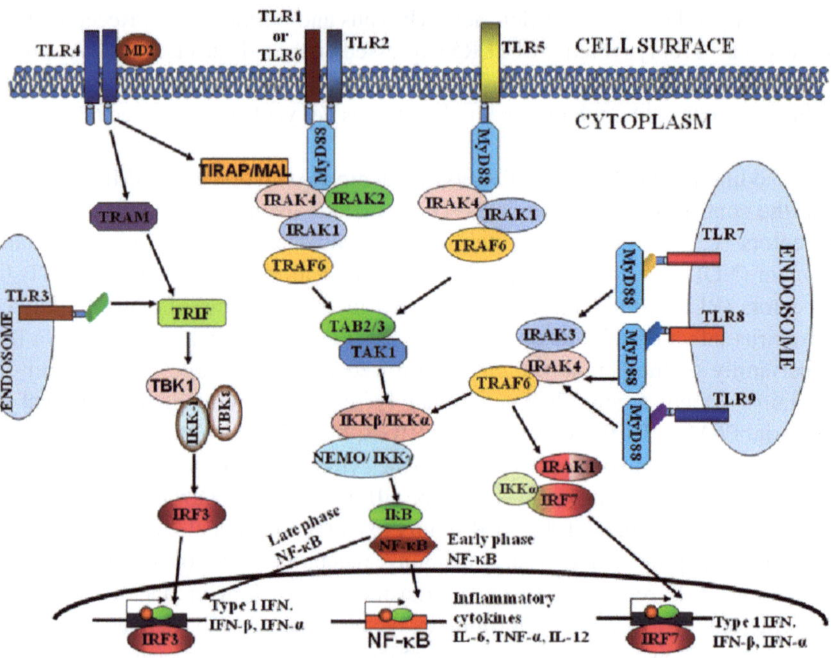

Fig. 8.1 Toll-like receptor (TLR) signalling pathways. Upon activation by ligands, TLRs recruit Toll/interleukin-1 receptor (TIR) adapter proteins MyD88, Mal, TRAM and TRIF, which lead to recruitment of IRAKs and consequently the induction of NF-κB-dependent genes, including TNF-α, IL-12 and IL-6. TLR3 and TLR4 also signal via TRAM and TRIF leading to IRF3-dependent gene expression. In addition, IRF7 is activated downstream of TLR7, TLR8 and TLR9, which leads to IRF7-dependent gene expression, including IFN-β and IFN-inducible genes

NF-κB to translocate into the nucleus and activate expression of pro-inflammatory cytokine genes. Activation of the MAP kinase cascade is responsible for the formation of another transcription factor complex, AP-1, that targets cytokine genes (Takeuchi and Akira 2010). A separate pathway to NF-κB and MAP kinase activation following TLR3 and TLR4 stimulation is mediated by TRIF independent of MyD88. TLR4 triggers both MyD88-dependent and TRIF-dependent signalling. TLR4, but not TLR3, requires another adaptor, TRAM, for activating TRIF (Takeuchi and Akira 2010).

8.3 Toll-Like Receptor Ligands

Of all PRRs in innate immunity, TLR2 recognises the structurally broadest range of bacterial compounds. This is possible because TLR2 forms heterodimers with either TLR1 or TLR6, thus broadening the spectrum of its ligands (Ozinsky et al. 2000; Takeuchi et al. 2002) and with the lipid scavenger receptor molecule

CD36 in response to diacylated lipoproteins (Hoebe et al. 2005). For example, TLR2 recognises peptidoglycan (PGN) from Gram-positive bacteria such as *Staphylococcus aureus*, lipoproteins and lipopeptides (LP) from several bacteria, glycophosphatidylinositol anchors from *Trypanosoma cruzi*, lipoarabinomannan from *M. tuberculosis*, porins from *Neisseria meningitidis* and zymosan from yeast cell wall (Akira 2003). TLR2 also recognises synthetic triacylated LP such as *N*-palmitoyl-*S*-[2,3-bis(palmitoyloxy)-(2RS)-propyl]-[R]-Cys-[S]-Ser-[S]-Lys (4) trihydrochloride (Pam3CSK4/Pam3Cys) that mimics the acylated amino terminus of bacterial LPs (Akira 2003). TLR10 is another candidate, which could form a heterodimer with TLR2 on B cells and plasmacytoid dendritic cells (pDCs) (Guan et al. 2010). Moreover, molecular modelling studies revealed that Pam3CysSK4, a potent agonist for the TLR2/1 heterodimer, may also be the ligand for the human (h) TLR10/2 complex, while Pam2CysPamSK4, a diacylated peptide, may activate hTLR10/1 heterodimer and hTLR10 homodimer (Govindaraj et al. 2010).

In addition to bacterial ligands, TLR2 has also been shown to recognise viral-derived ligands. For example, the envelope proteins from respiratory syncytial virus (RSV) have been shown to induce inflammatory cytokines and chemokines through TLR2 and TLR6 (Murawski et al. 2009). Furthermore, it was demonstrated that TLR2 and TLR6 played an essential role in controlling RSV infection in vivo. In addition to RSV, the haemagglutinin protein of the measles virus was also reported to be recognised by TLR2 (Kumar et al. 2009). Of note is that this recognition induced the production of type I IFNs by inflammatory monocytes (Kumar et al. 2009; Kawai and Akira 2010).

TLRs are also involved in sensing endogenous signals generated during tissue injury. One class of endogenous TLR2 ligands are the heat shock proteins (HSP), in particular HSP60, HSP70, HSP90, GP96 and HSP22 were reported to be recognised by TLR2 and TLR4 (Wallin et al. 2002; Roelofs et al. 2006; Warger et al. 2006). It has been shown that the high-mobility group box 1 (HMGB1), an alarmin protein released from necrotic cells, acts as an endogenous ligand for TLR2 and TLR4 to induce the production of pro-inflammatory cytokines (Takeuchi and Akira 2010). Reports have shown that small molecular weight fragments of hyaluronic acid (HA), biglycan and versican produced by tumour cells can trigger TLR2 and TLR4 activation (Jiang et al. 2005; Schaefer et al. 2005; Kim et al. 2009). Both biglycan and HA fragments accumulate during tissue injury and activate macrophages to produce inflammatory chemokines and cytokines via TLR2 and TLR4 (Jiang et al. 2005; Schaefer et al. 2005). It was reported that biglycan-deficient mice were less susceptible to death caused by TLR2 (Schaefer et al. 2005). These studies indicate that several endogenous ligands may provide signals through TLRs to initiate inflammatory diseases by non-microbial agents.

TLR3, an intracellular receptor, is activated by viral double-stranded (ds)RNA (Liu and Zhao 2007). dsRNA induces the production of IFN-α, IFN-β and IFN-inducible genes (Takeda and Akira 2005). TLR3 also recognises polyinosinic:polycytidylic acid (poly I:C), a synthetic analogue of viral dsRNA (O'Brien et al. 2008), which also activates the cytosolic receptor MDA-5.

TLR4, also referred to as CD284, detects LPS, which is one of the major constituent of the outer membrane of Gram-negative bacteria. LPS comprises polysaccharide side chains, core oligosaccharide and lipid A. Lipid A consists of unusual fatty acids such as hydroxymyristic acid (O'Brien et al. 2008). It is embedded into the outer membrane and is responsible for the toxicity of LPS. After being released into the bloodstream, LPS is captured immediately by LPS-binding protein, a specific lipid transfer protein that delivers LPS to CD14 present on the surfaces of mononuclear phagocytes. CD14 lacks a transmembrane domain therefore it is incapable of transducing signals, suggesting that other molecules are responsible for LPS signalling. The interaction of LPS with TLR4 requires MD-2, which associates with the extracellular domain of TLR4 (Akira 2003).

TLR5, a cell surface receptor, is activated by flagellin, a protein expressed on motile bacteria (Gewirtz et al. 2001). TLR7 and TLR8 are structurally highly conserved molecules. They are activated by single-stranded (ss)RNA from viruses. TLR7 has been shown to recognise synthetic compounds imidazoquinolines such as imiquimod. In addition, both TLR7 and human TLR8 recognise guanosine or uridine-rich ssRNA from viruses such as influenza virus and human immunodeficiency virus (HIV) (O'Brien et al. 2008).

TLR9 is essential for responses to bacterial and viral DNA. In addition, TLR9 recognises synthetic oligodeoxynucleotides-containing unmethylated CpG dinucleotides (CpG DNA). These oligonucleotides have been shown to stimulate the proliferation of B cells and to activate macrophages and DCs to secrete cytokines, especially Th1 cytokines such as IL-18 and IL-12 (Akira 2003; Liu and Zhao 2007). Both TLR7 and TLR9 are highly expressed in pDCs (O'Brien et al. 2008; O'Brien et al. 2010).

8.4 Toll-Like Receptor Expression and Function in T Cells

TLRs are widely distributed and are expressed at varying levels by immune cells including DCs, macrophages and B cells (Hornung et al. 2002; Erridge 2010; Mills 2011), but also in non-immune epithelial and endothelial cells (Cristofaro and Opal 2003; Hornef and Bogdan 2005). Interestingly, TLRs have also been shown to be expressed by T cells including, cytotoxic T lymphocytes (CTLs) and most excitingly, regulatory T cells (Tregs) (Caramalho et al. 2003; Caron et al. 2005; Nyirenda et al. 2011). The first studies focusing on TLR expression in human T cells reported the detectable production of nearly all TLR-encoding mRNAs (Hornung et al. 2002; Zarember and Godowski 2002). It has also been reported that high levels of TLR8 were expressed by human $CD25^{hi}CD4^{+}$ Tregs but not $CD25^{-}$ naïve $CD4^{+}$ T cells (Peng et al. 2005). Another group working on magnetically purified human Tregs described increased expression of TLR4 on $CD4^{+}CD25^{+}$ Tregs as compared to $CD4^{+}CD25^{-}$ T cells (Lewkowicz et al. 2006). Crellin et al. reported that Tregs expressed higher levels of TLR5 mRNA (Crellin et al. 2005). In another study, purified tonsillar T cells expressed mRNA for TLR1, TLR2, TLR3, TLR5, TLR9 and

TLR10, with distinct differences between $CD4^+$ and $CD8^+$ subsets (Mansson et al. 2006). TLR mRNA was also detected in purified murine T cells, again with substantial variability among different studies. Sorted naïve $CD45RB^{high}CD4^+$ T cells from C57/BL6 mice expressed TLR1, TLR2, TLR3, TLR6 and TLR7 but not TLR4, TLR5 and TLR9 mRNA as shown by reverse transcriptase polymerase chain reaction (PCR) or quantitative PCR (qPCR) (Caramalho et al. 2003; Sobek et al. 2004). By contrast, activated and memory $CD45RB^{low}CD4^+$ T cells, and particularly the $CD25^+$ subset, expressed TLR4 and TLR5 (Caramalho et al. 2003). However, Gelman et al. reported that TLR3, TLR4, TLR5 and TLR9 but not TLR2 was detected in naïve $CD4^+$ T cells from BALB/c mice (Gelman et al. 2004).

TLR expression has also been investigated in highly purified $CD8^+$ T cells from C57BL/6 and TCR-transgenic mice. These studies revealed the presence of TLR1, TLR2, TLR6, TLR7 and TLR9, yet little if any TLR3, TLR4, TLR5 and TLR8 in $CD8^+$ T cells (Cottalorda et al. 2006). Recently, we and others demonstrated the expression of TLR2 by subsets of human Tregs (Oberg et al. 2010; Nyirenda et al. 2011). TLR2 agonists have also been shown to promote the differentiation of mouse (Reynolds et al. 2010) and human (Nyirenda et al. 2011) Th17 cells in vitro. In addition, it has been reported that PAMP-induced secretion of pro-inflammatory cytokines from monocytes and DCs promotes the induction and proliferation of Th17 cells (Higgins et al. 2006; Evans et al. 2007; van Beelen et al. 2007; Mills 2011). For example, human monocytes stimulated with LPS, zymosan, flagellin or lipoteichoic acid promote IL-17 production by human $CD4^+$ T cells that are activated using a CD3-specific antibody (Evans et al. 2007). The TLR-induced signal was not identified, but addition of IL-6 or TGF-β inhibited IL-17 production in this setting. Another group showed that *Candida albicans* hyphae selectively promote Th17 cell induction by inducing IL-23 but not IL-12 production from human monocytes and DCs (Acosta-Rodriguez et al. 2007; Mills 2011). Furthermore, it has been shown that ligands for TLR3, TLR4 or TLR9 induce MyD88- dependent production of cytokines from DCs, and this promotes the differentiation of Th17 cells (Veldhoen et al. 2006; Mills 2011). Moreover, the TLR4 ligand LPS promotes IL-17 production by antigen-specific memory T cells in mice through the induction of IL-1 and IL-23 production by DCs (Higgins et al. 2006; Mills 2011).

Studies have also shown that Th17 cells can be induced independently of TLR and NLR activation through the activation of dectin 1 by the β-glucan curdlan, which promotes IL-6, TNF and IL-23 production by DCs (LeibundGut-Landmann et al. 2007; Mills 2011). In addition, bacterial ligands of NOD2, such as muramyl dipeptide (MDP), have been shown to drive IL-17 production by human memory T cells by stimulating IL-1 and IL-23 production by DCs (van Beelen et al. 2007). Furthermore, it has been reported that commensal microorganisms can promote the differentiation of Th17 cells in the lamina propria of mice that are deficient in MyD88 and TLR3, suggesting that TLR and IL-1R signalling is not essential for the induction of Th17 cells in the gut (Tigno-Aranjuez et al. 2009).

8.5 Modulation of Treg Functions by Toll-Like Receptors

Tregs play a central role in maintaining tolerance to self-antigens and preventing autoimmune responses harmful to the host. However, during acute infection, Tregs might hinder effector T cell (Teff) activity directed towards the elimination of the pathogenic challenge. Therefore, Treg-mediated suppression needs to be tightly controlled. Control of Treg function is known to occur through cytokines such as IL-1, IL-6 and IL-12, and multiple co-stimulatory molecules expressed by APCs (Kubo et al. 2004; Sutmuller et al. 2006b). Another key cytokine that supports Treg development and suppressive activity is IL-2 (Kubo et al. 2004; Scheffold et al. 2005). IL-15, which signals through the common IL-2 receptor β and γ chains, is able to substitute IL-2 as a growth factor in vitro, while IL-4 and IL-7 can act as growth and survival factors, respectively (Sutmuller et al. 2006b). These cytokines and co-stimulatory molecules are efficiently induced upon TLR stimulation of APCs and act either by direct stimulation of Treg proliferation and/or inhibition of Treg suppression or indirectly by rescuing Teffs from Treg-mediated suppression (Amiset et al. 2012).

Certain TLRs are expressed not only on APCs, but also on T cell subsets, including Tregs. Activation of TLRs has been reported to either increase or inhibit Treg functions, with opposite consequences depending on factors such as the specific TLRs involved and concentration of TLR agonists (Crellin et al. 2005; Liu et al. 2006; Zanin-Zhorov et al. 2006; Nyirenda et al. 2011). Several studies have shown that TLR activation can lead to reduced Treg function. Stimulation of TLR2 by the synthetic bacterial LP Pam3Cys-SK4 transiently reduced the suppressive function of murine and human Tregs (Liu et al. 2006; Sutmuller et al. 2006a, 2006b; Oberg et al. 2010; Nyirenda et al. 2011). We recently reported that Pam3Cys-SK4, an agonist of the TLR1/2 heterodimer, reduces the suppressive functions of human $CD4^{+}CD25^{+}CD127^{neg}FOXP3^{+}$ Tregs, whereas FSL-1 (a ligand for the TLR2/6 heterodimer) does not, suggesting a predominant role of TLR1/2 in modulating Treg functions. In addition, TLR2 stimulation reduced the suppressive functions of Tregs classified as naïve ($FOXP3^{low}CD45RA^{+}$) and effector-memory ($FOXP3^{hi}CD45RA^{-}$) (Ayyoub et al. 2009; Beriou et al. 2009; Miyara et al. 2009; Nyirenda et al. 2011). Furthermore, we showed that TLR2 stimulation induced Tregs to produce IL-17A/F and that neutralisation of IL-6-abrogated Pam3Cys-mediated reduction of Treg suppressive activity. Our data point to a mechanistic link between IL-6 production and reduced suppressive function of Tregs. Pam3Cys also led to increased production of IL-17, the neutralisation of which reversed the inhibition of suppression induced by TLR2. Data in our report are consistent with a model in which Tregs may become skewed towards a Th17 phenotype and effector function under inflammatory conditions in the presence of TLR2 stimuli. Such modulation of Treg phenotype and function may allow more effective protection against inflammation but may lead to increased susceptibility to autoimmune reactions (Viglietta et al. 2004; Nyirenda et al. 2009; Nyirenda et al. 2011) (Fig. 8.2).

Other TLRs have been shown also to reduce Treg function. Peng et al. reported that synthetic and natural ligands for human TLR8 can reverse the suppressive function

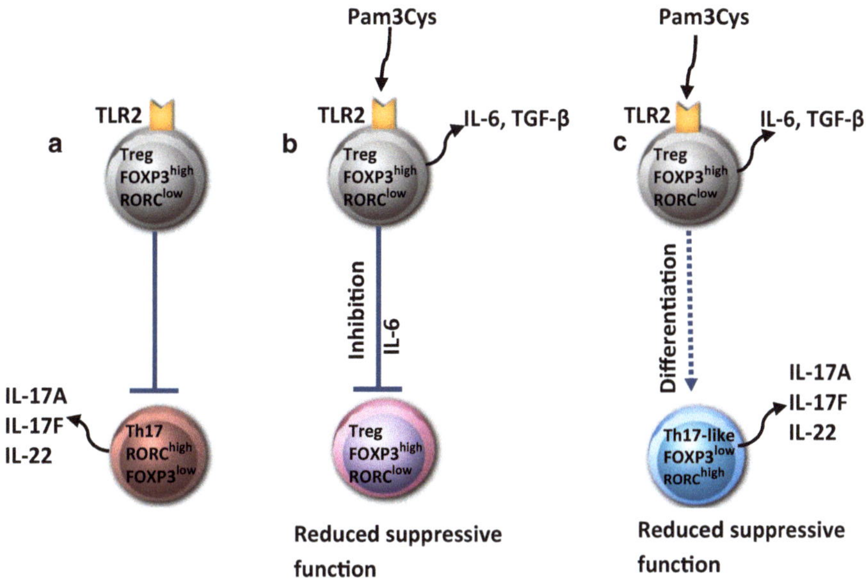

Fig. 8.2 Reduced suppressive function of Tregs and Th17 development after TLR2 stimulation. **a** Tregs suppress the proliferation of Th17 and effector cell proliferation. **b** TLR2 stimulation enhances the production and secretion of IL-6, which inhibits the suppressive functions of Tregs. **c** TLR2 stimulation also promotes the differentiation of Tregs towards a Th17-like phenotype with reduced suppressive function

of Tregs. They also demonstrated that transfer of TLR8 ligand-stimulated Tregs into tumour-bearing mice enhanced anti-tumour immunity (Peng et al. 2005). This was interpreted as the consequence of reduced Treg activity. Another group reported that stimulation with TLR9 ligands such as oligodeoxynucleotides-containing unmethylated CpG motifs (CpG ODN) reduced the suppressive functions of Tregs (Bach 2005). In this system, however, both reduced suppressive Treg function and direct co-stimulation of effector cells by CpG ODN were observed (Gelman et al. 2006).

TLR stimulation on Tregs can also enhance their suppressive function (Caramalho et al. 2003). It has been shown that the TLR4 agonist LPS enhanced the suppressive function of murine $CD4^+CD25^+$ Tregs (Caramalho et al. 2003). Specifically, the suppressive activity of naturally activated $CD45RB^{low}$ T cells was enhanced by culture with LPS whether these T cells were $CD25^+$ or $CD25^-$ (Caramalho et al. 2003). Engagement of TLR5 with the agonist flagellin enhanced the proliferation of Teffs and the suppressive function as well as Foxp3 expression of Tregs (Crellin et al. 2005). Another group reported increased suppressive function of human Tregs after stimulation with the TLR2 agonist HSP60 (Zanin-Zhorov et al. 2006). In co-cultures of Tregs and Teffs, they found that HSP60 and p277, a HSP60-derived peptide, enhanced Treg function through both contact-dependent and cytokine-dependent mechanisms. The effects of HSP60 on $CD4^+CD25^+$ T cells were specifically TLR2-dependent as demonstrated by experiments with neutralising antibodies (Zanin-Zhorov et al.

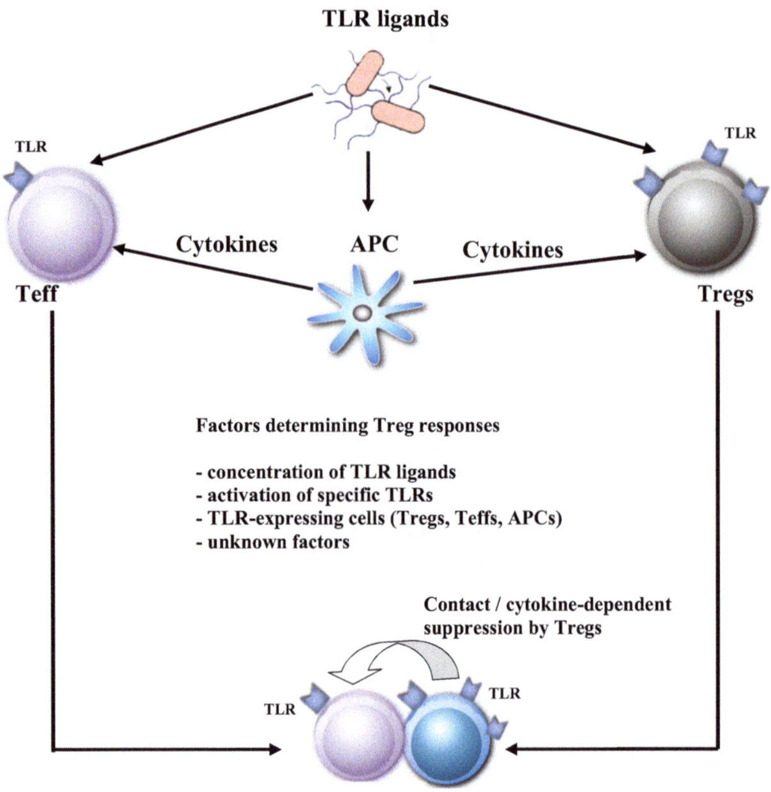

Fig. 8.3 Modulation of Treg function by Toll-like receptor (TLR) ligands. Microbial components can be recognised by TLRs expressed not only on APCs, but also on $CD4^{+}CD25^{hi}$ Tregs and, to a lesser extent, on $CD4^{+}CD25^{-}$ Teff. The figure shows both direct and APC-mediated effects of TLR activation on the functions of Tregs. Suppressive functions can be either decreased or enhanced depending on factors that include the concentration of TLR ligands and the specific TLRs involved

2006). The discrepancy between a report by Zanin-Zhorov et al. and those cited above could possibly be explained by concentrations of the ligands used or differences in the ways endogenous and exogenous ligands interact with TLR2. Enhancing Treg function with TLR stimuli could be used to enhance or restore immune tolerance to self-antigens. The previously cited studies suggest that several factors may be involved in the functional consequences of TLR activation on Tregs (Fig. 8.3).

8.6 Expression and Function of Toll-Like Receptors in B Cells

It is widely accepted that B cells play a role in the pathogenesis of MS and EAE (Racke 2008). This has been supported by the discovery of B cell germinal centre-like structures in the brains of MS patients with advanced secondary progressive disease (Magliozzi et al. 2007), however, the presence of cerebro spinal fluid (CSF) oligoclonal bands (IgG bands unique to the CSF) in over 90 % of people with MS had been known for decades (Kabat et al. 1942). In addition, the success of a clinical trial of rituximab, a monoclonal antibody that depletes B cells and reduces inflammatory disease activity without affecting immunoglobulin levels, pointed to an important role for B cells in relapsing forms of MS (Hauser et al. 2008).

Besides the production of autoantibodies, an additional concept of B cell involvement in MS emerged when Serafini et al. detected meningeal B cell aggregates in about 40 % of patients with late-stage secondary progressive-multiple sclerosis (SP-MS) (Serafini et al. 2004; Aloisi and Pujol-Borrell 2006). It was found that these patients had displayed an earlier onset and higher severity of disease, pointing to the potentially important role of B cells in the CNS itself. The authors observed that the aggregates were localised in cerebral sulci adjacent to subpial lesions, within structures reminiscent of germinal centres containing B cells, plasma cells, T cells, macrophages and a network of follicular dendritic cells (FDC) comparable to classical peripheral lymphoid follicles (Serafini et al. 2004; Aloisi and Pujol-Borrell 2006; Harp et al. 2007). Brains containing B cell aggregates exhibited more severe grey matter lesions with increased demyelination and neuronal damage while white matter lesions did not differ from other MS patients. It has therefore been suggested that ectopic B cell aggregates were responsible for grey matter pathology mediated by antibodies, cytokines or proteolytic enzymes (Magliozzi et al. 2007; Choi et al. 2012).

B cells have been shown to affect MS directly through the production of regulatory cytokines such as IL-10 and TGF-β and also have effect on the disease through the production of antibodies (Mizoguchi and Bhan 2006). TLR activation can also affect B cell function. It has been shown that stimulation of B cells with either TLR4 or TLR9 agonists resulted in production of IL-10 producing regulatory B cells, which were shown to reduce levels of inflammation and aid recovery in EAE (Fillatreau et al. 2002). Another study showed that MyD88-dependent stimulation of both TLR4 and TLR9 in B cells led to suppression of both Th1 and Th17 cells through the production of IL-10 and TGF-β (Lampropoulou et al. 2008).

Matsushita et al. reported that EAE induced with recombinant MOG antigen required B cells; whereas MOG peptide-induced EAE was independent of B cells (Matsushita et al. 2010). Depletion of B cell populations with anti-CD20 led to time-dependent outcomes in that prophylactic administration of anti-CD20 before EAE induction increased disease severity and therapeutic administration suppressed disease, suggesting that a regulatory B cell population may influence early stages of the disease (Matsushita et al. 2010; Dobson et al. 2011).

8.7 The Function of Toll-Like Receptors in Multiple Sclerosis

TLRs are expressed in the CNS and were shown to be increased during inflammation (Bsibsi et al. 2002). The involvement of TLRs in the pathogenesis of MS was further suggested by the enhanced TLR expression in microglia in active MS lesions

(Jack et al. 2005). In cultures of human microglia, it was shown that ligation of TLR3 and TLR4 by dsRNA and LPS, respectively, induced the secretion of the chemokine CXCL10, which is a potent chemoattractant for T cells and is thought to play a role in the MS lesion (Jack et al. 2005). Several endogenous TLR ligands have been identified in the MS lesions (Lassmann 2008). For example, HMGB1, a nuclear DNA-binding protein, has been identified in active lesions of MS and EAE (Andersson et al. 2008). HMGB1 is as a potent pro-inflammatory signal and its inflammatory effects occur through TLR2 or TLR4 activation (Sloane et al. 2010). In addition, it has been reported that the pro-inflammatory cytokine IL-23p19 was expressed in macrophages and microglia in human MS white matter lesions. Of note is that its expression in human microglia was induced via TLR2 and/or TLR4 signalling (Li et al. 2007). Baseline expression of TLR2 is increased in patients with MS (Correale and Farez 2009) and activation of TLR2 and its downstream PARP-1 pathway can have a therapeutic effect on the symptoms of patients with MS (Farez et al. 2009).

Of note, several reports have shown a relationship between infections and MS exacerbations (Sibley et al. 1985; Edwards et al. 1998; Buljevac et al. 2002; Levin et al. 2003; Correale et al. 2006). Available evidence suggests that clinical manifestations of exacerbation are the result of focal areas of CNS inflammation that block impulse conduction caused by direct effects of inflammatory mediators, the demyelination of axons or both (Edwards et al. 1998; Buljevac et al. 2002). In addition, an association between urinary tract infections (UTIs) and relapses in MS patients has been demonstrated (Metz et al. 1998). Urinary tract dysfunction affects up to 90 % of the MS population and UTIs were encountered in up to 74 % of the tested population (Metz et al. 1998; Hillman et al. 2000). An exacerbation of disease activity following manifestation of UTI, 80 % of which are caused by the Gram-negative bacteria, *Escherichia coli* and other pathogens such as the Gram-positive *Staphylococcus saprophyticus* have been reported (Correale et al. 2006; Nicolle 2008). Cell walls or membranes of these pathogens contain components such as LPs, lipoteichoic acid or PGN, all of which are either known or predicted TLR1/2 agonists (Schwandner et al. 1999; Yoshimura et al. 1999; Zahringer et al. 2008). Viral infections have also been associated with MS susceptibility and with clinical exacerbations. MS patients may be infected by measles, mumps and rubella at a later age than healthy individuals (Martyn et al. 1993). In the last 10 years, strong epidemiological data have linked Epstein-Barr virus (EBV) infection with MS (Martyn et al. 1993; Ascherio and Munch 2000; Levin et al. 2003; Thacker et al. 2006). Interestingly, induction of pro-inflammatory mediators in response to herpes simplex virus (HSV) infection has been shown to be mediated through TLR2-dependent mechanisms (Schachtele et al. 2010). That study demonstrated the importance of microglial cell TLR2 in inducing oxidative stress and neuronal damage in response to viral infection. In addition, others have reported that UV-inactivated EBV virions led to the activation of NF-κB through TLR2, suggesting that TLR2 may be an important PRR in the immune response against EBV infection (Gaudreault et al. 2007; Ariza et al. 2009). Moreover, it was reported that TLR2 was required for the production of inflammatory cytokines by microglial cells in response to HSV-1, thus supporting a role for TLR2 in the pathogenesis of HSV-1-induced encephalitis (Aravalli et al. 2005). In addition, varicella zoster virus (VZV) was found to induce the release of IL-6 in primary human monocytes in a TLR2-dependent manner (Wang et al. 2005). Our data suggest that the occurrence of relapses in relapsing-remitting-multiple sclerosis (RR-MS) patients following certain UTI or viral infections could be mediated by stimulation of TLR2 on Tregs, leading to loss of their suppressive functions and differentiation into a pathogenic Th17 lineage (Reynolds et al. 2010; Nyirenda et al. 2011; Amiset et al. 2012).

A recent study by Bustamante et al. showed that baseline expression of IRAK3, a negative regulator of TLR4 primarily expressed on monocytes, was reduced in patients that responded to IFN-β treatment compared with patients that did not respond. This suggests a role for TLR4 and its associated pathways in response to IFN-β treatment (Bustamante et al. 2011). It has also been shown that treatment with IFN-β causes an upregulation of TLR7 on DCs leading to reduction of IL-1 and IL-23 production and inhibition of Th17 differentiation (Zhang et al. 2009).

In relation to TLR9 function, treatment with IFN-β was shown to affect the function of pDCs through TLR9. pDCs from patients on IFN-β treatment produced lower levels of pro-inflammatory cytokines in response to TLR9 agonists than non-IFN-β-treated patients, suggesting that IFN-β may have an immunomodulatory effect on TLR9 function (Balashov et al. 2010). In addition, TLR9 has been proposed to have a protective effect in MS through the production of IL-10 from B cells. It has been shown that TLR9-mediated production of IL-10 was severely reduced in B cells from MS patients when stimulated with TLR9 agonist CpG compared to healthy controls, which was due to a reduced expression of TLR9 on B cells in MS patients (Hirotani et al. 2010).

8.8 Toll-Like Receptor Function in Experimental Autoimmune Encephalomyelitis

EAE develops similar clinical and pathological features to MS. To induce EAE, laboratory animals are immunised with myelin-derived peptides in CFA. CFA contains killed *M. tuberculosis* and PAMPs from these bacteria activate innate immune responses, which in turn promote pathogenic autoreactive T cell responses (Mills 2011). Immunisations are often supplemented with PT, which may promote CNS inflammatory infiltration through the activation of TLR4 (Kerfoot et al. 2004). Many variations of EAE have been developed including acute monophasic, relapsing–remitting and chronic progressive models as well as models for optic neuritis. Importantly, different EAE models mimic different aspects of MS (Steinman and Zamvil 2006). Each of these EAE models can be useful tools to address specific aspects of MS pathogenesis (O'Brien et al. 2008; Constantinescu et al. 2011; t Hart et al. 2011). So far, studies on EAE have led to significant breakthroughs in understanding the biology of MS and have contributed in the development and approval of at least three MS therapies, GA, mitoxantrone and natalizumab (Steinman and Zamvil 2006; O'Brien et al. 2008).

TLR signalling through the MyD88- dependent pathway has been suggested to play a significant role in regulating the development of EAE. Prinz et al. reported that MyD88 knockout mice were resistant to the development of active EAE, further supporting a role of MyD88-dependent signalling in disease development (Prinz et al. 2006). Interestingly, T cells derived from MyD88-deficient (−/−) mice did not significantly respond to their cognate antigen, suggesting that MyD88−/− mice did not develop active EAE, partly because of the inadequate T cell priming in the periphery (Prinz et al. 2006). However, bone marrow chimera studies indicated that MyD88 expression in the CNS also played a significant role in controlling the development of EAE. Adoptive transfer of myelin-specific T cells into MyD88−/− mice resulted in decreased severity of EAE relative to wild-type animals (Prinz et al. 2006).

8.8.1 The Role of Cell Surface Toll-Like Receptors

A number of studies have supported a role of TLR2 in modulating EAE. TLR2 serves as a ligand for Gram-positive bacteria including *Staphylococcus aureus* and *Streptococcus pneumoniae*. Molecules present in the cell wall of these organisms, such as PGN, serve as PAMPs that are capable of activating TLR2. *S. aureus* PGN added to incomplete Freund's adjuvant (IFA) was demonstrated to stimulate the development of EAE in C57BL/6 mice (Visser et al. 2005). In vitro studies showed that PGN-pulsed DCs stimulated T cell proliferation, drove T cell differentiation towards a Th1 phenotype and facilitated the development of EAE, suggesting that PGN signalling through TLR2 stimulated DC maturation, antigen presentation and production of effector molecules that resulted in Th1 cell differentiation and development of EAE. Other studies have demonstrated that infection of mice with *S. pneumoniae* was capable of increasing the severity of EAE, although this depended on the timing of infection relative to immunisation (Herrmann et al. 2006). Interestingly, these studies demonstrated that the effects of *S. pneumoniae* on EAE were TLR2-dependent, as TLR2−/− animals did not develop more severe EAE (Herrmann et al. 2006).

In addition, Laman et al. also demonstrated that PGN was observed in association with APCs in the CNS of MS patients as well as nonhuman primates (Visser et al. 2006). Furthermore, PGN-laden APCs were increased in the CNS of EAE animals, suggesting that PGN and possibly other TLR agonists were capable of accessing the CNS during EAE (Visser et al. 2006). This could facilitate the reactivation of myelin-reactive T cells in the target tissue in EAE and MS. Reynolds et al. reported that TLR2 promoted Th17 responses and mediated EAE. They observed that loss of TLR2 in $CD4^+$ T cells ameliorated EAE compared with wild-type controls (Reynolds et al. 2010). Adoptive transfer of TLR2-deficient T cells led to more dramatic reduction in disease severity and Th17 production, suggesting an important role of TLR2 in the induction of EAE (Reynolds et al. 2010).

It has also been shown in mouse models that TLR2 may play a role in the prevention of the remyelination of damaged axons. It has been proposed that activation of TLR2 on the surface of oligodendrocytes prevents the maturation of the cell rendering them unable to remyelinate damage axons (Sloane et al. 2010). It is reported that hyaluronan, a glycosaminoglycan present in the core of MS lesions, prevents maturation of oligodendrocytes through TLR2/MyD88 signalling and thus prevents the cell fulfilling its role in the remyelination of damaged axons within the lesion (Sloane et al. 2010). This effect was shown to be specific to TLR2 as the inhibitory action of hyaluronan on oligodendrocyte maturation was removed in the presence of neutralising antibodies to TLR2 but not to other hyaluronan-sensitive receptors TLR4 and CD44 (Hanafy and Sloane 2011). This effect was further proven when it was shown that TLR2−/− mice show a quicker and more efficient remyelination then wild-type mice (Hanafy and Sloane 2011).

EAE is commonly induced in susceptible mouse and rat strains by immunisation with myelin peptides emulsified in CFA. Importantly, *M. tuberculosis* present in CFA is known to activate a variety of TLRs, including TLR1, TLR2 and TLR4 (Hansen et al. 2006). Indeed, it was reported that mice immunised with myelin peptides in the presence of IFA did not develop EAE, but developed disease when *M. tuberculosis* was added to the adjuvant (Hansen et al. 2006). While agonists of most TLRs reconstituted the full adjuvant properties of IFA, the only exception were agonists of TLR3 (Hansen et al. 2006), confirming that the MyD88-independent, TRIF-dependent pathway has different properties as compared with the MyD88-dependent signalling pathway (Hansen et al. 2006; O'Brien et al. 2008) as they lead to preferential induction of endogenous type I interferons (O'Brien et al. 2008). Such properties of the TLR3-TRIF pathway underlie the observation that TLR3 activation can suppress EAE by the induction of endogenous IFN-β in both relapsing EAE in the SJL/J mouse and chronic EAE in the C57BL/6 mouse (Touil et al. 2006; Tzima et al. 2009). This demonstrates in principle the feasibility of inducing endogenous type I IFN as an alternative to the administration of recombinant-type IFN in patients with MS (Touil et al. 2006; O'Brien et al. 2008; O'Brien et al. 2010).

Studies have proven that TLR4-/- mice show an increased level of IL-6 and IL-23 and an expansion of the Th17 population due to an inhibition of the Th1 response (Marta et al. 2008). TLR4 is also vital in the induction of EAE due to its role in the effect of PT, which is typically given at the time of immunisation and 2 days later. PT is thought to promote the infiltration of inflammatory cells into the CNS. It has been shown that PT induces intracellular mechanisms through TLR4, one example being the induction of inflammatory adhesion molecules, such as p-selectin via NF-κB transcription (Kerfoot et al. 2004). PT was also shown to induce a proadhesive environment around the cerebrovascular endothelium causing an increase in the recruitment of leukocytes to the CNS in a TLR4-dependent manner (Kerfoot et al. 2004).

TLR6 has been related to EAE through the production of IFN-β- neutralising antibodies over long courses of IFN treatment. Polymorphisms within the TLR6 gene have a direct correlation to a production of anti-IFN-β antibodies, which can nullify the effect of IFN-β treatment (Enevold et al. 2010). In terms of direct action on EAE, TLR6 has been shown to be fairly redundant. Studies have shown that TLR6−/− mice have a very similar clinical disease course to wild-type C57BL/6 mice and therefore are seen to have little or no direct effect on the primary disease mechanisms (Marta et al. 2008).

8.8.2 The Role of Endosomal Toll-Like Receptors

Reports suggest that TLR signalling through the MyD88-independent pathway either does not support or suppresses the development of EAE. For example, the TLR3 agonist poly I:C does not support the development of active EAE when immunised with myelin antigens emulsified in IFA (Hansen et al. 2006). Furthermore, treatment of EAE mice with poly I:C suppressed the development of relapsing–remitting disease (Touil et al. 2006). In these studies, we showed that poly I:C treatment resulted in significant production of IFN-β, one of the critical products of the MyD88-independent signalling pathway, and that neutralisation of IFN-β reversed the inhibitory effect of poly I:C. In a later study, Tzima et al. showed that TLR3 activation could also inhibit the development of chronic EAE in a different mouse model (Tzima et al. 2009). IFN-β was the first disease-modifying immunotherapy approved for use in MS (The Interferon Study Group 1993). A report by Guo et al. further support a role of MyD88- independent signalling in suppression of EAE (Guo et al. 2008). In these studies, type I IFN receptor knockout mice developed more severe EAE than wild-type mice. Similarly, TRIF knockout mice lacking this critical adaptor molecule for MyD88-independent signalling also developed more severe disease. The studies further suggested that IFN-β-induced production of IL-27 by cells of the innate immune system played a critical role in suppressing the development of Th17 cells critical to disease development, and that this control was lost in type I IFN receptor and TRIF-deficient animals. Given the ability of the innate immune system to produce large amounts of endogenous type I IFN, these studies demonstrate in principle the possibility to induce the production of endogenous IFN-β as an alternative to the exogenous administration of recombinant molecule (Touil et al. 2006; O'Brien et al. 2008; O'Brien et al. 2010).

A small number of studies have been conducted into the role of TLR7 in EAE, one of which involved repeated inoculation with a low dose of TLR7 agonist to promote TLR7 tolerance (Hayashi et al. 2009) to subsequent activators of TLR7. This study showed that induction of TLR7 tolerance by a TLR7 agonist can cause hyposensitivity to not only TLR7 agonists, but also TLR2 and TLR9 agonists, with a positive effect on neural inflammation in mice induced with EAE. Other studies have shown that TLR7 can act via two different pathways, the pro-inflammatory NF-κB pathway and the anti-inflammatory IRF7 pathway. Both pathways start through the MyD88 molecule, with the pro-inflammatory arm running through NF-κB and the production of pro-inflammatory cytokines (O'Neill and Bowie 2007) whereas the anti-inflammatory pathway works through IRF7 and produces type I interferons such as IFN-α and IFN-β (Honda et al. 2005; O'Brien et al. 2010), which are protective against MS (The Interferon Study Group 1993; Durelli et al. 1994). These findings indicate that TLR7 can have both anti- and pro-inflammatory effects in EAE and suggest that its anti-inflammatory activity may be predominant.

TLR8 also recognises ssRNA. There are currently limited data on a potential role of TLR8 in inflammatory demyelination, except for its accumulation in the axons of EAE mice together with inflammasome protein NAcht leucine-rich repeat protein 1 (NALP1) (Soulika et al. 2009). TLR8 deficiency in the mouse was found to be associated with an overexpression of TLR7, increased levels of serum autoantibodies and the development of spontaneous glomerulonephritis (Demaria et al. 2010). In humans, but not in mice, TLR8 has been reported to recognise synthetic imidazoquinolines in addition to ssRNA (Jurk et al. 2002).

TLR signalling through the MyD88-dependent pathway has been suggested to play a significant role in regulating the development of EAE. Prinz et al. reported that MyD88 knockout mice were resistant to the development of active EAE, further supporting a role of MyD88-dependent signalling in disease development (Prinz et al. 2006). Interestingly, T cells derived from MyD88 knockout mice did not respond measurably to their cognate antigen, suggesting that MyD88 knockout mice did not develop active EAE, partly because of the inadequate T cell priming in the periphery (Prinz et al. 2006). However, bone marrow chimera studies indicated that MyD88 expression in the CNS also played a significant role in controlling the development of EAE. Adoptive transfer of myelin-specific T cells into MyD88 knockout mice resulted in decreased severity of EAE relative to wild-type animals (Prinz et al. 2006).

Another model for the regulatory effect of TLR9 activation is that it increases the production of tryptophan-catabolising enzyme Indoleamine 2,3 dioxygenase (IDO), which has immunoregulatory properties. Mice deficient in IDO develop more severe EAE than wild-type mice, with enhanced encephalitogenic Th1 and Th17 and reduced regulatory T cell responses (Yan et al. 2010). It has also been reported that TLR9 agonists can induce IDO-dependent protection against autoimmune responses in type 1 diabetes (Fallarino et al. 2009; Ciorba et al. 2010) and experimental colitis in (Ciorba et al. 2010) mouse models. We are currently investigating such TLR9/IDO axis in animal models of MS.

8.8.3 Toll-Like Receptors as Therapeutic Target for Inflammatory Diseases

As the evidence for the involvement of TLRs in multiple immune-mediated diseases has increased, so too have efforts to identify regulators of TLR-dependent signalling as therapeutic agents. Indeed, the possibility to downregulate immune responses with specific TLR agonists or antagonists and by inhibiting intracellular proteins involved in the cascade signalling pathways may provide a novel approach for the treatment of autoimmune diseases. For example, TLR2 could be a useful therapeutic target for the development of antagonists given the range of diseases that are associated with this receptor. Interestingly, the neutralising antibody T2.5, directed against

TLR2, has been shown to prevent sepsis induced by TLR2 ligands (Meng et al. 2004). In addition, recent data have shown that OPN-305, another TLR2-specific monoclonal antibody produced by Opsona Therapeutics, can inhibit TLR2-mediated pro-inflammatory cytokine production in the mouse model of myocardial ischaemia-reperfusion injury (Arslan et al. 2008; Dunne et al. 2011). The humanised version of OPN-305 entered phase I clinical trials for the treatment of inflammatory autoimmune diseases (Dunne et al. 2011).

The potential for the stimulation (rather than the inhibition) of TLR3 for the treatment of autoimmune inflammatory demyelination has been discussed in the previous section (Touil et al. 2006; O'Brien et al. 2008; Tzima et al. 2009). We took a similar approach with the stimulation of TLR7 using imiquimod, a therapeutic agent approved for use in human therapy for dermatologic conditions. Administration of Imiquimod induced the production of endogenous IFN-β and suppressed the development of EAE induced by MOG(35–55) in the C57BL/6 mouse (O'Brien et al. 2010). We are currently studying the potential of different agonists of TLR9 (CpGA and CpGB) to modulate EAE and interact with the immunoregulatory IDO pathway (Yan et al. 2010; Volpi et al. 2012).

A humanised TLR4-specific antibody (NI-0101), developed by NovImmune, interferes with the dimerisation of TLR4 by binding to an epitope on TLR4. The antibody is undergoing preclinical evaluation as a potential therapy for inflammatory bowel disease (IBD) (Hodgkinson 2010; Dunne et al. 2011). In addition, the lipid A mimetic CRX-526, a synthetic TLR4 antagonist, was reported to inhibit the development of dextran-sulphate sodium (DSS)-induced colitis and of colitis in mice deficient for multidrug resistance gene 1A100. It has also been shown that 1A6, a rat TLR4-specific monoclonal antibody, reduced inflammation in DSS-induced colitis in mice (Ungaro et al. 2009). Furthermore, the lipid A mimetic Eritoran (E5564), produced by Eisai Pharmaceuticals, interferes with the formation of the TLR4-MD2-LPS complex. The antibody was shown to be an effective inhibitor of LPS-induced shock in mice (Mills 2011). However, it did not meet its primary endpoint in patients with severe sepsis in a phase III clinical trial (Mills 2011).

Several other novel approaches have been devised to identify inhibitors of TLR2 and TLR4. A novel peptide inhibitor, VIPER, which is derived from vaccinia virus protein A46, has been described to inhibit TLR4-dependent signalling via blocking TIR–TIR domain interactions (Lysakova-Devine et al. 2010). In addition, using a conventional screening approach using TLR reporter cell lines, Zhou et al. identified a novel small molecule (E567), which inhibited lymphocytic choriomeningitis virus (LCMV)-induced TLR2-mediated signalling pathway (Zhou et al. 2010). The authors suggested that inhibiting TLR signalling in LCMV-infected cells could have great therapeutic potential in the treatment of viral diseases involving TLR activation, including HSV-1 and cytomegalovirus (CMV) (Zhou et al. 2010), which have been associated with MS.

Synthetic immunoregulatory sequences (IRS) have been used to modulate TLR-mediated responses. One such medication developed using this technique is CPG52364 (Pfizer), the antagonist of TLR7, TLR8 and TLR9. CPG52364 has shown efficacy in mouse models of systemic lupus erythematosus (SLE) and other autoimmune diseases, and it is in phase I clinical trials (Dunne et al. 2011). In addition, the TLR7/9 antagonist DV1179 (IRS945) developed by Dynavax Technologies, is currently being investigated for the potential treatment of autoimmune diseases. IRS945 was obtained by combining sequence elements from both IRS661 and IRS869 and removing non-essential nucleotides (Barrat et al. 2007). Furthermore, IMO-3100, an inhibitor for TLR7- and TLR9-mediated pathways, has been developed by Idera Pharmaceuticals. IMO-3100 has been shown to exert potent activity in reducing pathologic and immunologic manifestations in preclinical mouse models of SLE, rheumatoid arthritis (RA), psoriasis and hyperlipidemia. Results from humanised phase I clinical trials showed that IMO-3100 was well tolerated. It inhibited TLR7- and TLR9-mediated immune responses at all evaluated doses (Gambuzza et al. 2011). Of note, certain features of immune dysregulation in SLE are considered to be 'opposite' to those described in MS, for example, SLE is characterised by excessive production of endogenous type I IFNs, suggesting that stimulation of TLR7 and TLR9 may be valid alternative approaches to MS immunotherapy (O'Brien et al. 2010). However, others have proposed a TLR7 tolerance induction strategy to the treatment of EAE as a model of MS (Hayashi et al. 2009).

Agents that specifically modulate TLR signalling pathways may also be effective in the treatment of EAE and MS. Another study evaluated the effects of peroxisome proliferator-activated receptors (PPARs), which are members of the nuclear hormone receptor family, on the expression of TLR intermediates by cells of the CNS (Xu et al. 2007). The authors demonstrated that PPAR-α agonists suppressed the expression of critical MyD88-dependent signalling intermediates by primary microglia as well as in the CNS of mice with EAE (Xu et al. 2007). PPAR-γ agonists also suppressed the expression of MyD88 signalling intermediates by primary microglia (Xu and Drew 2007). In addition, these PPAR agonists suppressed glial production of IL-12 and IL-23, which were known to play important roles in the development of Th1 and Th17 cells that stimulated the development of EAE. Together, these suggested that PPAR agonists may be effective in the treatment of MS (Xu and Drew 2007).

Therapeutic approaches to the TLR and other immune pathways will need to take into account the complexity of such signalling pathways, in which activation or inhibition of specific innate receptors inevitably leads to interference with numerous molecules involved in inflammation and immune regulation (O'Brien et al. 2008; Nyirenda et al. 2009; O'Neill et al. 2009).

8.9 Summary

It is clear that TLRs can play a significant role in modulating MS and EAE. Studies to date suggest that TLRs, which activate MyD88- dependent signalling, may contribute to the development of MS, whereas MyD88-independent pathways may mitigate disease severity. TLRs present on cells of the innate immune system are thought to provide critical signals involved in the activation of cells of the adaptive immune system, including autoreactive lymphocytes. However, many questions concerning the role of TLRs in modulating MS remain unanswered. The complex pattern of TLR expression in the periphery and in the CNS, as well as by cells of both the innate and adaptive immune systems, is just beginning to be appreciated. Elucidation of the molecular mechanism of protein and nucleic acid recognition by different TLRs has provided the basis for the rational design of their specific agonists and antagonists. Small synthetic compounds, acting as TLR3 agonists and/or TLR2/TLR4, TLR7/9 and MyD88 antagonists, might favour the inhibition of signalling responsible for autoimmune responses in MS and EAE. Several immunomodulatory drugs influencing TLR signalling have already been approved for therapy or are currently undergoing clinical trials. Immunomodulatory compounds targeting innate immune system alone or in combination with other substances could represent advanced vaccine adjuvants and therapeutic drugs for MS. In addition, future studies are needed to understand the detailed mechanisms by which TLRs modulate MS and its experimental models. There is great potential for further advancement of knowledge and therapeutic opportunities.

Acknowledgments This work was supported by grants from the European Union FP6 Programme (Marie Curie International Reintegration Grant, Ref. 046527), the MS Society of Great Britain and Northern Ireland (Ref. 863/07), and the Italian MS Society (Ref. 2011/R/21).

References

Acosta-Rodriguez EV, Rivino L, Geginat J, Jarrossay D, Gattorno M, Lanzavecchia A, Sallusto F, Napolitani G (2007) Surface phenotype and antigenic specificity of human interleukin 17-producing T helper memory cells. Nat Immunol 8:639–646

Akira S (2003) Mammalian Toll-like receptors. Curr Opin Immunol 15:5–11

Akira S, Hemmi H (2003) Recognition of pathogen-associated molecular patterns by TLR family. Immunol Lett 85:85–95

Akira S, Uematsu S, Takeuchi O (2006) Pathogen recognition and innate immunity. Cell 124:783–801

Aloisi F, Pujol-Borrell R (2006) Lymphoid neogenesis in chronic inflammatory diseases. Nat Rev Immunol 6:205–217

Amiset L, Fend L, Gatard-Scheikl T, Rittner K, Duong V, Rooke R, Muller S, Bonnefoy JY, Preville X, Haegel H (2012) TLR2 ligation protects effector T cells from regulatory T-cell mediated suppression and repolarizes T helper responses following MVA-based cancer immunotherapy. Oncoimmunology 1:1271–1280

Anderson KV, Jurgens G, Nusslein-Volhard C (1985) Establishment of dorsal–ventral polarity in the Drosophila embryo: genetic studies on the role of the Toll gene product. Cell 42:779–789

Andersson A, Covacu R, Sunnemark D, Danilov AI, Bianco A D, Khademi M, Wallstrom E, Lobell A, Brundin L, Lassmann H, Harris RA (2008) Pivotal advance: HMGB1 expression in active lesions of human and experimental multiple sclerosis. J Leukoc Biol 84:1248–1255

Aravalli RN, Hu S, Rowen TN, Palmquist JM, Lokensgard JR (2005) Cutting edge: TLR2-mediated proinflammatory cytokine and chemokine production by microglial cells in response to herpes simplex virus. J Immunol 175:4189–4193

Ariza ME, Glaser R, Kaumaya PT, Jones C, Williams MV (2009) The EBV-encoded dUTPase activates NF-kappa B through the TLR2 and MyD88-dependent signaling pathway. J Immunol 182:851–859

Arslan F, Kleijn DP de, Timmers L, Doevendans PA, Pasterkamp G (2008) Bridging innate immunity and myocardial ischemia/reperfusion injury: the search for therapeutic targets. Curr Pharm Des 14:1205–1216

Ascherio A, Munch M (2000) Epstein-Barr virus and multiple sclerosis. Epidemiology 11:220–224

Ayyoub M, Deknuydt F, Raimbaud I, Dousset C, Leveque L, Bioley G, Valmori D (2009) Human memory FOXP3+ Tregs secrete IL-17 ex vivo and constitutively express the T(H)17 lineage-specific transcription factor RORgamma t. Proc Natl Acad Sci U S A 106:8635–8640

Bach JF (2005) Infections and autoimmune diseases. J Autoimmun 25 Suppl: 74–80

Balashov KE, Aung LL, Vaknin-Dembinsky A, Dhib-Jalbut S, Weiner HL (2010) Interferon-beta inhibits toll-like receptor 9 processing in multiple sclerosis. Ann Neurol 68:899–906

Barbalat R, Ewald SE, Mouchess ML, Barton GM (2011) Nucleic acid recognition by the innate immune system. Annu Rev Immunol 29:185–214

Barrat FJ, Meeker T, Chan JH, Guiducci C, Coffman RL (2007) Treatment of lupus-prone mice with a dual inhibitor of TLR7 and TLR9 leads to reduction of autoantibody production and amelioration of disease symptoms. Eur J Immunol 37:3582–3586

Beelen AJ van, Zelinkova Z, Taanman-Kueter EW, Muller FJ, Hommes DW, Zaat SA, Kapsenberg ML, Jong EC de (2007) Stimulation of the intracellular bacterial sensor NOD2 programs dendritic cells to promote interleukin-17 production in human memory T cells. Immunity 27:660–669

Beriou G, Costantino CM, Ashley CW, Yang L, Kuchroo VK, Baecher-Allan C, Hafler DA (2009) IL-17-producing human peripheral regulatory T cells retain suppressive function. Blood 113:4240–4249

Blasius AL, Beutler B (2010) Intracellular toll-like receptors. Immunity 32:305–315

Bsibsi M, Ravid R, Gveric D, Noort JM van (2002) Broad expression of Toll-like receptors in the human central nervous system. J Neuropathol Exp Neurol 61:1013–1021

Bsibsi M, Persoon-Deen C, Verwer RW, Meeuwsen S, Ravid R, Van Noort JM (2006) Toll-like receptor 3 on adult human astrocytes triggers production of neuroprotective mediators. Glia 53:688–695

Buljevac D, Flach HZ, Hop WC, Hijdra D, Laman JD, Savelkoul HF, Der Meche FG van, Doorn PA van, Hintzen RQ (2002) Prospective study on the relationship between infections and multiple sclerosis exacerbations. Brain 125:952–960

Bustamante MF, Fissolo N, Rio J, Espejo C, Costa C, Mansilla MJ, Lizasoain I, Moro MA, Carmen Edo M, Montalban X, Comabella M (2011) Implication of the Toll-like receptor 4 pathway in the response to interferon-beta in multiple sclerosis. Ann Neurol 70:634–645

Caramalho I, Lopes-Carvalho T, Ostler D, Zelenay S, Haury M, Demengeot J (2003) Regulatory T cells selectively express toll-like receptors and are activated by lipopolysaccharide. J Exp Med 197:403–411

Caron G, Duluc D, Fremaux I, Jeannin P, David C, Gascan H, Delneste Y (2005) Direct stimulation of human T cells via TLR5 and TLR7/8: flagellin and R-848 up-regulate proliferation and IFN-gamma production by memory CD4+ T cells. J Immunol 175:1551–1557

Chaturvedi A, Pierce SK (2009) How location governs toll-like receptor signaling. Traffic 10:621–628

Choi SR, Howell OW, Carassiti D, Magliozzi R, Gveric D, Muraro PA, Nicholas R, Roncaroli F, Reynolds R (2012) Meningeal inflammation plays a role in the pathology of primary progressive multiple sclerosis. Brain 135:2925–2937

Ciorba MA, Bettonville EE, McDonald KG, Metz R, Prendergast GC, Newberry RD, Stenson WF (2010) Induction of IDO-1 by immunostimulatory DNA limits severity of experimental colitis. J Immunol 184:3907–3916

Compston A, Coles A (2008) Multiple sclerosis. Lancet 372:1502–1517

Constantinescu CS, Farooqi N, O'Brien K, Gran B (2011) Experimental autoimmune encephalomyelitis (EAE) as a model for multiple sclerosis (MS). Br J Pharmacol 164:1079–1106

Correale J, Farez M (2009) Helminth antigens modulate immune responses in cells from multiple sclerosis patients through TLR2-dependent mechanisms. J Immunol 183:5999–6012

Correale J, Fiol M, Gilmore W (2006) The risk of relapses in multiple sclerosis during systemic infections. Neurology 67:652–659

Cottalorda A, Verschelde C, Marcais A, Tomkowiak M, Musette P, Uematsu S, Akira S, Marvel J, Bonnefoy-Berard N (2006) TLR2 engagement on CD8 T cells lowers the threshold for optimal antigen-induced T cell activation. Eur J Immunol 36:1684–1693

Crellin NK, Garcia RV, Hadisfar O, Allan SE, Steiner TS, Levings MK (2005) Human CD4+ T cells express TLR5 and its ligand flagellin enhances the suppressive capacity and expression of FOXP3 in CD4+ CD25+ T regulatory cells. J Immunol 175:8051–8059

Cristofaro P, Opal SM (2003) The Toll-like receptors and their role in septic shock. Expert Opin Ther Targets 7:603–612

Demaria O, Pagni PP, Traub S, Gassart A de, Branzk N, Murphy AJ, Valenzuela DM, Yancopoulos GD, Flavell RA, Alexopoulou L (2010) TLR8 deficiency leads to autoimmunity in mice. J Clin Invest 120:3651–3662

Dobson R, Meier UC, Giovannoni G (2011) More to come: humoral immune responses in MS. J Neuroimmunol 240–241:13–21

Dunne A, Marshall NA, Mills KH (2011) TLR based therapeutics. Curr Opin Pharmacol 11:404–411

Durelli L, Bongioanni MR, Cavallo R, Ferrero B, Ferri R, Ferrio MF, Bradac GB, Riva A, Vai S, Geuna M et al (1994) Chronic systemic high-dose recombinant interferon alfa-2a reduces exacerbation rate, MRI signs of disease activity, and lymphocyte interferon gamma production in relapsing-remitting multiple sclerosis. Neurology 44:406–413

Edwards S, Zvartau M, Clarke H, Irving W, Blumhardt LD (1998) Clinical relapses and disease activity on magnetic resonance imaging associated with viral upper respiratory tract infections in multiple sclerosis. J Neurol Neurosurg Psychiatry 64:736–741

Elinav E, Strowig T, Henao-Mejia J, Flavell RA (2011) Regulation of the antimicrobial response by NLR proteins. Immunity 34:665–679

Enevold C, Oturai AB, Sorensen PS, Ryder LP, Koch-Henriksen N, Bendtzen K (2010) Polymorphisms of innate pattern recognition receptors, response to interferon-beta and development of neutralizing antibodies in multiple sclerosis patients. Mult Scler 16:942–949

Erridge C (2010) Endogenous ligands of TLR2 and TLR4: agonists or assistants? J Leukoc Biol 87:989–999

Evans HG, Suddason T, Jackson I, Taams LS, Lord GM (2007) Optimal induction of T helper 17 cells in humans requires T cell receptor ligation in the context of Toll-like receptor-activated monocytes. Proc Natl Acad Sci U S A 104:17034–17039

Fallarino F, Volpi C, Zelante T, Vacca C, Calvitti M, Fioretti MC, Puccetti P, Romani L, Grohmann U (2009) IDO mediates TLR9-driven protection from experimental autoimmune diabetes. J Immunol 183:6303–6312

Farez MF, Quintana FJ, Gandhi R, Izquierdo G, Lucas M, Weiner HL (2009) Toll-like receptor 2 and poly(ADP-ribose) polymerase 1 promote central nervous system neuroinflammation in progressive EAE. Nat Immunol 10:958–964

Farooqi N, Gran B, Constantinescu CS (2010) Are current disease-modifying therapeutics in multiple sclerosis justified on the basis of studies in experimental autoimmune encephalomyelitis? J Neurochem 115:829–844

Fillatreau S, Sweenie CH, McGeachy MJ, Gray D, Anderton SM (2002) B cells regulate autoimmunity by provision of IL-10. Nat Immunol 3:944–950

Fischer M, Ehlers M (2008) Toll-like receptors in autoimmunity. Ann N Y Acad Sci 1143:21–34

Frohman EM, Filippi M, Stuve O, Waxman SG, Corboy J, Phillips JT, Lucchinetti C, Wilken J, Karandikar N, Hemmer B, Monson N, De Keyser J, Hartung H, Steinman L, Oksenberg JR, Cree BA, Hauser S, Racke MK (2005) Characterizing the mechanisms of progression in multiple sclerosis: evidence and new hypotheses for future directions. Arch Neurol 62:1345–1356

Frohman EM, Racke MK, Raine CS (2006) Multiple sclerosis–the plaque and its pathogenesis. N Engl J Med 354:942–955

Gambuzza M, Licata N, Palella E, Celi D, Foti Cuzzola V, Italiano D, Marino S, Bramanti P (2011) Targeting Toll-like receptors: emerging therapeutics for multiple sclerosis management. J Neuroimmunol 239:1–12

Gaudreault E, Fiola S, Olivier M, Gosselin J (2007) Epstein-Barr virus induces MCP-1 secretion by human monocytes via TLR2. J Virol 81:8016–8024
Gelman AE, Zhang J, Choi Y, Turka LA (2004) Toll-like receptor ligands directly promote activated CD4+ T cell survival. J Immunol 172:6065–6073
Gelman AE, LaRosa DF, Zhang J, Walsh PT, Choi Y, Sunyer JO, Turka LA (2006) The adaptor molecule MyD88 activates PI-3 kinase signaling in CD4+ T cells and enables CpG oligodeoxynucleotide-mediated costimulation. Immunity 25:783–793
Gewirtz AT, Navas TA, Lyons S, Godowski PJ, Madara JL (2001) Cutting edge: bacterial flagellin activates basolaterally expressed TLR5 to induce epithelial proinflammatory gene expression. J Immunol 167:1882–1885
Govindaraj RG, Manavalan B, Lee G, Choi S (2010) Molecular modeling-based evaluation of hTLR10 and identification of potential ligands in Toll-like receptor signaling. PLoS One 5:e12713
Guan Y, Ranoa DR, Jiang S, Mutha SK, Li X, Baudry J, Tapping RI (2010) Human TLRs 10 and 1 share common mechanisms of innate immune sensing but not signaling. J Immunol 184:5094–5103
Guo B, Chang EY, Cheng G (2008) The type I IFN induction pathway constrains Th17-mediated autoimmune inflammation in mice. J Clin Invest 118:1680–1690
Hanafy KA, Sloane JA (2011) Regulation of remyelination in multiple sclerosis. FEBS Lett 585:3821–3828
Hansen BS, Hussain RZ, Lovett-Racke AE, Thomas JA, Racke MK (2006) Multiple Toll-like receptor agonists act as potent adjuvants in the induction of autoimmunity. J Neuroimmunol 172:94–103
Harp C, Lee J, Lambracht-Washington D, Cameron E, Olsen G, Frohman E, Racke M, Monson N (2007) Cerebrospinal fluid B cells from multiple sclerosis patients are subject to normal germinal center selection. J Neuroimmunol 183:189–199
Hauser SL, Waubant E, Arnold DL, Vollmer T, Antel J, Fox RJ, Bar-Or A, Panzara M, Sarkar N, Agarwal S, Langer-Gould A, Smith CH (2008) B-cell depletion with rituximab in relapsing-remitting multiple sclerosis. N Engl J Med 358:676–688
Hayashi T, Gray CS, Chan M, Tawatao RI, Ronacher L, McGargill MA, Datta SK, Carson DA, Corr M (2009) Prevention of autoimmune disease by induction of tolerance to Toll-like receptor 7. Proc Natl Acad Sci U S A 106:2764–2769
Herrmann I, Kellert M, Schmidt H, Mildner A, Hanisch UK, Bruck W, Prinz M, Nau R (2006) Streptococcus pneumoniae Infection aggravates experimental autoimmune encephalomyelitis via toll-like receptor 2. Infect Immun 74:4841–4848
Higgins SC, Jarnicki AG, Lavelle EC, Mills KH (2006) TLR4 mediates vaccine-induced protective cellular immunity to Bordetella pertussis: role of IL-17-producing T cells. J Immunol 177:7980–7989
Hillman LJ, Burns SP, Kraft GH (2000) Neurological worsening due to infection from renal stones in a multiple sclerosis patient. Mult Scler 6:403–406
Hirotani M, Niino M, Fukazawa T, Kikuchi S, Yabe I, Hamada S, Tajima Y, Sasaki H (2010) Decreased IL-10 production mediated by Toll-like receptor 9 in B cells in multiple sclerosis. J Neuroimmunol 221:95–100
Hodgkinson L (2010) Digestive Disease Week 2010. Turning Science into Medicine–part 2. IDrugs 13:424–426
Hoebe K, Georgel P, Rutschmann S, Du X, Mudd S, Crozat K, Sovath S, Shamel L, Hartung T, Zahringer U, Beutler B (2005) CD36 is a sensor of diacylglycerides. Nature 433:523–527
Honda K, Yanai H, Negishi H, Asagiri M, Sato M, Mizutani T, Shimada N, Ohba Y, Takaoka A, Yoshida N, Taniguchi T (2005) IRF-7 is the master regulator of type-I interferon-dependent immune responses. Nature 434:772–777
Hornef MW, Bogdan C (2005) The role of epithelial Toll-like receptor expression in host defense and microbial tolerance. J Endotoxin Res 11:124–128

Hornung V, Rothenfusser S, Britsch S, Krug A, Jahrsdorfer B, Giese T, Endres S, Hartmann G (2002) Quantitative expression of toll-like receptor 1–10 mRNA in cellular subsets of human peripheral blood mononuclear cells and sensitivity to CpG oligodeoxynucleotides. J Immunol 168:4531–4537

Jack C, Ruffini F, Bar-Or A, Antel JP (2005) Microglia and multiple sclerosis. J Neurosci Res 81:363–373

Jiang D, Liang J, Fan J, Yu S, Chen S, Luo Y, Prestwich GD, Mascarenhas MM, Garg HG, Quinn DA, Homer RJ, Goldstein DR, Bucala R, Lee PJ, Medzhitov R, Noble PW (2005) Regulation of lung injury and repair by Toll-like receptors and hyaluronan. Nat Med 11:1173–1179

Johnson AJ, Suidan GL, McDole J, Pirko I (2007) The CD8T cell in multiple sclerosis: suppressor cell or mediator of neuropathology? Int Rev Neurobiol 79:73–97

Jurk M, Heil F, Vollmer J, Schetter C, Krieg AM, Wagner H, Lipford G, Bauer S (2002) Human TLR7 or TLR8 independently confer responsiveness to the antiviral compound R-848. Nat Immunol 3:499

Kabat EA, Moore DH, Landow H (1942) An electrophoretic study of the protein components in cerebrospinal fluid and their relationship to the serum proteins. J Clin Invest 21:571–577

Kabelitz D (2007) Expression and function of Toll-like receptors in T lymphocytes. Curr Opin Immunol 19:39–45

Kawagoe T, Sato S, Matsushita K, Kato H, Matsui K, Kumagai Y, Saitoh T, Kawai T, Takeuchi O, Akira S (2008) Sequential control of Toll-like receptor-dependent responses by IRAK1 and IRAK2. Nat Immunol 9:684–691

Kawai T, Akira S (2010) The role of pattern-recognition receptors in innate immunity: update on Toll-like receptors. Nat Immunol 11:373–384

Kawai T, Akira S (2011) Toll-like receptors and their crosstalk with other innate receptors in infection and immunity. Immunity 34:637–650

Kerfoot SM, Long EM, Hickey MJ, Andonegui G, Lapointe BM, Zanardo RC, Bonder C, James WG, Robbins SM, Kubes P (2004) TLR4 contributes to disease-inducing mechanisms resulting in central nervous system autoimmune disease. J Immunol 173:7070–7077

Kim S, Takahashi H, Lin WW, Descargues P, Grivennikov S, Kim Y, Luo JL, Karin M (2009) Carcinoma-produced factors activate myeloid cells through TLR2 to stimulate metastasis. Nature 457:102–106

Kubo T, Hatton RD, Oliver J, Liu X, Elson CO, Weaver CT (2004) Regulatory T cell suppression and anergy are differentially regulated by proinflammatory cytokines produced by TLR-activated dendritic cells. J Immunol 173:7249–7258

Kumar H, Kawai T, Akira S (2009) Toll-like receptors and innate immunity. Biochem Biophys Res Commun 388:621–625

Lampropoulou V, Hoehlig K, Roch T, Neves P, Calderon Gomez E, Sweenie CH, Hao Y, Freitas AA, Steinhoff U, Anderton SM, Fillatreau S (2008) TLR-activated B cells suppress T cell-mediated autoimmunity. J Immunol 180:4763–4773

Lassmann H (2008) Mechanisms of inflammation induced tissue injury in multiple sclerosis. J Neurol Sci 274:45–47

Lehnardt S, Massillon L, Follett P, Jensen FE, Ratan R, Rosenberg PA, Volpe JJ, Vartanian T (2003) Activation of innate immunity in the CNS triggers neurodegeneration through a Toll-like receptor 4-dependent pathway. Proc Natl Acad Sci U S A 100:8514–8519

LeibundGut-Landmann S, Gross O, Robinson MJ, Osorio F, Slack EC, Tsoni SV, Schweighoffer E, Tybulewicz V, Brown GD, Ruland J, Reis e Sousa C (2007) Syk- and CARD9-dependent coupling of innate immunity to the induction of T helper cells that produce interleukin 17. Nat Immunol 8:630–638

Lemaitre B, Nicolas E, Michaut L, Reichhart JM, Hoffmann JA (1996) The dorsoventral regulatory gene cassette spatzle/Toll/cactus controls the potent antifungal response in Drosophila adults. Cell 86:973–983

Levin LI, Munger KL, Rubertone MV, Peck CA, Lennette ET, Spiegelman D, Ascherio A (2003) Multiple sclerosis and Epstein-Barr virus. JAMA 289:1533–1536

Lewkowicz P, Lewkowicz N, Sasiak A, Tchorzewski H (2006) Lipopolysaccharide-activated CD4+ CD25+ T regulatory cells inhibit neutrophil function and promote their apoptosis and death. J Immunol 177:7155–7163
Li Y, Chu N, Hu A, Gran B, Rostami A, Zhang GX (2007) Increased IL-23p19 expression in multiple sclerosis lesions and its induction in microglia. Brain 130:490–501
Liu G, Zhao Y (2007) Toll-like receptors and immune regulation: their direct and indirect modulation on regulatory CD4+ CD25+ T cells. Immunology 122:149–156
Liu H, Komai-Koma M, Xu D, Liew FY (2006) Toll-like receptor 2 signaling modulates the functions of CD4+ CD25+ regulatory T cells. Proc Natl Acad Sci U S A 103:7048–7053
Lysakova-Devine T, Keogh B, Harrington B, Nagpal K, Halle A, Golenbock DT, Monie T, Bowie AG (2010) Viral inhibitory peptide of TLR4, a peptide derived from vaccinia protein A46, specifically inhibits TLR4 by directly targeting MyD88 adaptor-like and TRIF-related adaptor molecule. J Immunol 185:4261–4271
Magliozzi R, Howell O, Vora A, Serafini B, Nicholas R, Puopolo M, Reynolds R, Aloisi F (2007) Meningeal B-cell follicles in secondary progressive multiple sclerosis associate with early onset of disease and severe cortical pathology. Brain 130:1089–1104
Mansson A, Adner M, Cardell LO (2006) Toll-like receptors in cellular subsets of human tonsil T cells: altered expression during recurrent tonsillitis. Respir Res 7:36
Marta M, Andersson A, Isaksson M, Kampe O, Lobell A (2008) Unexpected regulatory roles of TLR4 and TLR9 in experimental autoimmune encephalomyelitis. Eur J Immunol 38:565–575
Martyn CN, Cruddas M, Compston DA (1993) Symptomatic Epstein-Barr virus infection and multiple sclerosis. J Neurol Neurosurg Psychiatry 56:167–168
Matsushita T, Horikawa M, Iwata Y, Tedder TF (2010) Regulatory B cells (B10 cells) and regulatory T cells have independent roles in controlling experimental autoimmune encephalomyelitis initiation and late-phase immunopathogenesis. J Immunol 185:2240–2252
Meng G, Rutz M, Schiemann M, Metzger J, Grabiec A, Schwandner R, Luppa PB, Ebel F, Busch DH, Bauer S, Wagner H, Kirschning CJ (2004) Antagonistic antibody prevents toll-like receptor 2-driven lethal shock-like syndromes. J Clin Invest 113:1473–1481
Metz LM, McGuinness SD, Harris C (1998) Urinary tract infections may trigger relapse in multiple sclerosis. Axone 19:67–70
Mills KH (2011) TLR-dependent T cell activation in autoimmunity. Nat Rev Immunol 11:807–822
Miyara M, Yoshioka Y, Kitoh A, Shima T, Wing K, Niwa A, Parizot C, Taflin C, Heike T, Valeyre D, Mathian A, Nakahata T, Yamaguchi T, Nomura T, Ono M, Amoura Z, Gorochov G, Sakaguchi S (2009) Functional delineation and differentiation dynamics of human CD4+ T cells expressing the FoxP3 transcription factor. Immunity 30:899–911
Mizoguchi A, Bhan AK (2006) A case for regulatory B cells. J Immunol 176:705–710
Murawski MR, Bowen GN, Cerny AM, Anderson LJ, Haynes LM, Tripp RA, Kurt-Jones EA, Finberg RW (2009) Respiratory syncytial virus activates innate immunity through Toll-like receptor 2. J Virol 83:1492–1500
Nair A, Frederick TJ, Miller SD (2008) Astrocytes in multiple sclerosis: a product of their environment. Cell Mol Life Sci 65:2702–2720
Nicolle LE (2008) Uncomplicated urinary tract infection in adults including uncomplicated pyelonephritis. Urol Clin North Am 35:1–12, v
Nyirenda MH, O'Brien K, Sanvito L, Constantinescu CS, Gran B (2009) Modulation of regulatory T cells in health and disease: role of toll-like receptors. Inflamm Allergy Drug Targets 8:124–129
Nyirenda MH, Sanvito L, Darlington PJ, O'Brien K, Zhang GX, Constantinescu CS, Bar-Or A, Gran B (2011) TLR2 stimulation drives human naive and effector regulatory T cells into a Th17-like phenotype with reduced suppressive function. J Immunol 187:2278–2290
O'Brien K, Fitzgerald DC, Naiken K, Alugupalli KR, Rostami AM, Gran B (2008) Role of the innate immune system in autoimmune inflammatory demyelination. Curr Med Chem 15:1105–1115
O'Brien K, Fitzgerald D, Rostami A, Gran B (2010) The TLR7 agonist, imiquimod, increases IFN-beta production and reduces the severity of experimental autoimmune encephalomyelitis. J Neuroimmunol 221:107–111

O'Neill LA, Bowie AG (2007) The family of five: TIR-domain-containing adaptors in Toll-like receptor signalling. Nat Rev Immunol 7:353–364
O'Neill LA, Bryant CE, Doyle SL (2009) Therapeutic targeting of Toll-like receptors for infectious and inflammatory diseases and cancer. Pharmacol Rev 61:177–197
Oberg HH, Ly TT, Ussat S, Meyer T, Kabelitz D, Wesch D (2010) Differential but direct abolishment of human regulatory T cell suppressive capacity by various TLR2 ligands. J Immunol 184:4733–4740
Ozinsky A, Underhill DM, Fontenot JD, Hajjar AM, Smith KD, Wilson CB, Schroeder L, Aderem A (2000) The repertoire for pattern recognition of pathogens by the innate immune system is defined by cooperation between toll-like receptors. Proc Natl Acad Sci U S A 97:13766–13771
Pasare C, Medzhitov R (2004) Toll-like receptors and acquired immunity. Semin Immunol 16:23–26
Peng G, Guo Z, Kiniwa Y, Voo KS, Peng W, Fu T, Wang DY, Li Y, Wang HY, Wang RF (2005) Toll-like receptor 8-mediated reversal of CD4+ regulatory T cell function. Science 309:1380–1384
Pifer R, Benson A, Sturge CR, Yarovinsky F (2011) UNC93B1 is essential for TLR11 activation and IL-12-dependent host resistance to Toxoplasma gondii. J Biol Chem 286:3307–3314
Prinz M, Garbe F, Schmidt H, Mildner A, Gutcher I, Wolter K, Piesche M, Schroers R, Weiss E, Kirschning CJ, Rochford CD, Bruck W, Becher B (2006) Innate immunity mediated by TLR9 modulates pathogenicity in an animal model of multiple sclerosis. J Clin Invest 116:456–464
Racke MK (2008) The role of B cells in multiple sclerosis: rationale for B-cell-targeted therapies. Curr Opin Neurol 21(Suppl 1):S9–S18
Racke MK, Drew PD (2009) Toll-like receptors in multiple sclerosis. Curr Top Microbiol Immunol 336:155–168
Reynolds JM, Pappu BP, Peng J, Martinez GJ, Zhang Y, Chung Y, Ma L, Yang XO, Nurieva RI, Tian Q, Dong C (2010) Toll-like receptor 2 signaling in CD4(+) T lymphocytes promotes T helper 17 responses and regulates the pathogenesis of autoimmune disease. Immunity 32:692–702
Rock FL, Hardiman G, Timans JC, Kastelein RA, Bazan JF (1998) A family of human receptors structurally related to Drosophila Toll. Proc Natl Acad Sci U S A 95:588–593
Roelofs MF, Boelens WC, Joosten LA, Abdollahi-Roodsaz S, Geurts J, Wunderink LU, Schreurs BW, den Berg WB van, Radstake TR (2006) Identification of small heat shock protein B8 (HSP22) as a novel TLR4 ligand and potential involvement in the pathogenesis of rheumatoid arthritis. J Immunol 176:7021–7027
Sanders P, Keyser J De (2007) Janus faces of microglia in multiple sclerosis. Brain Res Rev 54:274–285
Schachtele SJ, Hu S, Little MR, Lokensgard JR (2010) Herpes simplex virus induces neural oxidative damage via microglial cell Toll-like receptor-2. J Neuroinflammation 7:35
Schaefer L, Babelova A, Kiss E, Hausser HJ, Baliova M, Krzyzankova M, Marsche G, Young MF, Mihalik D, Gotte M, Malle E, Schaefer RM, Grone HJ (2005) The matrix component biglycan is proinflammatory and signals through Toll-like receptors 4 and 2 in macrophages. J Clin Invest 115:2223–2233
Scheffold A, Huhn J, Hofer T (2005) Regulation of CD4+ CD25+ regulatory T cell activity: it takes (IL-) two to tango. Eur J Immunol 35:1336–1341
Schwandner R, Dziarski R, Wesche H, Rothe M, Kirschning CJ (1999) Peptidoglycan- and lipoteichoic acid-induced cell activation is mediated by toll-like receptor 2. J Biol Chem 274:17406–17409
Serafini B, Rosicarelli B, Magliozzi R, Stigliano E, Aloisi F (2004) Detection of ectopic B-cell follicles with germinal centers in the meninges of patients with secondary progressive multiple sclerosis. Brain Pathol 14:164–174
Sibley WA, Bamford CR, Clark K (1985) Clinical viral infections and multiple sclerosis. Lancet 1:1313–1315
Sloane JA, Batt C, Ma Y, Harris ZM, Trapp B, Vartanian T (2010) Hyaluronan blocks oligodendrocyte progenitor maturation and remyelination through TLR2. Proc Natl Acad Sci U S A 107:11555–11560

Sobek V, Birkner N, Falk I, Wurch A, Kirschning CJ, Wagner H, Wallich R, Lamers MC, Simon MM (2004) Direct Toll-like receptor 2 mediated co-stimulation of T cells in the mouse system as a basis for chronic inflammatory joint disease. Arthritis Res Ther 6:R433–446
Soulika AM, Lee E, McCauley E, Miers L, Bannerman P, Pleasure D (2009) Initiation and progression of axonopathy in experimental autoimmune encephalomyelitis. J Neurosci 29:14965–14979
Steinman L, Zamvil SS (2006) How to successfully apply animal studies in experimental allergic encephalomyelitis to research on multiple sclerosis. Ann Neurol 60:12–21
Sutmuller RP, den Brok MH, Kramer M, Bennink EJ, Toonen LW, Kullberg BJ, Joosten LA, Akira S, Netea MG, Adema GJ (2006a) Toll-like receptor 2 controls expansion and function of regulatory T cells. J Clin Invest 116:485–494
Sutmuller RP, Morgan ME, Netea MG, Grauer O, Adema GJ (2006b) Toll-like receptors on regulatory T cells: expanding immune regulation. Trends Immunol 27:387–393
t Hart BA, Gran B, Weissert R (2011) EAE: imperfect but useful models of multiple sclerosis. Trends Mol Med 17:119–125
Takeda K, Akira S (2005) Toll-like receptors in innate immunity. Int Immunol 17:1–14
Takeuchi O, Akira S (2010) Pattern recognition receptors and inflammation. Cell 140:805–820
Takeuchi O, Sato S, Horiuchi T, Hoshino K, Takeda K, Dong Z, Modlin RL, Akira S (2002) Cutting edge: role of Toll-like receptor 1 in mediating immune response to microbial lipoproteins. J Immunol 169:10–14
Thacker EL, Mirzaei F, Ascherio A (2006) Infectious mononucleosis and risk for multiple sclerosis: A meta-analysis. Ann Neurol 59:499–503
The Interferon study group (1993) Interferon beta-1b is effective in relapsing-remitting multiple sclerosis. I. Clinical results of a multicenter, randomized, double-blind, placebo-controlled trial. Neurology 43:655–661
Tigno-Aranjuez JT, Jaini R, Tuohy VK, Lehmann PV, Tary-Lehmann M (2009) Encephalitogenicity of complete Freund's adjuvant relative to CpG is linked to induction of Th17 cells. J Immunol 183:5654–5661
Touil T, Fitzgerald D, Zhang GX, Rostami A, Gran B (2006) Cutting Edge: TLR3 stimulation suppresses experimental autoimmune encephalomyelitis by inducing endogenous IFN-beta. J Immunol 177:7505–7509
Tzima S, Victoratos P, Kranidioti K, Alexiou M, Kollias G (2009) Myeloid heme oxygenase-1 regulates innate immunity and autoimmunity by modulating IFN-beta production. J Exp Med 206:1167–1179
Ungaro R, Fukata M, Hsu D, Hernandez Y, Breglio K, Chen A, Xu R, Sotolongo J, Espana C, Zaias J, Elson G, Mayer L, Kosco-Vilbois M, Abreu MT (2009) A novel Toll-like receptor 4 antagonist antibody ameliorates inflammation but impairs mucosal healing in murine colitis. Am J Physiol Gastrointest Liver Physiol 296:G1167–1179
Veldhoen M, Hocking RJ, Atkins CJ, Locksley RM, Stockinger B (2006) TGFbeta in the context of an inflammatory cytokine milieu supports de novo differentiation of IL-17-producing T cells. Immunity 24:179–189
Viglietta V, Baecher-Allan C, Weiner HL, Hafler DA (2004) Loss of functional suppression by CD4+ CD25+ regulatory T cells in patients with multiple sclerosis. J Exp Med 199:971–979
Visser L, Jan de Heer H, Boven LA, Riel D van, Meurs M van, Melief MJ, Zahringer U, Strijp J van, Lambrecht BN, Nieuwenhuis EE, Laman JD (2005) Proinflammatory bacterial peptidoglycan as a cofactor for the development of central nervous system autoimmune disease. J Immunol 174:808–816
Visser L, Melief MJ, Riel D van, Meurs M van, Sick EA, Inamura S, Bajramovic JJ, Amor S, Hintzen RQ, Boven LA, t Hart BA, Laman JD (2006) Phagocytes containing a disease-promoting Toll-like receptor/Nod ligand are present in the brain during demyelinating disease in primates. Am J Pathol 169:1671–1685
Volpi C, Fallarino F, Bianchi R, Orabona C, De Luca A, Vacca C, Romani L, Gran B, Grohmann U, Puccetti P, Belladonna ML (2012) A GpC-rich oligonucleotide acts on plasmacytoid dendritic cells to promote immune suppression. J Immunol 189:2283–2289

Wallin RP, Lundqvist A, More SH, Bonin A von, Kiessling R, Ljunggren HG (2002) Heat-shock proteins as activators of the innate immune system. Trends Immunol 23:130–135

Wang JP, Kurt-Jones EA, Shin OS, Manchak MD, Levin MJ, Finberg RW (2005) Varicella-zoster virus activates inflammatory cytokines in human monocytes and macrophages via Toll-like receptor 2. J Virol 79:12658–12666

Warger T, Hilf N, Rechtsteiner G, Haselmayer P, Carrick DM, Jonuleit H, Landenberg P von, Rammensee HG, Nicchitta CV, Radsak MP, Schild H (2006) Interaction of TLR2 and TLR4 ligands with the N-terminal domain of Gp96 amplifies innate and adaptive immune responses. J Biol Chem 281:22545–22553

Xia ZP, Sun L, Chen X, Pineda G, Jiang X, Adhikari A, Zeng W, Chen ZJ (2009) Direct activation of protein kinases by unanchored polyubiquitin chains. Nature 461:114–119

Xu J, Drew PD (2007) Peroxisome proliferator-activated receptor-gamma agonists suppress the production of IL-12 family cytokines by activated glia. J Immunol 178:1904–1913

Xu J, Racke MK, Drew PD (2007) Peroxisome proliferator-activated receptor-alpha agonist fenofibrate regulates IL-12 family cytokine expression in the CNS: relevance to multiple sclerosis. J Neurochem 103:1801–1810

Yan Y, Zhang GX, Gran B, Fallarino F, Yu S, Li H, Cullimore ML, Rostami A, Xu H (2010) IDO upregulates regulatory T cells via tryptophan catabolite and suppresses encephalitogenic T cell responses in experimental autoimmune encephalomyelitis. J Immunol 185:5953–5961

Yoshimura A, Lien E, Ingalls RR, Tuomanen E, Dziarski R, Golenbock D (1999) Cutting edge: recognition of Gram-positive bacterial cell wall components by the innate immune system occurs via Toll-like receptor 2. J Immunol 163:1–5

Zahringer U, Lindner B, Inamura S, Heine H, Alexander C (2008) TLR2– promiscuous or specific? A critical re-evaluation of a receptor expressing apparent broad specificity. Immunobiology 213:205–224

Zanin-Zhorov A, Cahalon L, Tal G, Margalit R, Lider O, Cohen IR (2006) Heat shock protein 60 enhances CD4+ CD25+ regulatory T cell function via innate TLR2 signaling. J Clin Invest 116:2022–2032

Zarember KA, Godowski PJ (2002) Tissue expression of human Toll-like receptors and differential regulation of Toll-like receptor mRNAs in leukocytes in response to microbes, their products, and cytokines. J Immunol 168:554–561

Zhang X, Jin J, Tang Y, Speer D, Sujkowska D, Markovic-Plese S (2009) IFN-beta1a inhibits the secretion of Th17-polarizing cytokines in human dendritic cells via TLR7 up-regulation. J Immunol 182:3928–3936

Zhou S, Cerny AM, Bowen G, Chan M, Knipe DM, Kurt-Jones EA, Finberg RW (2010) Discovery of a novel TLR2 signaling inhibitor with anti-viral activity. Antiviral Res 87:295–306

Chapter 9
Macrophages and Microglia in Experimental Autoimmune Encephalomyelitis and Multiple Sclerosis

Manoj Kumar Mishra and V. Wee Yong

9.1 Introduction

Multiple Sclerosis (MS) is a complex inflammatory and demyelinating disease of the central nervous system (CNS) that is a leading cause of disability in young Caucasian adults. The pathogenesis of MS involves adaptive immune components such as T and B cells (McLaughlin and Wucherpfennig 2008; Goverman 2009; El-behi et al. 2010; Berer et al. 2011; Lovett-Racke et al. 2011) and innate immune cells including monocytes, macrophages, and microglia (Heppner et al. 2005; Gandhi et al. 2010; Ajami et al. 2011). Indeed, the predominant groups of inflammatory cells in active plaques are macrophages and microglia (Lucchinetti et al. 2000; Prineas et al. 2001; Howell et al. 2010), and these persist through secondary progressive MS (Prineas et al. 2001). In this chapter, we focus on the roles of macrophages and microglia in MS and its animal model experimental autoimmune encephalomyelitis (EAE).

9.2 Multiple Sclerosis

The etiology of MS is unclear but genetic predisposition and environmental factors contribute to its pathogenesis (Ontaneda et al. 2012). The result is that various immune cell types are activated and they enter the CNS in large numbers to produce injury. $CD8^+$ T cells, $CD4^+$ T helper (Th) cells (mainly Th1 and Th17 cells), B cells, macrophages, plasma cells, and other cells have been implicated in the pathogenesis of MS (Frohman et al. 2006; Nylander and Hafler 2012). The activation of these immune cell subsets may be the primary event in MS but some studies have suggested that MS may be initiated within the CNS prior to the activation and subsequent infiltration of immune cells (van Noort et al. 2011; Stys et al. 2012). The pathological

V. W. Yong (✉) · M. K. Mishra
Hotchkiss Brain Institute, University of Calgary, 3330 Hospital Drive,
Calgary, AB T2N 4N1, Canada
e-mail: vyong@ucalgary.ca

T. Yamamura, B. Gran (eds.), *Multiple Sclerosis Immunology*,
DOI 10.1007/978-1-4614-7953-6_9, © Springer Science+Business Media New York 2013

hallmark of an MS lesion is the presence of an MS plaque, which is characterized by demyelination, inflammation, and axonal loss (Lumsden 1972; Trapp et al. 1998; Compston and Coles 2008). The demyelination observed in MS results from damage to the myelin sheath and oligodendrocytes. Macrophages/microglia are the main cell types involved in myelin breakdown as they can produce proteases, lipases, proinflammatory cytokines, reactive oxygen species, and nitric oxide (NO). Phagocytosis of myelin components in lesions by these cells is an indication of ongoing demyelinating activity (Bauer et al. 1994; Sriram 2011).

9.3 EAE, An Animal Model for MS

EAE is a useful animal model of MS and it is induced by the immunization of animals with CNS antigens, such as spinal cord homogenates, proteins derived from myelin (commonly, myelin basic protein [MBP], proteolipid protein [PLP], or myelin oligodendrocyte glycoprotein [MOG]), or peptides of these myelin proteins (Kabat et al. 1950; Swanborg 1995; Steinman 1999). EAE models may be fine-tuned to reflect different courses of MS (Lassmann and Ransohoff 2004; Baker et al. 2011). MBP-immunized Lewis rats or B10.PL mice mimic an acute phase of MS characterized by monophasic outcomes; SJL mice injected with PLP model relapsing–remitting MS, with alternate stages of paralysis and recovery. The most commonly studied MOG-immunized C57Bl/6 mice produce signs that resemble the rapidly progressing and chronic phase of MS. EAE can be induced by active immunization, which consists of the subcutaneous injection of an emulsion containing CNS tissue homogenates or a peptide of myelin proteins together with an adjuvant, or passive immunization, based on the intravenous injection of T cells previously activated against myelin proteins. In all described models of EAE, the disease is characterized by perivascular infiltrates within the CNS and paralysis. The cells that infiltrate and initiate disease are thought to be predominantly myelin-reactive Th1 and Th17 cells that secrete their signature cytokines of interferon (IFN)-y and interleukin (IL)-17, respectively (Frohman et al. 2006; Jager et al. 2009; El-behi et al. 2010; Murphy et al. 2010), and antigen-presenting cells (APCs) including monocytes, macrophages, dendritic cells (DCs), and B lymphocytes (King et al. 2009; Mildner et al. 2009; Ajami et al. 2011).

9.4 Monocytes/Macrophages

9.4.1 Function and Origin

Elie Metchnikoff received the Nobel Prize in 1908 for the discovery of the macrophage and its phagocytic role. Tissue macrophages originate from circulating monocytes that patrol the body and are among the first cellular responders of the innate immune system. They play a critical role in host defense, wound healing, repair, and chronic inflammation (Mantovani et al. 2005; Flannagan et al. 2009). While monocytes and macrophages are derived from precursors in the bone marrow, some macrophages develop in the embryo before the appearance of definitive hematopoietic stem cells. The macrophages that derive from the yolk sac are genetically distinct from hematopoietic stem cell progenies (Schulz et al. 2012).

Monocytes are produced and maintained by hematopoietic stem cells that reside in specialized niches within bone marrow. Monocytes expressing CD115, Ly6C, and CCR2 receptor on their surface have been referred to as immature, proinflammatory, or M1 monocytes, and they enter the blood circulation from the bone marrow in response to chemokines (Gordon and Taylor 2005; Geissmann et al. 2010). These monocytes then circulate in the blood for 1–3 days. Circulating monocytes can home to an area of inflammation in response to a chemokine gradient, and they then utilize surface molecules such as integrins to adhere onto endothelium before migrating into tissues (Imhof and Aurrand-Lions 2004) where the local milieu promotes their differentiation into macrophages (Delneste et al. 2003). A subset of circulating monocytes that are Ly6C^{low}CCR2-CX3CR1^{hi} are referred to as M2 monocytes and they are available to become resident, tissue-specific macrophages (Gordon and Taylor 2005). Tissue-resident macrophages may maintain their numbers by local proliferation and by differentiation of blood-borne monocytes in strategic locations in different organs.

9.4.2 *Polarization of Macrophages*

The description of M1 and M2 monocytes above emphasizes that these cells can be subclassified. Similarly, macrophages are heterogeneous cells that are highly plastic in nature and they have also been subclassified (Gordon and Martinez 2010; Sica and Mantovani 2012). The two major subsets of macrophage-activation pathways are M1 (classical activation) and M2 (alternate activation; Gordon and Taylor 2005; Gordon and Martinez 2010). IFN-γ and lipopolysaccharide (LPS), generated during a proinflammatory response and bacterial infections, respectively, are activators of the M1 classical pathway for monocytes or resting macrophages. The M1 cells use arginine as a substrate for inducible nitric oxide synthase (iNOS) and result in high production of nitricoxide (NO; MacMicking et al. 1997). In contrast to classical activation, the alternative activation (M2) pathway is triggered in response to parasitic infestation or local tissue damage. The M2 phenotype is produced by IL-4 and IL-13 stimulation and cells use arginine as a substrate for arginase 1 to form ornithine, which is a precursor for polyamines, proline, and collagen needed in wound healing (Gordon and Martinez 2010). Besides iNOS and arginase 1 being differential markers for M1 and M2 cells, respectively, M1 cells also express CD 16, CD32, CD64 (Fc-γ receptor), CD80, and CD86 (costimulatory signal molecules) while M2 macrophages express CD23 (Fcε receptor II), CD163 (hemoglobin scavenger receptor), CD204 (macrophage scavenger receptor 1), and CD206 (mannose receptor). In mice, M2 macrophages are also characterized by their expression of Found in inflammatory

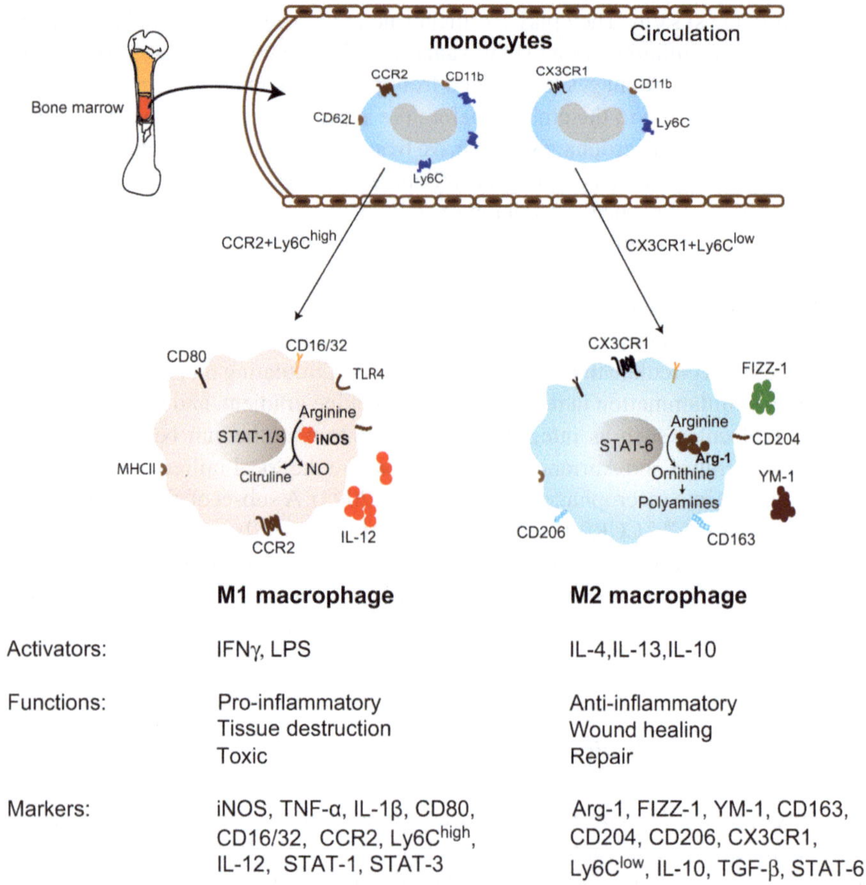

Fig. 9.1 A summary of M1 and M2 macrophages. Monocytes egress from the bone marrow and circulate in blood with a predominance of either the CCR2 or CX3CR1 receptor. Upon entering tissues including the CNS, an M1 or M2 macrophage subtype can be distinguished and some of the characteristics are listed

zone (FIZZ1) and YM1 (a protein from the chitinase family), although these are poorly expressed on human cells.

M1 and M2 macrophages are also characterized by the spectrum of cytokines that they produce (Fig. 9.1). The M1 cells produce high amounts of IL-1β, IL-12, and TNF-α that are largely proinflammatory, while the M2 subset secretes prominently regulatory/antiinflammatory cytokines including IL-4, IL-10, and IL-1 receptor antagonist. The differential cytokine profile helps promote the polarization of Th1/Th17 cells by M1 macrophages, and Th2 cells by M2 macrophages.

Iron toxicity is becoming topical in MS (Williams et al. 2012). Macrophage subsets may handle iron load differentially. The M1 subset has been reported to have iron retention capacity while the M2 subset can release iron and has the ability to recycle the metal (Corna et al. 2010). M1 macrophages express high levels of ferritin H, have low iron regulatory protein-binding activity, low levels of transferrin receptor 1 and take up iron with low efficiency, and only when the extracellular iron concentration is high. In contrast, M2 macrophages express low levels of ferritin H, have high iron regulatory protein-binding activity, and high levels of transferrin receptor 1. M2 macrophages have an intracellular labile iron pool and they take up iron effectively and spontaneously release iron at low concentrations; they have been reported to have limited storage ability for iron (Corna et al. 2010). M1 macrophages have the ability to present antigen even after iron depletion, a feature that allows them to maintain pathogen-specific T cells in conditions that are less permissive for microbe spreading. On the other hand, M2 macrophages play an important role in wound repair, resolution of inflammation, and tissue healing that requires nutrients including iron (Corna et al. 2010).

More recently, Schulz et al. (Schulz et al. 2012) used gene expression profiling and fate-mapping studies during early mouse development through adulthood to lend further understanding to the lineages of monocytes/macrophages. They concluded that tissue macrophages are derived from primitive embryonic precursors and that these are the resident macrophage populations that persist through life; in contrast, monocytes originate from bone marrow-derived hematopoietic stem cells throughout life.

9.5 Microglia

9.5.1 Origin and Function

Microglia are immune-competent cells of the CNS and they were originally described by del Rio-Hortega. Although generally considered CNS-resident macrophages, microglia and macrophages are now considered to have different lineages. In this regard, monocytes that originate from bone marrow enter the CNS from the circulation to become macrophages, particularly after an injury, while microglia are derived from the embryonic yolk sac early in development and they are not thought to be replenished by blood-derived monocytes after birth (Ginhoux et al. 2010; Prinz et al. 2011).

Microglia are distinguished from blood-derived macrophages by lower level of expression of CD45 (Ford et al. 1995; Agrawal et al. 2011) as detected by flow cytometry. Under basal "resting" conditions, microglia are highly dynamic and their processes constantly patrol the CNS microenvironment, a feature that is critical for maintaining CNS homeostasis (Nimmerjahn et al. 2005). Three states of microglia have been proposed based on pathophysiological studies: (1) the ramified microglia present in the normal adult CNS, (2) the activated, nonphagocytic microglia found in areas of secondary reaction due to nerve transection and CNS inflammation, and (3) the reactive or phagocytic microglia found in areas of trauma, infection, or neuronal degeneration (Hanisch and Kettenmann 2007). Microglia exhibit plasticity in their morphology and appearance, particularly during injury and disease. Resting microglia are highly branched (ramified) cells and express undetectable levels of MHC class I and II, CD80, CD86, and CD40 (Carson et al. 1998). Mechanisms that keep microglia quiescent include CD22, CD47, and CD200 expressed by neurons that interact with CD45, CD172, and CD200R on microglia, respectively (Mott et al. 2004; Ransohoff and Perry 2009; Saijo and Glass 2011), and by the release of fractalkine (CX3CL1) that interacts with CX3CR1 on microglia (Cardona et al. 2006). However, upon pathological insult, the ramified microglia become larger, retract their processes to become ameboid shaped cells, and they upregulate their expression of MHC and costimulatory molecules, and they increase their phagocytic ability (Aloisi 2001).

9.5.2 Microglia Polarization

Microglia also respond to the cytokine milieu to display markers of M1 and M2 polarization (Colton 2009). Microglia activation can be skewed similarly to that of macrophages. Treatment with M1 and M2 activators displays similar gene profiles (Colton et al. 2006; Colton and Wilcock 2010) in microglia and peripheral macrophages, indicating that Th1 and Th2 cytokines can drive microglial activation, which in turn can polarize Th1 and Th2 cells. Resting microglia also express the M2 markers arginase 1, YM1 and mannose receptor (CD206), and they express low/undetectable levels of TNF-α and NO (Kitamura et al. 2000; Ponomarev et al. 2007). Microglia are protected by the blood–brain barrier and not directly exposed to circulating cues such as proinflammatory cytokines in normal condition.

Adult human microglia in culture can also be polarized by appropriate cytokines. Interestingly, myelin phagocytosis was higher in M2 than in M1 human microglia, and this was elevated from that observed with macrophages (Durafourt et al. 2012).

9.6 Macrophages/Microglia in EAE and MS

9.6.1 Requirement of Monocytes/Macrophages, and Activation of Microglia, to Produce Disease

The rapid recruitment of blood-borne monocytes to become CNS macrophages, the activation of resident microglia and perivascular macrophages (PVMs), together with the recruitment of T cells, are among the most consistent alterations observed in MS and EAE (Bruck et al. 1995; Ford et al. 1995). In EAE, proinflammatory monocytes egress from the bone marrow and they accumulate in blood before entering into the CNS to produce pathology (King et al. 2009; Mildner et al. 2009). Mice deficient for the CCR2 receptor, which facilitates the trafficking of monocytes into inflamed tissues, are protected from EAE (Mildner et al. 2009). King et al. (2009) reported that granulocyte-macrophage colony-stimulating factor mobilized $CD11b^+$ $Ly6C^{high}$ proinflammatory monocytes from the bone marrow to produce an earlier onset and increased severity of EAE (King et al. 2009). Using a combination of irradiation and parabiosis, the infiltration of monocytes into the CNS was found to be necessary to drive the progression of clinical severity of EAE from mild to paralysis (Ajami et al. 2011).

Recently, we observed that $CD11b^{+}$ $Ly6C^{high}CCR2^{+}$ proinflammatory monocytes (similar to M1 cells described above) increase in numbers in the blood of mice by the next day following myelin peptide immunization for EAE, and that these cells accumulate for several days in blood prior to their entry into the CNS to produce pathology (Mishra et al. 2012). The migration of blood-accumulated monocytes into the CNS was correspondent with their elevated expression of the cell adhesion molecule, CD62L. Interestingly, we determined that the emerging MS medication, laquinimod, reduced the levels of CD62L and attenuated the migration of proinflammatory monocytes into the CNS correspondent with prevention of clinical manifestations of EAE (Mishra et al. 2012).

Prior to the description of proinflammatory monocytes, other authors have already reported on the essential role of migration of monocytes into the CNS to produce EAE. The depletion of monocytes/macrophages in rodents by treatment with silica dust or clodronate liposome reduced or prevented the clinical manifestations of EAE (Brosnan et al. 1981; Huitinga et al. 1990). Interestingly, clodronate liposomes eliminated only monocytes and peripheral blood-borne macrophages and PVMs but not the resident parenchymal microglia (Bauer et al. 1995; Fabriek et al. 2005). In addition, monocyte/macrophage depletion reduced the influx of $CD4^{+}$ T cells in the CNS, suggesting that they are critical for the subsequent infiltration of T cells into the CNS (Bauer et al. 1995; Tran et al. 1998). The depletion of infiltrating macrophages also resulted in inhibition of microglia activation (Bauer et al. 1995). These studies emphasize the requirement of monocytes/macrophages to orchestrate the immunological cascade that leads to EAE and MS.

Microglia activation is also important in the pathogenesis of MS and EAE. Microglial activation is a hallmark of demyelinating lesions in different models of EAE (Ponomarev et al. 2005; Rasmussen et al. 2007) and MS (Prineas et al. 2001). Microglial activation has been observed prior to demyelination in MS (Marik et al. 2007). In support, PET imaging data show that microglia activation was already apparent in the normal appearing white matter in MS, an area devoid of leukocyte infiltration, demyelination, or BBB disruption (van Noort et al. 2011).

The consequence of microglia activation was addressed by Heppner et al who ablated microglia in EAE by using transgenic CD11b-HSVTK mice, in which the CD11b promoter drove herpes simplex thymidine kinase expression (Heppner et al. 2005). When these CD11b-HSVTK mice were treated with ganciclovir, activated microglia were killed. The depletion of microglia resulted in attenuation of disease severity, inflammation, and demyelination in EAE (Heppner et al. 2005). Similar results were reported using another line of CD11b-HSVTK mice from another group (Guo et al. 2007). In support of these transgenic studies, the use of minocycline as an MMP inhibitor and with potent microglia inhibitory activity has been shown to ameliorate EAE severity (Brundula et al. 2002). Nonetheless, these studies have to be considered supportive but not definitive for a role of microglia in EAE and MS, since the CD11bHSVTK and minocycline approaches also affect macrophages and may have other activities.

9.6.2 *Antigen Presentation*

Th cells have been implicated in the pathogenesis of EAE and MS. Th1 and Th17 are thought to be the main pathogenic T cells in EAE and MS (Murphy et al. 2010). T cell activation requires antigen presentation by APCs. MHC class I and II molecules on APCs present the antigen to T cell receptor (TCR) and initiate T cell activation. The costimulatory signals between APCs (CD80, CD86, and CD40) and T cells (CD28, CTLA-4, and CD40L) are essential for complete T cell activation since MHC-TCR engagement without costimulatory signaling can lead to T cell death (Fletcher et al. 2010). DCs, the predominant APCs, normally initiate naive T cell activation (Raivich and Banati 2004; Becher et al. 2006). Macrophages express low level of MHC II and almost no expression of costimulatory molecules B7 in normal condition. It has been reported that macrophage and microglia acquire the ability of antigen presentation upon activation and that this activation favors the reactivation of primed T cells and regulates their differentiation (Raivich and Banati 2004). In the MS brain, activated microglia and macrophages present in all plaques express MHC II molecules (Raivich and Banati 2004), suggesting their role in T cell functions and lesion formation. Upon activation, macrophages/microglia have increased expression of MHC class II, CD40, CD80, and CD86. In EAE, macrophages and the majority of activated microglia express higher levels of MHC molecules at all stages (initiation, peak, and recovery) of disease, and their expression correlates with disease progression and T cell infiltration (Murphy et al. 2010). The expression of costimulatory molecules on macrophages/microglia elevates during EAE (Murphy et al. 2010). Along with professional APCs(DC), macrophages/microglia can present antigen to T cells and regulate T cell functions throughout the whole process of lesion formation in MS.

9.6.3 *Adhesion Molecules and Matrix-Degrading Enzymes*

9.6.3.1 Adhesion Molecules

The transmigration of lymphocytes and monocytes into the brain is a feature of MS and EAE (Owens et al. 1998; Ajami et al. 2011). Various approaches have been employed to block the entry of monocytes into the CNS (Bauer et al. 1995; Heppner et al. 2005). The mechanisms by which monocytes transmigrate into the CNS are not completely understood but are likely to involve a variety of adhesion molecules and chemokines (Owens et al. 1998).

Adhesion molecules that assist in the adherence of monocytes to endothelium include the β2-integrins MAC-1 (CD11b/CD18) and LFA-1 (CD11a/CD18), which are expressed on monocytes, and ICAM-1 (CD54), the receptor for both MAC-1 and LFA-1 that is expressed by activated endothelial cells (Bauer et al. 1995). An early study using antibodies to both MAC-1 and LFA-1 suppressed EAE clinical severity (Gordon et al. 1995), which is attributed to the blockade of infiltration of monocytes into the CNS. A recent study reported that Nerve injury-induced protein (Ninjurin)-1, a molecule involved in neuro–glia interaction, is present on immune cells and helps in the transmigration of immune cells into inflammatory lesions within the CNS. In EAE, Ninjurin-1 expression was increased particularly on monocytes/macrophages, neutrophils, and endothelial cells (Ifergan et al. 2011). Thus, inhibition of adhesion molecules on immune cells blocks the entry of monocytes into the CNS and subsequent neurological disease.

9.6.3.2 Matrix Metalloproteinase (MMPs)

Leukocytes enter into the CNS parenchyma in MS and EAE through several routes (Engelhardt and Ransohoff 2005). Leukocytes may enter via meningeal infiltration (Howell et al. 2011) and another route is through alpha 4 integrin-mediated leukocytes adhering to endothelial cells of postcapillary venules and transmigrating across them to enter the CNS (Engelhardt et al. 1994; Engelhardt 2008). Samples from both EAE and MS have two unique laminin-containing basement membranes surrounding the endothelial cells of venules within the CNS (Sixt et al. 2001; van Horssen et al. 2005); that proximal to endothelial cells is known as the endothelial basement membrane while that abutting the CNS parenchyma is the parenchymal basement membrane. Leukocytes including monocytes can cross the endothelial basement membrane but require MMPs to transmigrate the parenchymal basement membrane to enter the CNS parenchyma (Sixt et al. 2001; Agrawal et al. 2006; Toft-Hansen et al. 2006). MMPs are implicated in MS and EAE (Yong et al. 2001; Agrawal et al. 2006; Agrawal et al. 2011). In MS or EAE brains, and in vitro, monocytes, macrophages, and microglia express a variety of MMPs (Maeda and Sobel 1996; Yong et al. 2001; Toft-Hansen et al. 2004; Weaver et al. 2005); indeed, among immune cell subsets, the microglia produce the most abundant amount and spectrum of MMP members (Toft-Hansen et al. 2004). More recently, the upstream regulator of MMP expression, extracellular matrix metalloproteinase inducer (EMMPRIN), was found to be significantly elevated in leukocytes, including monocytes, and within the brains of EAE and MS specimens, on cells including macrophages/microglia (Agrawal et al. 2011). The EMMPRIN upregulation has pathological significance as an antibody to EMMPRIN diminished EAE severity (Agrawal et al. 2011).

Overall, the full activity of MMP and EMMPRIN expression by macrophages and microglia remains to be explored. In previous work, one role of the MMP members abundantly expressed on microglia is the regulation of the secretion of TNF-α (Nuttall et al. 2007). Additionally, MMP-3 from neurons has been implicated as a means to activate microglia (Kim et al. 2005) so the role of MMPs in cell–cell communication within the CNS remains to be further explored.

9.6.4 Macrophages/Microglia Produce Cytokines and Other Mediators

Macrophages/microglia upon activation produce many substances such as proteases, lipases, cytokines, glutamate, reactive oxygen species, and NO that can cause direct tissue injury (Takeuchi et al. 2006). Another relevant molecule produced by macrophage is osteopontin and it is highly expressed in MS (Chang et al. 2002). Osteopontin has been reported to stimulate monocyte recruitment, inhibit the apoptosis of proinflammatory T cells, and promote the production of proinflammatory cytokines from leukocytes.

Chemokines and cytokines mediate the recruitment and activation of leukocytes and other cells to sites of inflammation during an immune response. Activated macrophages/microglia secrete various cytokines/chemokines and have been extensively studied both *in vivo* and *in vitro* using different types of stimulation (Bauer et al. 1995; Hoarau et al. 2011). Classical activators such as LPS and IFN-γ induce macrophage/microglial expression of proinflammatory cytokines and mediators, including NO and TNF-α, to promote inflammation and antigen presentation. The majority of activated macrophages/microglia early in the course of lesion formation in MS and its animal models are thought to be of the proinflammatory M1 phenotype. M2 macrophages/microglia that are anti-inflammatory/regulatory and thought to help in tissue repair have been observed in both acute and chronic active lesions in MS patients (Mikita et al. 2011). Studies from EAE indicate that M1 monocytes or macrophages are present in onset or peak severity of the EAE disease course whereas during the recovery phase, M2 macrophages also exist. The administration of M2 monocytes through systemic injections ameliorates EAE disease severity in mice and rats (Weber et al. 2007; Mikita et al. 2011).

9.7 Neurotoxicity of Macrophages/Microglia of Relevance to MS

The chronic presence of activated macrophage/microglia in MS is likely undesirable for several reasons. First, a strong correlation is observed between macrophage/microglia activity and acute axonal injury (Ferguson et al. 1997; Kuhlmann et al. 2002) or loss of oligodendrocytes (Lucchinetti et al. 1999). Second, medium conditioned by microglia kills oligodendrocytes in culture (Merrill and Zimmerman 1991). In MS lesions, microglia in the process of stripping myelin can be found (Peterson et al. 2002). Third, there is persistent activation of microglia in relapsing–remitting EAE even after $CD4^+$ number wanes; the macrophage/microglia accumulation was correspondent with areas of synaptic pathology (Rasmussen et al. 2007). Fourth, products released from activated microglia impair neurogenesis (Ekdahl et al. 2003). The mechanisms of macrophage/microglia toxicity is likely related to the upregulation and release of the myriad of secretory products described above, including TNF-α, free radicals, and proteases (Graeber 2010; Lull and Block 2010; Rock and Peterson 2006).

That activated macrophages/microglia are toxic to neurons is amply demonstrated in tissue culture (Pang et al. 2000; Block et al. 2007; Qian et al. 2007). More recently, several groups have also reported that activated macrophages/microglia promote the death of oligodendrocyte precursor cells (Miller et al. 2007; Pang et al. 2010) or prevent their maturation into myelin-forming oligodendrocytes (Pang et al. 2010). The mechanisms of oligodendroglial injury include the secretion of free radicals and proteases, and the expression of CD137 ligand, along with reduced secretion of growth factors such as microglia-derived insulin like growth factor-1 (IGF-1) and ciliary neurotrophic factor (CNTF; Pang et al. 2010; Yeo et al. 2012).

Currently, there is no information on the potential outcomes of M1 and M2 cells on neurotoxicity in the context of MS. In spinal cord injury, M1 cells are thought to promote toxicity to neural structures in contrast to M2 cells that appear to lack the propensity to kill neurons (Kigerl et al. 2009). As noted above, the injection of EAE-afflicted rodents with M2 monocytes ameliorates disease severity (Weber et al. 2007; Mikita et al. 2011).

9.8 The Benefits of Macrophages/Microglia in MS

Although there is an extensive description of the potential detriments of activated macrophages/microglia as noted above, there are context in which these cells exert desirable properties including remyelination and neuroprotection. For remyelination, the depletion of macrophages by administration of clodronate liposomes retards the spontaneous repair that otherwise occurs robustly (Kotter et al. 2005); as well, promoting acute inflammation locally enhances remyelination in areas of chronic demyelination (Foote and Blakemore 2005) mainly due to the elevated response of macrophages/microglia. The use of LPS to stimulate microglia via TLR4 improves remyelination (Glezer et al. 2006; Setzu et al. 2006). The mechanisms for the usefulness of macrophages/microglia may be related to the observation that these cells are factories for a variety of neurotrophic factors; moreover, macrophages/microglia are required to clear the myelin debris, which inhibits remyelination (Kotter et al. 2006). The reader is referred elsewhere for the beneficial aspects of inflammation for the process of remyelination (Wee Yong 2010; Doring and Yong 2011).

It has been appreciated that there is an age-related decline in the capacity to remyelinate. This has been proposed to be due to a less robust recruitment of monocytes into lesions in older animals to become macrophages (Hinks and Franklin 2000; Shields et al. 2000). More recently, it was shown that the reduced remyelination with aging could be rejuvenated to juvenile levels through reconstituting in the aged mice the monocyte population from younger animals (Ruckh et al. 2012).

Besides remyelination, the facilitation of axonal regeneration by activated macrophages/microglia has also been noted. Benowitz and colleagues and others (Yin et al. 2006; Benowitz and Yin 2008; Yin et al. 2009) used a TLR-2 agonist to increase macrophage activity in the retina following optic nerve injury and demonstrated that axonal regeneration was improved. Moreover, they demonstrated that the beneficial macrophage activity was associated with a molecule called oncomodulin. As well, the transplantation of activated macrophages into a transected optic nerve increased axonal regrowth (Lazarov-Spiegler et al. 1998). These experiments support the results of David and colleagues who as early as 1990 reported that macrophages converted the nonpermissive nature of the CNS white matter into a permissible state for neurite growth (David et al. 1990; Prewitt et al. 1997).

The benefits of macrophages/microglia have also been reported in the context of neuroprotection. In spinal cord injury models, the implantation of activated macrophages depending on time and location of implants can be beneficial for wound repair (Rabchevsky and Streit 1997; Rapalino et al. 1998; Schwartz and Yoles 2006). In a model of Alzheimer' s disease, the clearance of beta-amyloid deposits (Malm et al. 2005; Simard et al. 2006) was facilitated by macrophages/microglia, with resultant improved functional recovery. The complex nature of macrophages/microglia in providing benefits or detriments to the CNS should now be obvious to the reader. The factors that regulate the neurotoxic or neurotrophic consequences of macrophages/microglia are beginning to be understood, and include the products that are predominantly produced at particular times, the balance of M1 versus M2 cells, the extent and chronicity of the insult, and the time period following the injury (Wee Yong 2010; Czeh et al. 2011).

9.9 Conclusion

An extensive literature implicates monocytes, macrophages, and microglia in lesion formation and propagation in MS. On the other hand, some aspects of the biology of these cells are useful for CNS outcomes. The complexities of the biology of these monocytoid cells are beginning to be revealed by factors such as their capacity to be polarized into different forms. Overall, preventing the transmigration of proinflammatory M1 monocytes into the CNS and the inhibition of activated microglia within the CNS could have therapeutic potential. In this regard, there is an increasing appreciation that several of the medications used in MS do affect monocytoid cells even if these were not the primary targets during drug development. For example, treatment with glatiramer acetate and dimethylfumarate (BG12; Weber et al. 2007; Ghoreschi et al. 2011) results in the generation of M2-polarized APCs. For the IFN-βs, the expression of the type 1 IFN-β receptor on myeloid cells is a key requirement for therapeutic efficacy (Prinz et al. 2008). In summary, a further understanding of the biology of monocytes, macrophages, and microglia, and the design of more effective therapies to inhibit the detrimental outcomes of these cells while sparing their beneficial aspects, could help improve the prognosis of MS and other neuroinflammatory disorders.

References

Agrawal S, Anderson P, Durbeej M, Rooijen N van, Ivars F, Opdenakker G, Sorokin LM (2006) Dystroglycan is selectively cleaved at the parenchymal basement membrane at sites of leukocyte extravasation in experimental autoimmune encephalomyelitis. J Exp Med 203:1007–1019

Agrawal SM, Silva C, Tourtellotte WW, Yong VW (2011) EMMPRIN: a novel regulator of leukocyte transmigration into the CNS in multiple sclerosis and experimental autoimmune encephalomyelitis. J neurosci 31:669–677

Ajami B, Bennett JL, Krieger C, McNagny KM, Rossi FM (2011) Infiltrating monocytes trigger EAE progression, but do not contribute to the resident microglia pool. Nat Neurosci 14(9):1142–1149

Aloisi F (2001) Immune function of microglia. Glia 36:165–179

Baker D, Gerritsen W, Rundle J, Amor S (2011) Critical appraisal of animal models of multiple sclerosis. Mult Scler 17:647–657

Bauer J, Sminia T, Wouterlood FG, Dijkstra CD (1994) Phagocytic activity of macrophages and microglial cells during the course of acute and chronic relapsing experimental autoimmune encephalomyelitis. J Neurosci Res 38:365–375

Bauer J, Huitinga I, Zhao W, Lassmann H, Hickey WF, Dijkstra CD (1995) The role of macrophages, perivascular cells, and microglial cells in the pathogenesis of experimental autoimmune encephalomyelitis. Glia 15:437–446

Becher B, Bechmann I, Greter M (2006) Antigen presentation in autoimmunity and CNS inflammation: how T lymphocytes recognize the brain. J Mol Med (Berl) 84:532–543

Benowitz L, Yin Y (2008) Rewiring the injured CNS: lessons from the optic nerve. Exp Neurol 209:389–398

Berer K, Wekerle H, Krishnamoorthy G (2011) B cells in spontaneous autoimmune diseases of the central nervous system. Mol Immunol 48:1332–1337

Block ML, Zecca L, Hong JS (2007) Microglia-mediated neurotoxicity: uncovering the molecular mechanisms. Nat Rev Neurosci 8:57–69

Brosnan CF, Bornstein MB, Bloom BR (1981) The effects of macrophage depletion on the clinical and pathologic expression of experimental allergic encephalomyelitis. J Immunol 126:614–620

Bruck W, Porada P, Poser S, Rieckmann P, Hanefeld F, Kretzschmar HA, Lassmann H (1995) Monocyte/macrophage differentiation in early multiple sclerosis lesions. Ann Neurol 38:788–796

Brundula V, Rewcastle NB, Metz LM, Bernard CC, Yong VW (2002) Targeting leukocyte MMPs and transmigration: minocycline as a potential therapy for multiple sclerosis. Brain 125:1297–1308

Cardona AE, Pioro EP, Sasse ME, Kostenko V, Cardona SM, Dijkstra IM, Huang D, Kidd G, Dombrowski S, Dutta R, Lee JC, Cook DN, Jung S, Lira SA, Littman DR, Ransohoff RM (2006) Control of microglial neurotoxicity by the fractalkine receptor. Nat Neurosci 9:917–924

Carson MJ, Reilly CR, Sutcliffe JG, Lo D (1998) Mature microglia resemble immature antigen-presenting cells. Glia 22:72–85

Chang A, Tourtellotte WW, Rudick R, Trapp BD (2002) Premyelinating oligodendrocytes in chronic lesions of multiple sclerosis. N Engl J Med 346:165–173

Colton CA (2009) Heterogeneity of microglial activation in the innate immune response in the brain. J Neuroimmune Pharmacol 4:399–418

Colton CA, Wilcock DM (2010) Assessing activation states in microglia. CNS Neurol Disord Drug Targets 9:174–191

Colton CA, Mott RT, Sharpe H, Xu Q, Van Nostrand WE, Vitek MP (2006) Expression profiles for macrophage alternative activation genes in AD and in mouse models of AD. J Neuroinflammation 3:27

Compston A, Coles A (2008) Multiple sclerosis. Lancet 372:1502–1517

Corna G, Campana L, Pignatti E, Castiglioni A, Tagliafico E, Bosurgi L, Campanella A, Brunelli S, Manfredi AA, Apostoli P, Silvestri L, Camaschella C, Rovere-Querini P (2010) Polarization dictates iron handling by inflammatory and alternatively activated macrophages. Haematologica 95:1814–1822

Czeh M, Gressens P, Kaindl AM (2011) The yin and yang of microglia. Dev Neurosc 33:199–209

David S, Bouchard C, Tsatas O, Giftochristos N (1990) Macrophages can modify the nonpermissive nature of the adult mammalian central nervous system. Neuron 5:463–469

Delneste Y, Charbonnier P, Herbault N, Magistrelli G, Caron G, Bonnefoy JY, Jeannin P (2003) Interferon-gamma switches monocyte differentiation from dendritic cells to macrophages. Blood 101:143–150

Doring A, Yong VW (2011) The good, the bad and the ugly. Macrophages/microglia with a focus on myelin repair. Front Biosci (Schol Ed) 3:846–856

Durafourt BA, Moore CS, Zammit DA, Johnson TA, Zaguia F, Guiot MC, Bar-Or A, Antel JP (2012) Comparison of polarization properties of human adult microglia and blood-derived macrophages. Glia 60:717–727

Ekdahl CT, Claasen JH, Bonde S, Kokaia Z, Lindvall O (2003) Inflammation is detrimental for neurogenesis in adult brain. Proc Natl Acad Sci U S A 100:13632–13637

El-behi M, Rostami A, Ciric B (2010) Current views on the roles of Th1 and Th17 cells in experimental autoimmune encephalomyelitis. J Neuroimmune Pharmacol 5:189–197

Engelhardt B (2008) The blood-central nervous system barriers actively control immune cell entry into the central nervous system. Curr Pharm Des 14:1555–1565

Engelhardt B, Ransohoff RM (2005) The ins and outs of T-lymphocyte trafficking to the CNS: anatomical sites and molecular mechanisms. Trends Immunol 26:485–495

Engelhardt B, Conley FK, Butcher EC (1994) Cell adhesion molecules on vessels during inflammation in the mouse central nervous system. J Neuroimmunol 51:199–208

Fabriek BO, Van Haastert ES, Galea I, Polfliet MM, Dopp ED, Van Den Heuvel MM, Van Den Berg TK, De Groot CJ, Van Der Valk P, Dijkstra CD (2005) CD163-positive perivascular macrophages in the human CNS express molecules for antigen recognition and presentation. Glia 51:297–305

Ferguson B, Matyszak MK, Esiri MM, Perry VH (1997) Axonal damage in acute multiple sclerosis lesions. Brain 120(Pt 3):393–399

Flannagan RS, Cosio G, Grinstein S (2009) Antimicrobial mechanisms of phagocytes and bacterial evasion strategies. Nat Rev Microbiol 7:355–366

Fletcher JM, Lalor SJ, Sweeney CM, Tubridy N, Mills KH (2010) T cells in multiple sclerosis and experimental autoimmune encephalomyelitis. Clin Exp Immunol 162:1–11

Foote AK, Blakemore WF (2005) Inflammation stimulates remyelination in areas of chronic demyelination. Brain: a journal of neurology 128:528–539

Ford AL, Goodsall AL, Hickey WF, Sedgwick JD (1995) Normal adult ramified microglia separated from other central nervous system macrophages by flow cytometric sorting. Phenotypic differences defined and direct ex vivo antigen presentation to myelin basic protein-reactive CD4 + T cells compared. J Immunol 154:4309–4321

Frohman EM, Racke MK, Raine CS (2006) Multiple sclerosis—the plaque and its pathogenesis. N Engl J Med 354:942–955

Gandhi R, Laroni A, Weiner HL (2010) Role of the innate immune system in the pathogenesis of multiple sclerosis. J Neuroimmunol 221:7–14

Geissmann F, Manz MG, Jung S, Sieweke MH, Merad M, Ley K (2010) Development of monocytes, macrophages, and dendritic cells. Science 327:656–661

Ghoreschi K, Bruck J, Kellerer C, Deng C, Peng H, Rothfuss O, Hussain RZ, Gocke AR, Respa A, Glocova I, Valtcheva N, Alexander E, Feil S, Feil R, Schulze-Osthoff K, Rupec RA, Lovett-Racke AE, Dringen R, Racke MK, Rocken M (2011) Fumarates improve psoriasis and multiple sclerosis by inducing type II dendritic cells. J Exp Med 208:2291–2303

Ginhoux F, Greter M, Leboeuf M, Nandi S, See P, Gokhan S, Mehler MF, Conway SJ, Ng LG, Stanley ER, Samokhvalov IM, Merad M (2010) Fate mapping analysis reveals that adult microglia derive from primitive macrophages. Science 330:841–845

Glezer I, Lapointe A, Rivest S (2006) Innate immunity triggers oligodendrocyte progenitor reactivity and confines damages to brain injuries. FASEB J 20:750–752

Gordon S, Taylor PR (2005) Monocyte and macrophage heterogeneity. Nat Rev Immunol 5:953–964

Gordon S, Martinez FO (2010) Alternative activation of macrophages: mechanism and functions. Immunity 32:593–604

Gordon EJ, Myers KJ, Dougherty JP, Rosen H, Ron Y (1995) Both anti-CD11a (LFA-1) and anti-CD11b (MAC-1) therapy delay the onset and diminish the severity of experimental autoimmune encephalomyelitis. J Neuroimmunol 62:153–160

Goverman J (2009) Autoimmune T cell responses in the central nervous system. Nat Rev Immunol 9:393–407
Graeber MB (2010) Changing face of microglia. Science 330:783–7880
Guo X, Nakamura K, Kohyama K, Harada C, Behanna HA, Watterson DM, Matsumoto Y, Harada T (2007) Inhibition of glial cell activation ameliorates the severity of experimental autoimmune encephalomyelitis. Neurosci Res 59:457–466
Hanisch UK, Kettenmann H (2007) Microglia: active sensor and versatile effector cells in the normal and pathologic brain. Nat Neurosci 10:1387–1394
Heppner FL, Greter M, Marino D, Falsig J, Raivich G, Hovelmeyer N, Waisman A, Rulicke T, Prinz M, Priller J, Becher B, Aguzzi A (2005) Experimental autoimmune encephalomyelitis repressed by microglial paralysis. Nat Med 11:146–152
Hinks GL, Franklin RJ (2000) Delayed changes in growth factor gene expression during slow remyelination in the CNS of aged rats. Mol Cell Neurosci 16:542–556
Hoarau JJ, Krejbich-Trotot P, Jaffar-Bandjee MC, Das T, Thon-Hon GV, Kumar S, Neal JW, Gasque P (2011) Activation and control of CNS innate immune responses in health and diseases: a balancing act finely tuned by neuroimmune regulators (NIReg). CNS Neurol Disord Drug Targets 10:25–43
Howell OW, Rundle JL, Garg A, Komada M, Brophy PJ, Reynolds R (2010) Activated microglia mediate axoglial disruption that contributes to axonal injury in multiple sclerosis. J Neuropathol Exp Neurol 69:1017–1033
Howell OW, Reeves CA, Nicholas R, Carassiti D, Radotra B, Gentleman SM, Serafini B, Aloisi F, Roncaroli F, Magliozzi R, Reynolds R (2011) Meningeal inflammation is widespread and linked to cortical pathology in multiple sclerosis. Brain 134:2755–2771
Huitinga I, Rooijen N van, Groot CJ de, Uitdehaag BM, Dijkstra CD (1990) Suppression of experimental allergic encephalomyelitis in Lewis rats after elimination of macrophages. J Exp Med 172:1025–1033
Ifergan I, Kebir H, Terouz S, Alvarez JI, Lecuyer MA, Gendron S, Bourbonniere L, Dunay IR, Bouthillier A, Moumdjian R, Fontana A, Haqqani A, Klopstein A, Prinz M, Lopez-Vales R, Birchler T, Prat A (2011) Role of Ninjurin-1 in the migration of myeloid cells to central nervous system inflammatory lesions. Ann Neurol 70:751–763
Imhof BA, Aurrand-Lions M (2004) Adhesion mechanisms regulating the migration of monocytes. Nat Rev Immunol 4:432–444
Jager A, Dardalhon V, Sobel RA, Bettelli E, Kuchroo VK (2009) Th1, Th17, and Th9 effector cells induce experimental autoimmune encephalomyelitis with different pathological phenotypes. J Immunol 183:7169–7177
Kabat EA, Wolf A, Bezer AE (1950) Experimental studies on acute disseminated encephalomyelitis in rhesus monkeys. Res Publ Assoc Res Nerv Ment Dis 28:113–132
Kigerl KA, Gensel JC, Ankeny DP, Alexander JK, Donnelly DJ, Popovich PG (2009) Identification of two distinct macrophage subsets with divergent effects causing either neurotoxicity or regeneration in the injured mouse spinal cord. J Neurosci 29:13435–13444
Kim YS, Kim SS, Cho JJ, Choi DH, Hwang O, Shin DH, Chun HS, Beal MF, Joh TH (2005) Matrix metalloproteinase-3: a novel signaling proteinase from apoptotic neuronal cells that activates microglia. J Neurosci 25:3701–3711
King IL, Dickendesher TL, Segal BM (2009) Circulating Ly-6C+ myeloid precursors migrate to the CNS and play a pathogenic role during autoimmune demyelinating disease. Blood 113:3190–3197
Kitamura Y, Taniguchi T, Kimura H, Nomura Y, Gebicke-Haerter PJ (2000) Interleukin- 4-inhibited mRNA expression in mixed rat glial and in isolated microglial cultures. J Neuroimmunol 106:95–104
Kotter MR, Zhao C, Rooijen N van, Franklin RJ (2005) Macrophage-depletion induced impairment of experimental CNS remyelination is associated with a reduced oligodendrocyte progenitor cell response and altered growth factor expression. Neurobiol Dis 18:166–175
Kotter MR, Li WW, Zhao C, Franklin RJ (2006) Myelin impairs CNS remyelination by inhibiting oligodendrocyte precursor cell differentiation. J Neurosci 26:328–332

Kuhlmann T, Lingfeld G, Bitsch A, Schuchardt J, Bruck W (2002) Acute axonal damage in multiple sclerosis is most extensive in early disease stages and decreases over time. Brain 125:2202–2212

Lassmann H, Ransohoff RM (2004) The CD4-Th1 model for multiple sclerosis: a critical [correction of crucial] re-appraisal. Trends Immunol 25:132–137

Lazarov-Spiegler O, Solomon AS, Schwartz M (1998) Peripheral nerve-stimulated macrophages simulate a peripheral nerve-like regenerative response in rat transected optic nerve. Glia 24:329–337

Lovett-Racke AE, Yang Y, Racke MK (2011) Th1 versus Th17: are T cell cytokines relevant in multiple sclerosis? Biochim Biophys Acta 1812:246–251

Lucchinetti C, Bruck W, Parisi J, Scheithauer B, Rodriguez M, Lassmann H (1999) A quantitative analysis of oligodendrocytes in multiple sclerosis lesions. A study of 113 cases. Brain 122(Pt 12):2279–2295

Lucchinetti C, Bruck W, Parisi J, Scheithauer B, Rodriguez M, Lassmann H (2000) Heterogeneity of multiple sclerosis lesions: implications for the pathogenesis of demyelination. Ann Neurol 47:707–717

Lull ME, Block ML (2010) Microglial activation and chronic neurodegeneration. Neurother 7:354–365

Lumsden CE (1972) Immunogenesis of demyelinizing plaque in multiple sclerosis. Rev Med Liege 27:521–537

MacMicking J, Xie QW, Nathan C (1997) Nitric oxide and macrophage function. Annu Rev Immunol 15:323–350

Maeda A, Sobel RA (1996) Matrix metalloproteinases in the normal human central nervous system, microglial nodules, and multiple sclerosis lesions. J Neuropathol Exp Neurol 55:300–309

Malm TM, Koistinaho M, Parepalo M, Vatanen T, Ooka A, Karlsson S, Koistinaho J (2005) Bone-marrow-derived cells contribute to the recruitment of microglial cells in response to beta-amyloid deposition in APP/PS1 double transgenic Alzheimer mice. Neurobiol Dis 18:134–142

Mantovani A, Sica A, Locati M (2005) Macrophage polarization comes of age. Immunity 23: 344–346

Marik C, Felts PA, Bauer J, Lassmann H, Smith KJ (2007) Lesion genesis in a subset of patients with multiple sclerosis: a role for innate immunity? Brain 130:2800–2815

McLaughlin KA, Wucherpfennig KW (2008) B cells and autoantibodies in the pathogenesis of multiple sclerosis and related inflammatory demyelinating diseases. Adv Immunol 98:121–149

Merrill JE, Zimmerman RP (1991) Natural and induced cytotoxicity of oligodendrocytes by microglia is inhibitable by TGF beta. Glia 4:327–331

Mikita J, Dubourdieu-Cassagno N, Deloire MS, Vekris A, Biran M, Raffard G, Brochet B, Canron MH, Franconi JM, Boiziau C, Petry KG (2011) Altered M1/M2 activation patterns of monocytes in severe relapsing experimental rat model of multiple sclerosis. Amelioration of clinical status by M2 activated monocyte administration. Mult Scler 17:2–15

Mildner A, Mack M, Schmidt H, Bruck W, Djukic M, Zabel MD, Hille A, Priller J, Prinz M (2009) CCR2+ Ly-6 Chi monocytes are crucial for the effector phase of autoimmunity in the central nervous system. Brain 132:2487–2500

Miller BA, Crum JM, Tovar CA, Ferguson AR, Bresnahan JC, Beattie MS (2007) Developmental stage of oligodendrocytes determines their response to activated microglia in vitro. J Neuroinflammation 4:28

Mishra MK, Wang J, Silva C, Mack M, Yong VW (2012) Kinetics of proinflammatory monocytes in a model of multiple sclerosis and its perturbation by laquinimod. Am J Pathol 181:642–651

Mott RT, Ait-Ghezala G, Town T, Mori T, Vendrame M, Zeng J, Ehrhart J, Mullan M, Tan J (2004) Neuronal expression of CD22: novel mechanism for inhibiting microglial proinflammatory cytokine production. Glia 46:369–379

Murphy AC, Lalor SJ, Lynch MA, Mills KH (2010) Infiltration of Th1 and Th17 cells and activation of microglia in the CNS during the course of experimental autoimmune encephalomyelitis. Brain Behav Immun 24:641–651

Nimmerjahn A, Kirchhoff F, Helmchen F (2005) Resting microglial cells are highly dynamic surveillants of brain parenchyma in vivo. Science 308:1314–1318

Nuttall RK, Silva C, Hader W, Bar-Or A, Patel KD, Edwards DR, Yong VW (2007) Metalloproteinases are enriched in microglia compared with leukocytes and they regulate cytokine levels in activated microglia. Glia 55:516–526
Nylander A, Hafler DA (2012) Multiple sclerosis. J Clin Invest 122:1180–1188
Ontaneda D, Hyland M, Cohen JA (2012) Multiple sclerosis: new insights in pathogenesis and novel therapeutics. Annu Rev Med 63:389–404
Owens T, Tran E, Hassan-Zahraee M, Krakowski M (1998) Immune cell entry to the CNS–a focus for immunoregulation of EAE. Res Immunol 149:781–789 (Discussion 844–786:855–760)
Pang Y, Cai Z, Rhodes PG (2000) Effects of lipopolysaccharide on oligodendrocyte progenitor cells are mediated by astrocytes and microglia. J Neurosci Res 62:510–520
Pang Y, Campbell L, Zheng B, Fan L, Cai Z, Rhodes P (2010) Lipopolysaccharide-activated microglia induce death of oligodendrocyte progenitor cells and impede their development. Neuroscience 166:464–475
Peterson JW, Bo L, Mork S, Chang A, Ransohoff RM, Trapp BD (2002) VCAM-1-positive microglia target oligodendrocytes at the border of multiple sclerosis lesions. J Neuropathol Exp Neurol 61:539–546
Ponomarev ED, Shriver LP, Maresz K, Dittel BN (2005) Microglial cell activation and proliferation precedes the onset of CNS autoimmunity. J Neurosci Res 81:374–389
Ponomarev ED, Maresz K, Tan Y, Dittel BN (2007) CNS-derived interleukin-4 is essential for the regulation of autoimmune inflammation and induces a state of alternative activation in microglial cells. J Neurosci 27:10714–10721
Prewitt CM, Niesman IR, Kane CJ, Houle JD (1997) Activated macrophage/microglial cells can promote the regeneration of sensory axons into the injured spinal cord. Exp Neurol 148:433–443
Prineas JW, Kwon EE, Cho ES, Sharer LR, Barnett MH, Oleszak EL, Hoffman B, Morgan BP (2001) Immunopathology of secondary-progressive multiple sclerosis. Ann Neurol 50:646–657
Prinz M, Schmidt H, Mildner A, Knobeloch KP, Hanisch UK, Raasch J, Merkler D, Detje C, Gutcher I, Mages J, Lang R, Martin R, Gold R, Becher B, Bruck W, Kalinke U (2008) Distinct and nonredundant in vivo functions of IFNAR on myeloid cells limit autoimmunity in the central nervous system. Immunity 28:675–686
Prinz M, Priller J, Sisodia SS, Ransohoff RM (2011) Heterogeneity of CNS myeloid cells and their roles in neurodegeneration. Nat Neurosci 14:1227–1235
Qian L, Tan KS, Wei SJ, Wu HM, Xu Z, Wilson B, Lu RB, Hong JS, Flood PM (2007) Microglia-mediated neurotoxicity is inhibited by morphine through an opioid receptor-independent reduction of NADPH oxidase activity. J Immunol 179:1198–1209
Rabchevsky AG, Streit WJ (1997) Grafting of cultured microglial cells into the lesioned spinal cord of adult rats enhances neurite outgrowth. J Neurosci Res 47:34–48
Raivich G, Banati R (2004) Brain microglia and blood-derived macrophages: molecular profiles and functional roles in multiple sclerosis and animal models of autoimmune demyelinating disease. Brain Res Rev 46:261–281
Ransohoff RM, Perry VH (2009) Microglial physiology: unique stimuli, specialized responses. Annu Rev Immunol 27:119–145
Rapalino O, Lazarov-Spiegler O, Agranov E, Velan GJ, Yoles E, Fraidakis M, Solomon A, Gepstein R, Katz A, Belkin M, Hadani M, Schwartz M (1998) Implantation of stimulated homologous macrophages results in partial recovery of paraplegic rats. Nat Med 4:814–821
Rasmussen S, Wang Y, Kivisakk P, Bronson RT, Meyer M, Imitola J, Khoury SJ (2007) Persistent activation of microglia is associated with neuronal dysfunction of callosal projecting pathways and multiple sclerosis-like lesions in relapsing-remitting experimental autoimmune encephalomyelitis. Brain 130:2816–2829
Rock RB, Peterson PK (2006) Microglia as a pharmacological target in infectious and inflammatory diseases of the brain. J Neuroimmune Pharmacol 1:117–126
Ruckh JM, Zhao JW, Shadrach JL, Wijngaarden P van, Rao TN, Wagers AJ, Franklin RJ (2012) Rejuvenation of regeneration in the aging central nervous system. Cell Stem Cell 10:96–103
Saijo K, Glass CK (2011) Microglial cell origin and phenotypes in health and disease. Nat Rev Immunol 11:775–787

Schulz C, Gomez Perdiguero E, Chorro L, Szabo-Rogers H, Cagnard N, Kierdorf K, Prinz M, Wu B, Jacobsen SE, Pollard JW, Frampton J, Liu KJ, Geissmann F (2012) A lineage of myeloid cells independent of Myb and hematopoietic stem cells. Science 336:86–90
Schwartz M, Yoles E (2006) Immune-based therapy for spinal cord repair: autologous macrophages and beyond. J Neurotrauma 23:360–370
Setzu A, Lathia JD, Zhao C, Wells K, Rao MS, Ffrench-Constant C, Franklin RJ (2006) Inflammation stimulates myelination by transplanted oligodendrocyte precursor cells. Glia 54:297–303
Shields S, Gilson J, Blakemore W, Franklin R (2000) Remyelination occurs as extensively but more slowly in old rats compared to young rats following fliotoxin-induced CNS demyelination. Glia 29:102
Sica A, Mantovani A (2012) Macrophage plasticity and polarization: in vivo veritas. J Clin Invest 122:787–795
Simard AR, Soulet D, Gowing G, Julien JP, Rivest S (2006) Bone marrow-derived microglia play a critical role in restricting senile plaque formation in Alzheimer's disease. Neuron 49:489–502
Sixt M, Engelhardt B, Pausch F, Hallmann R, Wendler O, Sorokin LM (2001) Endothelial cell laminin isoforms, laminins 8 and 10, play decisive roles in T cell recruitment across the blood-brain barrier in experimental autoimmune encephalomyelitis. J Cell Biol 153:933–946
Sriram S (2011) Role of glial cells in innate immunity and their role in CNS demyelination. J Neuroimmunol 239:13–20
Steinman L (1999) Assessment of animal models for MS and demyelinating disease in the design of rational therapy. Neuron 24:511–514
Stys PK, Zamponi GW, Minnen J van, Geurts JJ (2012) Will the real multiple sclerosis please stand up? Nat Rev Neurosci 13:507–514
Swanborg RH (1995) Experimental autoimmune encephalomyelitis in rodents as a model for human demyelinating disease. Clin Immunol Immunopathol 77:4–13
Takeuchi H, Jin S, Wang J, Zhang G, Kawanokuchi J, Kuno R, Sonobe Y, Mizuno T, Suzumura A (2006) Tumor necrosis factor-alpha induces neurotoxicity via glutamate release from hemichannels of activated microglia in an autocrine manner. J Biol Chem 281:21362–21368
Toft-Hansen H, Nuttall RK, Edwards DR, Owens T (2004) Key metalloproteinases are expressed by specific cell types in experimental autoimmune encephalomyelitis. J Immunol 173:5209–5218
Toft-Hansen H, Buist R, Sun XJ, Schellenberg A, Peeling J, Owens T (2006) Metalloproteinases control brain inflammation induced by pertussis toxin in miceoverexpressing the chemokine CCL2 in the central nervous system. J Immunol 177:7242–7249
Tran EH, Hoekstra K, Rooijen N van, Dijkstra CD, Owens T (1998) Immune invasion of the central nervous system parenchyma and experimental allergic encephalomyelitis, but not leukocyte extravasation from blood, are prevented in macrophage-depleted mice. J Immunol 161:3767–3775
Trapp BD, Peterson J, Ransohoff RM, Rudick R, Mork S, Bo L (1998) Axonal transection in the lesions of multiple sclerosis. N Engl J Med 338:278–285
Horssen J van, Bo L, Vos CM, Virtanen I, Vries HE de (2005) Basement membrane proteins in multiple sclerosis-associated inflammatory cuffs: potential role in influx and transport of leukocytes. J Neuropathol Exp Neurol 64:722–729
Noort JM van, den EPJ van, Horssen J van, Geurts JJ, Valk P van der, Amor S (2011) Preactive multiple sclerosis lesions offer novel clues for neuroprotective therapeutic strategies. CNS Neurol Disord Drug Targets 10:68–81
Weaver A, Goncalves daSA, Nuttall RK, Edwards DR, Shapiro SD, Rivest S, Yong VW (2005) An elevated matrix metalloproteinase (MMP) in an animal model of multiple sclerosis is protective by affecting Th1/Th2 polarization. FASEB J 19:1668–1670
Weber MS, Prod'homme T, Youssef S, Dunn SE, Rundle CD, Lee L, Patarroyo JC, Stuve O, Sobel RA, Steinman L, Zamvil SS (2007) Type II monocytes modulate T cell-mediated central nervous system autoimmune disease. Nat Med 13:935–943
Wee Yong V (2010) Inflammation in neurological disorders: a help or a hindrance? Neuroscientist 16:408–420

Williams R, Buchheit CL, Berman NE, LeVine SM (2012) Pathogenic implications of iron accumulation in multiple sclerosis. J Neurochem 120:7–25

Yeo YA, Martinez Gomez JM, Croxford JL, Gasser S, Ling EA, Schwarz H (2012) CD137 ligand activated microglia induces oligodendrocyte apoptosis via reactive oxygen species. J Neuroinflammation 9:173

Yin Y, Henzl MT, Lorber B, Nakazawa T, Thomas TT, Jiang F, Langer R, Benowitz LI (2006) Oncomodulin is a macrophage-derived signal for axon regeneration in retinal ganglion cells. Nat Neurosci 9:843–852

Yin Y, Cui Q, Gilbert HY, Yang Y, Yang Z, Berlinicke C, Li Z, Zaverucha-do-Valle C, He H, Petkova V, Zack DJ, Benowitz LI (2009) Oncomodulin links inflammation to optic nerve regeneration. Proc Natl Acad Sci U S A 106:19587–19592

Yong VW, Power C, Forsyth P, Edwards DR (2001) Metalloproteinases in biology and pathology of the nervous system. Nat Rev Neurosci 2:502–511

[illegible]

Chapter 10
Genetics of Multiple Sclerosis

Julia Y. Mescheriakova, Karim L. Kreft and Rogier Q. Hintzen

10.1 Genetic Epidemiology of Multiple Sclerosis

Multiple sclerosis (MS) is a presumed autoimmune disease of the central nervous system (CNS), triggered by environmental factors in genetically susceptible individuals. A genetic contribution to the pathogenesis of MS has already been suspected in 1896 with the discovery of familial aggregation of MS (Eichhorst 1896). It has been proven since the discovery of *HLA-DR2* locus and its association with MS in 1972 (Jersild et al. 1972). Epidemiological studies have measured disease risk in different types of relatives of MS patients, including monozygotic (MZ) and dizygotic (DZ) twins, siblings and half-siblings, parents and children, aunts, uncles, nephews, and nieces (Sadovnick et al. 1996; Ebers et al. 2004; Hoppenbrouwers et al. 2008; Hawkes and Macgregor 2009). The overall conclusion is that the higher the degree of relatedness, the higher the genetic burden and thereby the risk of MS. The risk to develop MS is about 3% in the first-degree relatives and 1% in second- and third-degree relatives of a MS patient compared to risk of 0.1% in general population (Sadovnick et al. 1988). In MZ twins, where the degree of relatedness is most extreme, the risk of MS is approximately 30 % (Hawkes and Macgregor 2009).

The female-to-male ratio was near 2:1 in the twentieth century. Orton and colleagues (Orton et al. 2006) reported a significant increase in incidence of MS in Canadian women, but not in men, over the past 30 years, causing a change in the female-to-male ratio to more than 3:1. Furthermore, the excess concordance of MZ twins for MS is almost entirely female-specific (Willer et al. 2003). On the basis of the apparent gender specificity, many studies attempted to examine the presence of

R. Q. Hintzen (✉)
Department of Neurology, Erasmus MC, Room Ba 4.92, P.O. Box 2040,
3000 CA, Rotterdam, The Netherlands
e-mail: r.hintzen@erasmusmc.nl

J. Y. Mescheriakova · K. L. Kreft
Department of Neurology, Erasmus University Medical Centre,
Dr. Molewaterplein 50, 3015 GE, Rotterdam, The Netherlands

T. Yamamura, B. Gran (eds.), *Multiple Sclerosis Immunology*,
DOI 10.1007/978-1-4614-7953-6_10, © Springer Science+Business Media New York 2013

parental origin-of-effect in MS. There is a tendency toward the maternal transmission of MS (Ebers et al. 2004; Herrera et al. 2008; Hoppenbrouwers et al. 2008). However, using a different approach the paternal origin-of-effect has been shown as well (Kantarci et al. 2006). Differences in family analysis may explain the lack of consensus regarding the parent-of-origin effect.

10.2 Human Leukocyte Antigen Class II

The earliest association between genes and MS was found in the human leucocyte antigen (HLA) region in 1972 (Jersild et al. 1972). The first association was with the HLA class I alleles *HLA-A*03* (Naito et al. 1972) and *HLA-B*07* (Jersild et al. 1972; Naito et al. 1972), which showed to be secondary to the *HLA-DR2* association (Batchelor 1977). Later, this has been fine-mapped to *the HLA-DRB5*0101-DRB1*1501-DQA1*0102-DQB1*0602* extended haplotype in the North European population with estimated risk ratios of approximately 3, and homozygozity for this haplotype increases MS risk sixfold (Dyment et al. 2004). This region is in a very strong linkage disequilibrium (LD), which makes it very difficult to distinguish the primary association (Spurkland et al. 1991). Several genetic studies have implicated *HLA-DRB1*1501* as the main susceptibility allele in MS (Oksenberg et al. 2004; Dyment et al. 2005; Lincoln et al. 2005). A recent genome-wide association (GWA) study (with 9,772 MS patients and ~ 17,000 controls) by the International Multiple Sclerosis Genetic Consortium (*IMSGC*) in collaboration with the Wellcome Trust Case Control Consortium 2 (WTCCC2) showed *DRB1*1501* to have the strongest association with MS with a p value of $< 1 \times 10^{-320}$ (International Multiple Sclerosis Genetics Consortium et al. 2011). However, in other ethnical populations, the risk allele or haplotype is different or does not contain DRB1*1501, such as in Sardinians where MS is associated with the *DRB1*0301–DQA1*0501–DQB1*0201* and *DRB1*0405–DQA1*0501–DQB1*0301* haplotypes (Marrosu et al. 1997), or in African–Brazilian MS patients where the strongest association was observed with *DQB1*0602* rather than *DRB1*1501*(Caballero et al. 1999).

There is evidence to assume that HLA-related susceptibility does not reflect the role of HLA *DRB1*1501* locus alone (Dyment et al. 2005). In Swedish and Canadian populations, *HLA-DRB1*17* allele has been associated with increased risk of MS, but to a lesser extent than *HLA-DRB1*1501* (Dyment et al. 2005; Modin et al. 2004). The recent GWA study revealed *DRB1*0301* ($p = 3.6 \times 10^{-10}$) and *DRB1*1303* ($p = 1.3 \times 10^{-11}$) alleles as risk alleles for MS (International Multiple Sclerosis Genetics Consortium et al. 2011).

Contrarily, *HLA-DRB1*14* was identified as strongly protective allele with an odds ratio (OR) of 0.31 (Dyment et al. 2005). This is a large effect considering the OR of *HLA-DRB1*15* being around 3 (Ramagopalan and Ebers 2009a). The effect of the *DRB1*14* allele might explain why the prevalence of MS is low in Asia where the frequency of this allele is very high (Ramagopalan et al. 2007). Interestingly, the *HLA-DRB1*14* allele has a strong protective role in type 1 diabetes (Erlich et al. 2008), possibly pointing at a common underlying mechanism of disease protection. The

*HLA-DRB1*11* and *HLA-DRB1*12* also showed a trend to significance as protective alleles against MS with OR of 0.75 and 0.55, respectively.

As stated previously, the prevalence of MS has been rising in women and there is a slight maternal parent-of-origin effect with higher number of affected mother–daughter pairs and few father–son pairs (Sadovnick et al. 1991). As the main genetic contribution in MS comes from HLA class II genes, Chao and colleagues (Chao et al. 2011) investigated in MS families whether reported gender predisposition could be HLA-mediated. Gender ratio analysis revealed that affected individuals with *HLA-DRB1*15* have a significantly higher female-to-male ratio as compared to those without. Five of six types of MS families (i.e., families with affected: sibling-pair, parent–child, sporadic cases, aunt/uncle–niece/nephew relationship and affected cousin; exception are multiplex families) seem to share the same trend of HLA- associated female predominance in MS susceptibility. Furthermore, significant difference in transmission of *HLADRB1*15* was observed in nuclear families (where first-degree relatives are affected) versus collateral families (affected second-degree and third-degree relatives) suggesting that the inheritance of supposed epigenetic alterations plays a role. Epigenetic markers will be explained later in this chapter.

10.3 Human Leucocyte Antigen Class I

As well as the established HLA class II associations, accumulating evidence has suggested that HLA class I loci may also influence MS susceptibility. The class I *HLA-A*03* allele was found to increase the risk to developing MS, while *HLA-A*02* and *HLA-C*05* alleles have protective effects independent of *HLA-DRB1*15* (Fogdell-Hahn et al. 2000; Yeo et al. 2007). Increased frequency of *B*0702* allele in MS patients was also significant, but this association was secondary to *DRB1*15–DQB1*06* and appeared to be in LD with these alleles (Fogdell-Hahn et al. 2000). Using transmission disequilibrium test (TDT) and haplotype analysis in families, Chao et al. have demonstrated that both *HLA-A*03* and *HLA-B*07* were significantly overtransmitted in families with *HLA-DRB1*15*-positive parents ($p = 0.0087$ and $p = 1.22 \times 10^{-6}$, respectively); the *HLA-C* allele was not studied (Chao et al. 2007). This indicates that the association with MS of both alleles, *HLA-A* and *HLA-B*, is HLA class II-dependent and secondary to LD with the HLA class II loci.

Cree at al. (2007) tagged 958 HLA spanning single nucleotide polymorphisms (SNPs) in two independent case-control data sets. They showed that 20 HLA class I SNPs were associated with MS susceptibility ($p \leq 1 \times 10^{-8}$). The most significant association was with SNP rs4959039 near the *HLA-G* gene (OR 1.59 with 95 % CI 1.40–1.81, $p = 8.45 \times 10^{-13}$). The MS susceptibility effect of this SNP was independent of *HLA-DRB1*1501*. Prior genetic studies of *HLA-G* in MS susceptibility found conflicting results. One study found no association between three *HLA-G* alleles and MS susceptibility (Kroner et al. 2007), whereas another study found an association of an *HLA-G*-promoter SNP with MS susceptibility by the transmission distortion test (Burfoot et al. 2008). Both studies were limited by relatively small sample sizes and few genetic markers studied. *HLA-G* is a biologically interesting candidate gene because of its prominent function in immune tolerance.

Using a combination of microsatellite, SNP, and HLA typing in family-based and case-control cohorts from two different populations, Yeo and colleagues have shown that *HLA-C*05* exerts a protective effect (RR $\sim 0.55, p = 3.3 \times 10^{-5}$) on MS susceptibility, independently of any effect attributable to the nearby *HLA-DRB1* gene (Yeo et al. 2007). An Italian study reported that the protective effect of *HLA-C*05* was possibly synergistic with that of *HLA-A2* (Bergamaschi et al. 2010). On the other hand, a Scandinavian study failed to confirm protection by this allele, but instead showed a positive association with *HLA-C*08* in *HLA-DRB1*15*-negative subjects (Link et al. 2010). HLA-C molecules, loaded with peptides, act as ligands for the killer cell immunoglobulin- like receptors (KIRs), which are important regulators of natural killer cell function.

The inhibitory KIRs have well-defined HLA class I ligands, the ligands for activating KIRs are yet poorly understood. *HLA-C*05* can be recognized by a variety of receptors such as KIR2DL1, KIR2DS1, and possibly also by KIR2DL2 and KIR2DL3 expressed on natural killer cells and/or a subpopulation of T cells, suggesting an increased potential for immune regulation via this HLA–KIR recognition pathway. (Parham 2005; Moesta et al. 2008). The protective association of *HLA-C*05* with other complex inflammatory disease such as psoriasis has been established earlier in Sardinian patients (Orru et al. 2005).

10.4 Risk Genes

GWA studies have become feasible in the last 5 years thanks to the development of new array technologies, analytical methods, improved central sample collection in MS centres and increased international collaborations. Array-based approach used in GWA study allows efficient genotyping of hundred thousands of SNPs throughout the genome simultaneously in a large number of patients and controls. A major highlight in the genetics of MS was the publication of the largest GWA study performed to date (International Multiple Sclerosis Genetics Consortium et al. 2011). This study confirmed the association of 23 previously reported loci and identified 29 novel loci plus 5 possible risk loci. It is important to realize that many of these risk loci are tagging SNPs and do not always locate to a certain gene. The majority of SNPs do not cause an amino acid change, since most of the MS risk SNPs are intronic SNPs. Furthermore, OR of these SNPs are in the range of 1.1–1.2 and thus much lower than those of the HLA class II loci. We will attempt to give an overview of these genetic discoveries by placing them in the context of their (presumed) function. However, some of these genes have multiple or unknown function (Table 10.1 and Fig. 10.1).

10.4.1 Risk Genes Exert Their Effect Probably via CNS Autoimmunity

Most of the SNPs, recently associated with an increased risk to develop MS in the large GWA study, are found in genes involved in immune development, functioning, and signaling.

Table 10.1 Overview of susceptibility genes for multiple sclerosis

Function	Genes
Neuronal molecules	*MMEL1, KIF21B*[a], *TAGAP, ZNF746, GALC, SOX8*
Vit. D metabolism	*CYP27B1, CYP21A1*
Ligands	*CD58*
Receptors	*MerTK, IL-7Rα, PTGER4, IL-2Rα, CXCR5, TNFRSF1a, TNFRSF6b, IL22Ra*[b]
Adhesion molecules	*VCAM-1, CD6*
Signaling	*RGS1, PTGER4, CBLB, TYK2, MALT1, MAPK1, RPS6KB1, DKKL1*[d], *PLEK, MerTK, BACH2*
Cytokines	*IL12A, IL12B, IL7*
Transport molecules	*EVI5, ARL61P4, KIF21B*
Transcription factors	*EOMES, NFKB1, MYC, HHEX, ZFP36L1, BATF, STAT3, MYB, ZMIZ1, IRF8, SOX8, MAPK1*
Transcriptional activity	*BACH2, ZMIZ1, ZFP36L1, BATF, Myb, Myc*
Costimulation	*CD40, CD86, CLECL1, TNFSF14*
Cell cycle	*MerTK, RPS6KB1*
Apoptosis	*BACH2, Myc, SOX8, ZFP31C1, ZNF36, TNFRSF6B*[c]
Proteolysis	*MALT, ZNF46*
Phagocytosis	*MerTK*
Endosomal maturation	*CLEC16A*
Autophagy	*CLEC16A*
Mitochondria	*SCO2*
Lymphoid development	*THEMIS*
Cytoskeleton remodeling	*PLEK*
Unknown	*PVT1, MPHOSPH9, MPV17L2, DKKL1, SP140*

Please note that some genes are categorized in more than one functional group

[a] The susceptibility SNP (rs12122721) that has been addressed to this gene lies actually nearby the open reading frame (C1orf106)

[b] IL-22Ra is a receptor antagonist

[c] Counteracts on TNFSF14 and FASL (CD154)-mediated cell death

[d] Inhibitor of WNT signaling

10.4.1.1 Lymphoid and Myeloid Cell Development

Already in the precursor state of lymphoid cells, SNPs with an increased risk to develop MS are found. In bone marrow, multiple polymorphisms are involved in lymphocyte and myeloid cell development. For example, Myb is an important regulator of hematopoiesis, especially for myeloid cells, but indispensable for yolk sack myeloid cells like microglia cells (Schulz et al. 2012). Moreover, HHEX is important for the development of B cells (Bogue et al. 2003). Interestingly, polymorphisms are also found in both *IL-7*, expressed by bone marrow stromal cells, and the *IL-7Rα* expressed on developing lymphoid cells. Signaling via the *IL-7/IL-7Rα* axis in the large pre-B cell stage is important for the rearrangement of the immunoglobulin κ light chain. Defects in this pathway lead to immunodeficiency, especially to severe combined immunodeficiency (SCID). Moreover, also for the development of mature T-lymphocytes, signaling via this pathway is important. In the thymus, IL-7 is expressed by stromal cells. The early T cell lineage progenitors (ETP) derived from the bone marrow migrate to the thymus where they mature into the double negative stage of thymocytes. The IL-7Rα is expressed on these cells and there it is important for the rearrangements of the T cell receptor. Thymocytes downregulate the IL-7Rα in the double positive state and when they mature into naive T cells, they reexpress the IL-7Rα (Mackall et al. 2011). The thymus is an important organ for the selection of antigen-specific T cells as well as for deletion and inactivation of auto-reactive T cells. *THEMIS*, another susceptibility gene, is important for late thymocyte development and is also involved in the positive selection of T cells (Gascoigne and Palmer 2011). It is thus intriguing to speculate that aberrancies in the development of lymphoid cells possibly caused by these polymorphisms are important for early development of enhanced autoreactive T and B cells, which might even after several years, contribute to the development of CNS autoimmunity.

10.4.1.2 Immune Cells in the Periphery

Mature naive T cells, which have left the thymus, are subsequently circulating in peripheral blood and are entering the secondary lymphoid tissues. Here, T cells encounter antigen-presenting cells (APCs) like monocytes, macrophages, and dendritic cells. In the interaction between APCs and T cells, multiple genes are associated with an increased risk to develop MS. First, there is the classical genetic association between HLA-II molecules and MS. These HLA-II molecules are important for the presentation of antigens to the T cell receptor. Second, multiple costimulatory molecules like CD40 and CD86 are able to give a second signal. Interaction between CD86 and CD28 on the T cells is important for T cell activation. The interaction between CD40L (also known as CD154) on T cells and CD40 on B cells is an important factor for B cell growth, differentiation, isotype switching of immunoglobulins, and cytokine production, which is in turn able to influence T cell polarization and functioning. Moreover, APCs are able to produce IL-12, which is a T helper-1 (Th1)-polarizing cytokine. Recently, it was shown in experimental autoimmune encephalomyelitis (EAE, the animal model of MS) that Th17 cells initiate breakdown and damage to the blood–brain barrier. Then Th1 cells are thought to sustain the damage to the CNS (Reboldi et al. 2009). Interestingly, the MS-associated risk gene *STAT3* is an important transcription factor for Th17 cells (Harris et al. 2007). *CLECL1*, expressed on B cells and APC is C-type lectin-like molecule involved in both costimulation to T cells, and in the polarization of T cells into IL-4-producing Th2 cells (Ryan et al. 2002). Moreover, it phosporylates MAP kinase and is involved in enhancing HLA-DR expression without affecting the expression of costimulatory molecules indicating that it might have a regulatory role in immunity (Ryan et al. 2009). Anti-inflammatory regulatory T cells (Tregs) are implicated in the immune pathogenesis of MS. One of the main features of Treg is the high expression of IL-2Rα (CD25) and low expression of the IL-7Rα (CD127), both genetically implicated in MS. The balance between different types of Th subsets is probably very important for the balance of tolerance and autoimmunity (Sakaguchi et al. 2010). One of the other interesting pathways important in this balance is the

IL-7/IL-7Rα axis. IL-7 is expressed in secondary lymphoid tissues by fibroblastic reticular cells (Mackall et al. 2011). For T cells in the periphery, signaling via the surface-bound IL-7Rα is important for the formation of immunological memory and homeostatic proliferation of potential autoreactive T cells. After activation of T cells by an APC, the T cells start to proliferate and differentiate into effector or memory cells. In this proces CD58, another risk gene associated with MS, is upregulated. CD58 is also known as LFA-3 and this is an activation and memory marker for T cells (De Jager et al. 2009a).

10.4.1.3 Lymphoid Cells in the Central Nervous System

After activation of T cells in the periphery, activated T cells express very late antigen-4 (VLA-4) enabling themselves to bind to VCAM-1, the product of eponymous gene which is associated with MS. After binding of VLA-4 to VCAM-1, which is expressed on endothelial cells in the brain, the T cells are able to migrate over the blood–brain barrier into the CNS. It is noteworthy that Natalizumab (Tysabri) is an effective and approved treatment for MS and this monoclonal-blocking antibody is directed against VLA-4 (Warnke et al. 2010). In the CNS, the activated T cells encounter APCs and might be reactivated after which they start to clonally expand and cause damage to the myelin sheets. Recently, it was shown that this mechanism is also applicable to CD8 T cells (Ifergan et al. 2011). Although much of the research on the immunology of MS has focused on CD4+ Th cells, it has already been noticed for a long time that CD8+ cytotoxic T cells outnumber CD4+ Th cells in MS brain. Moreover, it was shown that CD8 T cells are oligoclonally expanded in the brain of MS patients. Interestingly, *EOMES* was found in the recent GWA study. EOMES is the essential transcription factor for the effector function of CD8 T cells (Pearce et al. 2003). Moreover, in CD4+ Th cells, EOMES induces IFN-γ responses and suppresses IL-17 production by binding to the RORγC and IL-17 promoters.

Recently, in postmortem tissue, the occurence of B cell follicles in the meninges of MS patients has been described. These follicles are specialized tertiary lymphoid tissues, consisting of follicular helper T cells (Tfh), B cells, and plasma cells (Howell et al. 2011). Tfh have high expression of the chemokine receptor *CXCR5* (Breitfeld et al. 2000), another candidate gene for MS. Interestingly, B cells are able to produce CXCL13, the ligand for CXCR5. Moreover, it was shown that Tfh are expressing the TNF family member *TNFSF14* (also known as LIGHT), another MS susceptibility gene. LIGHT and lymphotoxin (LT) binds to the LTβR, which is an important factor for the formation of lymphoid follicles (Wu et al. 2001). The B cells and plasma cells might be the source of oligoclonal bands and raised IgG index, often observed in MS and often used as diagnostic tool for MS. Moreover, B cells are capable to present antigens to T cells and might thus serve as APCs in the brain to re-activate T cells, entering the brain after peripheral activation. It is noteworthy that a recent phase II trial with rituximab, a monoclonal-depleting antibody against CD20, a pan B cell marker was an effective treatment for MS compared to placebo

(Hauser et al. 2008). Validation of these results in phase III trials is expected. Moreover, it was shown that the mode of action of rituximab is mainly due to inhibition of the APC function of B cells thereby inhibiting T cell responses (Bar-Or et al. 2010; Piccio et al. 2010).

10.4.1.4 Immune Signaling

In multiple pathways and signaling cascades, MS risk genes are found. For example, in cytokine signaling, risk genes influence both receptors and ligands, and also adaptor proteins like STAT3 and Tyk2. In APC, multiple risk genes are involved in signaling for example MerTK. This is a tyrosine kinase receptor, which mediates phagocytosis of apoptotic materials and downregulates the activation of macrophages. Moreover, it is involved in homeostatic regulation of APC and is able to induce a tolerogenic phenotype in DC via blockade of NF-κB, one of the MS risk genes (Sen et al. 2007). Moreover, after binding of its ligand, protein S and GAS6, MerTK autophosphorylates and induces the phosphorylation of MAPK1 and MAPK2 among others. *MAPK1* is another MS risk gene. MAPK1 is involved in the regulation of the cell cycle (Coulthard et al. 2009). Moreover, it is a suppressor of gene transcription, including IFN-γ-inducible genes. Last, MAPK1 phosphorylates and regulates class II transactivator (CIITA), the master transcription factor for HLA class II expression and functioning (Paul et al. 2011). CBL-B belongs to the family of Cbl, which are molecular adaptors playing a key role in the regulation of tyrosin kinase-dependent signaling. CBL-B is described to inactivate NF-κB. Moreover, it inactivates T cells until the second signal for activation (first signal HLA-TCR interaction, second signal costimulation) is received (Paolino and Penninger 2010). Combination of these two mechanisms provides reduction of T cell activation. Moreover, it also reduces B cell functioning by negatively regulating B cell proliferation (Bachmaier et al. 2000).

10.4.1.5 Linking Multiple Sclerosis Risk Genes with Environmental Risk Factors

From epidemiological studies, it is well known that the etiology of MS probably consists of a combination of genetic susceptibility and environmental triggers. Infections are a well-known risk factor to develop MS. One of the strongest risk factors for the development of MS is a history of infectious mononucleosis (IM). Several studies have linked Epstein Barr virus (EBV) to MS (Thacker et al. 2006). Recently, it was demonstrated that gut microbiota in EAE are important for the development of dysfunction in mice (Berer et al. 2011). The SNP in *IL-22RA* is interesting, since IL-22 is important in the promotion of antimicrobial immunity, but also in the regulation of inflammation and tissue repair in the mucosal environment (Sonnenberg et al. 2011).

Other environmental risk factors have epidemiologically been linked to MS, such as vitamin D as a modulator of the immune response, both on APCs as well as on T cells. Interestingly, two SNP in the vitamin D metabolism were found associated with MS. One SNP is located in *CYP27B1* gene, which is involved in metabolizing the inactive form of vitamin D (25-hydroxy D3) into the bioactive vitamin D (1,25-dihydroxy D3). Another SNP is located in *CYP24A1* gene, which is involved in the inactivation of bioactive form into calcitroic acid. Aberrancies in this pathway, in combination with differences in sunlight exposure, might be an explanation for the observed latitude gradient of MS over the world, with the highest incidence of MS far away from the equator.

10.4.1.6 Genes with Functions Within the Central Nervous System

From the recent large-scale GWA study in MS, one of the observations is the relative lack of genes with known functions in the CNS. However, some genes have been described to have a function in the CNS.

GALC encodes the lysosomal enzyme galactocerebrosidase, which digest galactocerebroside. Galactocerebroside is the major substrate in Schwann cells and oligodendrocytes (ODCs), the myelinating cells of the nervous system (Kondo et al. 2005). Mutations leading to deficiencies in activity of galactocerebroside are found in globoid cell leukodystrophy (GLD, also known as Krabbe's disease), a devastating disease in young children leading to severe neurological complaints through progressive demyelination. Several studies have investigated whether MS patients have antibodies against GALC, but none of these studies have found anti-GALC antibodies (Lubetzki et al. 1986; Rostami et al. 1987). Moreover, incubation of primary human ODCs with the serum of MS patients did not result in ODC cytotoxicity nor morphological changes (Ruijs et al. 1990).

Membrane metalloendopeptidase like 1 (MMEL1), also known as neprilysin 2 (NEP2) is expressed in the brain in several neuronal populations, pituitary gland and testis (Ouimet et al. 2000). Relatively little is known about its function, but it is involved in the degradation of beta-amyloid (Huang et al. 2008). Decreased expression of MMEL1 is observed in the brain of Alzheimer's patients and inhibitors of MMEL1 peptidase activity leads to increased deposition of beta-amyloid depositions in mice (Huang et al. 2012).

ZNF746, also known as *PARIS*, is another MS risk gene which is associated with neurodegeneration. Recently, PARIS is implicated to be involved in the pathogenesis of Parkinson's disease. ZNF746 accumulates rather specifically in the striatum and substantia nigra, but not in the cerebellum or cortex. It suppresses the transcriptional activity of peroxisome proliferator-γ coactivator-1α (PGC-1α), by binding to its promoter and thereby inhibiting the transcription of NRF-1 (Shin et al. 2011), which is involved in cellular metabolism and mitochondrial biosynthesis (Castillo-Quan 2011). Overexpression of PARIS leads to dopaminergic neuronal cell death in the substantia nigra and thus to neurodegeneration (Shin et al. 2011). Mitochondrial dysfunction has also been implicated in the pathogenesis of MS. In active MS lesions, there is a loss of several important mitochondrial proteins. In chronic inactive lesions, the number and the activity of mitochondria increase (Mahad et al. 2008a, b). Recently, it was shown that there are extensive deletions in mitochondrial DNA (mtDNA) in neurons of MS patients. The cause of these deletions is currently unknown, although it is speculated that this occurs secondary to inflammation (Campbell et al. 2011). It should be mentioned that the inflammatory process in MS may cause damage to the mitochondria, for example, via reactive oxygen species and nitric oxide. Currently, from the GWA studies only one SNP in a mitochondrial gene (*SCO2* gene) is associated with MS. Moreover, some candidate gene studies regarding mtDNA SNP have been performed in MS. A SNP in the *mt-ND5* gene (nt13708G/A SNP) is associated with both adult (Yu et al. 2008) and pediatric MS (Venkateswaran et al. 2011). This SNP causes an amino acid change, but if this is affecting mitochondrial functioning is currently unclear. Another mtDNA SNP (rs659366 in the promoter of the *UCP2* gene) is associated with MS. The G-allele of this SNP has an increased prevalence in MS patients. This is associated with a decreased expression of *UPC2* gene, which increased ATP levels (Vogler et al. 2005). Increased ATP levels are associated with proinflammatory response via activation of the inflammasome. As the frequency of MS in females is increasing, it is worthwhile to further study mtDNA, as this is per definition maternally transmitted. Again, it should be noted that substantial evidence exist that MS is also maternally transmitted.

Lastly, several studies associated *KIF21B* with MS. However, in the latest GWA study, not *KIF21B*, but the nearby located open reading frame (ORF) (*C1orf106*) was found to give rise to this signal. It remains to be validated whether the association in this region comes from *KIF21B* or the ORF. Nevertheless, *KIF21B* is an interesting candidate. *KIF21B* belongs to the family of kinesins, which are responsible for intracellular transport of protein and organelles (Hirokawa et al. 2010). The exact cargo of the transporter *KIF21B* is currently unknown, but it is known that this kinesin is expressed in dendrites of neurons (Marszalek et al. 1999). Alterations in these important transport molecules might be related to neurodegeneration in MS. Moreover, *KIF1B* was also found in a GWA study (Aulchenko et al. 2008), although subsequent studies failed to replicate this finding (Booth et al. 2010). Also, candidate studies have implicated another kinesin, namely *KIF5A*, to be associated with MS (Alcina et al. 2010).

10.4.1.7 Functional Immunogenetics

A large number of SNPs associated with MS are SNPs in receptors and molecules with important functions in immune-related processes. Studying how these SNPs are affecting the expression and functioning of immune cells is an important step in improving our understanding of the immunopathogenesis of MS. Currently, only a minor number of studies is performed to unravel how these SNPs are affecting immune functioning.

CD6 is an adhesion molecule. Studies showed that the *CD6* risk allele is associated with impaired proliferation of long-term activated Th cells. The CD6 risk allele

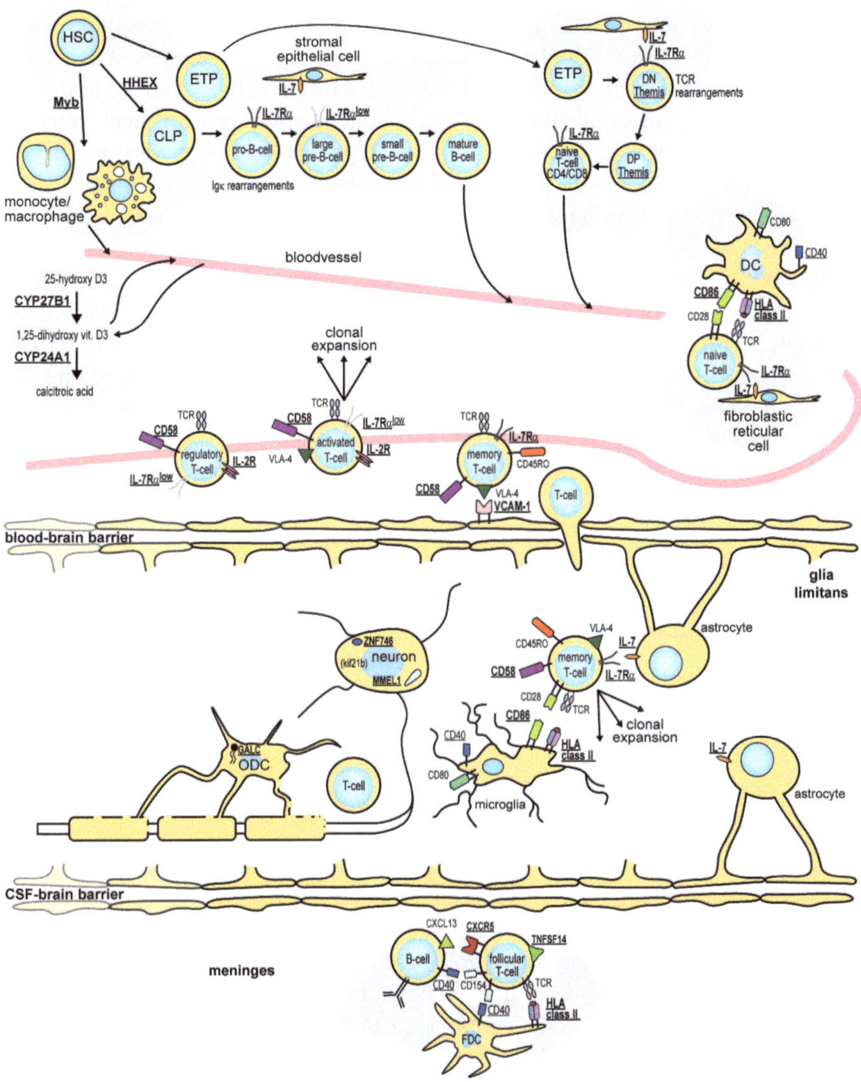

Fig. 10.1 Functions of single nucleotide polymorphism (SNP) in the development, activation of, and interaction between immune cells in the periphery and central nervous system (CNS). Model on presumed functions of the multiple sclerosis (MS) risk genes from the development in the bone marrow and thymus to activation of lymphoid cells in the secondary lymphoid tissue and the migration into the CNS and the formation of the B cell follicles in the meninges. Moreover, the vitamin D metabolism is shown in the kidney. *CLP* common lymphoid progenitor, *ETP* early thymic progenitor, *HSC* hematopoietic stem cell

(rs17824933) leads to consistent downregulation of expression of exon 5, which is the ALCAM-binding domain, the ligand for CD6, thereby, explaining the lower proliferative response (Kofler et al. 2011).

For *CD25*, the *IL-2Rα*, it was shown that the risk allele is associated with an increased expression of CD25 in naive T cells and a decreased expression in memory T cells. IL-2 has a double role in the immune system, namely it is a very potent proliferative stimulus after activation of naive T cells. It has an important role of induction and sustainability of Tregs in the memory compartment. Interestingly, it was shown that functionally active Tregs are expressing very low levels of the IL-7Rα. IL-2 and IL-7 are cytokines, which belong to the same family and have been shown to have similar as well as opposing functions (reviewed in Katzman et al. 2011). Functional studies in healthy controls have shown that the *IL-2R* SNP (rs2104286) risk carriership leads to increased expression of CD25 on naive CD4 T cells (Dendrou et al. 2009). Moreover, the *IL-7Rα* SNP (rs6897932) is associated with higher levels of the soluble form of the receptor (Hoe et al. 2010). Furthermore, it was shown that the surface expression was even increased on CD8 effector T cells, independent of the genotype (Kreft et al. 2012), as well as CD8 Tregs of MS patients (Kreft et al. 2011).

A polymorphism in *CD58* (rs2300747) is implicated to alter the expression of CD58 messenger RNA (mRNA) peripheral blood mononuclear cells (PBMC), which affects the functioning of Tregs (De Jager et al. 2009a). Another study assessed whether the SNP in *IRF8* (rs17445836) influenced the gene expression in PBMC. No association between the SNP and *IRF8* mRNA expression was found, although it should be noted that only one probe of the *IRF8* mRNA was present on the microarray chip used. Interestingly, in this study 16 genes were found to associate with the SNP in *IRF8* and eight of these genes are type I interferon-responding genes (De Jager et al. 2009b).

10.5 Gene–Gene Interaction

Many interactions with major MS susceptibility *HLA-DRB1*1501* allele have been studied, but not all of them have been validated yet. An Iranian study (Shahbazi et al. 2011) found that among *HLA-DRB1*1501*-positive individuals, association of *TNF*-α−308 G allele and G/G genotype with susceptibility to MS was more prominent (combined OR = 7.07, compared to OR = 1.57 for *HLA-DRB1*1501* alone, OR = 1.26 for only G-allele, and OR = 4.59 for GG genotype of *TNF*-α SNP). A recent meta-analysis showed that individuals carrying *TNF*-α−308A allele have indeed lower susceptibility to MS, and those with G allele, higher susceptibility to MS (Yang et al. 2011). This is not surprising because the G/A polymorphism of *TNF*-α−308 has direct effects on *TNF*-α gene regulation and the A allele is associated with a high level of TNF-α production (Wilson et al. 1997). A number of clinical studies suggested that decreased TNF-α activity is associated with CNS inflammatory lesions and treatment with monoclonal antibodies to TNF-α may trigger acute episodes of CNS inflammation in subjects with MS (van Oosten et al. 1996). Moreover, the anti-TNF-α therapy in some patients with Crohn's disease or rheumatoid arthritis is associated with inflammatory demyelinating events in the CNS and MS aggravation (Sicotte and Voskuhl 2001; Fromont et al. 2009).

Iranian study group has shown that the *IL-2*-330T allele and the G/T and T/T genotypes were associated with a higher risk of developing MS (Shahbazi et al. 2010). When combined with the *HLA-DRB1*1501* allele, the IL-2T allele was strongly associated with susceptibility to MS (OR = 16.0, CI 5.6–62.2, $p < 0.0001$). In literature, there are controversial findings in relation to which allele (T or G) is really responsible for higher susceptibility to MS (Matesanz et al. 2001; Amirzargar et al. 2007; Fedetz et al. 2009). Different cytokine production levels in the *IL-2*-330G and T allele carriers in vivo and in vitro were also reported (Hoffmann et al. 2001; Matesanz et al. 2004).

Bush et al. (2011) identified gene–gene interactions between genes *CHRM3* and *MYLK* ($p = 0.0002$), between *PLC-β 1* and *PLC-β 4* ($p = 0.0098$) and a modest interaction between *ACTN1* and *MYH9* ($p = 0.0326$), all localized to calcium-signaled cytoskeletal regulation. These are nonimmune susceptibility loci for MS suggestive for the neurodegenerative component to MS.

It has been observed that there are interactions between different HLA-loci in the *DRB1* gene. In the specific case of HLA-loci interactions, it is referred to as "epistatic interaction." A well-known *HLA-DRB1*15* allele is a major risk factor for the development of MS (OR ~ 3), but in combination with *HLA-DRB1*14*, the risk of *HLA-DRB1*15* is abrogated to an OR of 1. The *HLA-DRB1*08* allele modestly increases the risk of MS but when present in combination with *HLA-DRB1*15*, it more than doubles the risk associated with a single copy of *HLA-DRB1*15*. In addition, the *DRB1*01* and *DRB1*10* alleles protect against MS but only in the presence of *DRB1*15* (Ramagopalan and Ebers 2009b).

A significant interaction was shown between *HLA-DRB1*15* and *HLA-A*02*, in which the susceptibility risk of MS decreases in the presence of protective *HLA-A*02* allele (Hedstrom et al. 2011).

10.6 Gene–Environment Interaction

MS cannot be explained by any single known environmental or genetic factor alone. A combination of genes and environmental factors (including infections) is necessary for the development of MS (Ramagopalan and Giovannoni 2009). Their interaction appears to be required and this is now a main goal of many epidemiological studies.

10.6.1 Vitamin D and HLA-DRB1

Biological effect of the active form of vitamin D (1,25-dihydroxyvitamin D3) is mediated via the vitamin D receptor (VDR). This receptor is a member of steroid superfamily and influences the rate of transcription of vitamin D-responsive genes by binding to vitamin D-responsive elements (VDREs) in gene promoters across the genome. Ramagopalan et al. have shown that more than 2,700 binding sites (intragenic, intergenic, and intronic) across the genome are affected by vitamin D (Ramagopalan et al. 2010). Interestingly, a single VDRE exists in the *HLA-DRB1* promoter region, which showed haplotype- specific differences, being highly conserved in the major MS-associated haplotype *HLA-DRB1*15* dominant in North Europeans, but not conserved among other non-MS-associated haplotypes (Ramagopalan et al. 2009). This means that this region remained essentially unchanged throughout evolution in this specific HLA haplotype. B cells, transfected with the *HLA-DRB1*15* gene promoter, showed significantly increased gene expression on stimulation with 1,25-dihydroxyvitamin D3. This was not the case in cells with deleted VDRE site or cells with the homologous "VDRE" sequence found in non-MS-associated *HLA-DRB1* haplotypes. Flow cytometric analysis showed a specific increase in the cell surface expression of *HLA-DRB1* upon addition of vitamin D only in *HLA-DRB1*15* bearing lymphoblastoid cells. From this point of view, addressing SNPs in *VDR* region in MS patients is an interesting issue. There are four SNPs within the *VDR* gene, rs2228570 (Fok1), rs731236 (Taq1), rs1544410 (Bsm1), and rs7975232 (Apa1), of which the last three SNPS are in LD (Cox et al. 2012). Cox et al. (2012) found weak evidence for an association between the rs731236 (Taq1) C-allele and MS. There was a trend for a gene–gene interaction between *Taq1* and the *HLA-DRB1*1501*. However, this did not reach significance thresholds. In a recent meta-analysis, Handel could not find any significant association between the *VDR* SNPs and MS susceptibility (Handel and Ramagopalan 2012). More interesting was an observation that the ORs of these SNPs depend on the presence of *HLA-DRB1*1501* alleles (Handel and Ramagopalan 2012). This highlights the fact that functional interaction between VDR SNPs and *HLA-DRB1*1501* alleles may be concealing a considerable contribution to MS susceptibility.

Next to *HLA-DRB1* locus, VDR-binding sites were found near other autoimmune and cancer-associated genes identified from GWA studies, including *IRF8* associated with MS, and *PTPN2* associated with Crohn's disease (Wellcome Trust Case Control Consortium 2007), type I diabetes (T1D) (Todd et al. 2007), and rheumatoid arthritis (RA) (Okada et al. 2012). This evidence supports a role for vitamin D in susceptibility to MS and other autoimmune diseases through effects on a substantial number of associated genes and highlights a number of important candidate regions to be investigated further.

10.6.2 Infectious Mononucleosis and Human Leucocyte Antigen

A history of Infectious Mononucleosis (IM) increases the risk to develop MS. A meta-analysis (Thacker et al 2006) reported a combined relative risk of MS after IM of 2.3 (95 % CI 1.7–3.0). A suggested mechanism is a common genetic basis that predisposes to both diseases. Ramagopalan et al. (2011a) have failed to find any association with the strong MS risk allele *HLA-DRB1*1501*. Instead, they observed that *HLA-DRB1*01:01* allele was most significantly associated with IM, which has a protective role in MS (Ramagopalan et al. 2007). Jafari et al. (2010) showed that an *HLA-A* class I SNP rs6457110 associated with MI, was also associated with MS, independent of major class II allele, supporting the hypothesis that shared genetics may contribute to the association between IM and MS. Further research is thus necessary to assess whether the risk of IM on MS is genetically determined.

10.6.3 Smoking

There is an association between cigarette smoking and higher MS susceptibility (Biran and Steiner 2004; Riise et al. 2003). A recent meta-analysis, examining the effect of past or current smoking on MS susceptibility, reported a risk ratio of 1.57 (95 % CI 1.41–1.76, $p < 0.00001$) (Handel and Ramagopalan 2011) in sporadic MS. In MS multiplex family, no association was found between MS and smoking (Jafari et al. 2009).

Hedstrom et al. (2011) assessed interactions between smoking and the genetic risk factors *HLA-DRB1*15* and *HLA-A*02* in a Swedish case-control study. They found that the presence of susceptibility locus *HLA-DRB1*15* and absence of protective locus *HLA-A*02* in smokers rendered an OR of 13.5 (95 % CI 8.1–22.6), compared to OR of 4.9 (95 % CI 3.6–6.6) in nonsmokers. They hypothesized that smoking- related secondary lung infections and/or increased levels of posttranslational modified proteins in the lungs may provide cross-reactivity with CNS proteins, thus promoting autoreactive immune response (Hedstrom et al. 2011). Odoardi et al. (Nature 2012) showed in the EAE rat model that intravenoulsy transferred T-cell blasts gain the capacity to enter the CNS after residing transiently within the lung tissues.

10.7 Epigenetics

Several mechanisms exist which lead to epigenetic modifications, like DNA methylation, histone modification, noncoding RNA, and nucleosome positioning. The interplay between these factors leads to alterations of the chromatin structure and thereby altering the accessibility of the DNA to be transcribed into RNA and thus eventually protein. Importantly, epigenetical alterations are reversible and cell (type)-specific (Meda et al. 2011). For example, in Th1 cells the promoter of *IFN-γ* is demethylated, whereas in Tregs the *FoxP3* promoter must be fully demethylated for stable expression of FoxP3.

In MS, relatively little is known regarding epigenetical modifications compared with controls. One study compared the transciptome and epigenetical modification of CD4+ Th cells obtained from three pairs of disconcordant twins and unrelated controls. Surprisingly, they found no significant differences between the affected twin and the nonaffected twin. However, it should be noted that this first and very interesting study might be underpowered to detect differences given the very strict quality controls and corrections for multiple testing necessary to interpret the results

(Baranzini et al. 2010). Another study used postmortem normal-appearing white matter (NAWM) from four MS patients and four non-neurological controls for a chromatin immunoprecipitation (ChiP) assay. Their findings were subsequently validated in 19 other MS and 15 controls using quantitative polymerase chain reaction q-PCR immunohistochemistry, and blotting techniques to quantify protein levels, and also to compare different types of MS lesions. Interestingly, they found increased levels of deacetylation in early MS lesions whereas marked acetylation was observed in chronic lesions, indicating that during disease progression more transcriptional inhibitors of ODC differentiation genes are activated (Pedre et al. 2011). Moreover, histone deacetylase 1 (HDAC1), an important repressor of transcription, is found in damaged axons in the brain lesions of MS patients (Kim et al. 2010). In EAE, treatment with the histone deacetylase inhibitor trichostatin A reduces spinal cord inflammation, demyelination, neuronal and axonal loss, and ameliorates disability in the relapsing phase of this MS model (Camelo et al. 2005). Moreover, increased citrullinated myelin basic protein (MBP) is found in the NAWM of MS patients compared with other neurodegenerative diseases and non-neurological controls. This citrullinated MBP is less stable and might result in the observed myelin loss in MS brain. Citrullination of proteins is mediated by peptidylarginine deiminases family (PAD) and it was shown that PAD2 is increased in MS brain. In the NAWM of MS brains, there is hypomethylation of PAD2 promoter, possibly leading to aberrant PAD2 expression. However, in the thymus of the same patients, no alterations in methylation of the PAD2 promoter were found (Mastronardi et al. 2007). In addition to epigenetic alterations observed in different types of tissues in MS patients, it will be of interest to assess how environmental factors, like EBV and vitamin D, are able to alter the epigenome and how this might contribute to the risk of developing MS.

The increase in MS susceptibility mainly occurring in females might at least partially be explained with epigenetics. It is well known that epigenetical modifications can be inherited maternally. The classical epigenetical modification in females is X-chrosomal inactivation. Currently, studying X-chromosomal genetics is very challenging, because of the complex architecture of the X-chromosome.

10.7.1 Micro Ribonucleic Acid (miRNA)

As histone modifications and DNA methylation regulate the availability of DNA to be transcribed into mRNA, miRNA regulates the level of gene transcription at the posttranscriptional level. miRNA usually binds to the 3′-UTR of the mRNA and this binding might either lead to degradation or transcriptional repression, which depends on the level of sequence complementarity (Bartel 2004). A single miRNA can target hundreds of mRNAs and most of the currently known interactions between miRNA and mRNA are based on computational analysis and have yet not experimentally been validated (Angerstein et al. 2012).

Numerous studies have been performed to assess whether miRNA are upregulated or downregulated in MS patients. Similar to modifications in histones and methylation status of the DNA, it should be noted that miRNA expression profiles are cell type-and tissue-specific. Most of the miRNA studies performed in MS patients have focused on peripheral blood, either in whole blood samples or on sorted T cell subsets. A few studies have investigated the expression of miRNA in postmortem white matter brain materials of MS patients, whereas to our knowledge no study exists on gray matter brain lesions.

In total, 18 miRNA are found in at least two studies with MS patients or within EAE experiments. These were mostly upregulated in peripheral blood of MS patients (reviewed in Junker 2011). Using another approach, via a search using the miR2Disease database, Angerstein et al. (2012) found 16 miRNA differentially expressed in MS patients in at least four independent published studies. Five of these miRNA were also previously found in at least two MS or EAE studies. The discrepancy can be explained by the fact that the miR2Disease database does not contain the most recent miRNA profiling studies in MS patients. Several miRNA have consistently been shown to be upregulated in peripheral blood of MS patients. These include miR142-3p, miR146-5p, miR155-5p, and miR326. Interestingly, miR155-5p has also consistently been shown to be upregulated in MS brain. Experimentally validating the target genes of these miRNA will help to further understand the underlying mechanism and possibly the pathogenesis of MS.

10.8 Genetic Link to Other Autoimmune Diseases

Clinical and epidemiological observations imply that immune-mediated inflammatory and autoimmune diseases can occur simultaneously in a single person or in closely related family members. Many of the autoimmune diseases have a strong genetic component on the disease risk (Barrett et al. 2008; Hunt et al. 2008; Stahl et al. 2010; International Multiple Sclerosis Genetics Consortium et al. 2011) implicating that common causal genes and pathways may underlie the observed cosegregation of these diseases.

Through GWA studies, as many as 140 susceptibility loci have been identified for immune-mediated and autoimmune disorders (Cotsapas et al. 2011). There is evidence that genetic variations predisposing to one disease can have effect on risk of another disease (Smyth et al. 2008), for example, T1D susceptibility genes *CLEC16A* and *CD226*, also influence susceptibility to MS (International Multiple Sclerosis Genetics Consortium 2009).

Sometimes, a polymorphism can make an individual susceptible to one disease, but be protective of another (Sirota et al. 2009), for example, the HLA class II genes. Most autoimmune diseases show association with HLA genes. In MS, the disease risk is substantially increased in carriers of *HLA-DRB1*1501*. In T1D, this gene has a protective effect. In this light it may not be surprising why these two diseases segregate much often in Sardinia where *DRB1*1501* is uncommon in general

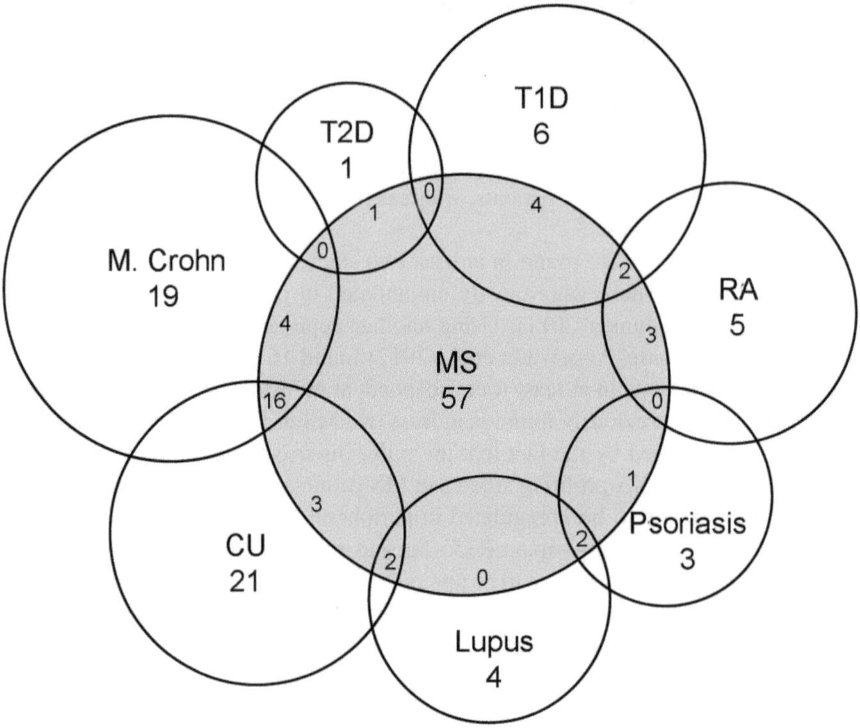

Fig. 10.2 Venn-diagram of genetic overlap between different autoimmune diseases. Increasing size of the circle represents more genetic overlap between autoimmune diseases. The number in the *outer circle* represents the number of genes shared between a given autoimmune disease and MS. In the *inner circles*, the genetic overlap between three autoimmune diseases is shown. Please note that these inner circles are not showing complete overlap between the diseases for the sake of clarity. *T1D* type 1 diabetes, *T2D* type 2 diabetes, *CU* colitis ulcerosa, *MS* multiple sclerosis, *RA* rheumatoid arthritis. (IMSGC Nature 2011 and www.genome.gov.)

population (Marrosu et al. 2004). When all known associated genes ($p < 10^{-7}$) for seven common autoimmune diseases are visualized together as a network, the extent of sharing can be clearly appreciated (Fig. 10.2). Visualization of such networks enables to inspect and understand the genetic similarity between the diseases.

10.9 Future Perspectives

The recent introduction of instruments and technologies, such as next-generation sequencing (NGS), is rapidly changing the landscape of genetics, providing the ability to answer questions with heretofore unimaginable speed. Here, we will elaborate some new techniques and discoveries made possible by these new technologies.

10.9.1 Next-Generation Sequencing and Rare Variants

Familial cases affected by MS seem to have higher risk allele frequencies than sporadic cases. They also exhibit a significant aggregation of susceptibility loci, resulting in increased disease susceptibility. Common susceptibility loci do not entirely explain the strong familial aggregation of MS. Attention should be drawn to rarer variants (minor allele frequencies of < 1 %), which might have larger effect on disease susceptibility and could possibility explain MS clustering in families. Different techniques are needed to be able to search for these rare variants, because most GWA studies are unable to detect them.

NGS techniques have allowed large-scale genomic sequencing to be used in genetic research. It can be used for whole-genome sequencing or more targeted discovery of mutations or polymorphisms, and also for mapping of structural rearrangements such as copy number variation, balanced translocation breakpoints, and chromosomal inversions. It can also be used for RNA sequencing, large-scale analysis of DNA methylation, and genome-wide mapping of DNA–protein interactions. Over the next few years, the list of applications in MS will undoubtedly grow.

Determining the sequence of the entire human genome is referred to as whole-genome sequencing. Whole-exome sequencing refers to the sequencing of the exome (all known protein-coding regions of the genome). An exome is less costly to sequence than a whole genome because the exome represents only about 1 % of the human genome. However, it should be noted that using only exome sequencing important SNP in regulatory regions remain undetected, while these might have important functions in the development of a disease, via the regulation of expression.

Whole-exome sequencing was for the first time carried out by Ramagopalan et al. (2011b) on probands from 43 multiplex MS families. They identified three rare variants in *CBLB*, *IL7R*, and *CYP27B1* genes. These were genotyped in 3,046 parents-affected child trios, but only one SNP (rs118204009) in *CYP27B1* showed evidence of association in this large MS cohort. Genotyping the variant in the original multiplex family showed that it was present in 100 % of affected family members and in one unaffected parent. The variant causes an arginine-to-histidine change at position 389 of the protein (R389H) and leads to complete loss of enzyme activity of CYP27B1, which converts 25-hydroxyvitamin D into bioactive 1,25-dihydroxyvitamin D3, and hereby induces low levels of vitamin D. The same study group has showed earlier that vitamin D regulates > 80 % of MS-associated genetic loci (Ramagopalan et al. 2010) and hypothesized that lower levels of calcitriol as a result of *CYP27B1* mutations lead to a violation of critical gene–environment interactions important for the development of MS.

Another study group (Dyment et al. 2012) performed sequencing in four members of a large MS family of German ancestry. After specific filtering conditions, an SNP (rs 55762744) in the *TYK2* gene on chromosome 19p13 was the only variant identified. This variant encodes a missense mutation in exon 3 that changes an alanine to threonine (A53T), predicted by PolyPhen and SIFT software to have an impact on protein function. Of the affected individuals with DNA available, a total of 10/14 (72 %) were positive for the *TYK2* mutation. The unaffected family members were also genotyped and a total of 28/60 (47 %) were positive for the variant. There was significant transmission disequilibrium from parents to affected offspring (16 times transmitted vs. 5 times not transmitted, $p = 0.016$). *TYK2* belongs to the JAK proteins. These are involved in phosphorylation of adaptor proteins after cytokine R signaling.

MS has previously been associated with another, nonsynonymous SNP (rs34536443) in *TYK2* (P1104A) (Mero et al. 2010), which lies over 25 kb downstream of rs55762744. SNP rs34536443 is considered as protective in MS, whereas evidence has been provided that rs55762744 confers risk to MS (Dyment et al. 2012). It is not strange to observe both, risk and protective SNP, together in susceptibility to MS. This has been shown previously for the HLA II genes (see HLA class II). Couturier et al. (Brain 2010) found no association of the rs34536554 polymorphism with responce to INF-β treatment in French MS patients. How the new identified variant in *TYK2* gene acts to increase MS risk is still to be verified through functional studies.

10.9.2 Expression Quantitative Trait Loci and Multiple Sclerosis

For many complex diseases such as MS, many susceptibility genes have been discovered through GWA studies. The association studies often report the most statistically significant hits and the suggested functionality is typically speculative, based on available annotation of genes in the vicinity of the variants. Furthermore, for the great majority of these variants, it is still unclear through which mechanisms they are associated with the disease (see also par. 10.4.1.7 Functional Immunogenetics). A conventional approach has been to assess disease-associated SNPs for associations with differential gene expression, since most of discovered susceptibility SNPs are situated in noncoding and regulatory regions of the genome. These are so-called expression quantitative trait loci (eQTLs). eQTLs can have local (*cis*) and distant (*trans*) effects, allowing the identification of pieces of biological network related to the disease. These networks might be the link between several different genetic variants that appeared to be associated with a disease in a GWA study.

Genome-wide eQTL analysis has proven fruitful in the study of diseases including obesity (Schadt et al. 2005), hypercholesterolemia (Goring et al. 2007), celiac disease (Dubois et al. 2010), late-onset Alzheimer disease (Webster et al. 2009), Crohn's disease (Fehrmann et al. 2011) and MS. As stated previously, the HLA region exerts the largest genetic contribution to MS susceptibility, but how it exactly alters the risk, is still unknown. By analyzing eQTLs in the HLA region, Alcina et al. (2012) found that the tagging SNP (rs3135388, A allele) of HLA-DRB1*1501 correlated with high expression of *DRB1*, *DRB5*, and *DQB1* genes in a Caucasion population with MS. The MS risk (AA) genotype carriers of rs3135388 were associated with 15.7-fold, 5.2-fold, and 8.3-fold higher mRNA expression of *DQB1*, *DRB5*, and *DRB1*, respectively, compared with the nonrisk (GG) carriers. In all populations studied, due to LD, the *DRB1*1501* allele correlated with higher expression of the *DRB1* gene. In a different study (Alcina et al. 2012) showed that a single SNP (rs10877013) could influence the enhancer acitivity of a regulatory element in the locus affecting the expression of several genes (*TSFM*, *TSPAN31*, *CYP27B1*, *AVIL* and *FAM119B*) which are located in the 12q13.3-12q14.1 chromosomal region associatied with MS.

The *CLEC16A* gene has previously been shown as a candidate gene for MS. It resides on chromosome 16 (16p13 region) together with other genes such as MHC class II transactivator (*CIITA*) and suppressor of cytokine signalling 1 (*SOCS1*) as well as *DEXI*, a gene of unknown function. Davison et al. (2012) found out that the increased expression of *DEXI* gene correlated with SNPs in intron 19 of *CLEC16A* gene, which are in high LD with each other, including SNP rs12708716, reported in several studies as most associated with T1D and MS (International Multiple Sclerosis Genetics Consortium 2009; Mero et al. 2011). These findings indicate a progression of our knowledge from disease-associated genetic regions identified in GWA study to more convincing evidence of causal genes in the pathogenesis of autoimmune disorders.

Further studies using the eQTL approach for other MS susceptibility genes are still yet to come.

10.9.3 Can Multiple Sclerosis Be Predicted by Susceptibility Genes?

An important goal in understanding the genetic basis of MS is predicting the disease risk using the genetics, so that environmental changes or therapeutic interventions can be initiated before inflammatory demyelination process starts. In high-risk population, such as first-degree family members and in individuals with an initial episode of neurological deficit, novel screening methods will be useful in order to determine which individuals will benefit most from early intervention. The early detection is important because early treatment in individuals with one episode is beneficial in reducing the accumulation of neurological disability (Kieseier et al. 2008).

De Jager et al. (2009c) have calculated the weighted genetic risk score (wGRS) using the OR of 16 MS susceptibility loci for the prediction of the diagnosis of MS in three independent cohorts. From the wGRS a C-statistic can be obtained which is used to compare the goodness-of-fit of logistic regression models. The discrimination between patients and controls is determined and the C-statistic value ranges from 0.5 to 1.0. A value of 0.5 indicates that the model is no better than a chance at making a prediction of person into a group (patients vs. controls) and a value of 1.0 indicates that the model perfectly differentiates between patients and controls. Models are typically considered reasonable when the C-statistic is higher than 0.7 and strong when C exceeds 0.8 (Hosmer andLemeshow 2000). For clinical prediction, a C-statistic greater than 0.8 is generally considered to be useful (Ramagopalan and Giovannoni 2009). De Jager and colleagues report a C-statistic of about 0.64 in two case-control validation populations. The C-statistic excluding the *HLA DRB1*15* allele in these cohorts was 0.56. When anti-EBNA1 (EBV) titres and smoking history were incorporated into the model, the C-statistic improved from 0.64 to 0.68, indicating the importance of including environmental factors in a prediction model. Their best C-statistic from the wGRS was 0.721 when gender was included as well. Gourraud et al. (2011) also investigated the accumulated genetic MS risk in affected individuals in multiple and single case families using 16 MS susceptibility loci, partly matching with those of de Jager et al. They showed that a greater genetic burden in siblings of MS patients was associated with an increased MS risk (OR 2.1, $p = 0.001$). However, the C-statistic for genetic burden difference between probands and siblings was only 0.57 (95 % CI 0.53–0.61), indicating that the available genetic data are not sufficient to achieve case-control prediction of MS. In another report, Jafari et al. used a model including 53 MS susceptibility loci but still achieving a C-statistic of only 0.69 (Jafari et al. 2011). They showed that theoretical inclusion of 50 newly found common genetic variants with OR of 1.4 or lesser number of rare variants with even higher OR, are needed to achieve a C-statistic of 0.85. Most of the susceptibility loci for MS risk identified so far, except *HLA-DRB1*, have only a modest effect on risk for MS with OR that ranges from 1.1 to 1.2

It can be summarized that the knowledge and the models available so far are not sufficient enough to be able to predict with reasonable accuracy, which individuals will develop MS and which individuals will not.

10.9.4 Pharmacogenetics and Multiple Sclerosis

Interferon-beta (IFN-β) is currently the most widely prescribed disease-modifying drug for relapsing–remitting MS and has been proven modestly effective in reducing the relapse rate and decreasing disease activity (Jacobs et al. 1996; Stone et al. 1997). About 20–50 % of patients do not respond to IFN-β treatment, depending on the development of neutralizing antibodies against IFN-β, or criteria used clinically and radiologically to evaluate treatment failure (Rio et al. 2002). INF-β signals through a cascade modulating cellular gene-expression. Affected pathways are antiviral activity, cell cycle, apoptosis, Th1 differentiation and other biological processes (Stark 2007). In order to provide predictive and accurate biomarkers for clinical use, different approaches have been used, such as candidate genes or whole-genome association scans and gene-expression/transcriptomic studies.

10.9.4.1 Candidate Gene Approach

The type I IFN system has been postulated to play a role in autoimmune diseases (Ronnblom et al. 1991). Increased expression of IFN-induced genes has been detected in several autoimmune diseases like systemic lupus erythematosus (SLE) (Baechler et al. 2003), Rheumatoid Arthritis (RA) (van der Pouw Kraan et al. 2007), and in MS patients (van Baarsen et al. 2006; Croze 2010; Hundeshagen et al. 2012). The interferon regulatory factors (IRFs) are major regulators of genes activated by the type I IFNs and a role in the regulation of the immune system is well established for the majority of the IRFs. Since the identification of the first

IRF, IRF-1, as a protein-binding to the *cis*-acting DNA elements of the IFN-β gene, a total of ten members has been identified in vertebrates with functions from activators (IRF-1, IRF-3, IRF-5, IRF-9, and IRF-10) to repressors (IRF-8); and some of them (IRF-2, IRF-4, and IRF-7) also exert both activating and repressing functions (Huang et al. 2010). IRF5 is a master regulator of IFN type 1 activity and it is involved in the toll-like receptor signaling pathways. In a candidate gene study, Vosslamber et al. (2011) found that patients with *IRF5* SNP rs2004640-TT and SNP rs47281420-AA genotype exerted a poor pharmacological response to IFN-β compared with patients carrying the respective G-alleles ($p = 0.0006$ and $p = 0.0023$, respectively). The rs2004640-TT genotype also correlated with development of more magnetic resonance imaging (MRI)-based T2 lesions during IFN-β treatment ($p = 0.003$). These findings were validated in a different cohort by the same group where they found a shorter time to first relapse ($p = 0.037$).

To date, only two whole-genome studies have been published investigating SNPs associated with INF-β therapy response (Byun et al. 2008; Comabella et al. 2009a). The results should be considered with caution because the studies are onderpowered and lack replication from other study groups. Buyn and colleagues have genotyped 99 responders (no relapses and no increase on Expanded Disability Status Scale (EDSS) during 2-year follow-up) and 107 nonresponders (two or more relapses or confirmed increase of at least one point on EDSS during 2-year follow-up) using Affimetrix 100 K SNP arrays (Byun et al. 2008). Top-scoring candidate SNPs were subsequently genotyped in 81 additional MS patients classified into responders and nonresponders. Using similar design, Comabella et al. genotyped 53 responders and 53 nonresponders using Affymetrix 500 K SNP arrays using the same criteria as Byun et al. (Byun et al. 2008), except for nonresponders both relapses and confirmed progression on EDSS scale were needed (Comabella et al. 2009a). Once again, the top 100 high-scoring candidate SNPs were validated in a different cohort of 94 responders and nonresponders. The most of the identified SNPs lie in brain-specific genes in both studies. Top-scoring intragenic SNPs that were found by Byun et al. are localized in the following genes *HAPLN1*, *GPC5*, *COL25A1*, *ERC2*, *FAM19A1*, and *NPAS3*. Comabella et al. identified *GRIA3*, *CIT*, *ADAR*, *ZFAT*, *STARD13*, *ZFHX4*, and *IFNAR2* genes. None of these genes are validated MS risk genes currently. Two of the genes have been associated with Parkinson's disease (*ERC2*) and Alzheimer's disease and Alzheimer's disease (*COL25AT*). *COL25AT* encodes a brain-specific membrane-bound collagen that is proteolytically cleaved to release a soluble form, which is associated with senile plaques in Alzheimer's patients. *ERC2* gene encodes a calpain inhibitor, which is part of the calpain/calpastatin system. This system is evolved in neural vesicle exocytosis, modulating cell adhesion, and migration (Hood et al. 2003). Furthermore, Comabella et al. have identified genes that belong to the type I IFN pathway among the group of responders. The genes included in this category are *IFNAR2a* and *ADAR*. Both have been replicated in the independent cohort by Comabella et al. *ADAR* encodes an RNA-editing enzyme that targets dsRNA and interferes with viral replication processes. *IFNAR2* encodes a type I membrane protein that forms one of the two subunits of the type I IFN receptor. Many more candidate gene studies have focused on the type I IFN receptor-responsive genes, providing conflicting evidence (Sriram et al. 2003; Cunningham et al. 2005;

Leyva et al. 2005; O'Doherty et al. 2009). A better understanding of their role in MS and response to INF-β therapy is needed.

The HLA class I and II genetic regions have been investigated in Spanish studies, but showed lack of association with response to IFN-β (Villoslada et al. 2002; Fernandez et al. 2005; Comabella et al. 2009b).

10.9.4.2 Expression Profiling

Transcriptional profiling studies have been performed in order to identify gene-expression patterns induced by IFN-β therapy. Stürzebecher et al. demonstrated ex vivo different gene-expression profiles between responders and nonresponders induced using PBMCs by IFN-β treatment (Sturzebecher et al. 2003). They also showed that responders to treatment experienced downregulation of IL-8 during treatment follow-up, while patients not fully responding to IFN-β treatment showed a lesser or no downregulation of IL-8. IL-8 is one of the important chemotactic mediators recruiting neutrophils to sites of inflammation and IFN-β has been shown to inhibit IL-8 expression *in vitro* via a nuclear factor-κB (NF-κB)- binding site (Oliveira et al. 1994). The role of neutrophils in the pathophysiology of MS is doubtful, but activated neutrophils can induce the chemotaxis of Th17 cell. Activated Th17 cells are capable of directly chemoattracting neutrophils via secretion of biologically active IL-8 (Pelletier et al. 2010). This is an important fact in view of evidence for an effector role of Th17 cells in MS. IL-8 also has an autocrine effect on monocytes (Browning et al. 2000) and triggers the adhesion of these cells to endothelial cells (Gerszten et al. 1999), suggesting that IL-8 may have a role in mediating the recruitment of monocytes into the CNS. High levels of Il-8 during the first trimester in pregnant women with history of MS are associated with high risk of postpartum relapse (Neuteboom et al. 2009). Comabella et al. found that IFN-β nonresponders express a substantial fraction of type I IFN-regulated genes at elevated levels prior to IFN-β treatment (Comabella et al. 2009c). In contrast, the expression of type I IFN genes was low in responders, but was inducible during treatment with IFN-β. Using eight best discriminating genes (*IFIT 3*, *RASGEF1B*, *OASl*, *IFI44*, *IFIT2*, *FADS1*, *OASL*, and *MARCKS*), where five genes are induced by type I IFNs, Comabella and colleagues calculated the predictive accuracy for response to IFN-β, ranging from 78 % (in original cohort) to 63 % (in replication cohort). They also assessed at the biomarkers for type I IFN response, such as phosphorylated STAT1 (p-STAT1) in monocytes. Significantly higher levels of p-STAT1 were found in monocytes, but not in T and B cells, of nonresponders compared to responders. These findings indicate that the type I IFN pathway in monocytes is fully activated prior to therapy with IFN-β and cannot be activated further in nonresponders (Comabella et al. 2009c). They also found a significantly elevated surface expression of IFNAR1, but not IFNAR2 on monocytes of nonresponders, increased serum type I IFN bioactivity, and elevated activity status of myeloid dendritic cells (increased expression of CD86). Furthermore, many other genes (*IL-1*β, *TNF-*α, *STAT1*, *CXCL10*, *PTX3*, and *CCR1*) were transcribed at higher levels in nonresponders, suggesting increased activation of the innate immune system. In conclusion, it seems to be counterintuitive to treat nonresponders with IFN-β, while their type I IFN genes are already overexpressed at the baseline. Clinically, it is questionable whether these patients will benefit from neutralization of type I IFNs, as proposed for other autoimmune diseases also characterized by the type I IFN signature (Stewart 2003). Approaches to idetify biomarkers associated with response to IFN-β treatment in MS are promising. However, before pharmacogenetics can be incorporated into clinical practice, majority of biomarkers needs to be validated in larger cohorts of responders and non-responders with long clinical follow-up.

10.10 Conclusions

Thanks to decreasing costs, increasing technological possibilities and improved collaborations between large academic MS centres, it became possible to investigate large numbers of genetic variants as well as gene expression in large groups of patients and controls. Currently, we are at the stage of discovering SNPs and risk genes, which up until now contribute only relatively little to the genetic burden of MS compared to HLA class II. It is now important to conduct functional studies to assess *how* these SNPs and genes are involved in the pathogenesis of MS and thus contribute to its susceptibility. It is of interest that the majority of these genes found unbiased have immunological functions, further supporting the assumption that MS is an autoimmune disease. Many of the genes found in MS, are also associated with other autoimmune diseases. This might implicate that there is a common mechanism, which increases the vulnerability to develop an autoimmune disease. From the very few neuronal genes found, only one has previously been associated with MS and two others have been implicated in other neurodegenerative diseases. Other important outstanding questions are how the environment may "modulate" the epigenetic landscape and thereby further contribute to the development of MS. Lastly, it will be of interest to assess whether the current MS risk genes can be used to predict response to treatment, as the number of treatment options for MS are increasing.

Acknowledgements Rotterdam MS centre is supported by the Dutch MS Research Foundation.

References

Alcina A et al (2010) The autoimmune disease-associated KIF5A, CD226 and SH2B3 gene variants confer susceptibility for multiple sclerosis. Genes Immun 11(5):439–445

Alcina A et al (2012) Multiple sclerosis risk variant HLA-DRB1*1501 associates with high expression of DRB1 gene in different human populations. PLoS One 7(1):e29819

Alcina et al (2013) Identification of a functional variant in the KIF5A-CYP27B1-METTL1-FAM119B locus association with MS. J Med Genet 50(1):25–33

Amirzargar A et al (2007) Profile of cytokine gene polymorphisms in Iranian multiple sclerosis patients. Mult Scler 13(2):253–255

Angerstein C et al (2012) Integration of MicroRNA databases to study microRNAs associated with multiple sclerosis. Mol Neurobiol 45(3):520–535

Aulchenko YS et al (2008) Genetic variation in the KIF1B locus influences susceptibility to multiple sclerosis. Nat Genet 40(12):1402–1403
Bachmaier K et al (2000) Negative regulation of lymphocyte activation and autoimmunity by the molecular adaptor Cbl-b. Nature 403(6766):211–216
Baechler EC et al (2003) Interferon-inducible gene expression signature in peripheral blood cells of patients with severe lupus. Proc Natl Acad Sci U S A 100(5):2610–2615
Baranzini SE et al (2010) Genome, epigenome and RNA sequences of monozygotic twins discordant for multiple sclerosis. Nature 464(7293):1351–1356
Bar-Or A et al (2010) Abnormal B-cell cytokine responses a trigger of T-cell-mediated disease in MS? Ann Neurol 67(4):452–461
Barrett JC et al (2008) Genome-wide association defines more than 30 distinct susceptibility loci for Crohn's disease. Nat Genet 40(8):955–962
Bartel DP (2004) MicroRNAs: genomics, biogenesis, mechanism, and function. Cell 116(2): 281–297
Batchelor JR (1977) Histocompatibility antigens and their relevance to multiple sclerosis. Br Med Bull 33(1):72–77
Berer K et al (2011) Commensal microbiota and myelin autoantigen cooperate to trigger autoimmune demyelination. Nature 479(7374):538–541
Bergamaschi L et al (2010) HLA-class I markers and multiple sclerosis susceptibility in the Italian population. Genes Immun 11(2):173–180
Biran I, Steiner I (2004) Smoking is a risk factor for multiple sclerosis. Neurology 63(4):763; author reply 763
Bogue CW et al (2003) Impaired B cell development and function in mice with a targeted disruption of the homeobox gene Hex. Proc Natl Acad Sci U S A 100(2):556–561
Booth DR et al (2010) Lack of support for association between the KIF1B rs10492972(C) variant and multiple sclerosis. Nat Genet 42(6):469–470; author reply 470–471
Breitfeld D et al (2000) Follicular B helper T cells express CXC chemokine receptor 5, localize to B cell follicles, and support immunoglobulin production. J Exp Med 192(11):1545–1552
Browning DD et al (2000) Autocrine regulation of interleukin-8 production in human monocytes. Am J Physiol Lung Cell Mol Physiol 279(6):L1129–1136
Bruder CE et al (2008) Phenotypically concordant and discordant monozygotic twins display different DNA copy-number-variation profiles. Am J Hum Genet 82(3):763–771
Burfoot RK et al (2008) SNP mapping and candidate gene sequencing in the class I region of the HLA complex: searching for multiple sclerosis susceptibility genes in Tasmanians. Tissue Antigens 71(1):42–50
Bush WS et al (2011) A knowledge-driven interaction analysis reveals potential neurodegenerative mechanism of multiple sclerosis susceptibility. Genes Immun 12(5):335–340
Byun E et al (2008) Genome-wide pharmacogenomic analysis of the response to interferon beta therapy in multiple sclerosis. Arch Neurol 65(3):337–344
Caballero A et al (1999) DQB1*0602 confers genetic susceptibility to multiple sclerosis in Afro-Brazilians. Tissue Antigens 54(5):524–526
Camelo S et al (2005) Transcriptional therapy with the histone deacetylase inhibitor trichostatin A ameliorates experimental autoimmune encephalomyelitis. J Neuroimmunol 164(1–2):10–21
Campbell GR et al (2011) Mitochondrial DNA deletions and neurodegeneration in multiple sclerosis. Ann Neurol 69(3):481–492
Castillo-Quan JI (2011) Parkin' control: regulation of PGC-1alpha through PARIS in Parkinson's disease. Dis Model Mech 4(4):427–429
Chao MJ et al (2007) Transmission of class I/II multi-locus MHC haplotypes and multiple sclerosis susceptibility: accounting for linkage disequilibrium. Hum Mol Genet 16(16):1951–1958
Chao MJ et al (2011) MHC transmission: insights into gender bias in MS susceptibility. Neurology 76(3):242–246
Comabella M et al (2009a) Genome-wide scan of 500,000 single-nucleotide polymorphisms among responders and nonresponders to interferon beta therapy in multiple sclerosis. Arch Neurol 66(8):972–978

Comabella M et al (2009b) HLA class I and II alleles and response to treatment with interferon-beta in relapsing-remitting multiple sclerosis. J Neuroimmunol 210(1–2):116–9
Comabella M et al (2009c) A type I interferon signature in monocytes is associated with poor response to interferon-beta in multiple sclerosis. Brain 132(Pt 12):3353–3365
Cotsapas C et al (2011) Pervasive sharing of genetic effects in autoimmune disease. PLoS Genet 7(8):e1002254
Coulthard LR et al (2009) p38(MAPK): stress responses from molecular mechanisms to therapeutics. Trends Mol Med 15(8):369–379
Couturier N et al (2011) Tyrosine kinase 2 variant influences T lymphocyte polarization and multiple sclerosis susceptibility. Brain 134(Pt 3):693–703
Cox MB et al (2012) Potential association of vitamin D receptor polymorphism Taq1 with multiple sclerosis. Mult Scler 18(1):16–22
Cree BA et al (2007) A major histocompatibility Class I locus contributes to multiple sclerosis susceptibility independently from HLA-DRB1*15:01. PLoS One 5(6):e11296
Croze E (2010) Differential gene expression and translational approaches to identify biomarkers of interferon beta activity in multiple sclerosis. J Interferon Cytokine Res 30(10):743–749
Cunningham S et al (2005) Pharmacogenomics of responsiveness to interferon IFN-beta treatment in multiple sclerosis: a genetic screen of 100 type I interferon-inducible genes. Clin Pharmacol Ther 78(6):635–646
Davison LJ et al (2012) Long-range DNA looping and gene expression analyses identify DEXI as an autoimmune disease candidate gene. Hum Mol Genet 21(2):322–333
De Jager PL et al (2009a) The role of the CD58 locus in multiple sclerosis. Proc Natl Acad Sci U S A 106(13):5264–5269
De Jager PL et al (2009b) Meta-analysis of genome scans and replication identify CD6, IRF8 and TNFRSF1A as new multiple sclerosis susceptibility loci. Nat Genet 41(7):776–782
De Jager PL et al (2009c) Integration of genetic risk factors into a clinical algorithm for multiple sclerosis susceptibility: a weighted genetic risk score. Lancet Neurol 8(12):1111–1119
Dendrou CA (2009) Cell-specific protein phenotypes for the autoimmune locus IL2RA using a genotype-selectable human bioresource. Nat Genet 41(9):1011–1015
Dubois PC et al (2010) Multiple common variants for celiac disease influencing immune gene expression. Nat Genet 42(4):295–302
Dyment DA, Ebers GC, Sadovnick AD (2004) Genetics of multiple sclerosis. Lancet Neurol 3(2):104–110
Dyment DA et al (2005) Complex interactions among MHC haplotypes in multiple sclerosis: susceptibility and resistance. Hum Mol Genet 14(14):2019–2026
Dyment DA et al (2012) Exome sequencing identifies a novel, multiple sclerosis susceptibility variant in the TYK2 gene. Neurology 79(5):406–411
Ebers GC et al (2000) Conjugal multiple sclerosis: population-based prevalence and recurrence risks in offspring. Canadian collaborative study group. Ann Neurol 48(6):927–931
Ebers GC et al (2004) Parent-of-origin effect in multiple sclerosis: observations in half-siblings. Lancet 363(9423):1773–1774
Eichhorst H (1896) Veber infantile und Hereditäre multiple sklerose. Arch Pathol Anat Physiol Klin Med 146:173–192
Erlich H et al (2008) HLA DR-DQ haplotypes and genotypes and type 1 diabetes risk: analysis of the type 1 diabetes genetics consortium families. Diabetes 57(4):1084–1092
Fedetz M et al (2009) Multiple sclerosis association study with the TENR-IL2-IL21 region in a Spanish population. Tissue Antigens 74(3):244–247
Fehrmann RS et al (2011) Trans-eQTLs reveal that independent genetic variants associated with a complex phenotype converge on intermediate genes, with a major role for the HLA. PLoS Genet 7(8):e1002197
Fernandez O et al (2005) HLA class II and response to interferon-beta in multiple sclerosis. Acta Neurol Scand 112(6):391–394

Fogdell-Hahn A et al (2000) Multiple sclerosis: a modifying influence of HLA class I genes in an HLA class II associated autoimmune disease. Tissue Antigens 55(2):140–148
Fromont A et al (2009) Inflammatory demyelinating events following treatment with anti-tumor necrosis factor. Cytokine 45(2):55–57
Gascoigne NR, Palmer E (2011) Signaling in thymic selection. Curr Opin Immunol 23(2):207–212
Gerszten RE et al (1999) MCP-1 and IL-8 trigger firm adhesion of monocytes to vascular endothelium under flow conditions. Nature 398(6729):718–723
Goring HH et al (2007) Discovery of expression QTLs using large-scale transcriptional profiling in human lymphocytes. Nat Genet 39(10):1208–1216
Gourraud PA et al (2011) Aggregation of multiple sclerosis genetic risk variants in multiple and single case families. Ann Neurol 69(1):65–74
Handel AE, Ramagopalan SV (2011) Smoking and multiple sclerosis: a matter of global importance. Neuroepidemiology 37(3–4):243–244
Handel AE, Ramagopalan SV (2012) Vitamin D and multiplesclerosis: an interaction between genes and environment. Mult Scler 18(1):2–4
Harris TJ et al (2007) Cutting edge: an in vivo requirement for STAT3 signaling in TH17 development and TH17-dependent autoimmunity. J Immunol 179(7):4313–4317
Hauser SL et al (2008) B-cell depletion with rituximab in relapsing-remitting multiple sclerosis. N Engl J Med 358(7):676–688
Hawkes CH, Macgregor AJ (2009) Twin studies and the heritability of MS: a conclusion. Mult Scler 15(6):661–667
Hedstrom AK et al (2011) Smoking and two human leukocyte antigen genes interact to increase the risk for multiple sclerosis. Brain 134(Pt 3):653–664
Herrera BM et al (2008) Parent-of-origin effects in MS: observations from avuncular pairs. Neurology 71(11):799–803
Hirokawa N, Niwa S, Tanaka Y (2010) Molecular motors in neurons: transport mechanisms and roles in brain function, development, and disease. Neuron 68(4):610–638
Hosmer DW, Lemeshow S (2000) Applied logistic regression. Wiley, New York
Hoe E et al (2010) Functionally significant differences in expression of disease-associated IL-7 receptor alpha haplotypes in CD4 T cells and dendritic cells. J Immunol 184(5):2512–2517
Hoffmann SC et al (2001) Association of cytokine polymorphic inheritance and in vitro cytokine production in anti-CD3/CD28-stimulated peripheral blood lymphocytes. Transplantation 72(8):1444–1450
Hood JL et al (2003) Association of the calpain/calpastatin network with subcellular organelles. Biochem Biophys Res Commun 310(4):1200–1212
Hoppenbrouwers IA et al (2008) Maternal transmission of multiple sclerosis in a dutch population. Arch Neurol 65(3):345–348
Howell OW et al (2011) Meningeal inflammation is widespread and linked to cortical pathology in multiple sclerosis. Brain 134(Pt 9):2755–2771
Huang JY et al (2008) Human membrane metallo-endopeptidase-like protein degrades both beta-amyloid 42 and beta-amyloid 40. Neuroscience 155(1):258–262
Huang B et al (2010) Global characterization of interferon regulatory factor (IRF) genes in vertebrates: glimpse of the diversification in evolution. BMC Immunol 11:22
Huang JY et al (2012) Altered NEP2 expression and activity in mild cognitive impairment and Alzheimer's disease. J Alzheimers Dis 28(2):433–441
Hundeshagen A et al (2012) Elevated type I interferon-like activity in a subset of multiple sclerosis patients: molecular basis and clinical relevance. J Neuroinflammation 9(1):140
Hunt KA et al (2008) Newly identified genetic risk variants for celiac disease related to the immune response. Nat Genet 40(4):395–402
Ifergan I et al (2011) Central nervous system recruitment of effector memory CD8+ T lymphocytes during neuroinflammation is dependent on alpha4 integrin. Brain 134(Pt 12):3560–3577
International Multiple Sclerosis Genetics Consortium (2009) The expanding genetic overlap between multiple sclerosis and type I diabetes. Genes Immun 10(1):11–14

International Multiple Sclerosis Genetics Consortium et al (2011) Genetic risk and a primary role for cell-mediated immune mechanisms in multiple sclerosis. Nature 476(7359):214–219

Jacobs LD et al (1996) Intramuscular interferon beta-1a for disease progression in relapsing multiple sclerosis. The multiple sclerosis collaborative research group (MSCRG). Ann Neurol 39(3):285–294

Jafari N et al (2009) Cigarette smoking and risk of MS in multiplex families. Mult Scler 15(11):1363–1367

Jafari N et al (2010) Infectious mononucleosis-linked HLA class I single nucleotide polymorphism is associated with multiple sclerosis. Mult Scler 16(11):1303–1307

Jafari N et al (2011) Perspectives on the use of multiple sclerosis risk genes for prediction. PLoS One 6(12):e26493

Jersild C, Svejgaard A, Fog T (1972) HL-A antigens and multiple sclerosis. Lancet 1(7762): 1240–1241

Junker A (2011) Pathophysiology of translational regulation by microRNAs in multiple sclerosis. FEBS Lett 585(23):3738–3746

Kantarci OH et al (2006) Men transmit MS more often to their children vs women: the carter effect. Neurology 67(2):305–310

Katzman SD et al (2011) Opposing functions of IL-2 and IL-7 in the regulation of immune responses. Cytokine 56(1):116–121

Kieseier BC et al (2008) Immunomodulatory treatment strategies in multiple sclerosis. J Neurol 255(Suppl 6):15–21

Kim JY et al (2010) HDAC1 nuclear export induced by pathological conditions is essential for the onset of axonal damage. Nat Neurosci 13(2):180–189

Kofler DM et al (2011) The CD6 multiple sclerosis susceptibility allele is associated with alterations in CD4+ T cell proliferation. J Immunol 187(6):3286–3291

Kondo Y et al (2005) Galactocerebrosidase-deficient oligodendrocytes maintain stable central myelin by exogenous replacement of the missing enzyme in mice. Proc Natl Acad Sci U S A 102(51):18670–18675

Kreft KL (2011) Role of CD8 regulatory T-cells in multiple sclerosis. Ann Neurol 69(3):593; author reply 593–594

Kreft KL et al (2012) The IL-7Ralpha pathway is quantitatively and functionally altered in CD8T cells in multiple sclerosis. J Immunol 188(4):1874–1883

Kroner A (2007) The genetic influence of the nonclassical MHC molecule HLA-G on multiple sclerosis. Hum Immunol 68(5):422–425

Leyva L et al (2005) IFNAR1 and IFNAR2 polymorphisms confer susceptibility to multiple sclerosis but not to interferon-beta treatment response. J Neuroimmunol 163(1–2):165–171

Lincoln MR et al (2005) A predominant role for the HLA class II region in the association of the MHC region with multiple sclerosis. Nat Genet 37(10):1108–1112

Link J et al (2010) Two HLA class I genes independently associated with multiple sclerosis. J Neuroimmunol 226(1–2):172–176

Lubetzki C et al (1986) Multiple sclerosis: rat and human oligodendrocytes are not the target for CSF immunoglobulins. Neurology 36(4):524–528

Mackall CL, Fry TJ, Gress RE (2011) Harnessing the biology of IL-7 for therapeutic application. Nat Rev Immunol 11(5):330–342

Mahad D, Lassmann H, Turnbull D (2008a) Review: mitochondria and disease progression in multiple sclerosis. Neuropathol Appl Neurobiol 34(6):577–589

Mahad D et al (2008b) Mitochondrial defects in acute multiple sclerosis lesions. Brain 131(Pt 7):1722–1735

Marrosu MG et al (1997) Multiple sclerosis in Sardinia is associated and in linkage disequilibrium with HLA-DR3 and -DR4 alleles. Am J Hum Genet 61(2):454–457

Marrosu MG et al (2004) The co-inheritance of type 1 diabetes and multiple sclerosis in Sardinia cannot be explained by genotype variation in the HLA region alone. Hum Mol Genet 13(23):2919–2924

Marszalek JR et al (1999) Novel dendritic kinesin sorting identified by different process targeting of two related kinesins: KIF21A and KIF21B. J Cell Biol 145(3):469–479
Mastronardi FG et al (2007) Peptidyl argininedeiminase 2 CpG island in multiple sclerosis white matter is hypomethylated. J Neurosci Res 85(9):2006–2016
Matesanz F et al (2001) Allelic expression and interleukin-2 polymorphisms in multiple sclerosis. J Neuroimmunol 119(1):101–105
Matesanz F et al (2004) Effects of the multiple sclerosis associated -330 promoter polymorphism in IL2 allelic expression. J Neuroimmunol 148(1–2):212–217
Meda F et al (2011) The epigenetics of autoimmunity. Cell Mol Immunol 8(3):226–236
Mero IL et al (2010) A rare variant of the TYK2 gene is confirmed to be associated with multiple sclerosis. Eur J Hum Genet 18(4):502–504
Mero IL et al (2011) Exploring the CLEC16A gene reveals a MS-associated variant with correlation to the relative expression of CLEC16A isoforms in thymus. Genes Immun 12(3):191–198
Modin H et al (2004) Modes of action of HLA-DR susceptibility specificities in multiple sclerosis. Am J Hum Genet 74(6):1321–1322
Moesta AK et al (2008) Synergistic polymorphism at two positions distal to the ligand-binding site makes KIR2DL2 a stronger receptor for HLA-C than KIR2DL3. J Immunol 180(6):3969–3979
Naito S et al (1972) Multiple sclerosis: association with HL-A3. Tissue Antigens 2(1):1–4
Neuteboom RF et al (2009) First trimester interleukin 8 levels are associated with postpartum relapse in multiple sclerosis. Mult Scler 15(11):1356–1358
O'Doherty C et al (2009) Genetic polymorphisms, their allele combinations and IFN-beta treatment response in Irish multiple sclerosis patients. Pharmacogenomics 10(7):1177–1186
Okada Y et al (2012) Meta-analysis identifies nine new loci associated with rheumatoid arthritis in the Japanese population. Nat Genet 44(5):511–516
Oksenberg JR et al (2004) Mapping multiple sclerosis susceptibility to the HLA-DR locus in African Americans. Am J Hum Genet 74(1):160–167
Oliveira IC et al (1994) Transcriptional inhibition of the interleukin-8 gene by interferon is mediated by the NF-kappa B site. Mol Cell Biol 14(8):5300–5308
Orru S et al (2005) Mapping of the major psoriasis-susceptibility locus (PSORS1) in a 70-Kb interval around the corneodesmosin gene (CDSN). Am J Hum Genet 76(1):164–171
Orton SM et al (2006) Sex ratio of multiple sclerosis in Canada: a longitudinal study. Lancet Neurol 5(11):932–936
Ouimet T et al (2000) Neprilysin II: a putative novel metalloprotease and its isoforms in CNS and testis. Biochem Biophys Res Commun 271(3):565–570
Paolino M, Penninger JM (2010) Cbl-b in T-cell activation. Semin Immunopathol 32(2):137–148
Parham P (2005) MHC class I molecules and KIRs in human history, health and survival. Nat Rev Immunol 5(3):201–214
Paul P et al (2011) A Genome-wide multidimensional RNAi screen reveals pathways controlling MHC class II antigen presentation. Cell 145(2):268–283
Pearce EL et al (2003) Control of effector CD8+ T cell function by the transcription factor Eomesodermin. Science 302(5647):1041–1043
Pedre X et al (2011) Changed histone acetylation patterns in normal-appearing white matter and early multiple sclerosis lesions. J Neurosci 31(9):3435–3445
Pelletier M et al (2010) Evidence for a cross-talk between human neutrophils and Th17 cells. Blood 115(2):335–343
Piccio L et al (2010) Changes in B- and T-lymphocyte and chemokine levels with rituximab treatment in multiple sclerosis. Arch Neurol 67(6):707–714
Ramagopalan SV, Ebers GC (2009a) Multiple sclerosis: major histocompatibility complexity and antigen presentation. Genome Med 1(11):105
Ramagopalan SV, Ebers GC (2009b) Epistasis: multiple sclerosis and the major histocompatibility complex. Neurology 72(6):566–567
Ramagopalan SV, Giovannoni G (2009) Can we predict multiple sclerosis? Lancet Neurol 8(12):1077–1079

Ramagopalan SV et al (2007) The inheritance of resistance alleles in multiple sclerosis. PLoS Genet 3(9):1607–1613
Ramagopalan SV et al (2009) Expression of the multiple sclerosis-associated MHC class II Allele HLA-DRB1*1501 is regulated by vitamin D. PLoS Genet 5(2):e1000369
Ramagopalan SV et al (2010) A ChIP-seq defined genome-wide map of vitamin D receptor binding: associations with disease and evolution. Genome Res 20(10):1352–1360
Ramagopalan SV et al (2011a) Role of the HLA system in the association between multiple sclerosis and infectious mononucleosis. Arch Neurol 68(4):469–472
Ramagopalan SV et al (2011b) Rare variants in the CYP27B1 gene are associated with multiple sclerosis. Ann Neurol 70(6):881–886
Reboldi A et al (2009) C-C chemokine receptor 6-regulated entry of TH-17 cells into the CNS through the choroid plexus is required for the initiation of EAE. Nat Immunol 10(5):514–523
Riise T, Nortvedt MW, Ascherio F (2003) Smoking is a risk factor for multiple sclerosis. Neurology 61(8):1122–1124
Rio J et al (2002) Assessment of different treatment failure criteria in a cohort of relapsing-remitting multiple sclerosis patients treated with interferon beta: implications for clinical trials. Ann Neurol 52(4):400–406
Ronnblom LE, Alm GV, Oberg KE (1991) Autoimmunity after alpha-interferon therapy for malignant carcinoid tumors. Ann Intern Med 115(3):178–183
Rostami AM et al (1987) Search for antibodies to galactocerebroside in the serum and cerebrospinal fluid in human demyelinating disorders. Ann Neurol 22(3):381–383
Ruijs TC, Olivier A, Antel JP (1990) Serum cytotoxicity to human and rat oligodendrocytes in culture. Brain Res 517(1–2):99–104
Ryan EJ et al (2002) Dendritic cell-associated lectin-1: a novel dendritic cell-associated, C-type lectin-like molecule enhances T cell secretion of IL-4. J Immunol 169(10):5638–5648
Ryan EJ et al (2009) Ligation of dendritic cell-associated lectin-1 induces partial maturation of human monocyte derived dendritic cells. Hum Immunol 70(1):1–5
Sadovnick AD, Baird PA, Ward RH (1988) Multiple sclerosis: updated risks for relatives. Am J Med Genet 29(3):533–541
Sadovnick AD, Bulman D, Ebers GC (1991) Parent-child concordance in multiple sclerosis. Ann Neurol 29(3):252–255
Sadovnick AD et al (1996) Evidence for genetic basis of multiple sclerosis. The Canadian collaborative study group. Lancet 347(9017):1728–1730
Sakaguchi S et al (2010) FOXP3+ regulatory T cells in the human immune system. Nat Rev Immunol 10(7):490–500
Schadt EE et al (2005) An integrative genomics approach to infer causal associations between gene expression and disease. Nat Genet 37(7):710–717
Schulz C et al (2012) A lineage of myeloid cells independent of Myb and hematopoietic stem cells. Science 336(6077):86–90
Sen P et al (2007) Apoptotic cells induce Mer tyrosine kinase-dependent blockade of NF-kappaB activation in dendritic cells. Blood 109(2):653–660
Shahbazi M et al (2010) High frequency of the IL-2 -330T/HLA-DRB1*1501 haplotype in patients with multiple sclerosis. Clin Immunol 137(1):134–138
Shahbazi M et al (2011) Interaction of HLA-DRB1*1501 allele and TNF-alpha -308 G/A single nucleotide polymorphism in the susceptibility to multiple sclerosis. Clin Immunol 139(3):277–281
Shin JH et al (2011) PARIS (ZNF746) repression of PGC-1alpha contributes to neurodegeneration in Parkinson's disease. Cell 144(5):689–702
Sicotte NL, Voskuhl RR (2001) Onset of multiple sclerosis associated with anti-TNF therapy. Neurology 57(10):1885–1888
Sirota M et al (2009) Autoimmune disease classification by inverse association with SNP alleles. PLoS Genet 5(12):e1000792
Smyth DJ et al (2008) Shared and distinct genetic variants in type 1 diabetes and celiac disease. N Engl J Med 359(26):2767–2777

Sonnenberg GF, Fouser LA, Artis D (2011) Border patrol: regulation of immunity, inflammation and tissue homeostasis at barrier surfaces by IL-22. Nat Immunol 12(5):383–390

Spurkland A et al (1991) HLA-DQA1 and HLA-DQB1 genes may jointly determine susceptibility to develop multiple sclerosis. Hum Immunol 30(1):69–75

Sriram U et al (2003) Pharmacogenomic analysis of interferon receptor polymorphisms in multiple sclerosis. Genes Immun 4(2):147–152

Stahl EA et al (2010) Genome-wide association study meta-analysis identifies seven new rheumatoid arthritis risk loci. Nat Genet 42(6):508–514

Stark GR (2007) How cells respond to interferons revisited: from early history to current complexity. Cytokine Growth Factor Rev 18(5–6):419–423

Stewart TA (2003) Neutralizing interferon alpha as a therapeutic approach to autoimmune diseases. Cytokine Growth Factor Rev 14(2):139–154

Stone LA et al (1997) Characterization of MRI response to treatment with interferon beta-1b: contrast-enhancing MRI lesion frequency as a primary outcome measure. Neurology 49(3):862–869

Sturzebecher S et al (2003) Expression profiling identifies responder and non-responder phenotypes to interferon-beta in multiple sclerosis. Brain 126(Pt 6):1419–29

Thacker EL, Mirzaei F, Ascherio A (2006) Infectious mononucleosis and risk for multiple sclerosis: a meta-analysis. Ann Neurol 59(3):499–503

Todd JA et al (2007) Robust associations of four new chromosome regions from genome-wide analyses of type 1 diabetes. Nat Genet 39(7):857–864

van Baarsen LG et al (2006) A subtype of multiple sclerosis defined by an activated immune defense program. Genes Immun 7(6):522–531

van der Pouw Kraan TC et al (2007) Rheumatoid arthritis subtypes identified by genomic profiling of peripheral blood cells: assignment of a type I interferon signature in a subpopulation of patients. Ann Rheum Dis 66(8):1008–1014

van Oosten BW et al (1996) Increased MRI activity and immune activation in two multiple sclerosis patients treated with the monoclonal anti-tumor necrosis factor antibody cA2. Neurology 47(6):1531–1534

Venkateswaran S et al (2011) Mitochondrial DNA haplogroups and mutations in children with acquired central demyelination. Neurology 76(9):774–780

Villoslada P et al (2002) The HLA locus and multiple sclerosis in Spain. Role in disease susceptibility, clinical course and response to interferon-beta. J Neuroimmunol 130(1–2):194–201

Vogler S et al (2005) Association of a common polymorphism in the promoter of UCP2 with susceptibility to multiple sclerosis. J Mol Med (Berl) 83(10):806–811

Vosslamber S et al (2011) Interferon regulatory factor 5 gene variants and pharmacological and clinical outcome of Interferonbeta therapy in multiple sclerosis. Genes Immun 12(6):466–472

Warnke C et al (2010) Natalizumab and progressive multifocal leukoencephalopathy: what are the causal factors and can it be avoided? Arch Neurol 67(8):923–930

Webster JA et al (2009) Genetic control of human brain transcript expression in Alzheimer disease. Am J Hum Genet 84(4):445–458

Wellcome Trust Case Control Consortium (2007) Genome-wide association study of 14,000 cases of seven common diseases and 3,000 shared controls. Nature 447(7145):661–678

Willer CJ et al (2003) Twin concordance and sibling recurrence rates in multiple sclerosis. Proc Natl Acad Sci U S A 100(22):12877–12882

Wilson AG et al (1997) Effects of a polymorphism in the human tumor necrosis factor alpha promoter on transcriptional activation. Proc Natl Acad Sci U S A 94(7):3195–3199

Wu Q et al (2001) Reversal of spontaneous autoimmune insulitis in nonobese diabetic mice by soluble lymphotoxin receptor. J Exp Med 193(11):1327–1332

Yang Y et al (2011) -308 G > A of TNF-alpha gene promoter decreases the risk of multiple sclerosis: a meta-analysis. Mult Scler 17(6):658–665

Yeo TW et al (2007) A second major histocompatibility complex susceptibility locus for multiple sclerosis. Ann Neurol 61(3):228–236

Yu X et al (2008) mtDNA nt13708A variant increases the risk of multiple sclerosis. PLoS One 3(2):e1530

Chapter 11
Gene Expression Profiling and Pathway Analysis for Identification of Molecular Targets in MS

Jun-ichi Satoh

11.1 Introduction

Multiple sclerosis (MS) is an inflammatory demyelinating disease affecting exclusively the central nervous system (CNS) white matter, mediated by an autoimmune process triggered by a complex interplay between genetic and environmental factors (Sospedra and Martin 2005). Although the precise immune mechanisms remain unknown, accumulating evidence indicates a pivotal role of proinflammatory T helper type 1 (Th1) and type 17 (Th17) lymphocytes in the pathogenesis of MS (Steinman 2007). MS shows a great range of phenotypic variability. In view of the clinical course, MS is classified into relapsing–remitting form (RRMS), secondary progressive form (SPMS), or primary progressive form (PPMS). Pathologically, MS lesions show a variable degree of inflammation, complement activation, antibody deposition, demyelination, remyelination, oligodendrocyte apoptosis, and axonal degeneration (Lucchinetti et al. 2000). The drugs currently used in clinical practice, including interferon-beta (IFN-β), glatiramer acetate, mitoxantrone, fingolimod (FTY720), and natalizumab, have shown limited efficacy in selected populations of patients (Rudick et al. 2004). Based on these observations, we could postulate that MS is a neurological syndrome, caused by different immunological mechanisms, leading to the final common pathway that triggers inflammatory demyelination. Therefore, the identification of molecular targets and biomarkers responsible for the complex phenotype of MS enables us to establish the molecular mechanism-based personalized therapy of MS.

After the completion of the Human Genome Project in 2003, the global analysis of the genome, transcriptome, proteome, and metabolome, collectively termed omics, enables us to characterize the genome-wide molecular mechanisms of the diseases, and helps us to identify disease-specific molecular signatures and biomarkers for

J.-i. Satoh (✉)
Department of Bioinformatics and Molecular Neuropathology,
Meiji Pharmaceutical University, 2–522-1 Noshio,
Kiyose, Tokyo 204–8588, Japan
e-mail: satoj@my-pharm.ac.jp

T. Yamamura, B. Gran (eds.), *Multiple Sclerosis Immunology*,
DOI 10.1007/978-1-4614-7953-6_11, © Springer Science+Business Media New York 2013

diagnosis and prediction of prognosis. Recently, the genome-wide association studies (GWAS) disclosed numerous risk alleles for the susceptibility of MS (International Multiple Sclerosis Genetics Consortium et al. 2007 and 2011). The comprehensive transcriptome and proteome profiling of disease-affected brain tissues elucidated key molecules whose role has not been previously predicted in the pathogenesis of MS (Lock et al. 2002; Han et al. 2008). Most recently, the next-generation sequencing (NGS) technology enables us to investigate the genetic basis of MS at the level of whole genome of individual patients (Baranzini et al. 2010).

As the omics study generally produces high-throughput data at one time, it is often difficult to extract the most important implications from such a huge data set. However, recent advances in bioinformatics and systems biology have made major breakthroughs by illustrating the cell-wide map of complex molecular interactions with the aid of the literature-based knowledgebase of molecular pathways (Satoh 2010). The logically arranged molecular networks construct the whole system characterized by robustness that maintains the proper function of the system in the face of genetic and environmental perturbations (Kitano 2007). In the scale-free molecular network, targeted disruption of limited numbers of critical components designated hubs, on which the biologically important molecular connections concentrate, disturbs the whole cellular function by destabilizing the network (Albert et al. 2000). From this point of view, the integration of "omics data" derived from disease-affected cells and tissues with underlying molecular networks may enable us to identify novel disease-relevant pathways and network-based effective drug targets for personalized therapy.

Increasing numbers of omics data have been deposited in public databases, such as the Gene Expression Omnibus (GEO) repository (www.ncbi.nlm.nih.gov/geo) and the ArrayExpress archive (www.ebi.ac.uk/arrayexpress). Importantly, they include the disease-oriented data that have potentially valuable information on molecular networks and biomarkers of the diseases, particularly when they are reanalyzed by means of appropriate bioinformatics tools (Satoh et al. 2009a). Here, this study would introduce our approach to establish the logical hypothesis of molecular mechanisms underlying MS, and to identify molecular targets and biomarkers from publicly accessible omics data of MS by effectively combining gene expression profiling and molecular network analysis.

11.2 From Global Gene Expression Profiling to Molecular Network Analysis

DNA microarray allows us to systematically monitor the genome-wide gene expression pattern of disease-affected cells and tissues. This technology enables us to illustrate most efficiently a global picture of cellular activity by quantification of the messenger RNA (mRNA) expression levels, although the mRNA levels do not always correlate with the protein levels, and the latter is more directly involved in cellular function. However, the use of DNA microarray is more convenient

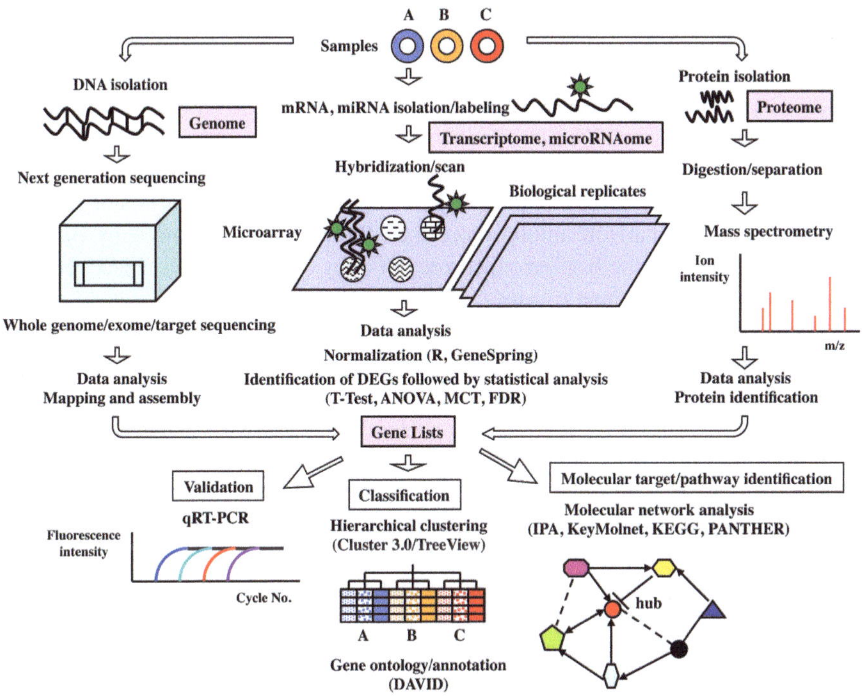

Fig. 11.1 The load map from global gene expression profiling to molecular network analysis. For transcriptome analysis, total RNA samples labeled with fluorescent dyes are processed for hybridization with oligonucleotide probes immobilized on the microarrays, which should include biological replicates. To identify the list of differentially expressed genes (DEGs) among the samples, the normalized data are processed for statistical analysis, followed by validation by quantitative RT-PCR (qRT-PCR). They are also processed for hierarchical clustering analysis, gene ontology, and function analysis. To identify biologically relevant molecular pathways, the list of DEGs is imported into pathway analysis tools of bioinformatics endowed with a comprehensive knowledgebase. They also accept the large-scale gene list derived from proteome analysis by mass spectrometry and genome analysis by deep sequencing on next-generation sequencers. *ANOVA* analysis of variance, *MCT* multiple comparison test, *FDR* false discovery rate, *DAVID* Database for Annotation, Visualization, and Integrated Discovery, *IPA* Ingenuity Pathways Analysis, *KEGG* Kyoto Encyclopedia of Genes and Genomes, *PANTHER* Protein Analysis through Evolutionary Relationships

to collect temporal and spatial snapshots of gene expression than the conventional mass spectrometry, which is often hampered by limited resolution of protein separation. We could logically assume that the set of coregulated genes identified in the transcriptome have similar biological functions within the cells.

Firstly, I would like to give a brief overview of the experimental procedure of global expression profiling and molecular network analysis (Fig. 11.1). For transcriptome analysis, various types of microarrays are currently available. The MicroArray Quality Control (MAQC) project has proven that the core results are well reproducible among different platforms employed (MAQC Consortium et al. 2006). Each experiment should contain biological replicates to validate reproducibility of the principal observations. The raw data are normalized by representative methods, such as the quantile normalization method and the Robust MultiChip Average (RMA) method by using the R software of the Bioconductor package (cran.r-project.org) or the GeneSpring software (Agilent Technology). To identify differentially expressed genes (DEGs) among distinct samples, the normalized data are processed for statistical analysis with *t*-test for comparison between two groups or analysis of variance (ANOVA) for comparison among more than three groups, followed by multiple comparison test with the Bonferroni correction or by controlling false discovery rate (FDR) below 0.05 to adjust *p*-values.

Then, the levels of expression of DEGs should be validated by quantitative RT-PCR (qRT-PCR). The normalized data are processed for hierarchical clustering analysis to classify the expression profile-based groups of genes and samples by using GeneSpring or the software named Cluster 3.0 (bonsai.ims.u-tokyo.ac.jp/~mdehoon/software/cluster) in combination with TreeView (sourceforge.net/projects/jtreeview). A large-scale gene list also comes from proteome analysis by mass spectrometry and genome analysis by deep sequencing on next-generation sequencers (Fig. 11.1).

To identify biologically relevant molecular pathways from large-scale data, we could analyze them by using a battery of pathway analysis tools endowed with a comprehensive knowledgebase curated and updated regularly by expert biologist. They include Kyoto Encyclopedia of Genes and Genomes (KEGG; www.kegg.jp), the Protein Analysis through Evolutionary Relationships (PANTHER) classification system (www.pantherdb.org), Ingenuity Pathways Analysis (IPA Ingenuity Systems, www.ingenuity.com), and KeyMolnet (Institute of Medicinal Molecular Design, www.immd.co.jp) (Fig. 11.1). The Gene ID Conversion tool of the Database for Annotation, Visualization, and Integrated Discovery (DAVID; david.abcc.ncifcrf.gov) converts the large-scale array-specific probe IDs into the corresponding Entrez Gene IDs, HUGO Gene Symbols, Ensembel Gene IDs, or UniProt IDs, which are convenient for application to the pathway analysis tools (Huang et al. 2009). DAVID also helps us to identify a set of enriched genes with a specified functional annotation in the entire list of genes. KEGG, PANTHER, and DAVID are open-access databases, while IPA and KeyMolnet are commercial ones.

KEGG systematically integrates genomic and chemical information to create the whole biological system *in silico* (Kanehisa et al. 2012). KEGG includes manually curated reference pathways that cover a wide range of metabolic, genetic, environmental and cellular processes, and human diseases. Currently, KEGG contains 253,252 pathways. PANTHER, operating on the computational algorithms that relate the evolution of protein sequences to the evolution of protein functions and biological roles, provides a structured representation of protein function in the context of biological reaction networks (Mi et al. 2010). PANTHER includes the information on 176 regulatory and metabolic pathways. By uploading the list of Gene IDs, the PANTHER gene expression data analysis tool identifies the genes in terms of over- or under-representation in canonical pathways, followed by statistical evaluation by multiple comparison test with the Bonferroni correction. IPA is a knowledgebase that contains approximately 3,000,000 biological and chemical interactions and functional annotations with definite scientific evidence. By uploading the list of Gene IDs and expression values, the network-generation algorithm identifies focused genes integrated in a global molecular network. IPA calculates the *p* value score, the statistical significance of association between the genes and the networks by the Fisher's exact test.

KeyMolnet contains knowledge-based contents on 157,700 relationships among human genes and proteins, small molecules, diseases, pathways, and drugs (Satoh 2010). They are categorized into the core contents collected from selected review articles with the highest reliability or the secondary contents extracted from abstracts of PubMed and Human Protein Reference database (HPRD). By importing the list of Gene ID and expression values, KeyMolnet automatically provides corresponding molecules as a node on networks. The "common upstream" network-search algorithm enables us to extract the most relevant molecular network composed of the genes coordinately regulated by putative common upstream transcription factors. The "neighboring" network-search algorithm selected one or more molecules as starting points to generate the network of all kinds of molecular interactions around starting molecules, including direct activation or inactivation, transcriptional activation or repression, and the complex formation within the designated number of paths from starting points. The "N-points to N-points" network-search algorithm identifies the molecular network constructed by the shortest route connecting the start point molecules and the end point molecules. The generated network was compared side by side with 459 human canonical pathways of the KeyMolnet library. The algorithm counting the number of overlapping molecular relations between the extracted network and the canonical pathway makes it possible to identify the canonical pathway showing the most significant contribution to the extracted network.

11.3 Molecular Network Analysis of Genome Data of MS

GWAS provide the most efficient approach to screening large numbers of disease-associated genetic variations, including single nucleotide polymorphisms (SNPs) and copy number variations (CNVs). Recently, GWAS identified numerous risk alleles for the susceptibility of MS, suggesting that the complex deregulation of variable genetic factors activates an autoimmune process in MS (International Multiple Sclerosis Genetics Consortium et al. 2007 and 2011). Accumulating data and the most recent large-scale collaborative GWAS involving 9,772 cases of European origin, taken together, discovered the collection of 102 MS risk SNPs outside the MHC region (Table 11.1; International Multiple Sclerosis Genetics Consortium et al. 2011). They validated 98 of the 102 SNPs overrepresented in MS patients versus the controls. By analyzing the relevant molecular network of the SNP genes with IPA, they found an enrichment of immunoregulatory genes involved in the T helper cell differentiation pathway. We studied the molecular network of the set of 98 genes by using KeyMolnet. By the neighboring network-search algorithm, it extracted a highly complex

Table 11.1 The list of 102 MS risk SNPs located outside the MHC. The list is modified from the recent GWAS of MS risk SNPs (International Multiple Sclerosis Genetics Consortium et al. 2011)

Chromosome	Reference SNP ID	Entrez gene ID	Gene symbol	Gene name	*p*-value	OR (95 % CI)
1	rs4648356	100287898	TTC34	Tetratricopeptide repeat domain 34	1.00E-14	1.14 (1.12–1.16)
1	rs233100	23576	DDAH1	Dimethylarginine dimethylaminohydrolase 1	1.00E-06	1.08 (1.07–1.1)
1	rs11810217	7813	EVI5	Ecotropic viral integration site 5	5.80E-15	1.15 (1.13–1.16)
1	rs11581062	148867	SLC30A7	Solute carrier family 30 (zinc transporter), member 7	2.50E-10	1.12 (1.1–1.13)
1	rs12048904	2135	EXTL2	Exostoses (multiple)-like 2	4.00E-08	1.09 (1.08–1.11)
1	rs1335532	965	CD58	CD58 molecule	3.20E-16	1.22 (1.19–1.24)
1	rs3761959	115352	FCRL3	Fc receptor-like 3	2.90E-06	1.08 (1.06–1.09)
1	rs1323292	5996	RGS1	Regulator of G-protein signaling 1	2.30E-08	1.12 (1.1–1.14)
1	rs7522462	55765	C1orf106	Chromosome 1 open reading frame 106	1.90E-09	1.11 (1.1–1.13)
2	rs12466022	100506047	LOC100506047	Uncharacterized LOC100506047	6.20E-10	1.11 (1.1–1.13)
2	rs7595037	5341	PLEK	Pleckstrin	5.10E-11	1.11 (1.1–1.12)
2	rs17174870	10461	MERTK	c-mer proto-oncogene tyrosine kinase	1.30E-08	1.11 (1.09–1.13)
2	rs281783	205327	C2orf69	Chromosome 2 open reading frame 69	0.00018	1.08 (1.06–1.1)
2	rs10201872	11262	SP140	SP140 nuclear body protein	1.80E-10	1.14 (1.12–1.16)
3	rs9821630	23228	PLCL2	Phospholipase C-like 2	3.90E-06	1.08 (1.07–1.1)
3	rs669607	152100	CMC1	COX assembly mitochondrial protein homolog (S. cerevisiae)	1.90E-15	1.13 (1.12–1.15)
3	rs11129295	8320	EOMES	Eomesodermin	1.20E-09	1.11 (1.09–1.12)
3	rs1500710	50650	ARHGEF3	Rho guanine nucleotide exchange factor (GEF) 3	5.20E-05	1.07 (1.05–1.08)
3	rs771767	152225	LOC152225	Uncharacterized LOC152225	8.60E-09	1.1 (1.09–1.12)
3	rs2293370	51300	TIMMDC1	Translocase of inner mitochondrial membrane domain containing 1	2.70E-09	1.13 (1.11–1.15)
3	rs9282641	942	CD86	CD86 molecule	1.00E-11	1.21 (1.18–1.24)
3	rs4308217	942	CD86	CD86 molecule	5.70E-08	1.1 (1.08–1.11)
3	rs4285028	6565	SLC15A2	Solute carrier family 15 (H + /peptide transporter), member 2	1.80E-08	1.1 (1.09–1.12)
3	rs2243123	3592	IL12A	Interleukin 12A (natural killer cell stimulatory factor 1, cytotoxic lymphocyte maturation factor 1, p35)	7.20E-06	1.08 (1.06–1.1)

Table 11.1 (continued)

Chromo-some	Reference SNP ID	Entrez gene ID	Gene symbol	Gene name	*p*-value	OR (95 % CI)
3	rs10936599	55892	MYNN	Myoneurin	7.00E-07	1.1 (1.08–1.11)
4	rs228614	4126	MANBA	Mannosidase, beta A, lysosomalp	1.40E-07	1.09 (1.07–1.1)
4	rs6821894	8470	SORBS2	Sorbin and SH3 domain containing 2	9.20E-05	1.07 (1.05–1.08)
5	rs6897932	3575	IL7R	Interleukin 7 receptor	1.70E-08	1.11 (1.09–1.13)
5	rs4613763	5734	PTGER4	Prostaglandin E receptor 4 (subtype EP4)	2.50E-16	1.2 (1.18–1.22)
5	rs350058	5734	PTGER4	Prostaglandin E receptor 4 (subtype EP4)	1.00E-04	1.11 (1.09–1.14)
5	rs756699	6932	TCF7	Transcription factor 7 (T-cell specific, HMG-box)	6.20E-07	1.12 (1.1–1.14)
5	rs1062158	80762	NDFIP1	Nedd4 family interacting protein 1	2.30E-06	1.08 (1.07–1.1)
5	rs2302103	1729	DIAPH1	Diaphanous homolog 1 (Drosophila)	0.00054	1.06 (1.04–1.07)
5	rs2546890	285626	LOC285626	Uncharacterized LOC285626	1.20E-11	1.11 (1.1–1.13)
5	rs4075958	10636	RGS14	Regulator of G-protein signaling 14	4.90E-07	1.09 (1.08–1.11)
6	rs11755724	6239	RREB1	Ras responsive element binding protein 1	2.60E-06	1.08 (1.06–1.09)
6	rs12212193	60468	BACH2	BTB and CNC homology 1, basic leucine zipper transcription factor 2	3.80E-08	1.09 (1.08–1.1)
6	rs854917	58528	RRAGD	Ras-related GTP binding D	0.00017	1.07 (1.05–1.09)
6	rs802734	5796	PTPRK	Protein tyrosine phosphatase, receptor type, K	5.50E-09	1.1 (1.09–1.12)
6	rs11154801	54806	AHI1	Abelson helper integration site 1	1.00E-13	1.13 (1.11–1.15)
6	rs9321490	4602	MYB	v-myb myeloblastosis viral oncogene homolog (avian)	1.60E-06	1.1 (1.08–1.11)
6	rs17066096	116379	IL22RA2	Interleukin 22 receptor, alpha 2	6.00E-13	1.14 (1.12–1.15)
6	rs13192841	100507406	LOC100507406	Uncharacterized LOC100507406	1.30E-08	1.1 (1.09–1.12)
6	rs1738074	117289	TAGAP	T-cell activation RhoGTPase activating protein	6.80E-15	1.13 (1.12–1.15)
7	rs1843938	84433	CARD11	Caspase recruitment Domain family, member 11	1.10E-05	1.07 (1.06–1.09)
7	rs6952809	55501	CHST12	Carbohydrate (chondroitin 4) sulfotransferase 12	3.60E-06	1.08 (1.06–1.09)
7	rs2214543	4697	NDUFA4	NADH dehydrogenase (ubiquinone) 1 alpha subcomplex, 4, 9kDa	0.00016	1.07 (1.05–1.09)
7	rs2066992	3569	IL6	Interleukin 6 (interferon, beta 2)	6.30E-05	1.15 (1.12–1.18)
7	rs11984075	9844	ELMO1	Engulfment and cell motility 1	1.10E-05	1.11 (1.09–1.14)
7	rs354033	79970	ZNF767	Zinc finger family member 767	4.70E-09	1.11 (1.1–1.13)
8	rs6986386	8658	TNKS	Tankyrase, TRF1-interacting ankyrin-related ADP-ribose polymerase	1.60E-05	1.08 (1.06–1.1)

Table 11.1 (continued)

Chromosome	Reference SNP ID	Entrez gene ID	Gene symbol	Gene name	*p*-value	OR (95 % CI)
8	rs1520333	5569	PKIA	Protein kinase (cAMP-dependent, catalytic) inhibitor alpha	1.60E-07	1.1 (1.08–1.11)
8	rs4410871	5820	PVT1	Pvt1 oncogene (non-protein coding)	7.70E-09	1.11 (1.09–1.12)
8	rs2019960	100302281	MIR1208	MicroRNA 1208	5.20E-09	1.12 (1.1–1.13)
9	rs290986	6850	SYK	Spleen tyrosine kinase	9.10E-07	1.1 (1.08–1.12)
10	rs3118470	3559	IL2RA	Interleukin 2 receptor, alpha	3.20E-11	1.12 (1.1–1.13)
10	rs7090512	3559	IL2RA	Interleukin 2 receptor, alpha	4.60E-20	1.19 (1.17–1.21)
10	rs793108	220929	ZNF438	Zinc finger protein 438	2.60E-06	1.08 (1.06–1.09)
10	rs7912269	3778	KCNMA1	Potassium large conductance calcium-activated channel, subfamily M, alpha member 1	1.40E-05	1.14 (1.12–1.17)
10	rs1250550	57178	ZMIZ1	Zinc finger, MIZ-type containing 1	6.30E-09	1.1 (1.09–1.12)
10	rs7923837	3087	HHEX	Hematopoietically expressed homeobox	4.90E-09	1.1 (1.08–1.11)
11	rs650258	923	CD6	CD6 molecule	2.00E-11	1.12 (1.1–1.13)
11	rs694739	25824	PRDX5	Peroxiredoxin 5	0.00014	1.06 (1.05–1.08)
11	rs4409785	143684	FAM76B	Family with sequence similarity 76, member B	6.30E-07	1.1 (1.09–1.12)
11	rs491111	84811	BUD13	BUD13 homolog (S. cerevisiae)	0.00048	1.06 (1.04–1.07)
11	rs630923	643	CXCR5	Chemokine (C-X-C motif) receptor 5	2.80E-07	1.12 (1.1–1.14)
11	rs7941030	84959	UBASH3B	Ubiquitin associated and SH3 domain containing B	1.60E-05	1.07 (1.06–1.09)
12	rs1800693	7132	TNFRSF1A	Tumor necrosis factor receptor superfamily, member 1A	4.10E-14	1.12 (1.11–1.14)
12	rs10466829	160365	CLECL1	C-type lectin-like 1	1.40E-08	1.09 (1.08–1.11)
12	rs12368653	116986	AGAP2	ArfGAP with GTPase domain, ankyrin repeat and PH domain 2	1.70E-09	1.1 (1.09–1.12)
13	rs17594362	23078	KIAA0564	KIAA0564	3.70E-06	1.11 (1.09–1.13)
13	rs806321	8847	DLEU2	Deleted in lymphocytic leukemia 2 (nonprotein coding)	5.00E-07	1.08 (1.07–1.1)
14	rs4902647	677	ZFP36L1	Zinc finger protein 36, C3H type-like 1	9.30E-12	1.11 (1.1–1.13)
14	rs2300603	10538	BATF	Basic leucine zipper transcription factor, ATF-like	2.00E-08	1.11 (1.09–1.12)
14	rs2119704	8477	GPR65	G protein-coupled receptor 65	2.20E-10	1.22 (1.19–1.25)
16	rs2744148	30812	SOX8	SRY (sex determining region Y)-box 8	8.40E-08	1.12 (1.1–1.14)
16	rs7200786	23274	CLEC16A	C-type lectin domain family 16, member A	8.50E-17	1.15 (1.13–1.16)

Table 11.1 (continued)

Chromosome	Reference SNP ID	Entrez gene ID	Gene symbol	Gene name	*p*-value	OR (95 % CI)
16	rs11864333	388210	LOC388210	Apolipophorins-like	3.60E-05	1.07 (1.05–1.08)
16	rs386965	4094	MAF	v-maf musculoaponeurotic fibrosarcoma oncogene homolog (avian)	3.90E-06	1.09 (1.07–1.11)
16	rs13333054	3394	IRF8	Interferon regulatory factor 8	1.30E-08	1.11 (1.1–1.13)
17	rs9891119	6774	STAT3	Signal transducer and activator of transcription 3 (acute-phase response factor)	1.80E-10	1.11 (1.09–1.12)
17	rs4792814	9020	MAP3K14	Mitogen-activated protein kinase kinase kinase 14	3.00E-06	1.08 (1.06–1.09)
17	rs1373089	7484	WNT9B	Wingless-type MMTV integration site family, member 9B	4.00E-05	1.07 (1.05–1.08)
17	rs180515	6198	RPS6KB1	Ribosomal protein S6 kinase, 70 kDa, polypeptide 1	8.80E-08	1.09 (1.08–1.11)
17	rs8081176	57674	RNF213	Ring finger protein 213	1.50E-05	1.07 (1.06–1.09)
18	rs7238078	10892	MALT1	Mucosa associated lymphoid tissue lymphoma translocation gene 1	2.50E-09	1.12 (1.1–1.14)
18	rs12456021	115701	ALPK2	Alpha-kinase 2	3.60E-06	1.1 (1.08–1.12)
19	rs1077667	8740	TNFSF14	Tumor necrosis factor (ligand) superfamily, member 14	9.40E-14	1.16 (1.14–1.18)
19	rs8112449	11140	CDC37	Cell division cycle 37 homolog (S. cerevisiae)	1.20E-06	1.08 (1.07–1.1)
19	rs2278442	3385	ICAM3	Intercellular adhesion molecule 3	0.00012	1.07 (1.05–1.08)
19	rs874628	84769	MPV17L2	MPV17 mitochondrial membrane protein-like 2	1.30E-08	1.11 (1.09–1.12)
19	rs7255066	5817	PVR	Poliovirus receptor	1.20E-06	1.09 (1.07–1.11)
19	rs307896	10055	SAE1	SUMO1 activating enzyme subunit 1	4.60E-07	1.09 (1.08–1.11)
19	rs2303759	27120	DKKL1	Dickkopf-like 1	5.20E-09	1.11 (1.09–1.13)
19	rs281380	284358	MAMSTR	MEF2 activating motif and SAP domain containing transcriptional regulator	1.90E-06	1.08 (1.07–1.09)
20	rs2425752	57727	NCOA5	Nuclear receptor coactivator 5	5.10E-10	1.11 (1.1–1.13)
20	rs2248359	1591	CYP24A1	Cytochrome P450, family 24, subfamily A, polypeptide 1	2.50E-11	1.12 (1.1–1.13)
20	rs2762932	1591	CYP24A1	Cytochrome P450, family 24, subfamily A, polypeptide 1	8.10E-07	1.12 (1.09–1.14)
20	rs6062314	140685	ZBTB46	Zinc finger and BTB domain containing 46	1.30E-07	1.16 (1.14–1.19)
22	rs2283792	5594	MAPK1	Mitogen-activated protein kinase 1	4.70E-09	1.1 (1.08–1.11)
22	rs2072711	4689	NCF4	Neutrophil cytosolic factor 4, 40 kDa	6.30E-05	1.09 (1.07–1.11)
22	rs140522	440836	ODF3B	Outer dense fiber of sperm tails 3B	1.70E-08	1.1 (1.09–1.12)

Four genes, such as CD86, PTGER4, IL2RA, and CYP24A1, are repeatedly listed with different reference SNP IDs molecular network composed of 607 molecules and 728 molecular relations, showing the most significant relationship with transcriptional regulation by Myb ($p = 4.755E\text{-}176$), followed by AP-1 ($p = 3.162E\text{-}90$) and STAT ($p = 2.683E\text{-}71$; Fig. 11.2). Thus, Myb, a key transcription factor for hematopoietic cell proliferation and differentiation, acts as a hub molecule in the network of MS risk SNP genes. Myb expression is induced in neurons by apoptotic stimuli and in reactive astrocytes by excitotoxic stress, and it plays a pivotal role in neural progenitor cell proliferation (Jeon et al. 2004; Malaterre et al. 2008). It is noteworthy that intravenous administration of human neural stem cells ameliorates experimental autoimmune encephalomyelitis (EAE) in a primate model of MS via an immune regulatory mechanism (Pluchino et al. 2009). Based on these observations, further studies are warranted to investigate an unpredicted role of Myb in the pathogenesis of MS.

11.4 Molecular Network Analysis of Transcriptome Data of MS

Recombinant IFN-β therapy is widely used as the gold standard to reduce disease activity of MS, although up to 50 % of the patients under the treatment continue to have relapses, followed by progression of disability. If molecular biomarkers for IFN-β responsiveness are identified, we could adopt the best treatment options depending on the patients, being invaluable to establish the personalized therapy of MS.

By gene expression profiling on Human Genome U133 A Plus 2.0 arrays (Affymetrix), a previous study showed that IFN-β nonresponders (NR) of RRMS patients following a 2-year treatment are characterized by overexpression of type I IFN-induced genes in peripheral blood mononuclear cells (PBMC), associated with increased endogenous production of type I IFN by monocytes at pretreatment (Comabella et al. 2009). These observations suggest that a preactivated type I IFN signaling pathway contributes to IFN-β nonresponsiveness in MS. By gene expression profiling on Human Genome Focus arrays (Affymetrix), different study revealed that *in vivo* injection of IFN-β rapidly induces elevation of IFI27, CCL2, and CXCL10 in PBMC of MS patients even after 6 months of the treatment, and the induction of IFN-responsive genes is greatly reduced in the patients with neutralizing antibodies (NAbs) against IFN-β (Sellebjerg et al. 2009). By gene expression profiling on a custom microarray, we found that IFN-β immediately induces a burst of expression of chemokine genes with potential relevance to IFN-β-related early adverse effects in MS (Satoh et al. 2006b). Furthermore, T cell gene expression profiling classifies a heterogeneous population of Japanese MS patients into four distinct subgroups that differ in the disease activity and therapeutic response to IFN-β (Satoh et al. 2006a). In the latter study, we identified 286 DEGs expressed between 72 untreated Japanese MS patients and 22 age- and sex-matched healthy subjects. From these DEGs, KeyMolnet by the common upstream network-search algorithm extracted the molecular network, showing the most significant relationship with transcriptional regulation by NF-κB, a central transcription factor that regulates diverse immune responses (Satoh et al. 2007). An active role of NF-κB was also found in the MS relapse-related gene network (Satoh et al. 2008).

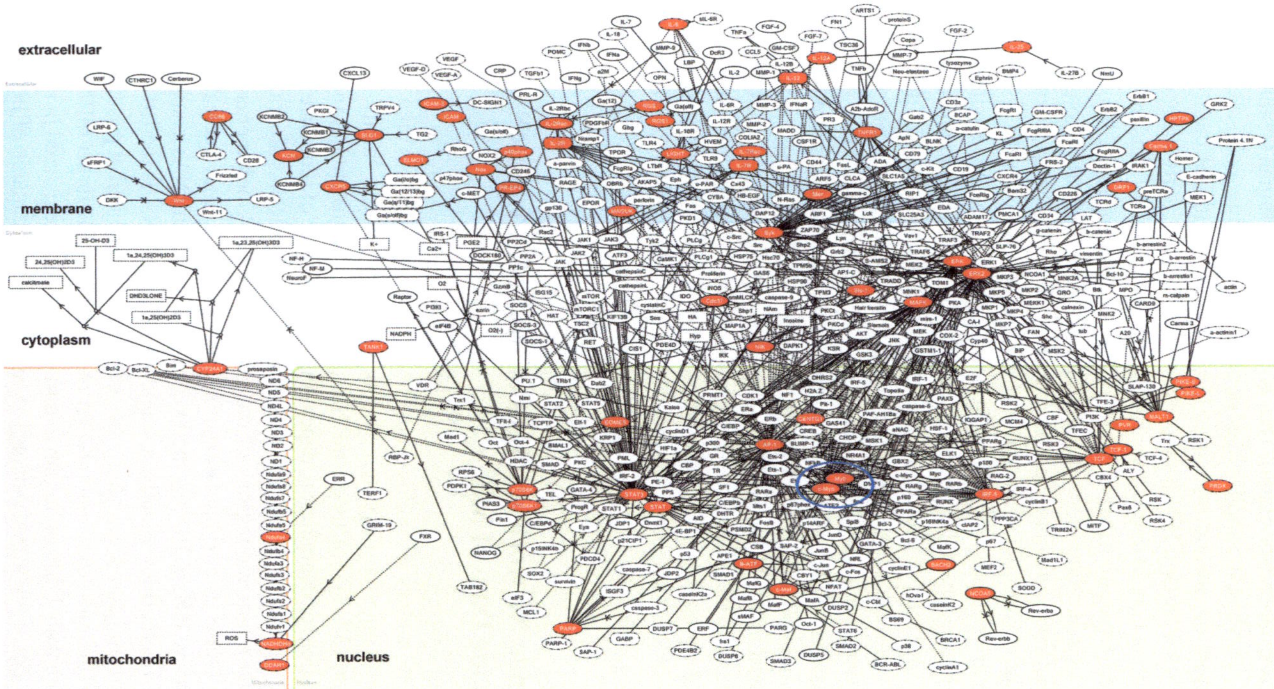

Fig. 11.2 Molecular network of MS risk SNP genes. The recent largest GWAS identified 102 MS risk SNPs outside the MHC region (Table 11.1; International Multiple Sclerosis Genetics Consortium et al. 2011). From these genes, KeyMolnet by the neighboring network-search algorithm extracted a highly complex molecular network, showing the significant relationship with transcriptional regulation by Myb, AP-1, and STAT. *Red* nodes represent MS risk SNP genes, whereas *white* nodes exhibit additional nodes extracted automatically from the core contents of KeyMolnet to establish molecular connections. The molecular relation is indicated by *solid line with arrow* (direct activation), *solid line with arrow* and stop (direct inactivation), *solid line without arrow* (direct interaction or complex formation), *dash line with arrow* (transcriptional activation), and *dash line with arrow and stop* (transcriptional repression). The transcription factor Myb is highlighted by a *blue circle*

Recently, we studied a large-scale GEO data set numbered GSE33464, composed of PBMC transcriptome derived from 12 RRMS patients following a 2-year treatment with IFN-β1a (Rebif; unpublished data). They were studied on Human Genome U133 A Plus 2.0 arrays. The blood sampling was performed at the time points before the first injection, before the second injection, 1, 12, and 24 months of the treatment. From these data, we identified IFN-β-responsive genes significantly upregulated at 1 month after treatment compared with pretreatment ($p < 0.001$ by Student's t-test). Top 25 upregulated genes are listed in Table 11.2. Among them, 20 are known IFN-responsive genes by searching them on Interferome (www.interferome.org). At 24 months of the treatment, we classified the patients into IFN-β responders (R) as those without relapses during 2 years and with the interval between the start of the treatment and the first relapse longer than 24 months, and NR as those with two or more relapses during 2 years of the treatment and with the interval between the start of treatment and the first relapse shorter than 12 months. Those who do not meet with these definitions were categorized into the unclassified (UC) group. Surprisingly, hierarchical clustering analysis with the set of 25 genes as a discriminator indicated that two R are clustered in the pretreatment-type gene expression signature, whereas four NR are accumulated in the IFN-β-responsive gene signature (Fig. 11.3). These observations suggest that IFN-β R and NR of MS are not clearly separated by gene expression signature of IFN-β-responsive genes in PBMC. This is consistent with the recent study showing that there exist no global differences in gene expression profiles of PBMC of RRMS patients between NAb-negative IFN-β NR and R (Hesse et al. 2010).

11.5 Molecular Network Analysis of MicroRNA (miRNA) Targetome Data of MS

miRNAs constitute a class of endogenous small noncoding RNAs that mediate posttranscriptional regulation of protein-coding genes by binding chiefly to the 3′ untranslated region (3′UTR) of target mRNAs, leading to translational inhibition, mRNA destabilization, or degradation, depending on the degree of sequence complementarity. During the process of miRNA biogenesis, the pri-miRNAs are transcribed from the intra- and intergenic regions of the genome by RNA polymerase II, and processed by the RNase III enzyme Drosha into pre-miRNAs. After nuclear export, they are processed by RNase III enzyme Dicer into mature miRNAs consisting of approximately 22 nucleotides. Finally, a single-stranded miRNA is loaded onto the RNA-induced silencing complex, where the seed sequence located at positions 2–8 from the 5′ end of the miRNA is essential for recognition of the target mRNA.

At present, more than 2,500 of human mature miRNAs are registered in miRBase Release 20 (June 2013; www.mirbase.org). A single miRNA capable of binding to numerous target mRNAs concurrently reduces production of hundreds of proteins, whereas the 3′UTR of a single mRNA is often targeted by multiple different miRNAs, providing the complexity of miRNA-regulated gene expression (Selbach et al.

Table 11.2 The list of top 25 genes upregulated in PBMC of RRMS patients folowing treatment with IFN-β

Entrez Gene ID	Gene Symbol	Gene Name	Fold Change	Known IFN-Responsive Genes (Interferome)
3429	IFI27	Interferon, alpha-inducible protein 27	27.36	Yes
6347	CCL2	Chemokine (C-C motif) ligand 2	7.62	Yes
10964	IFI44L	Interferon-induced protein 44-like	7.44	Yes
91543	RSAD2	Radical S-adenosyl methionine domain containing 2	7.31	Yes
8820	HESX1	HESX homeobox 1	7.20	
6614	SIGLEC1	Sialic acid binding Ig-like lectin 1, sialoadhesin	6.86	
3434	IFIT1	Interferon-induced protein with tetratricopeptide repeats 1	6.47	Yes
9381	OTOF	Otoferlin	6.37	
6355	CCL8	Chemokine (C-C motif) ligand 8	6.11	Yes
3437	IFIT3	Interferon-induced protein with tetratricopeptide repeats 3	3.89	Yes
9636	ISG15	ISG15 ubiquitin-like modifier	3.88	Yes
129607	CMPK2	Cytidine monophosphate (UMP-CMP) kinase 2, mitochondrial	3.67	Yes
10561	IFI44	interferon-induced protein 44	3.57	Yes
4599	MX1	Myxovirus (influenza virus) resistance 1	3.54	Yes
57801	HES4	Hairy and enhancer of split 4 (Drosophila)	3.48	Yes
51191	HERC5	Hect domain and RLD 5	3.26	Yes
8638	OASL	2′–5′-oligoadenylate synthetase-like	3.17	Yes
3433	IFIT2	Interferon-induced protein with tetratricopeptide repeats 2	2.97	Yes
55026	FAM70A	Family with sequence similarity 70, member A	2.92	
4061	LY6E	Lymphocyte antigen 6 complex, locus E	2.88	Yes
27074	LAMP3	Lysosomal-associated membrane protein 3	2.71	Yes
94240	EPSTI1	Epithelial stromal interaction 1 (breast)	2.66	Yes
55008	HERC6	Hect domain and RLD 6	2.52	Yes
54739	XAF1	XIAP associated factor 1	2.32	Yes
6712	SPTBN2	Spectrin, beta, nonerythrocytic 2	2.30	

We studied the transcriptome dataset GSE33464 of PBMC derived from 12 RRMS patients following a 2 year-treatment with IFN-β. Top 25 genes significantly upregulated at 1 month of the treatment are listed

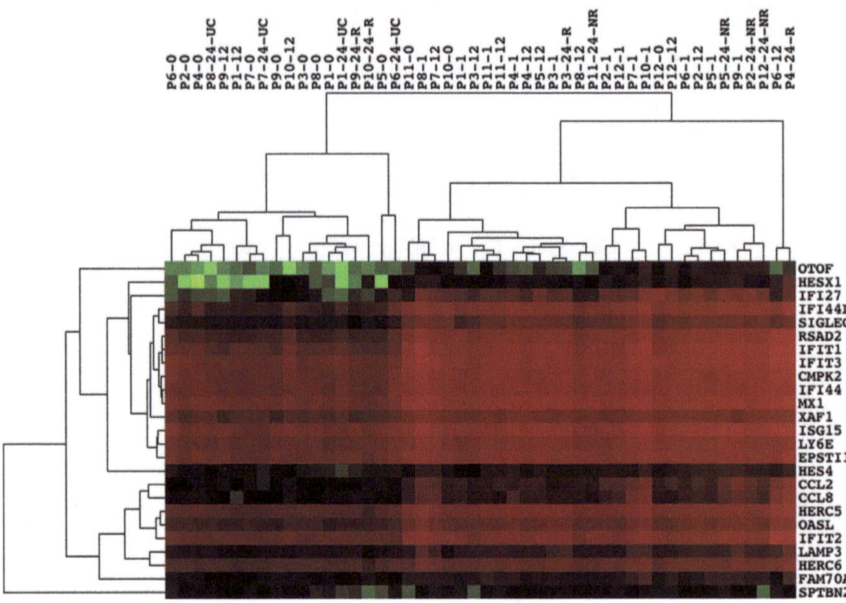

Fig. 11.3 Hierarchical clustering analysis of transcriptome of PBMC derived from 12 RRMS patients following a 2-year treatment with IFN-β. We studied the GEO data set GSE33464, composed of transcriptome of PBMC derived from 12 RRMS patients (P1–P12). The blood sampling was performed at the time points before the first injection (time 0), 1, 12, and 24 months of the treatment. We identified top 25 IFN-β-responsive genes upregulated at 1 month (Table 11.2). Based on the clinical disease activity, the patients were classified into R, NR, or unclassified (UC). Hierarchical clustering analysis was performed by Cluster 3.0 and TreeView with the set of 25 genes as a discriminator

2008). The set of miRNA target genes coregulated by an individual miRNA termed "the miRNA targetome" generally constitutes the biologically integrated network of functionally associated molecules (Satoh and Tabunoki 2011). Consequently, the whole human miRNA system termed "the microRNAome" regulates greater than 60 % of all protein-coding genes essential for cellular development, differentiation, proliferation, apoptosis, and immune response (Friedman et al. 2009). Furthermore, approximately 70 % of presently identified miRNAs are expressed in the brain in a spatially and temporally controlled manner, where they fine-tune diverse neuronal and glial functions (Fineberg et al. 2009). Increasing evidence indicates that miRNA-regulated gene expression is deregulated in MS (Junker et al. 2011). The levels of expression of miR-326 that targets Ets-1, a negative regulator of Th17 differentiation, are elevated substantially in PBMC of RRMS patients and in active MS lesions (Du et al. 2009; Junker et al. 2009). Clinical relapses of MS are closely associated with upregulation of miR-326 in purified $CD4^+$ T cells. By miRNA microarray analysis of peripheral blood samples derived from 59 treatment-free MS patients and 37 healthy controls, a recent study showed that both miR-17 and miR-20a that target T cell-activation genes are significantly downregulated in MS (Cox et al. 2010). We reanalyzed their data set GEO GSE21079. The MS group is composed of 24 RRMS, 17 SPMS, and 18 PPMS patients. We identified the set of 11 miRNAs, such as let-7f, miR-17–5p, 20b, 27a, 98, 106a, 126*, 140–5p, 374a, 454, and 624*, showing greater than a 0.8-fold decrease in MS patients versus controls ($p < 0.05$ by Student's t-test).

Recently, various bioinformatics programs have been established for the *in silico* prediction of miRNA target genes. They include TargetScan 6.0 (www.targetscan.org), PicTar (pictar.mdc-berlin.de), MicroCosm (www.ebi.ac.uk/enright-srv/microcosm/htdocs/targets/v5), miRanda (www.microrna.org), and Diana-microT 3.0 (diana.cslab.ece.ntua.gr/microT; Satoh and Tabunoki 2011). However, the miRNA target prediction by these programs is often hampered by detection of numerous false positive targets. To avoid this problem, we imported the set of 11 miRNAs described above into the miRTarBase (mirtarbase.mbc.nctu.edu.tw), the largest collection of more than 3,500 manually curated miRNA–target interactions from 985 articles, all of which are validated by luciferase reporter assay, Western blot, qRT-PCR, microarray experiments with overexpression or knockdown of miRNAs, or pulsed stable isotope labeling with amino acids in culture (pSILAC) experiments (Hsu et al. 2011). As a result, we identified 56 targets for the imported set of miRNAs, except for miR-454 and miR-624* that lack the experimentally validated targets (Table 11.3). We assume that these miRNA targetome molecules are potentially upregulated in MS due to reduction of the corresponding miRNAs. From 56 targets, IPA identified three molecular networks defined by "Gene Expression, Cell Cycle, and Cellular Development" ($p = 1E\text{-}27$), "Cellular Movement, Cellular Development, Cellular Growth and Proliferation" ($p = 1E\text{-}22$), and "Connective Tissue Disorders, Genetic Disorder, Inflammatory Disease" ($p = 1E\text{-}22$). Importantly, they are enriched in the canonical pathway termed "Cell Cycle: G1/S Checkpoint Regulation" ($p = 4.12E\text{-}10$; Fig. 11.4). Supporting these observations, previous transcriptome studies of PBMC showed that the expression of cell cycle and DNA damage regulators is aberrantly regulated in MS, having possible relevance to development of autoimmune T lymphocytes (Bomprezzi et al. 2003; Satoh et al. 2005).

11.6 Molecular Network Analysis of Proteome Data of MS

A previous study investigated a comprehensive proteome of MS brain lesions (Han et al. 2008). Protein samples were prepared from small pieces of frozen brain tissues derived from six MS patients isolated by laser-captured microdissection (LCM), and their histopathology was classified into acute plaques (AP), chronic active plaques (CAP), or chronic plaques (CP) based on the disease activity. They were then separated on one-dimensional SDS-PADE gels, digested in-gel with trypsin, and peptide fragments were processed for mass spectrometry analysis. Among 2,574 proteins determined with high confidence, the INTERSECT/INTERACT program identified 158, 416, and 236 lesion-specific proteins detected exclusively in AP, CAP, and CP, respectively. They found that five molecules, including tissue factor and protein C inhibitor, involved in the coagulation cascade were enriched in CAP, and they play

Table 11.3 The list of 56 targets for microRNAs downregulated in the peripheral blood of MS

Enterez gene ID	Gene symbol of target	Gene name	Corresponding microRNA	Validation methods
34	ACADM	Acyl-Coenzyme A dehydrogenase, C-4 to C-12 straight chain	hsa-miR-98	qRT-PCR
9949	AMMECR1	Alport syndrome, mental retardation, midface hypoplasia and elliptocytosis chromosomal region gene 1	hsa-miR-98	qRT-PCR
351	APP	Amyloid beta (A4) precursor protein	hsa-miR-17-5p, hsa-miR-106a	Luciferase reporter assay, Western blot, qRT-PCR
51742	ARID4B	AT rich interactive domain 4B (RBP1-like)	hsa-miR-20b, hsa-miR-106a	Luciferase reporter assay
472	ATM	Ataxia telangiectasia mutated	hsa-miR-374a	Immunoblot, Luciferase reporter assay, qRT-PCR
25805	BAMBI	BMP and activin membrane-bound inhibitor homolog (Xenopus laevis)	hsa-miR-20b	Luciferase reporter assay, qRT-PCR
659	BMPR2	Bone morphogenetic protein receptor, type II (serine/threonine kinase)	hsa-miR-17-5p	Luciferase reporter assay, qRT-PCR, Western blot
23468	CBX5	chromobox homolog 5 (HP1 alpha homolog, Drosophila)	hsa-miR-98	qRT-PCR
1026	CDKN1A	Cyclin-dependent kinase inhibitor 1A (p21, Cip1)	hsa-miR-20b, hsa-miR-106a	qRT-PCR, Luciferase reporter assay, Western blot, Microarray
1140	CHRNB1	Cholinergic receptor, nicotinic, beta 1 (muscle)	hsa-miR-98	qRT-PCR
4850	CNOT4	CCR4-NOT transcription complex, subunit 4	hsa-miR-98	qRT-PCR
51232	CRIM1	Cysteine rich transmembrane BMP regulator 1 (chordin-like)	hsa-miR-20b	Luciferase reporter assay, qRT-PCR
23405	DICER1	Dicer 1, ribonuclease type III	hsa-miR-374a	Immunoblot, Luciferase reporter assay, qRT-PCR

Table 11.3 (continued)

Enterez gene ID	Gene symbol of target	Gene name	Corresponding microRNA	Validation methods
1869	E2F1	E2F transcription factor 1	hsa-miR-17-5p, hsa-miR-98, hsa-miR-106a	qRT-PCR, Western blot, Luciferase reporter assay, Northern blot, Immunohistochemistry, Microarray
1870	E2F2	E2F transcription factor 2	hsa-miR-98	Northern blot, Western blot, qRT-PCR, ChIP, Luciferase reporter assay
2099	ESR1	Estrogen receptor 1	hsa-miR-20b	Western blot, qRT-PCR, Luciferase reporter assay
2308	FOXO1	Forkhead box O1	hsa-miR-27a	qRT-PCR, Luciferase reporter assay, Western blot, Immunohistochemistry, Northern blot
1647	GADD45A	Growth arrest and DNA-damage-inducible, alpha	hsa-miR-374a	Immunoblot, Luciferase reporter assay, qRT-PCR
9759	HDAC4	Histone deacetylase 4	hsa-miR-140-5p	qRT-PCR, Western blot, Luciferase reporter assay
3091	HIF1A	Hypoxia inducible factor 1, alpha subunit (basic helix-loop-helix transcription factor)	hsa-miR-20b	qRT-PCR, ELISA, ChIP, Western blot
28996	HIPK2	Homeodomain interacting protein kinase 2	hsa-miR-27a	qRT-PCR, Western blot
10114	HIPK3	Homeodomain interacting protein kinase 3	hsa-miR-20b, hsa-miR-106a	Luciferase reporter assay
8091	HMGA2	High mobility group AT-hook 2	hsa-miR-98	Northern blot, qRT-PCR
9987	HNRPDL	Heterogeneous nuclear ribonucleoprotein D-like	hsa-miR-98	qRT-PCR
3586	IL10	Interleukin 10	hsa-miR-106a	Luciferase reporter assay, qRT-PCR
5655	KLK10	Kallikrein-related peptidase 10	hsa-let-7f	qRT-PCR, Luciferase reporter assay, ELISA
5653	KLK6	Kallikrein-related peptidase 6	hsa-let-7f	ELISA, Luciferase reporter assay, qRT-PCR

Table 11.3 (continued)

Enterez gene ID	Gene symbol of target	Gene name	Corresponding microRNA	Validation methods
5601	MAPK9	Mitogen-activated protein kinase 9	hsa-miR-17-5p	qRT-PCR, Luciferase reporter assay, Western blot
4211	MEIS1	Meis homeobox 1	hsa-miR-98	qRT-PCR
140453	MUC17	Mucin 17, cell surface associated	hsa-miR-20b	Immunohistochemistry, Microarray, qRT-PCR
4609	MYC	v-myc myelocytomatosis viral oncogene homolog (avian)	hsa-miR-17-5p, hsa-miR-98	Western blot, Luciferase reporter assay, Northern blot, qRT-PCR, ChIP
29116	MYLIP	Myosin regulatory light chain interacting protein	hsa-miR-20b, hsa-miR-106a	Luciferase reporter assay
4661	MYT1	Myelin transcription factor 1	hsa-miR-27a	Western blot, Luciferase reporter assay
8202	NCOA3	Nuclear receptor coactivator 3	hsa-miR-17-5p, hsa-miR-98	Luciferase reporter assay, Northern blot, qRT-PCR, Western blot
5245	PHB	Prohibitin	hsa-miR-27a	qRT-PCR, GFP reporter assay, Western blot
5468	PPARG	Peroxisome proliferator-activated receptor gamma	hsa-miR-20b	Luciferase reporter assay, qRT-PCR
639	PRDM1	PR domain containing 1, with ZNF domain	hsa-let-7f	Immunohistochemistry, Luciferase reporter assay, qRT-PCR, Western blot
5925	RB1	Retinoblastoma 1	hsa-miR-106a	Microarray, immuno-histochemistry, Immunohistochem-istry, Western blot, Luciferase reporter assay
861	RUNX1	Runt-related transcription factor 1	hsa-miR-106a	Luciferase reporter assay, qRT-PCR, Western blot
27230	SERP1	Stress-associated endoplasmic reticulum protein 1	hsa-miR-98	qRT-PCR
6574	SLC20A1	Solute carrier family 20 (phosphate transporter), member 1	hsa-miR-98	qRT-PCR
85414	SLC45A3	Solute carrier family 45, member 3	hsa-miR-126*	Western blot, Luciferase reporter assay

Table 11.3 (continued)

Enterez gene ID	Gene symbol of target	Gene name	Corresponding microRNA	Validation methods
122809	SOCS4	Suppressor of cytokine signaling 4	hsa-miR-98	Luciferase reporter assay, Northern blot, qRT-PCR, Western blot
6667	SP1	Sp1 transcription factor	hsa-miR-27a	Western blot
6670	SP3	Sp3 transcription factor	hsa-miR-27a	Western blot
6671	SP4	Sp4 transcription factor	hsa-miR-27a	Western blot
10253	SPRY2	Sprouty homolog 2 (Drosophila)	hsa-miR-27a	Immunohistochemistry, Luciferase reporter assay, Microarray, qRT-PCR, Western blot
6774	STAT3	Signal transducer and activator of transcription 3 (acute-phase response factor)	hsa-miR-20b	qRT-PCR, ELISA, ChIP, Western blot
7057	THBS1	Thrombospondin 1	hsa-miR-17-5p, hsa-miR-98	Microarray, qRT-PCR
7068	THRB	Thyroid hormone receptor, beta (erythroblastic leukemia viral (v-erb-a) oncogene homolog 2, avian)	hsa-miR-27a	Luciferase reporter assay, Northern blot, Western blot
8742	TNFSF12	Tumor necrosis factor (ligand) superfamily, member 12	hsa-miR-17-5p	Luciferase reporter assay
11334	TUSC2	Tumor suppressor candidate 2	hsa-miR-98	Luciferase reporter assay, Western blot, qRT-PCR
7422	VEGFA	Vascular endothelial growth factor A	hsa-miR-17-5p, hsa-miR-20b, hsa-miR-106a	ELISA, Luciferase reporter assay
65986	ZBTB10	Zinc finger and BTB domain containing 10	hsa-miR-27a	Western blot, Luciferase reporter assay
677	ZFP36L1	Zinc finger protein 36, C3H type-like 1	hsa-miR-98	qRT-PCR
10269	ZMPSTE24	Zinc metallopeptidase (STE24 homolog, S. cerevisiae)	hsa-miR-98	qRT-PCR

The set of 11 miRNAs whose expression is reduced in peripheral blood samples of 59 treatment-free MS patients were imported into the miRTarBase to identify the miRNA targetome. The set of 56 experimentally validated targets are identified.

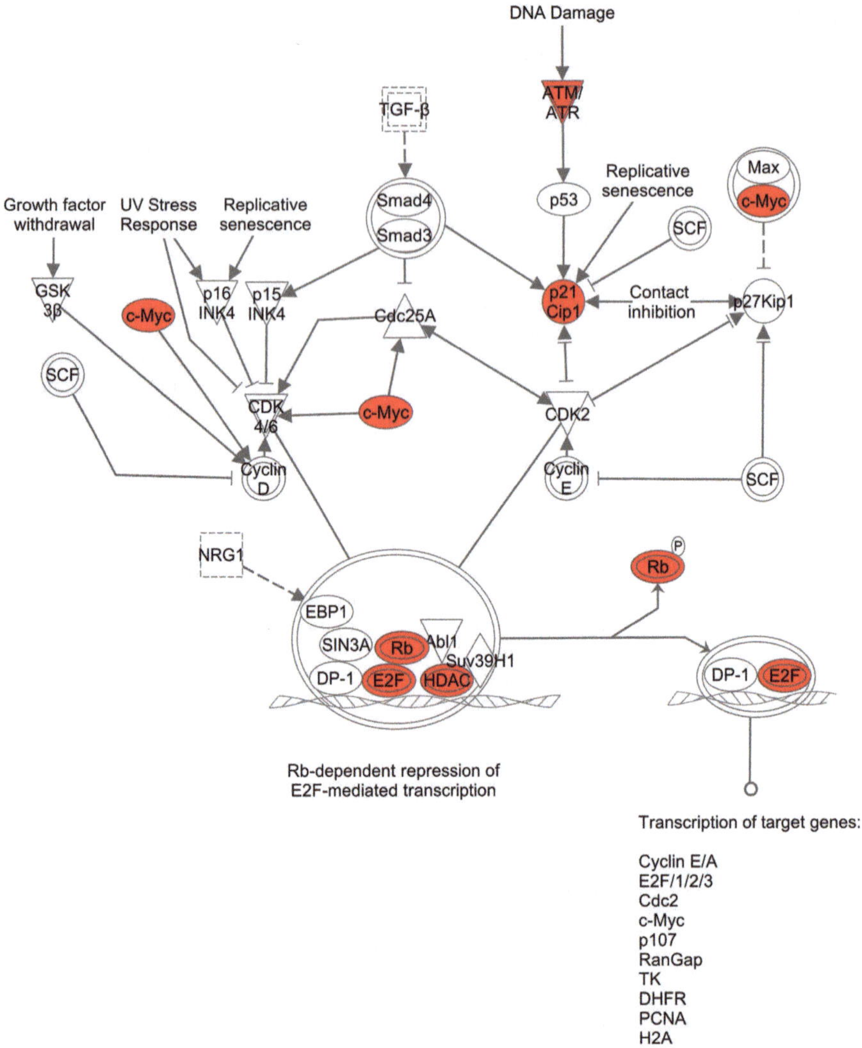

Fig. 11.4 Molecular network of miRNA targetome of peripheral blood samples derived from 59 treatment-free MS patients. We studied the GEO data set GSE21079, composed of miRNA microarray analysis of peripheral blood samples derived from 59 treatment-free MS patients and 37 healthy controls. The set of 11 miRNAs downregulated in MS were imported into the miRTarBase to identify the miRNA targetome (Table 11.3). From 56 experimentally validated targets, IPA identified three relevant molecular networks, which are enriched in the canonical pathway termed "Cell Cycle: G1/S Checkpoint Regulation." *Red* nodes indicate miRNA target genes potentially upregulated in MS

a central role in molecular events ongoing in CAP. Furthermore, *in vivo* administration of coagulation cascade inhibitors ameliorated EAE, supporting the view that the blockade of the coagulation cascade would be indeed promising for treatment of MS. However, nearly all proteins except the five molecules remain uncharacterized in terms of their implications in MS brain lesion development.

We studied molecular networks and pathways of the whole proteome set from the Han's data set by using KEGG, PANTHER, KeyMolnet, and IPA (Satoh et al. 2009b). KEGG and PANTHER indicated the relevance of extracellular matrix (ECM)-mediated focal adhesion and integrin signaling to the CAP and CP proteome sets. KeyMolnet by the N-points to N-points network-search algorithm disclosed a central role of the complex interaction among diverse cytokine signaling pathways in brain lesion development at all disease stages, as well as a role of integrin signaling in CAP and CP. IPA identified the network constructed with a wide range of ECM components, such as COL1A1, COL1A2, COL6A2, COL6A3, FN1, FBLN2, LAMA1, VTN, and HSPG2, as one of the networks highly relevant to the CAP proteome. Thus, four distinct tools commonly suggested a role of ECM and integrin signaling in development of chronic MS lesions. These observations suggest that the selective blockade of the interaction between ECM and integrin molecules in brain lesions *in situ* would be a target for therapeutic intervention to terminate ongoing events responsible for persistent inflammatory demyelination.

A recent study investigated a large-scale proteome of highly purified myelin and axogliasome proteins isolated from surgically resected human white matter tissues (Dhaunchak et al. 2010). The axogliasome is the specialized structure immediately flanking the nodes of Ranvier, composed of the overlying and attached paranodal loops. By multidimensional protein identification technology (MudPIT)-based mass spectrometry analysis, they identified total 1,022 proteins, including 568 proteins isolated exclusively from the compact myelin, 211 proteins only from the axogliasome, and 243 proteins from both fractions. By using the PANTHER database, they found that cytoskeletal proteins and nucleic acid-binding proteins are more enriched in the axogliasome, suggesting that cytoskeletal remodeling actively takes place in this site.

The acute stage pathology of MS is characterized by inflammatory demyelination, resulting in substantial leakage of myelin constituents, such as myelin basic protein (MBP), proteolipid protein (PLP), and myelin oligodendrocyte glycoprotein (MOG), into the cerebrospinal fluid (CSF). They potentially serve as an autoantigen that amplifies the immune response and these molecules and corresponding autoantibodies are utilized as a biomarker for diagnosis of MS (Lamers et al. 1998; Lalive et al. 2006). However, none of them are useful for accurate evaluation of MS disease activity. We studied the molecular network of the whole set of 1,022 myelin and axogliasomal proteins by using IPA. It identified the complex molecular network defined by "protein synthesis, carbohydrate metabolism, RNA posttranscriptional modification" ($p = 1E\text{-}146$). To identify a novel CSF biomarker candidate for detection of demyelination, the list of the proteins were filtered by evidence of detection in the CSF supported by the knowledgebase of IPA. We identified a set of 74 CSF biomarker candidate proteins (Table 11.4). They were enriched in three molecular networks defined by "lipid metabolism, small molecule biochemistry, and cell-to-cell signaling and interaction" ($p = 1E\text{-}36$), "cell death, posttranslational modification, protein folding, and organismal injury" ($p = 1E\text{-}33$), and abnormalities, inflammatory response, and cardiovascular disease ($p = 1E\text{-}29$; Fig. 11.5). It is possible that even minor perturbation in neuronal–glial interactions causes uncoupling of the glial

Table 11.4 The list of 74 CSF biomarker candidate proteins for detection of demyelination

Entrez gene ID	Gene symbol	Gene name	Protein-isolated fraction
39	ACAT2	Acetyl-CoA acetyltransferase 2	M
47	ACLY	ATP citrate lyase	M
102	ADAM10	ADAM metallopeptidase domain 10	M
161	AP2A2	Adaptor-related protein complex 2, alpha 2 subunit	M
335	APOA1	Apolipoprotein A-I	M
347	APOD	Apolipoprotein D	M
348	APOE	Apolipoprotein E	M
350	APOH	Apolipoprotein H (beta-2-glycoprotein I)	M
351	APP	Amyloid beta (A4) precursor protein	M
63827	BCAN	Brevican	M, Ax
718	C3	Complement component 3	M
721	C4B	Complement component 4B (Chido blood group)	M
821	CANX	Calnexin	M, Ax
22948	CCT5	Chaperonin containing TCP1, subunit 5 (epsilon)	M
960	CD44	CD44 molecule (Indian blood group)	M
966	CD59	CD59 molecule, complement regulatory protein	M
1000	CDH2	Cadherin 2, type 1, N-cadherin (neuronal)	Ax
1191	CLU	Clusterin	M, Ax
6900	CNTN2	Contactin 2 (axonal)	M
1501	CTNND2	Catenin (cadherin-associated protein), delta 2 (neural plakophilin-related arm-repeat protein)	Ax
1508	CTSB	Cathepsin B	Ax
51596	CUTA	CutA divalent cation tolerance homolog (E. coli)	M
27122	DKK3	Dickkopf homolog 3 (Xenopus laevis)	Ax
1937	EEF1G	Eukaryotic translation elongation factor 1 gamma	M
1984	EIF5A	Eukaryotic translation initiation factor 5A	M, Ax
2023	ENO1	Enolase 1, (alpha)	M, Ax
2194	FASN	Fatty acid synthase	M
6624	FSCN1	Fascin homolog 1, actin-bundling protein (Strongylocentrotus purpuratus)	M, Ax
2934	GSN	Gelsolin	M, Ax
3312	HSPA8	Heat shock 70 kDa protein 8	M, Ax
3303	HSPA1A	Heat shock 70 kDa protein 1A	M, Ax
3493	IGHA1	Immunoglobulin heavy constant alpha 1	M
3514	IGKC	Immunoglobulin kappa constant	M
93185	IGSF8	Immunoglobulin superfamily, member 8	M, Ax
3848	KRT1	Keratin 1	M, Ax
3849	KRT2	Keratin 2	M, Ax
3857	KRT9	Keratin 9	Ax
3939	LDHA	Lactate dehydrogenase A	M
3945	LDHB	Lactate dehydrogenase B	M
3956	LGALS1	Lectin, galactoside-binding, soluble, 1	Ax
4045	LSAMP	Limbic system-associated membrane protein	M
4062	LY6H	Lymphocyte antigen 6 complex, locus H	M
4190	MDH1	Malate dehydrogenase 1, NAD (soluble)	M
4282	MIF	Macrophage migration inhibitory factor (glycosylation-inhibiting factor)	M, Ax
4684	NCAM1	Neural cell adhesion molecule 1	M, Ax
4897	NRCAM	Neuronal cell adhesion molecule	M
4974	OMG	Oligodendrocyte myelin glycoprotein	M, Ax

Table 11.4 (continued)

Entrez gene ID	Gene symbol	Gene name	Protein-isolated fraction
11315	PARK7	Parkinson protein 7	M
27344	PCSK1N	Proprotein convertase subtilisin/kexin type 1 inhibitor	M
10130	PDIA6	Protein disulfide isomerase family A, member 6	M
5037	PEBP1	Phosphatidylethanolamine binding protein 1	M, Ax
5315	PKM2	Pyruvate kinase, muscle	M, Ax
5358	PLS3	Plastin 3	M
5478	PPIA	Peptidylprolyl isomerase A (cyclophilin A)	M, Ax
5500	PPP1CB	Protein phosphatase 1, catalytic subunit, beta isozyme	M
5052	PRDX1	Peroxiredoxin 1	M, Ax
7001	PRDX2	Peroxiredoxin 2	M, Ax
5589	PRKCSH	Protein kinase C substrate 80K-H	M
5621	PRNP	Prion protein	M
5660	PSAP	Prosaposin	M
6136	RPL12	Ribosomal protein L12	Ax
6193	RPS5	Ribosomal protein S5	M
6189	RPS3A	Ribosomal protein S3A	Ax
140885	SIRPA	Signal-regulatory protein alpha	M
6647	SOD1	Superoxide dismutase 1, soluble	M
8878	SQSTM1	Sequestosome 1	Ax
7018	TF	Transferrin	M, Ax
7070	THY1	Thy-1 cell surface antigen	M, Ax
7114	TMSB4X	Thymosin beta 4, X-linked	M
7345	UCHL1	Ubiquitin carboxyl-terminal esterase L1 (ubiquitin thiolesterase)	M, Ax
7384	UQCRC1	Ubiquinol-cytochrome c reductase core protein I	M
7425	VGF	VGF nerve growth factor inducible	M
7531	YWHAE	Tyrosine 3-monooxygenase/tryptophan 5-monooxygenase activation protein, epsilon polypeptide	M, Ax
7534	YWHAZ	Tyrosine 3-monooxygenase or tryptophan 5-monooxygenase activation protein, zeta polypeptide	Ax

The set of 1,022 human myelin (M) and axogliasome (Ax) proteins (Dhaunchak et al. 2010) were filtered by evidence of detection in the CSF supported by the knowledgebase of IPA.

support of axons. Therefore, we classified CSF biomarker candidates into two groups differentially expressed at the specialized myelin structures, i.e., ACAT2, ACLY, CD59, FASN, LDHA, LDHB, LSAM, MDH1, PARK7, PLS3, PPP1CB, PSAP, and VGF as a group of the compact myelin-derived biomarkers, and LGALS1, CTNND2, CDH2, CTSB, KRT9, and 14–3-3ς(YWHAZ) as a group of the axogliasome-derived biomarkers (Table 11.4; Fig. 11.5). We assume that detection of the latter in the CSF of MS patients reflects the very early sign of axonal damage. Importantly, these molecules may serve as a novel encephalitogen that provokes the relapses of MS. It is worthy to note that the levels of PARK7, alternatively named DJ-1, are significantly elevated in the CSF of RRMS patients, and are correlated with the severity of the

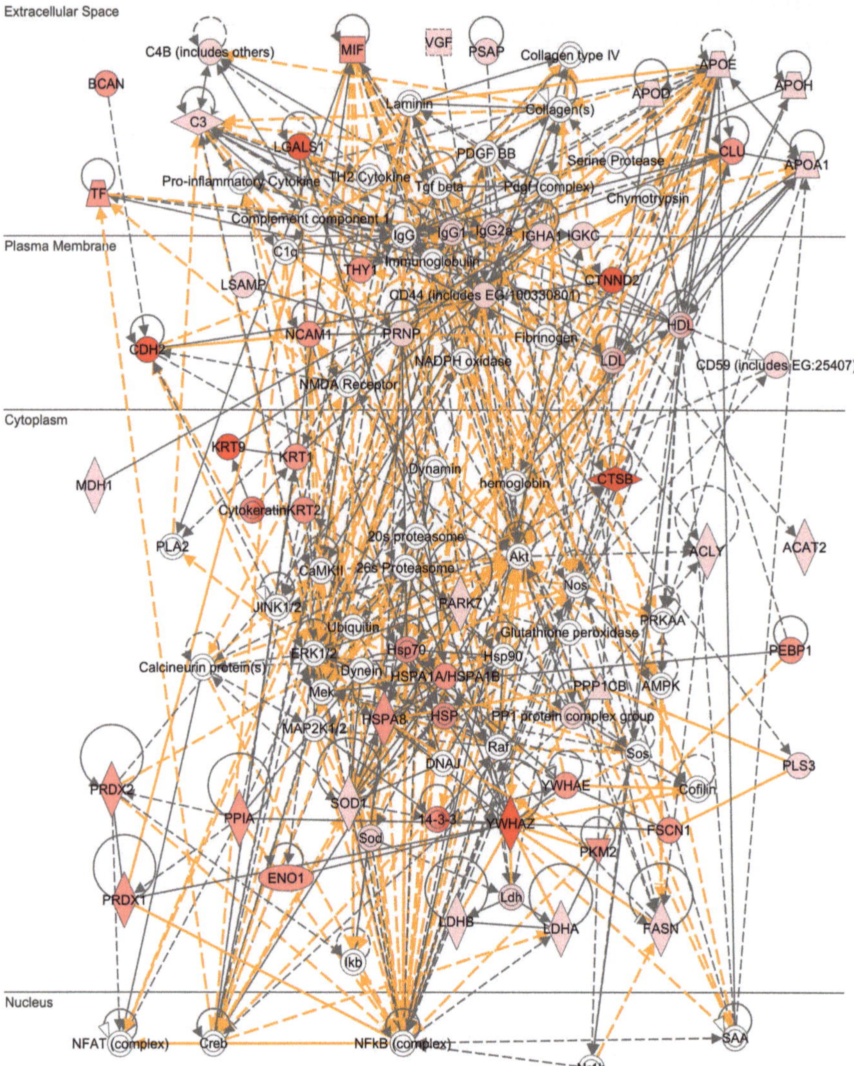

Fig. 11.5 Molecular network of human myelin proteome detectable in the CSF. By using IPA, we identified a set of 74 CSF protein biomarker candidates (Table 11.4) from 1,022 human myelin and axogliasome proteins identified by mass spectrometry (Dhaunchak et al. 2010). They were enriched in three molecular networks defined by "lipid metabolism, small molecule biochemistry, cell-to-cell signaling and interaction," "cell death, posttranslational modification, protein folding, and organismal injury," and "abnormalities, inflammatory response, and cardiovascular disease." The molecular networks were merged by additional molecular relations colored by *orange* and intervening *white* nodes. *Pink* nodes indicate the compact myelin proteins, while the most intense *red* nodes (LGALS1, CTNND2, CDH2, KRT9, CTSB, and YWHAZ) indicate the axogliosomal proteins, and other *red* nodes represent the proteins isolated from both fractions

disease (Hirotani et al. 2008). The 14-3-3 proteins are detectable in the CSF of MS patients presenting with severe inflammation-induced CNS tissue damage (Satoh et al. 2003).

11.7 Concluding Remarks

Recently, the global analysis of the genome, transcriptome, proteome, and metabolome promotes us to characterize the genome-wide molecular mechanisms of MS. The identification of biomarkers responsible for the complex disease phenotype of MS enables us to establish the molecular mechanism-based personalized therapy of MS. As omics studies produce high-throughput experimental data, it often hampers identification of the most important biological implications from the data. Recent advances in bioinformatics and systems biology have made major breakthroughs by illustrating the cell-wide map of complex molecular interactions with the aid of the literature-based knowledgebase of molecular pathways. By molecular network analysis of publicly accessible omics data with bioinformatics tools composed of the knowledgebase, we identified the transcription factor Myb as a central player in the MS risk SNP gene network, and found possible upregulation of cell cycle regulators in the miRNA targetome network of MS peripheral blood, and characterized the novel CSF biomarker candidates for detection of demyelination from the network of the human myelin proteome. We also found that IFN-β R and NR of MS are indistinguishable in view of gene expression signature of IFN-β-responsive genes in PBMC. These observations suggest that molecular network analysis of large-scale omics data provides a rational approach to establish the logical hypothesis of molecular mechanisms underlying MS, and to identify molecular targets and biomarkers for personalized therapy of MS.

Acknowledgements This work was supported by grants from the Research on Intractable Diseases (H21-Nanchi-Ippan-201; H22-Nanchi-Ippan-136), the Ministry of Health, Labour and Welfare (MHLW), Japan and the High-Tech Research Center Project (S0801043) and the Grant-in-Aid (C22500322, C25430054), the Ministry of Education, Culture, Sports, Science and Technology (MEXT), Japan.

References

Albert R, Jeong H, Barabasi AL (2000) Error and attack tolerance of complex networks. Nature 406:378–382

Baranzini SE, Mudge J, van Velkinburgh JC et al (2010) Genome, epigenome and RNA sequences of monozygotic twins discordant for multiple sclerosis. Nature 464:1351–1356

Bomprezzi R, Ringnér M, Kim S et al (2003) Gene expression profile in multiple sclerosis patients and healthy controls: identifying pathways relevant to disease. Hum Mol Genet 12:2191–2199

Comabella M, Lünemann JD, Rào J et al (2009) A type I interferon signature in monocytes is associated with poor response to interferon-β in multiple sclerosis. Brain 132:3353–3365

Consortium MAQC, Shi L, Reid LH et al (2006) The MicroArray Quality Control (MAQC) project shows inter- and intraplatform reproducibility of gene expression measurements. Nat Biotechnol 24:1151–1161

Cox MB, Cairns MJ, Gandhi KS et al (2010) MicroRNAs miR-17 and miR-20a inhibit T cell activation genes and are under-expressed in MS whole blood. PLoS One 5:e12132

Dhaunchak AS, Huang JK, De FJuniorOetal (2010) A proteome map of axoglial specializations isolated and purified from human central nervous system. Glia 58:1949–1960

Du C, Liu C, Kang J et al (2009) MicroRNA miR-326 regulates T_H-17 differentiation and is associated with the pathogenesis of multiple sclerosis. Nat Immunol 10:1252–1259

Fineberg SK, Kosik KS, Davidson BL (2009) MicroRNAs potentiate neural development. Neuron 64:303–309

Friedman RC, Farh KK, Burge CB et al (2009) Most mammalian mRNAs are conserved targets of microRNAs. Genome Res 19:92–105

Han MH, Hwang SI, Roy DB et al (2008) Proteomic analysis of active multiple sclerosis lesions reveals therapeutic targets. Nature 451:1076–1081

Hesse D, Krakauer M, Lund H et al (2010) Breakthrough disease during interferon-β therapy in MS: No signs of impaired biologic response. Neurology 74:1455–1462

Hirotani M, Maita C, Niino M et al (2008) Correlation between DJ-1 levels in the cerebrospinal fluid and the progression of disabilities in multiple sclerosis patients. Mult Scler 14:1056–1060

Hsu SD, Lin FM, Wu WY et al (2011) miRTarBase: a database curates experimentally validated microRNA-target interactions. Nucleic Acids Res 39:D163–D169

Huang da W, Sherman BT, Lempicki RA (2009) Systematic and integrative analysis of large gene lists using DAVID bioinformatics resources. Nat Protoc 4:44–57

International Multiple Sclerosis Genetics Consortium, Hafler DA, Compston A et al (2007) Risk alleles for multiple sclerosis identified by a genomewide study. N Engl J Med 357:851–862

International Multiple Sclerosis Genetics Consortium, Wellcome Trust Case Control Consortium 2, Sawcer S et al (2011) Genetic risk and a primary role for cell-mediated immune mechanisms in multiple sclerosis. Nature 476:214–219

Jeon GS, Shin DH, Cho SS (2004) Induction of transcription factor c-myb expression in reactive astrocytes following intracerebroventricular kainic acid injection in mouse hippocampus. Neurosci Lett 360:13–16

Junker A, Hohlfeld R, Meinl E (2011) The emerging role of microRNAs in multiple sclerosis. Nat Rev Neurol 7:56–59

Junker A, Krumbholz M, Eisele S et al (2009) MicroRNA profiling of multiple sclerosis lesions identifies modulators of the regulatory protein CD47. Brain 132:3342–3352

Kanehisa M, Goto S, Sato Y et al (2012) KEGG for integration and interpretation of large-scale molecular data sets. Nucleic Acids Res 40:D109–114

Kitano H (2007) A robustness-based approach to systems-oriented drug design. Nat Rev Drug Discov 6:202–210

Lalive PH, Menge T, Delarasse C et al (2006) Antibodies to native myelin oligodendrocyte glycoprotein are serologic markers of early inflammation in multiple sclerosis. Proc Natl Acad Sci USA 103:2280–2285

Lamers KJ, Reus HP de, Jongen PJ (1998) Myelin basic protein in CSF as indicator of disease activity in multiple sclerosis. Mult Scler 4:124–126

Lock C, Hermans G, Pedotti R et al (2002) Gene-microarray analysis of multiple sclerosis lesions yields new targets validated in autoimmune encephalomyelitis. Nature Med 8:500–508

Lucchinetti C, Brück W, Parisi J et al (2000) Heterogeneity of multiple sclerosis lesions: implications for the pathogenesis of demyelination. Ann Neurol 47:707–717

Malaterre J, Mantamadiotis T, Dworkin S et al (2008) c-Myb is required for neural progenitor cell proliferation and maintenance of the neural stem cell niche in adult brain. Stem Cells 26:173–181

Mi H, Dong Q, Muruganujan A et al (2010) PANTHER version 7: improved phylogenetic trees, orthologs and collaboration with the Gene Ontology Consortium. Nucleic Acids Res 38:D204–D210

Pluchino S, Gritti A, Blezer E et al (2009) Human neural stem cells ameliorate autoimmune encephalomyelitis in non-human primates. Ann Neurol 66:343–354
Rudick RA, Lee JC, Simon J et al (2004) Defining interferon β response status in multiple sclerosis patients. Ann Neurol 56:548–555
Satoh J (2010) Bioinformatics approach to identifying molecular biomarkers and networks in multiple sclerosis. Clin Exp Neuroimmunol 1:127–140
Satoh J, Illes Z, Peterfalvi A et al (2007) Aberrant transcriptional regulatory network in T cells of multiple sclerosis. Neurosci Lett 422:30–33
Satoh J, Misawa T, Tabunoki H et al (2008) Molecular network analysis of T-cell transcriptome suggests aberrant regulation of gene expression by NF-κB as a biomarker for relapse of multiple sclerosis. Dis Markers 25:27–35
Satoh J, Nakanishi M, Koike F et al (2005) Microarray analysis identifies an aberrant expression of apoptosis and DNA damage-regulatory genes in multiple sclerosis. Neurobiol Dis 18:537–550
Satoh J, Nakanishi M, Koike F et al (2006a) T cell gene expression profiling identifies distinct subgroups of Japanese multiple sclerosis patients. J Neuroimmunol 174:108–118
Satoh J, Nanri Y, Tabunoki H et al (2006b) Microarray analysis identifies a set of CXCR3 and CCR2 ligand chemokines as early IFNβ-responsive genes in peripheral blood lymphocytes in vitro: an implication for IFNβ-related adverse effects in multiple sclerosis. BMC Neurol 6:18
Satoh J, Tabunoki H (2011) Comprehensive analysis of human microRNA target networks. BioData Min 4:17
Satoh J, Tabunoki H, Arima K (2009a) Molecular network analysis suggests aberrant CREB-mediated gene regulation in the Alzheimer disease hippocampus. Dis Markers 27:239–252
Satoh J, Yukitake M, Kurohara K et al (2003) Detection of the 14–3-3 protein in the cerebrospinal fluid of Japanese multiple sclerosis patients presenting with severe myelitis. J Neurol Sci 212:11–20
Satoh JI, Tabunoki H, Yamamura T (2009b) Molecular network of the comprehensive multiple sclerosis brain-lesion proteome. Mult Scler 15:531–541
Selbach M, Schwanhäusser B, Thierfelder N et al (2008) Widespread changes in protein synthesis induced by microRNAs. Nature 455:58–63
Sellebjerg F, Krakauer M, Hesse D et al (2009) Identification of new sensitive biomarkers for the in vivo response to interferon-β treatment in multiple sclerosis using DNA-array evaluation. Eur J Neurol 16:1291–1298
Sospedra M, Martin R (2005) Immunology of multiple sclerosis. Annu Rev Immunol 23:683–747
Steinman L (2007) A brief history of T_H17, the first major revision in the T_H1/T_H2 hypothesis of T cell-mediated tissue damage. Nat Med 13:139–145

Chapter 12
Systems Biology for the Study of Multiple Sclerosis

Pablo Villoslada and Lawrence Steinman

Understanding complex diseases such as multiple sclerosis (MS) requires the integration of information from different levels at various times. Key information that must be integrated includes genetic background, environmental exposure, the state of sensitization of the immune system, and the state of cross-talk between the immune system and central nervous system (CNS). In order to achieve this goal, it will be necessary to relate all cellular and molecular events to changes in the tissue and organs and to map these changes on to imaging studies and on to assessment of the clinical course. This represents a difficult challenge for brain diseases because of the practical difficulties in obtaining accurate molecular and cellular information from the CNS in different diseases. In the study of MS, cellular and molecular biology and the new "omics" (genomics, transcriptomics, proteomics, lipidomics, metabolomics, etc.) have identified possible pathways involved in the course of disease; yet an integrative understanding of the pathogenesis is still lacking (Baranzini 2006; Noorbakhsh et al. 2009).

Systems biology applied to MS aims to understand the pathobiology of the disease as a process, from an integrative perspective, considering all paths involved and including the dynamics of the events (Foster 2011; Barabasi et al. 2011; Villoslada et al. 2009). For this reason, systems biology address problems by integrating all data generated by clinical, imaging, cellular, and molecular biology studies and using computational tools for modeling biological processes (Villoslada et al. 2009). The integration of molecular data generated by "omics" studies in

---

P. Villoslada (✉)
Department of Neurology, Center of Neuroimmunology,
Institute of Biomedical Research August Pi Sunyer (IDIBAPS)—Hospital Clinic
of Barcelona, Villarroel 170, 08036 Barcelona, Spain
e-mail: pvilloslada@clinic.ub.es

L. Steinman
Department of Neurology and Neurological Sciences, Stanford University,
Stanford, CA 94305, USA
e-mail: steinman@stanford.edu

Beckman Center for Molecular Medicine, 279 Campus Drive, Room B002,
Stanford University, Stanford, CA 94305, USA

T. Yamamura, B. Gran (eds.), *Multiple Sclerosis Immunology*,
DOI 10.1007/978-1-4614-7953-6_12, © Springer Science+Business Media New York 2013

models of the disease pathogenesis, signaling pathways, and biological networks is pursued in order to provide a physiological explanation of the findings and to relate them across the different levels of biological complexity (genes, molecules, cells, tissues, and the organisms) and, finally, to the clinical phenotype (Baranzini 2006; Noorbakhsh et al. 2009; Villoslada et al. 2009; Villoslada and Baranzini 2012; Han and Steinman 2009; Quintana et al. 2008). In this chapter, we review several attempts at modeling the pathogenesis of MS using the most common tools from systems biology such as network analysis or mathematical modeling. The review of previous omics studies including genomics, transcriptomics, or proteomics studies, including pathway analysis, is covered elsewhere in this book. For a detailed introduction to the theory and concepts of systems biology and the possible applications to brain diseases, we suggest our previous review (Villoslada et al. 2009).

Deciphering the pathogenesis of MS requires integrating in a comprehensive way the knowledge about the role of immune activation, the generation of autoimmune responses, the peripheral immune tolerance, the maintenance of the CNS immune privilege, the immunopathology within the CNS, and the degeneration and regeneration of the CNS. In order to achieve such a goal, the main approaches are the analysis of networks of the immune system and CNS and the modeling of its dynamics relating both the immune and nervous systems using computational tools based on differential equations or algorithms (Quintana et al. 2008; Villoslada and Oksenberg 2006; van der Greef et al. 2007). Although modeling biological process by means of mathematical equations has been the basis of quantitative biology and has provided significant success in some areas such as ecology, current application to MS is still limited. For this reason and on the basis of the success of network theory, the analysis of gene, protein, and pathway interactions may indicate common properties of optimal candidates to be targeted by therapy (Barabasi et al. 2011; Barabasi and Oltvai 2004). In addition, understanding the emergent properties of a system may help identify new targets that will be missed by a reductionist approach (Kitano 2007).

Network biology has emerged as a powerful theory and tool to analyze large data sets in novel ways (Barabasi and Oltvai 2004). Recent applications of this approach have enabled a comprehensive view of the genetic landscape of human phenotypes and diseases (Ideker and Sharan 2008; Goh et al. 2007; Schadt et al. 2009; Sieberts and Schadt 2007). For example, identification of genetic similarities among complex diseases, particularly autoimmune diseases, has been analyzed (Cotsapas et al. 2011; Gutierrez-Achury et al. 2011; Zhernakova et al. 2009). Recently, the group of Sergio Baranzini at UCSF has developed iCTNet (http://flux.cs.queensu.ca/ictnet), a new analytical tool that allows integrating data from disparate sources (Wang et al. 2011). iCTNet helps in indentifying relationships between diseases and genes and DNA and proteins; among proteins, genes, and tissues; and between therapeutic drugs and their targets were joined into a common database and visualized together in a network environment (using Cytoscape, a popular software for network visualization). This tool permits identifying patterns that may not be obvious, such as the extent of the genetic similarity between MS and other autoimmune diseases, and the number of MS-associated genes expressed in the brain.

Another approach focused on the properties that complex networks exhibit, such as centrality (degree, clustering, betweenness, etc. (Barabasi and Oltvai 2004; Barabasi et al. 2011)). A previous analysis assessed the centrality-related features of proteins whose genes were differentially expressed (seed proteins) in MS with respect to their protein neighbors, comparing the degree and the betweenness of these seed proteins and its comparison to their neighbors in the human protein–protein interaction (PPI) network (Goñi et al. 2008). The MS PPI network from blood tissue (Fig. 12.1a) contains 28 out of the 42 seed proteins and 177 neighbors, forming a giant component of 180 proteins. The MS PPI network from brain tissue (Fig. 12.1b) contains 38 out of the 99 seed proteins and 96 neighbors, with a giant component of 109 proteins. Accordingly, it was found that the degree and betweenness of seed proteins was lower than that of the PPI neighbors, situating seed proteins in peripheral regions of the network. The pathway analysis using gene ontology (GO) showed that such peripheral regions are distributed among many pathways, pointing toward heterogeneity of the processes involved. Thus, these findings show differential centrality properties of proteins whose gene expression is modulated in MS. Therefore, our results support the application of therapeutic strategies other than those previously applied, whereby only hubs that may compromise the robustness of networks were generally searched (Barabasi and Oltvai 2004; He and Zhang 2006). This may be the case of current immunomodulatory therapies for MS, such as interferon beta (IFN-beta) that modulates multiple pathways to certain degree without significantly abrogating certain hubs such as NFκB or p53, which are critical in the immune response.

Another network study aimed to identify causal relationship between key genes controlling the T cell activation, differentiation, and effectors' functions. We developed a network model of T cell activation in MS by integrating gene expression data from 20 genes quantified by real-time polymerase chain reaction (PCR) in patients and controls, with literature and coexpression information available at Ingenuity database using Bayesian networks (Fig. 12.2) (Palacios et al. 2007). This approach identified gene interactions (links within the network) that were upregulated or downregulated in MS, instead of single gene expression differences. Comparisons of the gene interactions (links) between patients and control networks identified differences suggestive of the involvement of common pathways as well as new therapeutic targets such as Jagged-1 that were validated in vitro and in vivo thereafter. Also, the network analysis was used for discovering and testing the efficacy of combination therapy. The combination of the in vitro treatment with Jagged-1 peptide and IFN-beta revealed gene interactions that were associated with the response of both therapies, suggesting a synergistic efficacy. Thus, we can generalize from this approach that by performing the comparison between cases and controls or before and after treatment, network analysis allows to identify genes, gene interactions, cluster of genes or pathways associated with the pathogenesis of the disease, or the response to therapy. This approach can even be used to analyze the complexity of studying combination therapy.

As explained before, dynamic/mathematical models of biological process using differential equations have been extensively used in biology. Such models benefit from the precise mathematical analysis that allow very precise predictions, but they are limited in the case of MS and many other complex diseases because of lack of quantitative information from the majority of cellular and molecular events involved as well as by the complexity of biological process that prevents simplification. Even

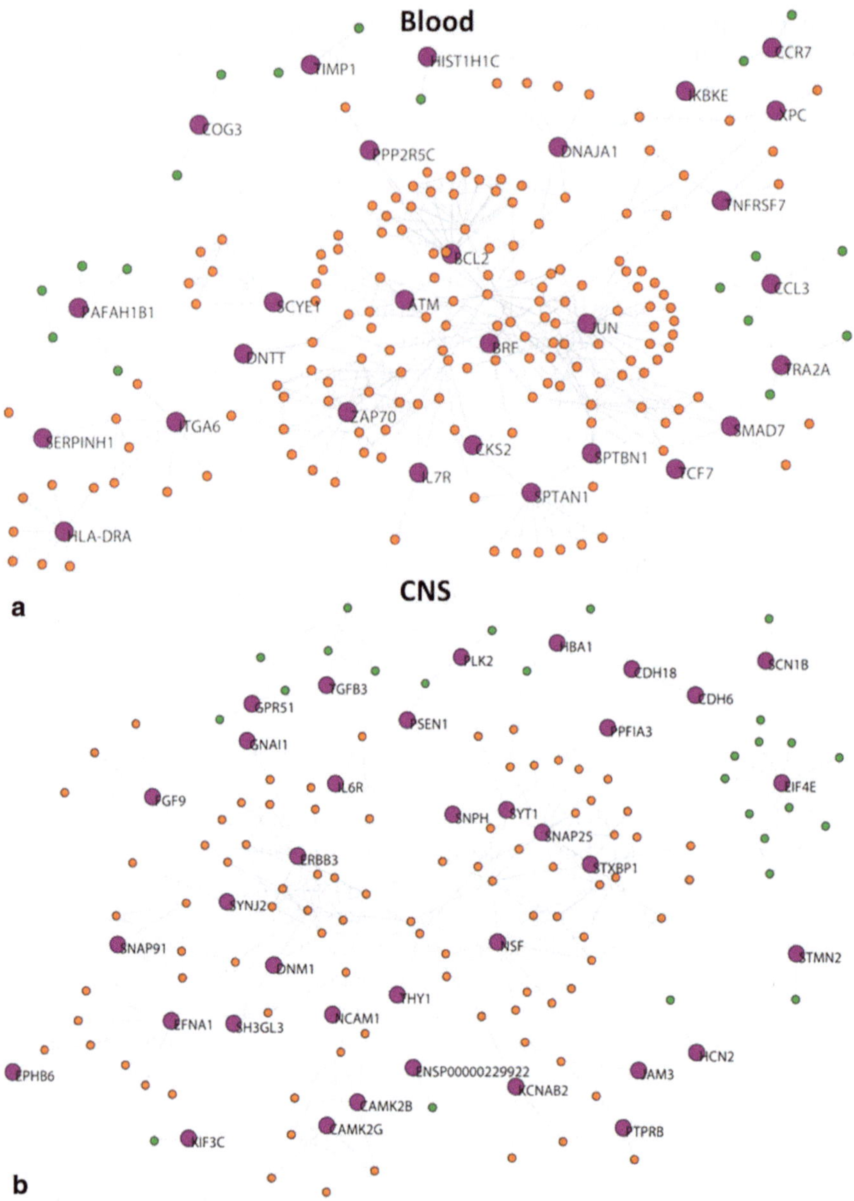

Fig. 12.1 Protein–protein interaction (PPI) network in multiple sclerosis (MS). PPI network from blood (**a**) and the central nervous system (CNS) (**b**) from patients with MS. PPI networks were built on the basis of corresponding differentially expressed genes (seed genes) identified in gene expression studies embedded in the human PPI network. *Purple* nodes indicate the seed proteins with their names. *Orange* nodes indicate neighboring proteins belonging to the giant component. *Green* nodes indicate neighbors that do not belong to the giant component. Visual inspection reveals that seed proteins are not hubs and are located in the periphery of the network, which would have implications for targeting the disease with new therapies. (Reproduced from Goñi et al. 2008)

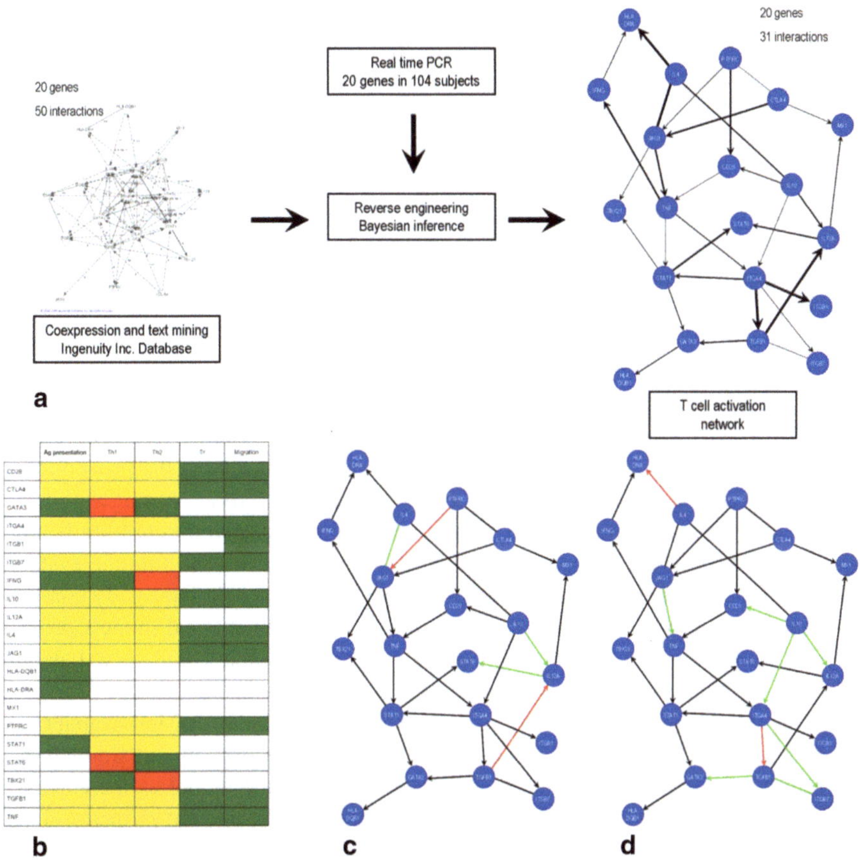

Fig. 12.2 Modeling T cell activation network for the study of multiple sclerosis (MS). **a** The structural network (*left*) was obtained from coexpression analysis using the Ingenuity database. The structural network has 20 genes and 50 links. Using the structural network as a template and the experimental data set (gene expression levels of the 20 genes from 104 subjects quantified by real-time polymerase chain reaction (PCR)), the T cell activation network was reconstructed (*right*). The network contains 20 genes and 31 functional links. **b** Dependence matrix: the role of each gene in every T cell activation function (antigen (Ag) presentation; Th1 differentiation; Th2 differentiation; regulatory lymphocyte (Treg) function; migration) based on the topology of the network (**a**, *right*) is displayed using the following color code: *yellow*, dual role (activator or inhibitor); *green*, full activator; *red*, full inhibitor; *white*, no influence. Dependence matrix revealed that the topology of the network maintains the relationship between genes defined by logic rules based on biological knowledge. Comparison of the T cell activation network between MS patients and controls (**c**), and untreated MS patients versus MS patients treated with IFN-beta (**d**). Comparisons between gene interaction weights are described using the following color code: *black*, no change; *green*, decreased; *red*, increased. The comparisons revealed differences in gene interactions in MS and in response to therapy. (Reproduced from Palacios et al. 2007)

with these limitations, several models reproducing different aspects of MS pathogenesis have been developed that can provide some insights on the pathogenesis of MS (Broome and Coleman 2011; Velez de Mendizabal et al. 2011). As such, we addressed the question of the dynamics of the disease. Relapsing–remitting (oscillatory) behavior is a hallmark of autoimmune diseases such as MS (Hauser and Oksenberg 2006; Sospedra and Martin 2005). At the clinical level, the presence of relapses defines the subtypes of MS. At the pathological level, a relapse is the result of an acute inflammatory process within the CNS, which produces myelin and axonal damage and impairs neural conduction, leading to clinical symptoms. It is not known what triggers relapse onset, although one-third of the relapses are preceded by common infections or stressful events (Buljevac et al. 2002, 2003). Understanding the biological basis of relapses in MS may have implications for immunotherapy. In autoimmune diseases, the balance between the proinflammatory response and regulatory factors is disrupted: antigen-specific effector T cells (Teff) are overactivated, whereas the function of regulatory lymphocytes (Treg) is altered (Martin et al. 1992; Viglietta et al. 2004; Martinez-Forero et al. 2008), indicating impairment of peripheral tolerance. It could be expected that this impaired immune response would produce a chronic inflammatory process leading to a progressive clinical course. However, in MS and other autoimmune diseases, the predominant behavior is oscillatory, with periods of T cell activation and tissue damage followed by deactivation and repair. We have postulated that the relapsing–remitting behavior of the autoimmune response is intrinsic to the design of the immune system, with several control mechanisms providing a negative feedback that tightly controls T cell activation (Velez de Mendizabal et al. 2011). Mathematical models predict that cross-regulation of Teff and Treg cells generates a stable oscillatory dynamic of both populations that not only maintains homeostasis in health but also promotes relapsing–remitting flares under autoimmune conditions (Velez de Mendizabal et al. 2011; Leon et al. 2001; Carneiro et al. 2007). On the basis of model simulations, we found that peripheral immune tolerance, defined in the model as the capacity to suppress or cap the activation of effector T cells, is an emergent property of the Teff–Treg cross-regulation (Fig. 12.3). This indicates that the Teff–Treg loop is a powerful control module that regulates the adaptive immune system when activated by stochastic environmental factors. A pathological dynamic regime of the Teff–Treg loop created a pulsing dynamic in which the expansion of the Teff population transiently escapes control of the Treg population, creating the relapses typical of autoimmune diseases such as MS. In the model, relapses mainly arise because of the failure in the Treg response and were mainly driven by stochastic process that may correspond either to thymic production of new self-reacting T cells or because of random sporadic infections. Interestingly, the frequency of such stochastic events was not the main factor producing relapses, but the severity in the dysfunction of the Teff–Treg cross-regulation was the main factor responsible for relapse frequency and severity. This finding can explain why the relapse activity in patients with MS is quite stable during the relapsing–remitting phase, because it would mainly depend on the dysfunction of the immune system. This, however, makes relapses very difficult to predict. Also, we modeled the effect of a therapy aimed to increase the activity and number of Treg cells. We found that depending on the doses and timing of such interventions, the outcome deviated from beneficial to even detrimental because of a rebound effect in the immune response (Velez de Mendizabal 2011). In summary, modeling biological process involved in the pathogenesis of MS process

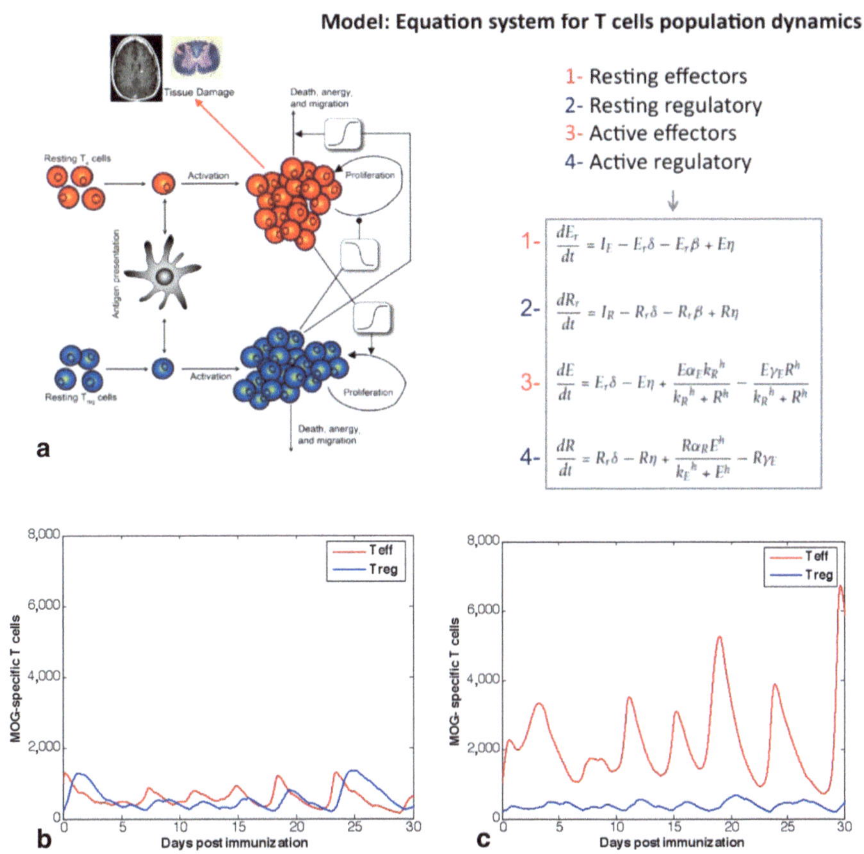

Fig. 12.3 Modeling the peripheral immune tolerance of autoimmune T cells in MS. **a** Graphical representation and the equations of the T cell cross-regulation model as described in Velez de Mendizabal et al. (2011). Simulation of the time course of the number of myelin oligodendrocyte glycoprotein (MOG)-specific effector T cells (Teff; *red*) or regulatory lymphocytes (Treg; *blue*) cells in the spleen after immunization in healthy state (**b**) and in autoimmune state (**c**). In both cases, cell populations oscillate, but in the case of MS simulations, peaks of Teff escape from the negative feedback of Treg and would translate to target tissue (central nervous system (CNS)) inflammation and clinical relapses

provides a theoretical framework for the understanding of the pathogenesis of MS or for predicting the response to immunotherapies.

Another promising area provided by systems biology is the study of networks dynamics. Although this area still requires significant development of the theory and tools, the case of chemical network reactions (CNR) is pioneering the development of this approach. The study of metabolites (metabolomics) and its reactions (metabonomics) or fluxes (fluxomics) has been developed by biochemistry for more than one century. Metabolism is in the basis of the functioning of all cell functions and, although less popular in the recent years than macromolecules such as DNA or proteins, there are suitable tools for its analysis in detail. This is based on characterization of metabolites, enzymes, and the reaction kinetics based on Michaelis–Menten equilibrium that permits studying the metabolic dynamics in detail. The introduction of the CNR theory and several mathematical tools for managing significant amounts of metabolic reactions provide a framework for modeling in detail the metabolic pathways related with the pathogenesis of complex diseases (Conradi et al. 2005; Martinez-Forero et al. 2010). The analysis of the metabolism may provide significant insights for MS considering that several metabolites have been implicated in the pathogenesis of the disease or as therapies for treating MS. We have abundant evidence for this with fumarate, kynurenines, and methylthioadenosine (Linker et al. 2011; Moreno et al. 2006; Platten et al. 2005). Then, the use of metabolomics tools for discovering metabolites associated with MS in combination with metabolomic analysis using CNR analysis is providing a new avenue for improving our understanding of the disease. Moreover, CNR analysis can be applied not only to metabolomics but also to the field of cell signaling, considering that phosphorylation of signaling molecules is a biochemical reaction involving kinases and phosphatases as enzymes and signaling molecules as substrates. Following the CNR theory, we have developed a model of type 1 interferon (IFN) pathway. Type 1 IFN are involved both in the pathogenesis of the MS as well as in the therapy because of the use of IFN-beta for treating patients with MS (Comabella et al. 2009a, b; O'Doherty 2007). The model of type 1 IFN pathway contains seven reactions (Eq. 1), modeling the phosphorylation of STAT1 and STAT2 in order to activate IFN-responding elements (ISRE), which mediate the gene expression pattern triggered by type 1 IFN (Fig. 12.4).

$$\begin{aligned}
\dot{x}_1 &= -k_1x_1x_2 + k_2x_3 + k_6x_7 - k_7x_1x_4 + k_8x_5 \\
\dot{x}_2 &= -k_1x_1x_2 + k_2x_3 + k_3x_3 \\
\dot{x}_3 &= k_1x_1x_2 - k_2x_3 - k_3x_3 \\
\dot{x}_4 &= k_3x_3 - k_4x_4x_6 + k_5x_7k_7x_1x_4 + k_8x_5 + 2k_9x_5 \\
\dot{x}_5 &= k_7x_1x_4 - k_8x_5 - k_9x_5 \\
\dot{x}_6 &= -k_4x_4x_6 + k_5x_7 + k_6x_7 \\
\dot{x}_7 &= k_4x_4x_6 - k_5x_7 - k_6x_7
\end{aligned} \tag{12.1}$$

x_1 JAK protein
x_2 STAT1
x_3 JAK–STAT1 complex
x_4 Phosphorylated STAT1
x_5 Unphosphorylated STA1–phosphorylated STAT1
x_6 Complex phosphatase
x_7 Phosphorylated STAT1–phosphatase complex

The solution at equilibrium shows a bistable state in which the pathway can be either switched on or off (Fig. 12.4c, d), which is critical for defining the activation of the cells in response to IFN-beta. This behavior is not obvious because in a linear

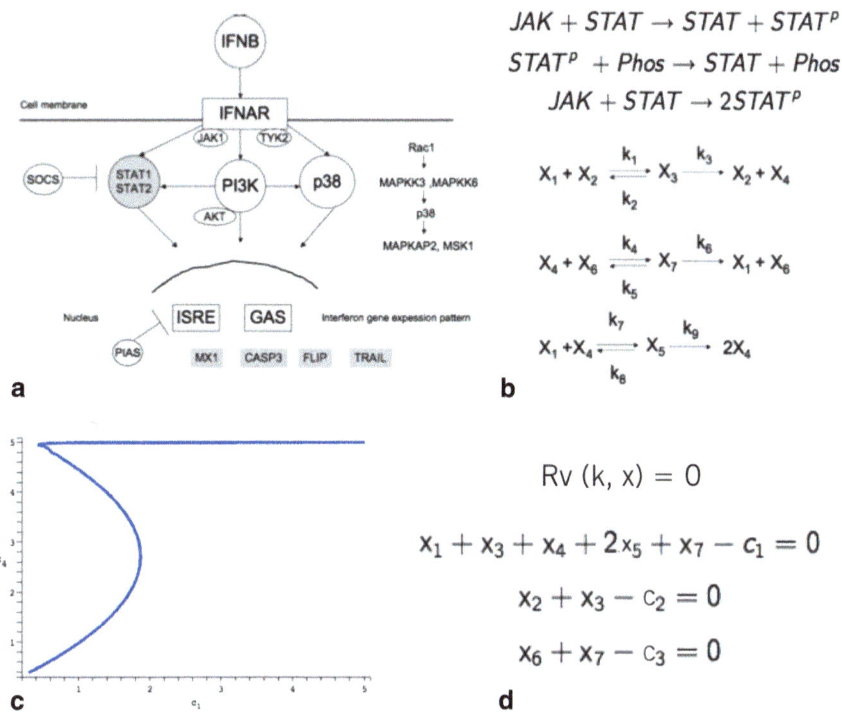

Fig. 12.4 Type 1 interferon (IFN) pathway analysis using chemical network reactions (CNR). **a** The type 1 IFN pathway signals through STAT1–STAT2, PI3K, and MAPK-P38 pathways in order to activate IFN-responding elements (ISRE) and/or gamma-IFN-activated sequence (GAS) transcription factors that mediate the gene expression pattern triggered by IFNs. **b** The model is composed of seven reactions modeling STAT1 activation (phosphorylation). JAK protein $= x_1$; STAT1 $= x_2$; JAK–STAT1 complex $= x_3$; phosphorylated STAT1 $= x_4$; unphosphorylated STA1–phosphorylated STAT1 complex $= x_5$; phosphatase $= x_6$; and phosphorylated STAT1–phosphatase complex $= x_7$. **c** Bifurcation diagram for total STAT (c_1) and phosphorylated STAT1 (x_4): by raising the levels of STAT1, the systems switch from low (off) to high (on) levels of phosphoSTAT1, indicating the activation of the type 1 IFN pathway. **d** Equilibrium solution of the CNR model of type 1 IFN pathway, where c_1, c_2, and c_3 represent total STAT, total JAK, and total phosphatase, respectively

model we would expect a direct rise of ISRE levels based on the number of IFN-beta molecules binding to the receptor. However, biological studies as well as our model support the concept that signaling pathways are able to analyze the signal and provide a qualitative response such as activating the gene and protein response to type 1 IFN. Bistability and other properties of complex dynamics in networks of reactions provide the building blocks for cells to analyze the environment and adapt to it by producing a response such as changes in gene expression. Therefore, this kind of quantitative model can be used for measuring the kinetics of signaling pathway in order to obtain functional information of its activity in health and disease and in response to therapy.

In conclusion, the conjunction between the high-throughput generation of data by omics technologies applied to MS, as well as the realization that a reductionist approach may not be sufficient to provide a clear explanation for the pathogenesis of complex diseases such as MS, has motivated the interest in applying systems biology for the study of the disease. However, systems biology still requires development of new theories and models of complex biological systems, identification of almost all the molecules and pathways participating in the disease, as well as the development of new computational tools for managing this amount of complex data in order to obtain knowledge from information. Models used in systems biology will be useful if they are applied to answer well-defined questions that a reductionist approach cannot approach and for which data and theoretical framework are available. Here, we have provided some examples of several approaches in this direction, probing that they provide new insights in the disease that would not be captured with previous methods. However, we need to recognize that answers provided by systems biology models are limited at present because the field still requires development of new theories, tools, and access to quantitative data. Overall, different approaches for dynamic analysis of MS offer the opportunity for integrating quantitative and temporal information and provide a theoretical framework for explaining the pathogenesis of MS.

References

Barabasi AL, Oltvai ZN (2004) Network biology: understanding the cell's functional organization. Nat Rev Genet 5:101–113

Barabasi AL, Gulbahce N, Loscalzo J (2011) Network medicine: a network-based approach to human disease. Nat Rev Genet 12:56–68

Baranzini SE (2006) Systems-based medicine approaches to understand and treat complex diseases. The example of multiple sclerosis. Autoimmunity 39:651–662

Broome TM, Coleman RA (2011) A mathematical model of cell death in multiple sclerosis. J Neurosci Methods 201:420–425

Buljevac D, Flach HZ, Hop WC et al (2002) Prospective study on the relationship between infections and multiple sclerosis exacerbations. Brain 125:952–960

Buljevac D, Hop WC, Reedeker W et al (2003) Self reported stressful life events and exacerbations in multiple sclerosis: prospective study. BMJ 327:646

Carneiro J, Leon K, Caramalho I et al (2007) When three is not a crowd: a Crossregulation model of the dynamics and repertoire selection of regulatory CD4(+) T cells. Immunol Rev 216:48–68

Conradi C, Saez-Rodriguez J, Gilles ED, Raisch J (2005) Using chemical reaction network theory to discard a kinetic mechanism hypothesis. Syst Biol (Stevenage) 152:243–248

Comabella M, Lunemann JD, Rio J et al (2009a) A type I interferon signature in monocytes is associated with poor response to interferon-beta in multiple sclerosis. Brain 132:3353–3365

Comabella M, Craig DW, Morcillo-Suarez C et al (2009b) Genome-wide scan of 500,000 single-nucleotide polymorphisms among responders and nonresponders to interferon beta therapy in multiple sclerosis. Arch Neurol 66:972–978

Cotsapas C, Voight BF, Rossin E et al (2011) Pervasive sharing of genetic effects in autoimmune disease. PLoS Genet 7:e1002254

Foster KR (2011) The sociobiology of molecular systems. Nat Rev Genet 12:193–203

Goh KI, Cusick ME, Valle D, Childs B, Vidal M, Barabasi AL (2007) The human disease network. Proc Natl Acad Sci U S A 104:8685–8690

Goñi J, Esteban FJ, Velez N, Sepulcre J, Ardanza-Trevijano S, Villoslada P (2008) A computational analysis of protein-protein interaction networks in neurodegenerative diseases. BMC Sys Biol 2:52
Gutierrez-Achury J, Coutinho de Almeida R, Wijmenga C (2011) Shared genetics in coeliac disease and other immune-mediated diseases. J Intern Med 269:591–603
Han MH, Steinman L (2009) Systems biology for identification of molecular networks in multiple sclerosis. Mult Scler 15:529–530
Hauser SL, Oksenberg JR (2006) The neurobiology of multiple sclerosis: genes, inflammation, and neurodegeneration. Neuron 52:61–76
He X, Zhang J. Why do hubs tend to be essential in protein networks? PLoS Genet 2:e88
Ideker T, Sharan R (2008) Protein networks in disease. Genome Res 18:644–652
Kitano H (2007) A robustness-based approach to systems-oriented drug design. Nat Rev Drug Discov 6:202–210
Leon K, Perez R, Lage A, Carneiro J (2001) Three-cell interactions in T cell-mediated suppression? A mathematical analysis of its quantitative implications. J Immunol 166:5356–5365
Linker RA, Lee DH, Ryan S et al (2011) Fumaric acid esters exert neuroprotective effects in neuroinflammation via activation of the Nrf2 antioxidant pathway. Brain 134:678–692
Martin R, McFarland HF, McFarlin DE (1992) Immunological aspects of demyelinating diseases. Annu Rev Immunol 10:153–87
Martinez-Forero I, Garcia-Munoz R, Martinez-Pasamar S et al (2008) IL-10 suppressor activity and ex vivo Tr1 cell function are impaired in multiple sclerosis. Eur J Immunol 38:576–586
Martinez-Forero I, Pelaez-Lopez A, Villoslada P (2010) Steady state detection of chemical reaction networks using a simplified analytical method. PloS One 5:e10823
Moreno B, Hevia H, Santamaria M et al (2006) Methylthioadenosine reverses brain autoimmune disease. Ann Neurol 60:323–334
Noorbakhsh F, Overall CM, Power C (2009) Deciphering complex mechanisms in neurodegenerative diseases: the advent of systems biology. Trends Neurosci 32:88–100
O'Doherty C, Villoslada P, Vandenbroeck K (2007) Pharmacogenomics of Type I interferon therapy: a survey of response-modifying genes. Cytokine Growth Factor Rev 18:211–222
Palacios R, Goni J, Martinez-Forero I et al (2007) A network analysis of the human T-cell activation gene network identifies JAGGED1 as a therapeutic target for autoimmune diseases. PloS One 2:e1222
Platten M, Ho PP, Youssef S et al (2005) Treatment of autoimmune neuroinflammation with a synthetic tryptophan metabolite. Science 310:850–855
Quintana FJ, Farez MF, Weiner HL (2008) Systems biology approaches for the study of multiple sclerosis. J Cell Mol Med 12:1087–1093
Schadt EE, Friend SH, Shaywitz DA (2009) A network view of disease and compound screening. Nat Rev Drug Discov 8:286–295
Sieberts SK, Schadt EE (2007) Moving toward a system genetics view of disease. Mamm Genome 18:389–401
Sospedra M, Martin R (2005) Immunology of multiple sclerosis. Annu Rev Immunol 23:683–747
van der Greef J, Martin S, Juhasz P et al. (2007) The art and practice of systems biology in medicine: mapping patterns of relationships. J Proteome Res 6:1540–1559
Velez de Mendizabal N, Carneiro J, Sole RV et al (2011) Modeling the effector—regulatory T cell cross-regulation reveals the intrinsic character of relapses in multiple sclerosis. BMC Syst Biol 5:114
Viglietta V, Baecher-Allan C, Weiner HL, Hafler DA (2004) Loss of functional suppression by CD4 + CD25 + regulatory T cells in patients with multiple sclerosis. J Exp Med 199:971–979
Villoslada P, Oksenberg J (2006) Neuroinformatics in clinical practice: are computers going to help neurological patients and their physicians? Future Neurology 1:1–12
Villoslada P, Baranzini S (2012) Data integration and systems biology approaches for biomarker discovery: challenges and opportunities for multiple sclerosis. J Neuroimmunol 248(1–2):58–65

Villoslada P, Steinman L, Baranzini SE (2009) Systems biology and its application to the understanding of neurological diseases. Ann Neurol 65:124–139
Wang L, Khankhanian P, Baranzini SE, Mousavi P (2011) iCTNet: a Cytoscape plugin to produce and analyze integrative complex traits networks. BMC Bioinformatics 12:380
Zhernakova A, van Diemen CC, Wijmenga C (2009) Detecting shared pathogenesis from the shared genetics of immune-related diseases. Nat Rev Genet 10:43–55

Chapter 13
Checkpoints in the Development of Pathogenic and Regulatory T Cells in Experimental Autoimmune Encephalomyelitis—A Basis for Current and Future Interventions in MS

Denise C. Fitzgerald and Stephen M. Anderton

13.1 Introduction

Given the relative inaccessibility of the target tissue—the Central Nervous System (CNS)—to experimental exploration, a wide range of in vivo experimental models are employed to study multiple sclerosis (MS), each of which affords particular suitability to studying different aspects of the disease. Individual models exhibit similarities to different types of histopathological lesions (type I–IV) described in MS (Lucchinetti et al. 1996, 2000). Most commonly, rodent models are used with mice being the most frequent choice, due in part to the range of reagents and genetically modified (GM) lines available as well as the reduced cost and breeding time of this species compared to larger mammals. While this chapter will primarily focus on the range of experimental autoimmune encephalomyelitis (EAE) models, it is important to summarise other approaches taken to model CNS demyelination. Aside of EAE, which will be discussed in detail later, three other main categories of models are frequently used: toxin-induced demyelination, viral-induced demyelination and genetic manipulation resulting in de-/dysmyelination. These models have been reviewed in depth elsewhere (Uschkureit et al. 2000; Matthews et al. 2002; Oleszak et al. 2004; Ercolini and Miller 2006; Blakemore and Franklin 2008; Kipp et al. 2009).

Several toxins have been used to induce demyelination experimentally including cuprizone, lysolecithin and ethidium bromide. Feeding of cuprizone, a copper-chelating agent induces demyelination in a number of CNS regions; however, it is most frequently studied in the corpus callosum (Carlton 1966, 1967; Hoffmann et al. 2008; Torkildsen et al. 2008; Skripuletz et al. 2010). Partial remyelination can be detectable by 3 weeks post-feeding and as such, this model is particularly useful for studies investigating concurrent de- and re-myelination (Stidworthy et al. 2003;

D. C. Fitzgerald (✉)
Centre for Infection and Immunity, Queen's University Belfast, Belfast, UK
e-mail: d.fitzgerald@qub.ac.uk

S. M. Anderton
Centre for Inflammation Research, Centre for Multiple Sclerosis Research and Centre for Immunity Infection and Evolution, University of Edinburgh, Edinburgh, UK

T. Yamamura, B. Gran (eds.), *Multiple Sclerosis Immunology*,
DOI 10.1007/978-1-4614-7953-6_13, © Springer Science+Business Media New York 2013

Armstrong et al. 2006; Lindner et al. 2008). Lysolecithin and ethidium bromide are injected directly into CNS tissue and induce focal lesions of demyelination, which also exhibit remyelination in general; however, this occurs subsequent to the process of demyelination (Yajima and Suzuki 1979; Woodruff and Franklin 1999; Blakemore and Franklin 2008). These distinct phases of de- and re-myelination facilitate studies on individual mechanisms at play in each process. In general, there is a localised immune response to toxin-induced demyelination, dominated by infiltrating monocyte/macrophage and microglial reactivity (Pavelko et al. 1998; Remington et al. 2007). However, in contrast to EAE models, immunopathogenesis is not thought to be a feature of demyelination in these models, rather, the immune response appears to be important for efficient resolution and repair of the lesion in toxin-induced CNS demyelination (Pavelko et al. 1998; Kotter et al. 2001; Setzu et al. 2006; Li et al. 2005).

Demyelination can be induced following infection of mice with a range of viruses including Theiler's Murine Encephalitis Virus, Mouse Hepatitis Virus (MHV) and Semliki Forest Virus (Croxford et al. 2002; Bender and Weiss 2010; Fazakerley 2004). These models are useful for interrogating the hypothesis of a viral basis to MS. For example, MHV infection results in acute encephalitis within a week post-infection, which generally resolves but is followed by chronic demyelination up to a month later (Bender and Weiss 2010). This type of experimental model facilitates investigations of pre-disposition of individuals to CNS demyelination by viral infection early in life, resulting in delayed onset of demyelinating illness later in life. Mechanisms of demyelination induced by viruses can be studied by molecular manipulation of viral strains. For example, Das Sarma et al. showed that mutation of the gene encoding the spike protein of MHV rendered this virus nondemyelinating despite the fact that it retained the capability to induce hepatitis and encephalitis (Das et al. 2000). Such studies allow detailed dissection of viral mechanisms of demyelination in the CNS. As the aetiology of MS remains unknown, and indeed may vary in different groups of patients, utilisation of these differing types of experimental models in testing of potential MS therapies can increase the chance of translation to the clinic as well as reveal mechanistic aspects of potential therapeutics in different pathological settings.

The most commonly used model of the inflammatory component of MS is EAE. Arising as it did from a human clinical scenario over a century ago, EAE is the prototypic animal model of autoimmune disease, provoked by immunisation with defined myelin autoantigens and transferrable to nonimmunised syngeneic animals with $CD4^+$ T cells. However, there are now a variety of experimental options available to the investigator, from the straightforward immunisation of standard laboratory strains of mice with autoantigen plus complete Freund's adjuvant (CFA) to more complex GM models that can develop spontaneous disease (Krishnamoorthy et al. 2006; Pollinger et al. 2009). These more complex models also include humanised mouse models involving the combined transgenic expression of a T cell receptor (TCR) derived from an MS patient, the relevant HLA class II molecule and human CD4 (Madsen et al. 1999). EAE can follow a range of clinical courses from acute/monophasic, through relapsing–remitting to chronic–progressive, depending on the precise model used. The same model can also show different courses in different laboratories. This variety allows different questions to be asked, such as what triggers resolution of acute disease and what drives relapses? It also allows the efficacy of potential drugs to be tested in different phases of disease.

13.2 Cellular Interactions Leading to Antimyelin Immunity in the Periphery—An Outline

The standard protocol for the active induction of EAE involves immunisation with myelin autoantigen in CFA (Stromnes and Goverman 2006a). Myelin-reactive $CD4^{+}$ T cells become activated in the draining lymph nodes in response to peptide MHC class II complexes presented on the surface of antigen-presenting cells (APC). This provides "signal 1" for T cell activation (ligation of the TCR). Signal 2 is provided by costimulation. Classically, costimulation is the interaction of CD28 on the T cell with CD80/CD86 on the APC, but full signal 2 is now appreciated to involve a temporal dialogue between the T cell and the APC involving several receptor/ligand pairs (Sharpe 2009). Interruption of this process through blockade of a variety receptors or ligands can disrupt T cell activation and prevent/abrogate EAE (Grewal 1996; Perrin et al. 1999; Weinberg et al. 1999). Signals 1 and 2 act in concert to drive clonal expansion of the myelin-responsive T cells, but the qualitative function of those cells (the inflammatory mediators they secrete and cell surface molecules they express) is shaped by "signal 3", the cytokine milieu generated chiefly by the APC (these will be discussed further in the following text). Signal 3 is, in turn, shaped by "signal 0", activation of the APC via pattern recognition receptors (PRRs) that bind to pathogen-associated molecular patterns (PAMPs). This also strengthens signals 1 and 2. CFA contains heat-killed mycobacterium tuberculosis, which provides a range of PAMPs for APC activation. Incomplete Freund's adjuvant (IFA) lacks mycobacteria and the lack of sufficient APC activation means that autoantigen in IFA is not a successful immunogen for EAE induction. Because CFA contains so many PAMPs, a series of studies have attempted to clarify the minimal requirements for APC activation leading to EAE. These have either used gene knockout mice lacking individual PRR, notably toll-like receptors (TLR; Kerfoot et al. 2004; Miranda-Hernandez 2011), or have substituted CFA for more defined microbial products, known to stimulate individual (or a more limited set of) TLR (Segal et al. 2000; Visser 2005; Wolf et al. 2007). The rationale for these studies clearly is to identify novel target pathways for therapy. However, although some success has been reported with more limited adjuvants, these have not been adopted widely for EAE induction and data on the susceptibility of individual TLR knockout mice to EAE are often contradictory between investigators.

The dendritic cell (DC), armed with a battery of PRRs and the capacity to greatly increase provision of signals 1–3, is viewed as the key initiating APC for T cell immunity. Experimental manipulation of DC functions is therefore an area of intense interest. The search goes on for a "tolerogenic DC", either naturally occurring, or the result of manipulation in vitro or pharmacological modification in vivo (Steinman et al. 2003). This includes comparative analyses of plasmacytoid DC versus myeloid DC. A series of reports have described successful prevention or amelioration of EAE by targeting DC (Hawiger et al. 2004; Loschko 2011). It must also be noted that other APC can also play key early roles in modulating T cell clonal expansion and function during EAE development, including B cells (see the following text), macrophages and subsets thereof. The fact that different APC populations (B cells vs. DC/macrophages) can show different cytokine responses to the same PAMP (Lampropoulou et al. 2008) is likely to be of importance when considering when and how it might be best to therapeutically intervene in autoimmune disease by targeting signal 0.

Although activated APC provide costimulation to boost T cell responses, they can also keep clonal expansion in check through coinhibition. The classical coinhibitory molecule is CTLA-4 (Lenschow et al. 1996), a homolog of CD28 that also binds to CD80/86. Further control is provided by iPD-1, which binds to PD-L1 and PD-L2 (Francisco et al. 2010). Both CTLA-4 and PD-1 are upregulated on the surface of T cells following TCR stimulation and serve as brakes on clonal expansion and, in the case of PD-1, cytokine production. Manipulations of each of these pathways can modify the development of EAE (Hurwitz et al. 1997; Carter et al. 2007). The components of the initial priming phase of EAE outlined in the previous text can therefore be interrogated to therapeutic effect, limiting either the size of the myelin-responsive T cell cohort generated, or its functional quality.

The experiments that identified EAE as a $CD4^{+}$ T cell- mediated disease used T cell clones cultivated from Lewis rats that had been immunised with myelin basic protein (the host rats were unimmunised, receiving only an infusion of T cells; Ben-Nun 1981). This approach is now widely adopted in mouse passive transfer models, usually with a brief (3–5 days) in vitro TCR stimulation in the presence of a selected cytokine cocktail (Stromnes and Goverman 2006b). These approaches are often used when studying the effects of gene deficiency; i.e., placing gene-deficient T cells into wild-type hosts and vice versa. Given that the donor animals for these experiments are still immunised with autoantigen in CFA, the complex in vivo cellular interactions outlined above can still have a strong bearing on the eventual clinical outcome. This complication can be circumvented using TCR transgenic mice, from which naive T cells can be isolated and TCR stimulated in vitro for the first time in the presence of defined cytokines. However, the net effect of either active or passive EAE is to provide a cohort of autoaggressive T cells in the circulation. Their next task is to enter the CNS.

13.3 Leukocyte Migration—Traversing the Blood–Brain Barrier (BBB)

In order to reach the target organ in EAE and MS, autoreactive T cells must exit lymph nodes and transmigrate across the BBB or blood–CSF barrier into the CNS via the CNS microvasculature. As the CNS is an immunologically specialised site with tight regulation of immune responses relative to other parts of the body, such cellular migration involves highly regulated and complex processes. Studies of EAE have helped to shed light on many molecular aspects of these sequential processes and indeed, greatly supported the development of therapeutic candidates that interfere with T cell migration to the CNS. Such migration is a coordinated process involving expression of chemokines, chemokine receptors, adhesion molecules and factors that increase the permeability of the BBB. The first oral therapy for MS, fingolimod (Gilenya®), targets the first phase of this process. By binding sphingosine-1-phosphate receptors on lymphocytes, fingolimod limits lymphocyte egress from lymph nodes. An earlier therapeutic, natalizumab (Tysabri®) binds to and blocks the $\alpha 4\beta 1$ integrin on the surface of lymphocytes, a molecule that is required for adhesion to endothelial cells to facilitate BBB transmigration. By blocking this interaction, lymphocyte migration into the CNS is inhibited. Both these therapies exemplify how leukocyte migration to the CNS can be inhibited for therapeutic gain and will be discussed in greater detail later.

Activated lymphocytes are recruited from the bloodstream to the CNS via chemokine gradients, however, circulating lymphocytes must first slow down to facilitate chemokine–chemokine receptor interactions. Endothelial cells are critical to this process of drawing lymphocytes from the swift flow of the bloodstream. Upon activation by inflammatory stimuli such as cytokines (e.g., TNF-α), endothelial cells express high levels of cell adhesion molecules such as ICAM-1 and VCAM-1. These cell adhesion molecules bind dimeric molecules of integrin family expressed on lymphocytes such as LFA-1 and VLA-4, thereby drawing them from the rapid flow of the blood stream (reviewed in (Engelhardt 2006)). Arrest and attachment of lymphocytes to the endothelium in the face of the shear forces of blood flow is accomplished by high-avidity binding between these cell adhesion molecule partnerships. Indeed, such may be the avidity of binding that lymphocytes have recently been shown to be capable of crawling against the direction of blood flow at the BBB in EAE (Bartholomaus et al. 2009). However, the type of EAE model used influences the rolling behaviour of such cells as in vitro-activated encephalitogenic T cells can abruptly cross the BBB without the need for rolling (Vajkoczy et al 2001). This is likely due to differential activation status of in vitro and in vivo primed T cells resulting in different patterns of cell adhesion molecule expression.

Adherence of lymphocytes to BBB endothelia facilitates efficient lymphocyte detection of local chemokines, which serves to augment lymphocyte tethering and eventual diapedesis. T cell subsets express distinct chemokine receptors and as such the profile of chemokine production influences the type of T cell population that is recruited at a particular site. For example, Th1 cells predominantly express the chemokine receptors CXCR3 and CCR5, which bind the chemokines CXCL9/CXCL10/CXCL11 and CCL3/CCL4/CCL5, respectively, while Th17 cells express CCR6, which recognises CCL20 (Bromley et al. 2008). In response to adhesion molecule and chemokine signalling, lymphocytes can migrate across endothelia in the CNS tissue either via paracellular or transcellular routes. Paracellular migration of lymphocytes in EAE involves disruption of endothelial tight junctions by dephosphorylation or relocalisation of tight junctional proteins such as ZO-1 and occludin

(Bennett 2010; Morgan et al. 2007). Conversely, in transcellular lymphocyte migration, interendothelial tight junctions remain intact as lymphocytes migrate directly through endothelial cells into the CNS tissue. Transcellular migration appears to be more common at the BBB than at other anatomical sites; such maintenance of BBB tight junction integrity may serve to maximise the highly selective permeability of this important barrier (reviewed in (Engelhardt and Wolburg 2004)). Once through the BBB, myelin-specific lymphocytes orchestrate and potentiate local inflammatory responses as a result of reactivation by local antigen presentation. In EAE, the type and location of inflammatory lesions and immune cell infiltration is heavily influenced by the T lymphocyte phenotype.

13.4 Heterogeneity of Demyelinating Lesions in EAE

In MS, there is considerable lesion heterogeneity (Lucchinetti et al. 1996, 2000) and a criticism of EAE is that such heterogeneity is not a feature of any single model. This is a valid criticism of individual models. However, EAE is now a range of models that collectively recapitulate some of the lesion variability observed in MS such as anatomical distribution, cellular composition and importance of antibody in immunopathogenesis.

Recently, it has emerged that the helper T cell phenotype, or more specifically the ratio of Th1:Th17 cells influences the predominant anatomical site of lesion development. Stromnes et al. (2008) used varying myelin epitopes to generate models of EAE in which lesions occurred in anatomically restricted sites. Myelin oligodendrocyte glycoprotein $(MOG)_{(35-55)}$ and $MOG_{(79-90)}$ induced lesion development in the spinal cord but not in the brain and presented clinically as ascending flaccid paralysis, which is considered "classical/typical" EAE. However, $MOG_{(97-144)}$ induced lesions in the brain rather than spinal cord and presented clinically as "nonclassical/atypical" EAE characterised by ataxia, proprioceptive impairment and hyper-reflexia. Using cytokine-polarised models of adoptively transferred EAE, it was shown that Th1 cells predominantly induce spinal cord lesions and classical EAE while Th17 cells induced inflammation in the brain with relative sparing of the spinal cord, resulting in nonclassical/atypical EAE. Furthermore, it was shown that the ratio of Th17 to Th1 cells was critical to the development of brain lesions. Using the MOG epitopes that induce spinal cord lesions and classical EAE in active immunisation, these investigators showed that brain lesions and nonclassical/atypical EAE could actually be induced with these antigens when the Th17:Th1 ratio was > 1. These studies showed that the balance, rather than the absolute number of Th17 and Th1 cells, influences the site of lesion development in the CNS. Another dichotomous feature of Th1- and Th17-biased EAE models is lesion composition. Lesions in IL-12-driven Th1-biased EAE feature monocyte infiltration and a dominance of activated macrophages. However, lesions in IL-23-driven Th17-biased EAE preferentially show recruitment of neutrophils. In both cases, distinct chemokine expression profiles in lesions accounted for the differential immune cell recruitment (Kroenke et al. 2008).

Recent developments in modelling CNS inflammatory demyelination have expanded the repertoire of EAE to models with strong B cell/autoantibody involvement, an aspect that is a prominent feature of MS lesions but limited in classical murine EAE models induced with short myelin peptides. Krishnamoorthy et al. developed a novel double transgenic mouse model of EAE, which spontaneously developed CNS lesions and clinical disease similar to opticospinal MS (Devic's disease, neuromyelitis optica; Krishnamoorthy et al. 2006). This model features T and B cell autoreactivity to $MOG_{(35-55)}$ and MOG protein, respectively, and lesions consisted mainly of $CD4^{+}$ T cells, macrophages and eosinophils with a low presence of $B220^{+}$ B cells and $CD8^{+}$ T cells (Krishnamoorthy et al. 2006). More recently, Pollinger et al. reported a TCR transgenic mouse model that also exhibits both T and B cell autoreactivity (Pollinger et al. 2009). These mice express a TCR specific for $MOG_{(92-106)}$ and develop spontaneous, relapsing–remitting EAE. Critically, disease did not develop in B cell-depleted mice and autoantibodies generated in this transgenic model potentiate demyelinating episodes. Mice developed inflammatory lesions in several CNS sites such as the spinal cord, cerebellum and optic nerve, which consequentially presented with differing clinical signs as discussed earlier. Lesions mainly consisted of $CD4^{+}$ T cells, B cells and activated macrophages and both demyelination and axonal destruction occurred.

In this very limited set of models discussed, a wide range of heterogeneous aspects of CNS inflammatory demyelination can be investigated, such as multiple anatomical sites of lesions, pathology driven by individual T cell subsets and B cells, effector mechanism of tissue destruction induced by macrophages, neutrophils, eosinophils or $CD8^{+}$ T cells and the role of autoantibodies in potentiating demyelination. Models of EAE in other species and indeed other murine models expand the heterogeneity of lesion development and clinical disease and as such, collectively, represent a valuable research tool for inflammatory demyelinating diseases. Indeed, murine EAE has, in recent years, facilitated major advances in our fundamental knowledge of immunology, particularly $CD4^{+}$ T cell biology and this has, in turn, advanced our understanding of autoimmune mechanisms in CNS inflammatory demyelination. Much of this discovery arose from apparent paradoxical findings in studies investigating the functions and requirement of specific cytokines in murine EAE

13.5 The Effects of Genetic Manipulation on the Development of the Pathogenic T Cell Cohort—Towards a Working Model

Although standard laboratory strains of rat are susceptible to EAE, for many years, the study of murine EAE was confined to the specialist labs that held the "unusual" strains of mice required (SJL, PL/J, B10.PL, Biozzi/ABH). This limited progress into the essential immune genes required for the development of EAE, because gene-deficient mice are routinely generated in the $H\text{-}2^{b}$ strains, C57BL/6 and 129. In 1995, this limitation was removed by the description by Ben-Nun's group of the typical clinical signs of EAE in H-2^b mice that had been immunised with the 35–55 peptide of $MOG_{(35-55)}$ (Mendel et al. 1995). Since then, the increase in reports on EAE sensitivity of gene-deficient mice has been exponential, with often startling results that have forced major revisions of our view of the pathogenic and protective processes that underlie the development and resolution of the disease. The most striking of these revisions involved a sea change in the view of the pathogenic T cell subset from Th1 to Th17. Although this is covered in more details elsewhere (Chaps. 1 and 3), it warrants reiteration here as it leads us to a working model for the generation and evolution of the pathogenic T cell response with implications for therapeutic intervention.

The end-stage cellular agents of EAE pathology (i.e., those cells that directly damage the myelin sheath and kill oligodendrocytes) are activated mononuclear phagocytes; the resident microglia and/or infiltrating inflammatory macrophages. Macrophage depletion experiments performed by Celia Brosnan and Barry Bloom suggested this some three decades ago (Brosnan et al. 1981) and the subsequent work of Christine Dijkstra cemented this view (Huitinga et al. 1990, 1995). IFN-γ is a key cytokine capable of activating macrophages and it therefore made perfect sense for $CD4^+$ T cells of the Th1 type to be the orchestrators of EAE pathology. Indeed, many studies have reported the passive transfer of EAE with Th1-like cells. It therefore came as some surprise when IFN-$\gamma^{-/-}$ and IFN-$\gamma R^{-/-}$ mice were reported to develop EAE of greater severity, rather than to be protected from EAE as was predicted (Willenborg et al. 1996). Despite this, mice lacking the p40 chain of IL-12, or treated with a neutralising anti-p40, were protected from EAE (Segal et al. 1998). The first step in understanding this disconnect between the need for the Th1-promoting IL-12 to drive disease and the need for the Th1 signature cytokine IFN-γ to promote resolution of EAE came from the realisation that p40 is not only a component of IL-12, but also the related cytokine IL-23 (Oppmann et al. 2000). Based on this, a seminal study by Dan Cua performed the necessary comparison of EAE susceptibility in $p40^{-/-}$ mice (lacking both IL-12 and IL-23), $p35^{-/-}$ mice (lacking IL-12, but not IL-23) and $p19^{-/-}$ mice (lacking IL-23, but not IL-12). Resistance to EAE was seen in $p40^{-/-}$ and $p19^{-/-}$, but not in $p35^{-/-}$, leading to the conclusion that it is IL-23 and not IL-12 that is essential for EAE development (Cua et al. 2003). This was supported by similar reports that p35 was dispensable for EAE development (Becher et al. 2002; Gran et al. 2002).

How IL-23 contributes to EAE was not unearthed by that study, and this remains the subject of active investigation (see the following text), but the next advance was to implicate IL-23 in the generation of Th17 cells. Although IL-17 had been reported some years earlier (interestingly, as a cytokine that could be produced by Th1 cells), Cua's group suggested that a separate lineage of $CD4^+$ cells existed that could produce IL-17, but not IFN-γ, under the influence of IL-23 and that such T cells (first termed ThIL-17 cells, later shortened to Th17) were more efficient than Th1 cells at transferring EAE (Langrish et al. 2005). Subsequent work has shown that IL-23 is in fact not the key driver of IL-17 production and Th17 differentiation, this is a function of IL-6-driven, STAT-3-dependent expression of the RORγt transcription factor (Korn et al. 2009). One consequence of this is the de novo expression of IL-23R, which is not expressed on naive $CD4^+$ T cells, and therefore Th17 cells are acutely sensitive to IL-23. This can enhance their ability to produce IL-17, but also has other effects, including improving their capacity for migration into the tissues. Alternative roles for IL-23 shall be revisited later.

So by this stage, the paradigm had switched from EAE being a Th1-mediated disease to a Th17-mediated. This made some sense based on the accumulating data from studies of gene knockout mice using the $MOG_{(35-55)}$. These data had shown that lack of IL-6, ROR-γt and IL-23 all resulted in resistance (Samoilova et al. 1998; Cua et al. 2003; Ivanov et al. 2006). Moreover, neither IFN-γ nor IL-12 (both intimately associated with Th1 responses) were required; in fact disease is exacerbated/nonremitting in the absence of IFN-γ-signalling and, to a lesser extent, when IL-12 is absent (Willenborg et al. 1996; Cua et al. 2003). A simple interpretation of this would be that Th17 differentiation is exaggerated in the absence of IFN-γ or IL-12 (both of which have been shown to inhibit Th17 responses; Korn et al. 2009). This is most likely an oversimplification, however. IFN-γ has complex effects on immune responses, such as boosting T cell sensitivity to apoptotic signals. It should also be noted that $p35^{-/-}$ mice, originally described as specifically lacking IL-12, also lack IL-35. This novel cytokine (a heterodimer of p35 and EBI3) has been implicated in immunosuppressive function of $Foxp3^+$ Treg (Collison et al. 2007). Although a protective role for IL-35 in EAE has yet to be reported, this possibility should be considered when interpreting previous data using $p35^{-/-}$ mice. Another contradiction to the idea that Th17 cells and not Th1 cells were the key mediators of EAE comes from reports that T-bet, the master regulator transcription factor of Th1 cell function, is required for EAE pathology (Bettelli et al. 2004). Furthermore, using passive transfer models, it has been reported that Th17 cells in which T-bet expression is suppressed by RNA interference have an impaired pathogenic function (Yang et al. 2009). T-bet has many genetic targets, but the two most pronounced effects are upregulation of IFN-γ (not required for EAE) and the chemokine receptor CXCR3. Again, a simple explanation for the need for T-bet would be that Th17 cells need to upregulate CXCR3 to enter the CNS. However, CXCR3 expression is generally viewed as a Th1-amplification mechanism, allowing cells to migrate to sites of existing Th1 inflammation. Where would this come from in the CNS of a mouse that received Th17 cell transfer? Moreover, CXCR3 is not absolutely required for EAE development (Liu et al. 2006a; Sporici and Issekutz 2010), and other studies have suggested a (controversial) role for Th17-associated receptor CCR6 in CNS entry via the choroids plexus (Elhofy 2009; Liston et al. 2009; Reboldi et al. 2009).

Therefore, our current knowledge cannot easily explain a requirement for T cell expression of T-bet in the processes that ultimately leads to EAE pathology. However, together with a series of important observations, this demands a reconsideration of the description of EAE as a "Th17-mediated disease". First, highly pure Th1 cells are perfectly capable of transferring aggressive pathology (O'Connor et al. 2008). Second, IL-17 is not required for development of EAE (Haak et al. 2009). Third, many authors favour focusing on the relatively low numbers of $CD4^+$ T cells producing IL-17 in the inflamed CNS (and the effects of experimental manipulation thereof), often choosing to ignore the larger population that produces IFN-γ, rather than IL-17. At this stage, it is also worth noting that the IFN-γ^+ IL-17^+ cells are also seen in the CNS and these have been suggested to be the most potently autoaggressive T cells. Fourth, the most efficient passive EAE models often supplement the in vitro cultures prior to cell transfer with the Th1-driving cytokines IL-12 and IL-18 (O'Connor et al. 2008). We reported that highly pure Th17 cells, generated in vitro from naive myelin basic protein (MBP)-responsive TCR transgenic T cells by exposure to MBP in the presence of TGF-β, IL-6 and IL-23, were only poorly pathogenic in contrast to their Th1 counterparts. This may have been a consequence of the use of suboptimal "Th17 conditions", as a more effective protocol was subsequently reported (Jager et al. 2009). However, using either Th17 protocol, the interesting observation was that, when Th17 cells could transfer disease, those cells showed evidence of a differentiation away from IL-17 production towards IFN-γ production (O'Connor et al. 2008). The idea of Th17→Th1 "transdifferentiation" was subsequently strengthened by reports from in vitro studies and perhaps most clearly shown in a T cell transfer model of autoimmune diabetes (in that model the de novo production of IFN-γ was required for disease development; Bending et al. 2009).

A clearer picture of this process has recently been presented by Gitta Stockinger's group, using an elegant fate-mapping technology in which IL-17 expression renders cells identifiable by flow cytometry (Hirota et al. 2011). The striking observation was that, following immunisation for EAE induction, the majority of T-bet$^+$ and IFN-γ^+ cells had previously expressed IL-17. This was already true in the lymph nodes by the time clinical signs of EAE were evident, but became exaggerated in the inflamed CNS. Therefore, this technology revealed that cells that would have been considered as Th1 cells had passed through a phase of Th17-like activity. What drives this process is not fully clear as yet, but it was not observed in a more acute inflammation driven by infection.

However, neither IL-17 nor IFN-γ is required for EAE (Willenborg 1996, Haak et al. 2009). Are there additional T cell-derived factors that had so far been overlooked and could a key role be identified for IL-23 in driving their production? Mice lacking GM-CSF were shown to be resistant to EAE over a decade ago (McQualter et al. 2001) and it was later shown that CD4$^+$ T cells were the critical cellular source of pathogenic GM-CSF (Ponomarev et al. 2007). Given the importance of inflammatory macrophages to the aetiopathology of EAE and the role of GM-CSF in the mobilisation and recruitment of these cells, this was not a surprising result. Two recent reports, however, have focused on the relative pathogenicity of CD4$^+$ T cell subsets based on their profile of GM-CSF production relative to IFN-γ and IL-17 production. GM-CSF-deficient T cells cannot transfer disease and both Th1 and Th17 cells can produce GM-CSF. Moreover, T cells that produced GM-CSF but not IL-17 or IFN-γ were shown to be highly pathogenic upon transfer, resulting in accelerated onset and increased severity compared to Th1- or Th17-driven EAE (Codarri et al. 2011). Of note, culture conditions that maximised T cell production of GM-CSF at the expense of IFN-γ and IL-17 were found to require IL-23. GM-CSF also appeared to enhance IL-23 production by innate immune cells and this could

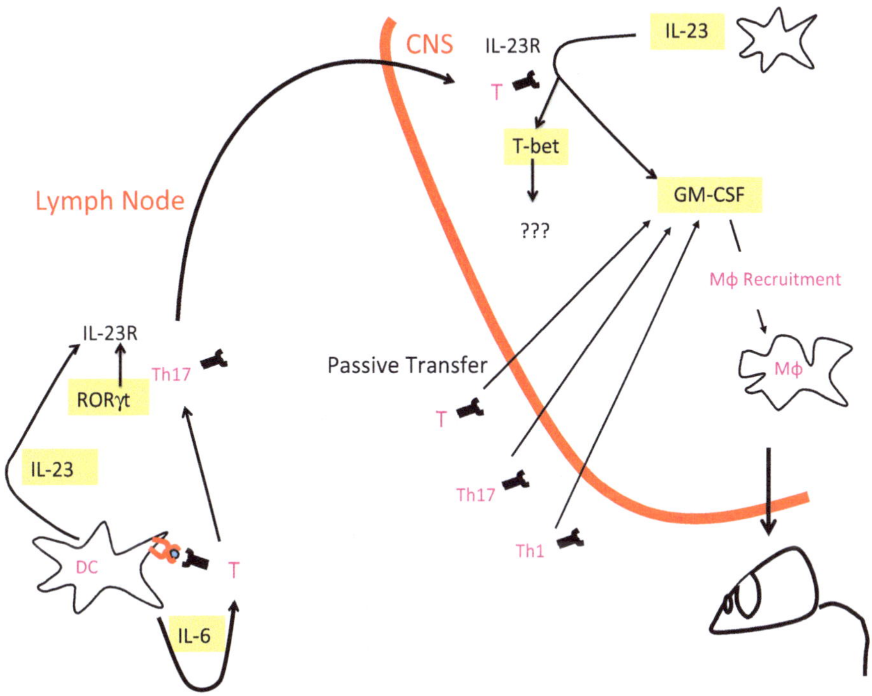

Fig. 13.1 Generating the pathogenic CD4$^+$ T cell population in EAE—a model. Myelin-responsive T cells are initially activated in the lymph nodes draining the site of immunisation. CFA promotes IL-6 production by innate immune cells, driving STAT3-dependent RORγt expression and leading to IL-17 production (not required for EAE) and IL-23R expression (required). T cells begin to lose IL-17 production and gain T-bet expression (required, but function uncertain), leading to expression of IFN-γ (not required) and CXCR3 (not required). Exposure to IL-23 (required) promotes T cell ability to enter the CNS (key molecules uncertain—CCR6?) and to produce GM-CSF (this latter effect may be boosted by further exposure to IL-23 within the CNS). GM-CSF recruits and activates macrophages/microglia to form the EAE lesions. T cells can be deliberately driven to produce high levels of GM-CSF (Codarri et al. 2011). However, Th1 and Th17 cells can also make GM-CSF. This would explain why all three populations have been shown to be encephalitogenic in passive transfer models of EAE

therefore allow a positive feedback mechanism to develop in the inflamed CNS (El-Behi 2011). In contrast, both IFN-γ and IL-12 were found to lower, but not totally ablate GM-CSF production (Codarri et al. 2011). These observations now allow a reconciliation of the data showing that either Th1 or Th17 cells can be pathogenic on transfer, because both these populations can produce GM-CSF and, in the case of Th17 cells, this is greatly enhanced by prolonged exposure to IL-23.

These recent reports now allow us to develop a working model for the progression towards pathogenic T cell function and clinical in EAE following immunisation with myelin autoantigen in CFA as follows (Fig. 13.1):

1. Antigen presentation in the draining lymph nodes triggers naive myelin-responsive T cells.
2. PAMPs present in the CFA drive APC production of IL-6, this drives STAT3-dependent RORγt expression, leading to IL-17 production (not required) and IL-23R expression (required).
3. T cells begin to lose IL-17 production and gain T-bet expression (required, but function uncertain), which drives expression of IFN-γ (not required) and CXCR3 (not required).
4. Exposure to IL-23 (required) promotes T cell ability to enter the CNS (key molecules uncertain—CCR6?) and to produce GM-CSF.
5. GM-CSF draws macrophages into the CNS to establish the inflammatory lesion.

Clearly, there are gaps that need to be filled in this model, for example, the exact role of T-bet and the key molecules required for entry into the CNS. On this latter point, the importance of α4 integrin was described some years ago in EAE, leading to the development of natalizumab/Tysabri, which can be a highly potent treatment for MS. Recent work in EAE has suggested that Th1 cells are more likely to use α4 integrin with Th17 cells more reliant on LFA-1/ICAM1 interactions (Rothhammer et al. 2011).

13.6 T Cell-mediated Regulation of EAE

The evidence for T-cell-mediated immune regulation in EAE stretches back to Swanborg's early work and we have recently reviewed the field from the historical perspective (O'Connor and Anderton 2008). Here, we shall therefore restrict ourselves to discussing some advances in understanding of the immunoregulation of EAE over the past decade.

13.7 Regulation During the Induction Phase of EAE

The key regulatory T cell population essential for immune homeostasis is, of course, the Foxp3^{+} CD4^{+} Treg population (Wing and Sakaguchi 2010). These arise as a fraction of preformed natural (n)Treg during thymic development or can be induced (iTreg) from Foxp3− naive T cell precursors in vivo, or in vitro. As discussed in the following text, there is clear evidence of that Foxp3^{+} Treg accumulate in the inflamed CNS and positively influence in the natural resolution of EAE. However, it seems that the balance between these and the autoaggressive T effector cell population is very precise (Anderton 2010). Thus, if the effector response is too strong, the Treg are unable to resolve the inflammation leading to chronic degenerative disease to which T cells might not be required to contribute (Hoehlig et al. 2012). By extension, the idea that early, and often subtle, alterations in the quality and magnitude of the T effector response can have gross effects on the long-term disease outcome has some credence. Clearly, Treg are present within the lymph nodes during the priming phase of EAE and have the opportunity to limit the size of the encephalitogenic T cell cohort at this point. Indeed, one of the effects of pertussis toxin on the EAE was proposed to be a transient reduction in Treg, thereby enhancing the initial expansion of the pathogenic T cell cohort (Cassan et al. 2006). Furthermore, deliberate depletion of Treg before EAE induction causes severe/nonresolving disease (McGeachy et al. 2005). There is evidence that autoantigen-responsive Treg are activated in the lymph node, although a little later than their pathogenic counterparts (Korn et al. 2007). Treg are not the only cells able to influence the early expansion of the pathogenic T cell population. B cells will be discussed in the following text and in more detail elsewhere (Chap. 5), as are NKT cells and mucosal-associated invariant T cells (Chap. 6).

13.8 Therapeutic Use of Foxp3$^+$ Treg in EAE

Early experiments transferring very high numbers of Treg (sorted as CD4$^+$ CD25$^+$ cells) from naive donors into host mice immediately prior to immunisation showed some protection against EAE, but not if the donor Treg were from IL-10−/− mice (Zhang et al. 2004). A series of studies have compared the transfer of polyclonal Treg with myelin antigen-responsive Treg (either nTreg or iTreg derived from TCR transgenic mice) and have found that the latter are far more potent on a per cell basis (Selvaraj and Geiger 2008; Stephens et al. 2009; O'Connor et al. 2010). Although there is evidence that myelin-responsive Treg can "cure" ongoing EAE (Stephens et al. 2009), the relative difficulty in tracking these cells after transfer makes it uncertain that they are acting to directly suppress inflammation in the CNS, rather than having an (undefined) effect in the periphery that promotes resolution. Many recent studies using existing drugs or novel therapeutic compounds have associated positive effects on EAE with a shift in the Treg/T effector cell balance towards the Treg.

13.9 Treg in the CNS During the Natural Resolution of Acute EAE

Treg are essentially absent from the CNS of healthy mice and appear at only very low frequencies during the first phases of clinical EAE. There is then a rapid accumulation of highly activated and suppressive Treg specifically within the CNS (not mirrored in the peripheral lymphoid organs), which correlates with entry into the resolution phase (McGeachy et al. 2005, O'Connor et al. 2007). Mice depleted of Treg do not recover (McGeachy et al. 2005), indicating an obligate role for Treg in the resolution process. TGF-β, the key cytokine required to drive Foxp3 expression in naive T cells to generate iTreg, is available in the CNS and one study suggested that effector T cells could differentiate into iTreg in the CNS (Liu et al. 2006b). However, no other study has provided any evidence for such a process. Rather, the Foxp3$^+$ cells that accumulate in the CNS appear to be from a pre-existing nTreg pool, based on differential cell transfer studies and epigenetic analysis (Korn et al. 2007; O'Connor et al. 2012).

Whether CNS Treg are truly suppressive has been questioned, with the suggestion that the pro-inflammatory environment within the CNS during EAE (notably, high levels of IL-6 and TNF-α) can abrogate their suppressive function (Korn et al. 2007). However, Treg from the inflamed CNS are highly capable of suppressing pro-inflammatory cytokine production by CNS T-effector cells in vitro, a suppressive function that "resting" Treg, taken from healthy mice, are not able to perform (McGeachy et al. 2005; O'Connor et al. 2007). A further complicating issue is the idea that Foxp3$^+$ Treg can be prompted to transdifferentiate in vitro, losing Foxp3 expression and gaining the ability to produce pro-inflammatory cytokines. This is particularly notable in the presence of IL-6 when splenic nTreg from healthy mice can develop the ability to produce IL-17, analogous to that seen with Th17 development from naive Foxp3$-$ T cells. The use of Foxp3 reporter mice allowed the isolation of highly pure Foxp3$^+$ and Foxp3$-$ CD4$^+$ populations from the CNS during EAE. TCR stimulation revealed that while Foxp3$-$ cells could produce a range of pro-inflammatory cytokines, Foxp3$^+$ cells could not (but could produce IL-10). Moreover, when exposed to IL-6 in vitro, CNS Treg did not switch on production of IL-17 (O'Connor et al. 2012). The IL-6 receptor is a heterodimer of the IL-6Rα chain (CD126) and the gp130 chain, which is responsible for STAT3- phosphorylation and intracellular signalling. While naive T cells expressed both CD126 and gp130, all CNS CD4$^+$ T cells were found to have lost expression of CD126 and gp130 (O'Connor et al. 2012). This therefore explained why CNS Treg could not be driven to produce IL-17 by exposure to IL-6. Thus, despite being in a highly inflammatory environment, CNS Treg seem to be locked in suppressive mode and do not deviate towards a pathogenic function. This is, of course, desirable. Furthermore, Foxp3$-$ cells were also insensitive to IL-6. Whether this process was involved in their relative loss of IL-17 production is unknown, but it is likely that IL-17 production could be maintained on T effector cells in the CNS by their sustained expression of the IL-23R (which is not expressed by Treg). The lack of sensitivity to IL-6 in CNS T cells makes it difficult to see how the previously proposed role of IL-6 in preventing CNS Treg from functioning could actually work at the T cell level (Korn et al. 2007). Of note, however, innate immune cells in the CNS do maintain IL-6 receptors, so it remains possible that IL-6 might exert effects via these cells.

The above observations on IL-6 receptor expression fit well with data from previous studies using antibody blockade of IL-6 signalling in EAE. These showed that blockade was highly effective at preventing EAE when given for the first week after immunisation (i.e., when T cells express IL-6 receptors) but did not modulate ongoing EAE (when CNS T cells have lost their IL-6-sensitivity; Serada et al. 2008). These blocking data would therefore also suggest no major role for IL-6 signalling in CNS innate immune cells. Taken together, the key time for IL-6 to impact on EAE seems to be at the initial point of T cell differentiation after immunisation. Although one study has concluded that the major effect of IL-6 at this point is to ensure generation of autoantigen-responsive Th17 cells (rather than autoantigen-responsive iTreg; Korn et al. 2008), IL-6 would also be needed to drive IL-23R and maximise

GM-CSF production (Fig. 13.1). Despite these recent advances in understanding the functional stability of CNS Treg, the key question—precisely how do CNS Treg actually lead to the resolution of EAE—remains unanswered.

13.10 B Cells As a Source of Cytokines Modulating CNS Autoaggression

B cells can produce autoantibodies and despite the inability to transfer EAE with serum or purified autoantibodies alone, such transfer can exaggerate pathology primarily driven by $CD4^{+}$ T cells, particularly when using demyelinating antibodies directed against MOG (Linington et al. 1988). However, B cells can also influence pathology in other ways (Berer et al. 2011), notably by acting as APC (Weber et al. 2010) and by being a major source of cytokines, which can modulate the T cell response. B cell-deficient mice are not protected from EAE. In fact, these mice show an exacerbated, non-remitting clinical profile (Wolf 1996; Fillatreau et al. 2002). Development of a novel bone marrow chimeric technology that allows restriction of gene deficiency to only the B cell compartment identified that to allow the natural resolution of EAE B cells needed to produce IL-10 (Fillatreau et al. 2002). To identify the time at which B cells were required, Tedder's group administered B cell-depleting antibodies at different stages of the disease (Matsushita et al. 2008). Consistent with the studies in B cell-deficient mice, B cell depletion at an early time point led to non-remitting disease. In contrast, depleting B cells once disease was established did not exaggerate the disease, but instead accelerated resolution. More recent data have indicated that in addition to producing IL-10, B cells can also be an important source of IL-6 (Lampropoulou et al. 2008). They are not an essential source because mice in which only B cells cannot make IL-6 do still develop EAE, but the disease is less severe in these mice (Barr et al. 2012). In addition, the late-stage depletion of B cells does not accelerate recovery in these mice. B cell depletion has proved remarkably successful as a therapy in some MS patients. B cells from MS patients showed elevated IL-6 production compared to healthy controls and this difference was removed in patients whose B cell population had recovered, post-depletion (Barr et al. 2012). This ability of B cells to contribute an inflammatory cytokine may therefore go some way to explain the paradoxical observation that B cell depletion can be clinically effective without significant loss of autoantibody titres (Hauser et al. 2008). The full scope of pro-inflammatory cytokines that might be produced by B cells in a range of inflammatory contexts therefore warrants investigation. An obvious contradiction in the B cell IL-6 story is that, as described in the previous text, T cells in the CNS are insensitive to IL-6 and IL-6 blockade does not modulate ongoing disease. Therefore, this also requires further investigation.

13.11 B Cells and Treg—Working in Series or in Parallel?

Mice can therefore show exacerbated, non-remitting pathology in the absence of either Treg, or IL-10-producing B cells (McGeachy et al. 2005; Fillatreau et al. 2002). This begs the question, do these two immune populations interact to deliver a coordinated regulatory function? B cell-deficient mice do show a reduced frequency of Foxp3$^+$ cells in their peripheral CD4$^+$ T cell compartment (Hoehlig et al. 2012). Moreover, mice transgenic for B cell activation factor of the TNF family (BAFF) show an elevated Treg frequency, a phenomenon that was reported to be dependent on the presence of B cells, rather than BAFF acting directly on the Treg population (Walters et al. 2009). However, there is no reduction in the ability of Treg to accumulate within the CNS in B cell-deficient mice (Hoehlig et al. 2012). Dittel's group has reported that B cells do play a role in the expansion/maintenance of the Treg population through expression of B7 (Mann et al. 2007) and, more recently, GITR (Ray et al. 2012). However, this idea contrasts with studies from the groups of Tedder and Fillatreau, which both concluded that there was a requirement for B cells and Treg in controlling EAE, but that these were essentially separable (Hoehlig et al. 2012; Matsushita et al. 2010). B cell-derived IL-10 was required at an early stage, to limit the initial expansion of pathogenic T cells, whereas Treg function in the CNS was important later, to drive the resolution of inflammation in the target organ. These insights provide impetus for the design of new therapeutic options to boost the immunoregulatory function of these two independent, but apparently synergistic, lymphocyte populations.

13.12 Development and Mechanistic Investigation of MS Therapies in EAE Models

EAE has been used to test the therapeutic efficacy of a wide range of agents over several decades. A criticism frequently levelled against the use of EAE in MS research is that the vast majority of agents that have successfully ameliorated EAE have failed to translate to the clinic (Sriram and Steiner 2005). However, it is important to note that most of the current pharmacologic/biologic therapies for MS were either developed, or have since been shown to be effective, in EAE. Steroids have been used for several decades to treat exacerbations of MS (Durelli et al. 1986), a therapeutic approach that is also effective in EAE. Indeed, subsequent studies of steroid administration in EAE models have contributed to our understanding of mechanisms of action of steroids in inflammatory disease (Schmidt et al. 2000; Chen et al. 2006; Donia et al. 2010). Mitoxantrone is used as a second-line therapy for aggressive MS and has also demonstrated efficacy in EAE (Ridge et al. 1985).

In 1993, Interferon-β (IFN-β) became the first approved drug specifically indicated for MS (Connelly 1994), however, at that time, its mechanism of action was poorly understood. IFN-β has since been shown to suppress EAE in a number of models and associated mechanisms including inhibition of pro-inflammatory cytokines such as

IL-6, IL-17 and IL-18 as well as upregulation of anti-inflammatory cytokines such as IL-10, IL-4, TGF-β and IL-27 (Yasuda et al. 1999; Guo et al. 2008; Galligan et al. 2010; Sweeney et al. 2011). IFN-β has also been shown to inhibit effector T cell proliferation in EAE as well as the function of APC (Galligan et al. 2010; Prinz et al. 2008). Recent studies have demonstrated a dichotomy in the types of EAE that are responsive to IFN-β therapy. Axtell and colleagues identified a protective effect of IFN-β in EAE that was driven by Th1-biased immunopathology while Th17-biased EAE was exacerbated by IFN-β (Axtell et al. 2010). In 2012, Inoue showed that only EAE that is induced via the NLRP3 inflammasome is sensitive to IFN-β therapy (Inoue et al. 2012). These EAE studies may inform some of the reasons that only a subset of MS patients respond to IFN-β clinically and aid patient stratification for strategic therapeutic decision making.

EAE has also been used to identify agents to take forward to clinical trials for MS. In 1996, Glatiramer acetate (GA) became the second type of therapeutic agent that was approved for MS treatment. This compound consists of a polymer of amino acids found in MBP and was originally developed to induce EAE. However, GA was found to potently suppress EAE and was taken through to clinical trials for MS. Its mechanisms of action are not completely understood but shifts in $CD4^+$ T cell polarisation from pathogenic Th1/Th17 phenotypes towards immunoregulatory Th2/Th3/Treg responses have been shown (Aharoni et al. 1997, 2008; Begum-Haque et al. 2008). Effects of GA on APC have also been reported and it had been suggested that binding of MHC II on APC by GA inhibits the orchestration of pathogenic effector T cells' responses. Modulation of cytokine production by GA-treated APC, such as increased IL-10 and TGF-β and decreased IL-12p70 has also been proposed to mediate its suppressive effect on autoimmune inflammation (Jung et al. 2004; Weber et al. 2007).

Natalizumab represents another MS therapy that was developed using EAE models. Natalizumab is a monoclonal antibody that binds α4β1 integrin on the surface of lymphocytes, thereby inhibiting adhesion to endothelial cells via VCAM-1 (Rice et al. 2005). By inhibiting this interaction, transmigration of T lymphocytes across the BBB is blocked, which effectively inhibits the development of inflammatory lesions in the CNS resulting in a reduction in relapse rate by approximately two-thirds. The use of natalizumab clinically is hampered by the risk of the development of JC virus- induced Progressive Multifocal Leukoencephalopathy, a potentially fatal CNS infection (Vermersch et al. 2011). Notwithstanding this limitation, the concept of blocking migration of inflammatory T cells across the BBB into the CNS was a paradigm that could readily be tested and demonstrated potent efficacy in EAE models (Yednock et al. 1992).

The most recently approved and first-in-class oral therapy for MS, Fingolimod, was initially developed for its immunomodulatory effects in transplantation. However, in a rat model of acute EAE, Fujino et al. demonstrated potent suppression of clinical EAE when fingolimod was administered from the time of immunisation (Fujino et al. 2003). Webb et al. went on to test fingolimod in the SJL models of relapsing–remitting EAE and observed potent suppression of clinical disease when administered after disease onset (Webb et al. 2004), a critical aspect for translational consideration. As fingolimod binds sphingosine-1-phosphate receptors in vivo, it inhibits lymphocyte egress from lymph nodes, which is thought to be the primary mechanism of action of this drug. However, studies in EAE have also pointed towards previously unappreciated additional functions of fingolimod such as neuroprotection (Rossi et al. 2012) and other in vitro and in vivo models have provided evidence of a beneficial effect of fingolimod in oligodendrocyte lineage cell protection and possibly CNS remyelination although this is currently contentious (Miron et al. 2010; Kim et al. 2011; Hu et al. 2011).

Despite the criticism of the low translational rate of therapeutically effective agents in EAE to the clinic (Sriram and Steiner 2005), it is important to bear in mind that all seven FDA-approved treatments for MS (three variants of IFN-β, GA, mitoxantrone, natalizumab and fingolimod) have been shown to effectively suppress clinical disease in EAE models. Translation of therapeutic successes in EAE models can be impeded by the relative cost of human clinical trials, particularly when one considers the complexities of decisions regarding stages of interventions, dosing and testing new candidate drugs in add-on trials, given the ethical implications of access to approved treatments. Such variables are easily tested in the EAE models at a fraction of the cost and mechanistic and pathological insight can be gained to a level of detail not currently possibly in human studies. The most crucial aspect that will ensure appropriate use of this range of models to develop future therapies for MS is the continual refinement and characterisation of these models such that researchers can select the model and mode of treatment most suitable to the question being asked. With this approach, inherent limitations of the model can be accounted for such that overinterpretation of findings is minimised.

References

Aharoni R, Teitelbaum D, Sela M, Arnon R (1997) Copolymer 1 induces T cells of the T helper type 2 that crossreact with myelin basic protein and suppress experimental autoimmune encephalomyelitis. Proc Natl Acad Sci USA 94:10821–10826

Aharoni R, Herschkovitz A, Eilam R, Blumberg-Hazan M, Sela M, Bruck W, Arnon R (2008) Demyelination arrest and remyelination induced by glatiramer acetate treatment of experimental autoimmune encephalomyelitis. Proc Natl Acad Sci USA 105:11358–11363

Anderton SM (2010) Treg and T-effector cells in autoimmune CNS inflammation: a delicate balance, easily disturbed. Eur J Immunol 40:3321–3324

Armstrong RC, Le TQ, Flint NC, Vana AC, Zhou YX (2006) Endogenous cell repair of chronic demyelination. J Neuropathol Exp Neurol 65:245–256

Axtell RC, Jong BA de, Boniface K, Voort LF van der, Bhat R, De Sarno P, Naves R, Han M, Zhong F, Castellanos JG, Mair R, Christakos A, Kolkowitz I, Katz L, Killestein J, Polman CH, Waal Malefyt R de, Steinman L, Raman C (2010) T helper type 1 and 17 cells determine efficacy of interferon-beta in multiple sclerosis and experimental encephalomyelitis. Nat Med 16:406–412

Barr TA, Shen P, Brown S, Lampropoulou V, Roch T, Lawrie S, Fan B, O'Connor RA, Anderton SM, Bar-Or A, Fillatreau S, Gray D (2012) B cell depletion therapy ameliorates autoimmune disease through ablation of IL-6-producing B cells. J Exp Med 209:1001–1010

Bartholomaus I, Kawakami N, Odoardi F, Schlager C, Miljkovic D, Ellwart JW, Klinkert WE, Flugel-Koch C, Issekutz TB, Wekerle H, Flugel A (2009) Effector T cell interactions with meningeal vascular structures in nascent autoimmune CNS lesions. Nature 462:94–98

Becher B, Durell BG, Noelle RJ (2002) Experimental autoimmune encephalitis and inflammation in the absence of interleukin-12. J Clin Invest 110:493–497
Begum-Haque S, Sharma A, Kasper IR, Foureau DM, Mielcarz DW, Haque A, Kasper LH (2008) Downregulation of IL-17 and IL-6 in the central nervous system by glatiramer acetate in experimental autoimmune encephalomyelitis. J Neuroimmunol 204:58–65
Ben-Nun A, Wekerle H, Cohen IR (1981) The rapid isolation of clonable antigen-specific T lymphocyte lines capable of mediating autoimmune encephalomyelitis. Eur J Immunol 11:195–199
Bender SJ, Weiss SR (2010) Pathogenesis of murine coronavirus in the central nervous system. J Neuroimmune Pharmacol 5:336–354
Bending D, De la Pena H, Veldhoen M, Phillips JM, Uyttenhove C, Stockinger B, Cooke A (2009) Highly purified Th17 cells from BDC2.5NOD mice convert into Th1-like cells in NOD/SCID recipient mice. J Clin Invest 119:565–572
Bennett J, Basivireddy J, Kollar A, Biron KE, Reickmann P, Jefferies WA, McQuaid S (2010) Blood-brain barrier disruption and enhanced vascular permeability in the multiple sclerosis model EAE. J Neuroimmunol 229:180–191
Berer K, Wekerle H, Krishnamoorthy G (2011) B cells in spontaneous autoimmune diseases of the central nervous system. Mol Immunol 48:1332–1337
Bettelli E, Sullivan B, Szabo SJ, Sobel RA, Glimcher LH, Kuchroo VK (2004) Loss of T-bet, but not STAT1, prevents the development of experimental autoimmune encephalomyelitis. J Exp Med 200:79–87
Blakemore WF, Franklin RJ (2008) Remyelination in experimental models of toxin-induced demyelination. Curr Top Microbiol Immunol 318:193–212
Bromley SK, Mempel TR, Luster AD (2008) Orchestrating the orchestrators: chemokines in control of T cell traffic. Nat Immunol 9:970–980
Brosnan CF, Bornstein MB, Bloom BR (1981) The effects of macrophage depletion on the clinical and pathologic expression of experimental allergic encephalomyelitis. J Immunol 126:614–620
Carlton WW (1966) Response of mice to the chelating agents sodium diethyldithiocarbamate, alpha-benzoinoxime, and biscyclohexanone oxaldihydrazone. Toxicol Appl Pharmacol 8:512–521
Carlton WW (1967) Studies on the induction of hydrocephalus and spongy degeneration by cuprizone feeding and attempts to antidote the toxicity. Life Sci 6:11–19
Carter LL, Leach MW, Azoitei ML, Cui J, Pelker JW, Jussif J, Benoit S, Ireland G, Luxenberg D, Askew GR, Milarski KL, Groves C, Brown T, Carito BA, Percival K, Carreno BM, Collins M, Marusic S (2007) PD-1/PD-L1, but not PD-1/PD-L2, interactions regulate the severity of experimental autoimmune encephalomyelitis. J Neuroimmunol 182:124–134
Cassan C, Piaggio E, Zappulla JP, Mars LT, Couturier N, Bucciarelli F, Desbois S, Bauer J, Gonzalez-Dunia D, Liblau RS (2006) Pertussis toxin reduces the number of splenic Foxp3+ regulatory T cells. J Immunol 177:1552–1560
Chen X, Oppenheim JJ, Winkler-Pickett RT, Ortaldo JR, Howard OM (2006) Glucocorticoid amplifies IL-2-dependent expansion of functional FoxP3(+)CD4(+)CD25(+) T regulatory cells in vivo and enhances their capacity to suppress EAE. Eur J Immunol 36:2139–2149
Codarri L, Gyulveszi G, Tosevski V, Hesske L, Fontana A, Magnenat L, Suter T, Becher B (2011) RORgammat drives production of the cytokine GM-CSF in helper T cells, which is essential for the effector phase of autoimmune neuroinflammation. Nat Immunol 12:560–567
Collison LW, Workman CJ, Kuo TT, Boyd K, Wang Y, Vignali KM, Cross R, Sehy D, Blumberg RS, Vignali DA (2007) The inhibitory cytokine IL-35 contributes to regulatory T-cell function. Nature 450:566–569
Connelly JF (1994) Interferon beta for multiple sclerosis. Ann Pharmacother 28:610–616
Croxford JL, Olson JK, Miller SD (2002) Epitope spreading and molecular mimicry as triggers of autoimmunity in the Theiler's virus-induced demyelinating disease model of multiple sclerosis. Autoimmun Rev 1:251–260
Cua DJ, Sherlock J, Chen Y, Murphy CA, Joyce B, Seymour B, Lucian L, To W, Kwan S, Churakova T, Zurawski S, Wiekowski M, Lira SA, Gorman D, Kastelein RA, Sedgwick JD (2003) Interleukin-23 rather than interleukin-12 is the critical cytokine for autoimmune inflammation of the brain. Nature 421:744–748
Das SJ, Fu L, Tsai JC, Weiss SR, Lavi E (2000) Demyelination determinants map to the spike glycoprotein gene of coronavirus mouse hepatitis virus. J Virol 74:9206–9213

Donia M, Mangano K, Quattrocchi C, Fagone P, Signorelli S, Magro G, Sfacteria A, Bendtzen K, Nicoletti F (2010) Specific and strain-independent effects of dexamethasone in the prevention and treatment of experimental autoimmune encephalomyelitis in rodents. Scand J Immunol 72:396–407

Durelli L, Cocito D, Riccio A, Barile C, Bergamasco B, Baggio GF, Perla F, Delsedime M, Gusmaroli G, Bergamini L (1986) High-dose intravenous methylprednisolone in the treatment of multiple sclerosis: clinical-immunologic correlations. Neurology 36:238–243

El-Behi M, Ciric B, Dai H, Yan Y, Cullimore M, Safavi F, Zhang GX, Dittel BN, Rostami A (2011) The encephalitogenicity of T(H)17 cells is dependent on IL-1- and IL-23-induced production of the cytokine GM-CSF. Nat Immunol 12:568–575

Elhofy A, Depaolo RW, Lira SA, Lukacs NW, Karpus WJ (2009) Mice deficient for CCR6 fail to control chronic experimental autoimmune encephalomyelitis. J Neuroimmunol 213:91–99

Engelhardt B, Wolburg H (2004) Mini-review: Transendothelial migration of leukocytes: through the front door or around the side of the house? Eur J Immunol 34:2955–2963

Engelhardt B (2006) Molecular mechanisms involved in T cell migration across the blood-brain barrier. J Neural Transm 113:477–485

Ercolini AM, Miller SD (2006) Mechanisms of immunopathology in murine models of central nervous system demyelinating disease. J Immunol 176:3293–3298

Fazakerley JK (2004) Semliki forest virus infection of laboratory mice: a model to study the pathogenesis of viral encephalitis. Arch Virol Suppl:179–190

Fillatreau S, Sweenie CH, McGeachy MJ, Gray D, Anderton SM (2002) B cells regulate autoimmunity by provision of IL-10. Nat Immunol 3:944–950

Francisco LM, Sage PT, Sharpe AH (2010) The PD-1 pathway in tolerance and autoimmunity. Immunol Rev 236:219–242

Fujino M, Funeshima N, Kitazawa Y, Kimura H, Amemiya H, Suzuki S, Li XK (2003) Amelioration of experimental autoimmune encephalomyelitis in Lewis rats by FTY720 treatment. J Pharmacol Exp Ther 305:70–77

Galligan CL, Pennell LM, Murooka TT, Baig E, Majchrzak-Kita B, Rahbar R, Fish EN (2010) Interferon-beta is a key regulator of proinflammatory events in experimental autoimmune encephalomyelitis. Mult Scler 16:1458–1473

Gran B, Zhang GX, Yu S, Li J, Chen XH, Ventura ES, Kamoun M, Rostami A (2002) IL-12p35-deficient mice are susceptible to experimental autoimmune encephalomyelitis: evidence for redundancy in the IL-12 system in the induction of central nervous system autoimmune demyelination. J Immunol 169:7104–7110

Grewal IS, Foellmer HG, Grewal KD, Xu J, Hardardottir F, Baron JL, Janeway CA Jr, Flavell RA (1996) Requirement for CD40 ligand in costimulation induction, T cell activation, and experimental allergic encephalomyelitis. Science 273:1864–1867

Guo B, Chang EY, Cheng G (2008) The type I IFN induction pathway constrains Th17-mediated autoimmune inflammation in mice. J Clin Invest 118:1680–1690

Haak S, Croxford AL, Kreymborg K, Heppner FL, Pouly S, Becher B, Waisman A (2009) IL-17 A and IL-17 F do not contribute vitally to autoimmune neuro-inflammation in mice. J Clin Invest 119:61–69

Hauser SL, Waubant E, Arnold DL, Vollmer T, Antel J, Fox RJ, Bar-Or A, Panzara M, Sarkar N, Agarwal S, Langer-Gould A, Smith CH (2008) B-cell depletion with rituximab in relapsing-remitting multiple sclerosis. N Engl J Med 358:676–688

Hawiger D, Masilamani RF, Bettelli E, Kuchroo VK, Nussenzweig MC (2004) Immunological unresponsiveness characterized by increased expression of CD5 on peripheral T cells induced by dendritic cells in vivo. Immunity 20:695–705

Hirota K, Duarte JH, Veldhoen M, Hornsby E, Li Y, Cua DJ, Ahlfors H, Wilhelm C, Tolaini M, Menzel U, Garefalaki A, Potocnik AJ, Stockinger B (2011) Fate mapping of IL-17-producing T cells in inflammatory responses. Nat Immunol 12:255–263

Hoehlig K, Shen P, Lampropoulou V, Roch T, Malissen B, O'Connor R, Ries S, Hilgenberg E, Anderton SM, Fillatreau S (2012) Activation of CD4(+) Foxp3(+) regulatory T cells proceeds normally in the absence of B cells during EAE. Eur J Immunol 42:1164–1173

Hoffmann K, Lindner M, Groticke I, Stangel M, Loscher W (2008) Epileptic seizures and hippocampal damage after cuprizone-induced demyelination in C57BL/6 mice. Exp Neurol 210:308–321

Hu Y, Lee X, Ji B, Guckian K, Apicco D, Pepinsky RB, Miller RH, Mi S (2011) Sphingosine 1-phosphate receptor modulator fingolimod (FTY720) does not promote remyelination in vivo. Mol Cell Neurosci 48:72–81

Huitinga I, Rooijen N van, Groot CJ de, Uitdehaag BM, Dijkstra CD (1990) Suppression of experimental allergic encephalomyelitis in Lewis rats after elimination of macrophages. J Exp Med 172:1025–1033

Huitinga I, Ruuls SR, Jung S, Van Rooijen N, Hartung HP, Dijkstra CD (1995) Macrophages in T cell line-mediated, demyelinating, and chronic relapsing experimental autoimmune encephalomyelitis in Lewis rats. Clin Exp Immunol 100:344–351

Hurwitz AA, Sullivan TJ, Krummel MF, Sobel RA, Allison JP (1997) Specific blockade of CTLA-4/B7 interactions results in exacerbated clinical and histologic disease in an actively-induced model of experimental allergic encephalomyelitis. J Neuroimmunol 73:57–62

Inoue M, Williams KL, Oliver T, Vandenabeele P, Rajan JV, Miao EA, Shinohara ML (2012) Interferon-beta therapy against EAE Is effective only when development of the disease depends on the NLRP3 inflammasome. Sci Signal 5:ra38

Ivanov II, McKenzie BS, Zhou L, Tadokoro CE, Lepelley A, Lafaille JJ, Cua DJ, Littman DR (2006) The orphan nuclear receptor RORgammat directs the differentiation program of proinflammatory IL-17 + T helper cells. Cell 126:1121–1133

Jager A, Dardalhon V, Sobel RA, Bettelli E, Kuchroo VK (2009) Th1, Th17, and Th9 effector cells induce experimental autoimmune encephalomyelitis with different pathological phenotypes. J Immunol 183:7169–7177

Jung S, Siglienti I, Grauer O, Magnus T, Scarlato G, Toyka K (2004) Induction of IL-10 in rat peritoneal macrophages and dendritic cells by glatiramer acetate. J Neuroimmunol 148:63–73

Kerfoot SM, Long EM, Hickey MJ, Andonegui G, Lapointe BM, Zanardo RC, Bonder C, James WG, Robbins SM, Kubes P (2004) TLR4 contributes to disease-inducing mechanisms resulting in central nervous system autoimmune disease. J Immunol 173:7070–7077

Kim HJ, Miron VE, Dukala D, Proia RL, Ludwin SK, Traka M, Antel JP, Soliven B (2011) Neurobiological effects of sphingosine 1-phosphate receptor modulation in the cuprizone model. FASEB J 25:1509–1518

Kipp M, Clarner T, Dang J, Copray S, Beyer C (2009) The cuprizone animal model: new insights into an old story. Acta Neuropathol 118:723–736

Korn T, Reddy J, Gao W, Bettelli E, Awasthi A, Petersen TR, Backstrom BT, Sobel RA, Wucherpfennig KW, Strom TB, Oukka M, Kuchroo VK (2007) Myelin-specific regulatory T cells accumulate in the CNS but fail to control autoimmune inflammation. Nat Med 13:423–431

Korn T, Mitsdoerffer M, Croxford AL, Awasthi A, Dardalhon VA, Galileos G, Vollmar P, Stritesky GL, Kaplan MH, Waisman A, Kuchroo VK, Oukka M (2008) IL-6 controls Th17 immunity in vivo by inhibiting the conversion of conventional T cells into Foxp3 + regulatory T cells. Proc Natl Acad Sci U S A 105:18460–18465

Korn T, Bettelli E, Oukka M, Kuchroo VK (2009) IL-17 and Th17 Cells. Annu Rev Immunol 27:485–517

Kotter MR, Setzu A, Sim FJ, Van Rooijen N, Franklin RJ (2001) Macrophage depletion impairs oligodendrocyte remyelination following lysolecithin-induced demyelination. Glia 35:204–212

Krishnamoorthy G, Lassmann H, Wekerle H, Holz A (2006) Spontaneous opticospinal encephalomyelitis in a double-transgenic mouse model of autoimmune T cell/B cell cooperation. J Clin Invest 116:2385–2392

Kroenke MA, Carlson TJ, Andjelkovic AV, Segal BM (2008) IL-12- and IL-23-modulated T cells induce distinct types of EAE based on histology, CNS chemokine profile, and response to cytokine inhibition. J Exp Med 205:1535–1541

Lampropoulou V, Hoehlig K, Roch T, Neves P, Calderon GE, Sweenie CH, Hao Y, Freitas AA, Steinhoff U, Anderton SM, Fillatreau S (2008) TLR-activated B cells suppress T cell-mediated autoimmunity. J Immunol 180:4763–4773

Langrish CL, Chen Y, Blumenschein WM, Mattson J, Basham B, Sedgwick JD, McClanahan T, Kastelein RA, Cua DJ (2005) IL-23 drives a pathogenic T cell population that induces autoimmune inflammation. J Exp Med 201:233–240

Lenschow DJ, Walunas TL, Bluestone JA (1996) CD28/B7 system of T cell costimulation. Annu Rev of Immunol 14:233–258
Li WW, Setzu A, Zhao C, Franklin RJ (2005) Minocycline-mediated inhibition of microglia activation impairs oligodendrocyte progenitor cell responses and remyelination in a non-immune model of demyelination. J Neuroimmunol 158:58–66
Lindner M, Heine S, Haastert K, Garde N, Fokuhl J, Linsmeier F, Grothe C, Baumgartner W, Stangel M (2008) Sequential myelin protein expression during remyelination reveals fast and efficient repair after central nervous system demyelination. Neuropathol Appl Neurobiol 34:105–114
Linington C, Bradl M, Lassmann H, Brunner C, Vass K (1988) Augmentation of demyelination in rat acute allergic encephalomyelitis by circulating mouse monoclonal antibodies directed against a myelin/oligodendrocyte glycoprotein. Am J Pathol 130:443–454
Liston A, Kohler RE, Townley S, Haylock-Jacobs S, Comerford I, Caon AC, Webster J, Harrison JM, Swann J, Clark-Lewis I, Korner H, McColl SR (2009) Inhibition of CCR6 function reduces the severity of experimental autoimmune encephalomyelitis via effects on the priming phase of the immune response. J Immunol 182:3121–3130
Liu L, Huang D, Matsui M, He TT, Hu T, Demartino J, Lu B, Gerard C, Ransohoff RM (2006a) Severe disease, unaltered leukocyte migration, and reduced IFN-gamma production in CXCR3 –/– mice with experimental autoimmune encephalomyelitis. J Immunol 176:4399–4409
Liu Y, Teige I, Birnir B, Issazadeh-Navikas S (2006b) Neuron-mediated generation of regulatory T cells from encephalitogenic T cells suppresses EAE. Nat Med 12:518–525
Loschko J, Heink S, Hackl D, Dudziak D, Reindl W, Korn T, Krug AB (2011) Antigen targeting to plasmacytoid dendritic cells via Siglec-H inhibits Th cell-dependent autoimmunity. J Immunol 187:6346–6356
Lucchinetti CF, Bruck W, Rodriguez M, Lassmann H (1996) Distinct patterns of multiple sclerosis pathology indicates heterogeneity on pathogenesis. Brain Pathol 6:259–274
Lucchinetti C, Bruck W, Parisi J, Scheithauer B, Rodriguez M, Lassmann H (2000) Heterogeneity of multiple sclerosis lesions: implications for the pathogenesis of demyelination. Ann Neurol 47:707–717
Madsen LS, Andersson EC, Jansson L, krogsgaard M, Andersen CB, Engberg J, Strominger JL, Svejgaard A, Hjorth JP, Holmdahl R, Wucherpfennig KW, Fugger L (1999) A humanized model for multiple sclerosis using HLA-DR2 and a human T-cell receptor. Nat Genet 23:343–347
Mann MK, Maresz K, Shriver LP, Tan Y, Dittel BN (2007) B cell regulation of CD4+ CD25+ T regulatory cells and IL-10 via B7 is essential for recovery from experimental autoimmune encephalomyelitis. J Immunol 178:3447–3456
Matsushita T, Yanaba K, Bouaziz JD, Fujimoto M, Tedder TF (2008) Regulatory B cells inhibit EAE initiation in mice while other B cells promote disease progression. J Clin Invest 118:3420–3430
Matsushita T, Horikawa M, Iwata Y, Tedder TF (2010) Regulatory B cells (B10 cells) and regulatory T cells have independent roles in controlling experimental autoimmune encephalomyelitis initiation and late-phase immunopathogenesis. J Immunol 185:2240–2252
Matthews AE, Weiss SR, Paterson Y (2002) Murine hepatitis virus–a model for virus-induced CNS demyelination. J Neurovirol 8:76–85
McGeachy MJ, Stephens LA, Anderton SM (2005) Natural recovery and protection from autoimmune encephalomyelitis: contribution of CD4 +CD25 + regulatory cells within the central nervous system. J Immunol 175:3025–3032
McQualter JL, Darwiche R, Ewing C, Onuki M, Kay TW, Hamilton JA, Reid HH, Bernard CC (2001) Granulocyte macrophage colony-stimulating factor: a new putative therapeutic target in multiple sclerosis. J Exp Med 194:873–882
Mendel I, Kerlero de Rosbo N, Ben-Nun A (1995) A myelin oligodendrocyte glycoprotein peptide induces typical chronic experimental autoimmune encephalomyelitis in H-2b mice: fine specificity and T cell receptor V beta expression of encephalitogenic T cells. Eur J Immunol 25:1951–1959
Miranda-Hernandez S, Gerlach N, Fletcher JM, Biros E, Mack M, Korner H, Baxter AG (2011) Role for MyD88, TLR2 and TLR9 but not TLR1, TLR4 or TLR6 in experimental autoimmune encephalomyelitis. J Immunol 187:791–804

Miron VE, Ludwin SK, Darlington PJ, Jarjour AA, Soliven B, Kennedy TE, Antel JP (2010) Fingolimod (FTY720) enhances remyelination following demyelination of organotypic cerebellar slices. Am J Pathol 176:2682–2694
Morgan L, Shah B, Rivers LE, Barden L, Groom AJ, Chung R, Higazi D, Desmond H, Smith T, Staddon JM (2007) Inflammation and dephosphorylation of the tight junction protein occludin in an experimental model of multiple sclerosis. Neuroscience 147:664–673
O'Connor RA, Anderton SM (2008) Foxp3 + regulatory T cells in the control of experimental CNS autoimmune disease. J Neuroimmunol 193:1–11
O'Connor RA, Malpass KH, Anderton SM (2007) The inflamed central nervous system drives the activation and rapid proliferation of Foxp3 + regulatory T cells. J Immunol 179:958–966
O'Connor RA, Prendergast CT, Sabatos CA, Lau CW, Leech MD, Wraith DC, Anderton SM (2008) Cutting edge: Th1 cells facilitate the entry of Th17 cells to the central nervous system during experimental autoimmune encephalomyelitis. J Immunol 181:3750–3754
O'Connor RA, Leech MD, Suffner J, Hammerling GJ, Anderton SM (2010) Myelin-reactive, TGF-beta-induced regulatory T cells can be programmed to develop Th1-like effector function but remain less proinflammatory than myelin-reactive Th1 effectors and can suppress pathogenic T cell clonal expansion in vivo. J Immunol 185:7235–7243
O'Connor RA, Floess S, Huehn J, Jones SA, Anderton SM (2012) Foxp3(+) Treg cells in the inflamed CNS are insensitive to IL-6-driven IL-17 production. Eur J Immunol 42:1174–1179
Oleszak EL, Chang JR, Friedman H, Katsetos CD, Platsoucas CD (2004) Theiler's virus infection: a model for multiple sclerosis. Clin Microbiol Rev 17:174–207
Oppmann B, Lesley R, Blom B, Timans JC, Xu Y, Hunte B, Vega F, Yu N, Wang J, Singh K, Zonin F, Vaisberg E, Churakova T, Liu M, Gorman D, Wagner J, Zurawski S, Liu Y, Abrams JS, Moore KW, Rennick D, Waal-Malefyt R de, Hannum C, Bazan JF, Kastelein RA (2000) Novel p19 protein engages IL-12p40 to form a cytokine, IL-23, with biological activities similar as well as distinct from IL-12. Immunity 13:715–725
Pavelko KD, Engelen BG van, Rodriguez M (1998) Acceleration in the rate of CNS remyelination in lysolecithin-induced demyelination. J Neurosci 18:2498–2505
Perrin PJ, June CH, Maldonado JH, Ratts RB, Racke MK (1999) Blockade of CD28 during in vitro activation of encephalitogenic T cells or after disease onset ameliorates experimental autoimmune encephalomyelitis. J Immunol 163:1704–1710
Pollinger B, Krishnamoorthy G, Berer K, Lassmann H, Bosl MR, Dunn R, Domingues HS, Holz A, Kurschus FC, Wekerle H (2009) Spontaneous relapsing-remitting EAE in the SJL/J mouse: MOG-reactive transgenic T cells recruit endogenous MOG-specific B cells. J Exp Med 206:1303–1316
Ponomarev ED, Shriver LP, Maresz K, Pedras-Vasconcelos J, Verthelyi D, Dittel BN (2007) GM-CSF production by autoreactive T cells is required for the activation of microglial cells and the onset of experimental autoimmune encephalomyelitis. J Immunol 178:39–48
Prinz M, Schmidt H, Mildner A, Knobeloch KP, Hanisch UK, Raasch J, Merkler D, Detje C, Gutcher I, Mages J, Lang R, Martin R, Gold R, Becher B, Bruck W, Kalinke U (2008) Distinct and nonredundant in vivo functions of IFNAR on myeloid cells limit autoimmunity in the central nervous system. Immunity 28:675–686
Ray A, Basu S, Williams CB, Salzman NH, Dittel BN (2012) A novel IL-10-independent regulatory role for B cells in suppressing autoimmunity by maintenance of regulatory T cells via GITR ligand. J Immunol 188:3188–3198
Reboldi A, Coisne C, Baumjohann D, Benvenuto F, Bottinelli D, Lira S, Uccelli A, Lanzavecchia A, Engelhardt B, Sallusto F (2009) C-C chemokine receptor 6-regulated entry of TH-17 cells into the CNS through the choroid plexus is required for the initiation of EAE. Nat Immunol 10:514–523
Remington LT, Babcock AA, Zehntner SP, Owens T (2007) Microglial recruitment, activation, and proliferation in response to primary demyelination. Am J Pathol 170:1713–1724
Rice GP, Hartung HP, Calabresi PA (2005) Anti-alpha4 integrin therapy for multiple sclerosis: mechanisms and rationale. Neurology 64:1336–1342
Ridge SC, Sloboda AE, McReynolds RA, Levine S, Oronsky AL, Kerwar SS (1985) Suppression of experimental allergic encephalomyelitis by mitoxantrone. Clin Immunol Immunopathol 35:35–42

Rossi S, Lo Giudice T, De Chiara V, Musella A, Studer V, Motta C, Bernardi G, Martino G, Furlan R, Martorana A, Centonze D (2012) Oral fingolimod rescues the functional deficits of synapses in experimental autoimmune encephalomyelitis. Br J Pharmacol 165:861–869

Rothhammer V, Heink S, Petermann F, Srivastava R, Claussen MC, Hemmer B, Korn T (2011) Th17 lymphocytes traffic to the central nervous system independently of alpha4 integrin expression during EAE. J Exp Med 208:2465–2476

Samoilova EB, Horton JL, Hilliard B, Liu TS, Chen Y (1998) IL-6-deficient mice are resistant to experimental autoimmune encephalomyelitis: roles of IL-6 in the activation and differentiation of autoreactive T cells. J Immunol 161:6480–6486

Schmidt J, Gold R, Schonrock L, Zettl UK, Hartung HP, Toyka KV (2000) T-cell apoptosis in situ in experimental autoimmune encephalomyelitis following methylprednisolone pulse therapy. Brain 123(Pt 7):1431–1441

Segal BM, Dwyer BK, Shevach EM (1998) An interleukin (IL)-10/IL-12 immunoregulatory circuit controls susceptibility to autoimmune disease. J Exp Med 187:537–546

Segal BM, Chang JT, Shevach EM (2000) CpG oligonucleotides are potent adjuvants for the activation of autoreactive encephalitogenic T cells in vivo. J Immunol 164:5683–5688

Selvaraj RK, Geiger TL (2008) Mitigation of experimental allergic encephalomyelitis by TGF-beta induced Foxp3 + regulatory T lymphocytes through the induction of anergy and infectious tolerance. J Immunol 180:2830–2838

Serada S, Fujimoto M, Mihara M, Koike N, Ohsugi Y, Nomura S, Yoshida H, Nishikawa T, Terabe F, Ohkawara T, Takahashi T, Ripley B, Kimura A, Kishimoto T, Naka T (2008) IL-6 blockade inhibits the induction of myelin antigen-specific Th17 cells and Th1 cells in experimental autoimmune encephalomyelitis. Proc Nat Acad Sci U S A 105:9041–9046

Setzu A, Lathia JD, Zhao C, Wells K, Rao MS, Ffrench-Constant C, Franklin RJ (2006) Inflammation stimulates myelination by transplanted oligodendrocyte precursor cells. Glia 54:297–303

Sharpe AH (2009) Mechanisms of costimulation. Immunol Rev 229:5–11

Skripuletz T, Bussmann JH, Gudi V, Koutsoudaki PN, Pul R, Moharregh-Khiabani D, Lindner M, Stangel M (2010) Cerebellar cortical demyelination in the murine cuprizone model. Brain Pathol 20:301–312

Sporici R, Issekutz TB (2010) CXCR3 blockade inhibits T-cell migration into the CNS during EAE and prevents development of adoptively transferred, but not actively induced, disease. Eur J Immunol 40:2751–2761

Sriram S, Steiner I (2005) Experimental allergic encephalomyelitis: a misleading model of multiple sclerosis. Ann Neurol 58:939–945

Steinman RM, Hawiger D, Nussenzweig MC (2003) Tolerogenic dendritic cells. Annu Rev Immunol 21:685–711

Stephens LA, Malpass KH, Anderton SM (2009) Curing CNS autoimmune disease with myelin-reactive Foxp3 + Treg. Eur J Immunol 39:1108–1117

Stidworthy MF, Genoud S, Suter U, Mantei N, Franklin RJ (2003) Quantifying the early stages of remyelination following cuprizone-induced demyelination. Brain Pathol 13:329–339

Stromnes IM, Goverman JM (2006a) Active induction of experimental allergic encephalomyelitis. Nat protoc 1:1810–1819

Stromnes IM, Goverman JM (2006b) Passive induction of experimental allergic encephalomyelitis. Nat protoc 1:1952–1960

Stromnes IM, Cerretti LM, Liggitt D, Harris RA, Goverman JM (2008) Differential regulation of central nervous system autoimmunity by T(H)1 and T(H)17 cells. Nat Med 14:337–342

Sweeney CM, Lonergan R, Basdeo SA, Kinsella K, Dungan LS, Higgins SC, Kelly PJ, Costelloe L, Tubridy N, Mills KH, Fletcher JM (2011) IL-27 mediates the response to IFN-beta therapy in multiple sclerosis patients by inhibiting Th17 cells. Brain Behav Immun 25:1170–1181

Torkildsen O, Brunborg LA, Myhr KM, Bo L (2008) The cuprizone model for demyelination. Acta Neurol Scand Suppl 188:72–76

Uschkureit T, Sporkel O, Stracke J, Bussow H, Stoffel W (2000) Early onset of axonal degeneration in double (plp-/-mag-/-) and hypomyelinosis in triple (plp–/–mbp–/–mag–/–) mutant mice. J Neurosci 20:5225–5233

Vajkoczy P, Laschinger M, Engelhardt B (2001) Alpha4-integrin-VCAM-1 binding mediates G protein-independent capture of encephalitogenic T cell blasts to CNS white matter microvessels. J Clin Invest 108:557–565

Vermersch P, Kappos L, Gold R, Foley JF, Olsson T, Cadavid D, Bozic C, Richman S (2011) Clinical outcomes of natalizumab-associated progressive multifocal leukoencephalopathy. Neurology 76:1697–1704

Visser L, Jan de Heer H, Boven LA, Riel D van, Meurs M van, Melief MJ, Zahringer U, Strijp J van, Lambrecht BN, Nieuwenhuis EE, Laman JD (2005) Proinflammatory bacterial peptidoglycan as a cofactor for the development of central nervous system autoimmune disease. J Immunol 174:808–816

Walters S, Webster KE, Sutherland A, Gardam S, Groom J, Liuwantara D, Marino E, Thaxton J, Weinberg A, Mackay F, Brink R, Sprent J, Grey ST (2009) Increased CD4 + Foxp3 + T cells in BAFF-transgenic mice suppress T cell effector responses. J Immunol 182:793–801

Webb M, Tham CS, Lin FF, Lariosa-Willingham K, Yu N, Hale J, Mandala S, Chun J, Rao TS (2004) Sphingosine 1-phosphate receptor agonists attenuate relapsing-remitting experimental autoimmune encephalitis in SJL mice. J Neuroimmunol 153:108–121

Weber MS, Prod'homme T, Youssef S, Dunn SE, Rundle CD, Lee L, Patarroyo JC, Stuve O, Sobel RA, Steinman L, Zamvil SS (2007) Type II monocytes modulate T cell-mediated central nervous system autoimmune disease. Nat Med 13:935–943

Weber MS, Prod'homme T, Patarroyo JC, Molnarfi N, Karnezis T, Lehmann-Horn K, Danilenko DM, Eastham-Anderson J, Slavin AJ, Linington C, Bernard CC, Martin F, Zamvil SS (2010) B-cell activation influences T-cell polarization and outcome of anti-CD20 B-cell depletion in central nervous system autoimmunity. Ann Neurol 68:369–383

Weinberg AD, Wegmann KW, Funatake C, Whitham RH (1999) Blocking OX-40/OX-40 ligand interaction in vitro and in vivo leads to decreased T cell function and amelioration of experimental allergic encephalomyelitis. J Immunol 162:1818–1826

Willenborg DO, Fordham S, Bernard CC, Cowden WB, Ramshaw IA (1996) IFN-gamma plays a critical down-regulatory role in the induction and effector phase of myelin oligodendrocyte glycoprotein-induced autoimmune encephalomyelitis. J Immunol 157:3223–3227

Wing K, Sakaguchi S (2010) Regulatory T cells exert checks and balances on self tolerance and autoimmunity. Nat Immunol 11:7–13

Wolf SD, Dittel BN, Hardardottir F, Janeway CA Jr (1996) Experimental autoimmune encephalomyelitis induction in genetically B cell-deficient mice. J Exp Med 184:2271–2278

Wolf NA, Amouzegar TK, Swanborg RH (2007) Synergistic interaction between Toll-like receptor agonists is required for induction of experimental autoimmune encephalomyelitis in Lewis rats. J Neuroimmunol 185:115–122

Woodruff RH, Franklin RJ (1999) Demyelination and remyelination of the caudal cerebellar peduncle of adult rats following stereotaxic injections of lysolecithin, ethidium bromide, and complement/anti-galactocerebroside: a comparative study. Glia 25:216–228

Yajima K, Suzuki K (1979) Demyelination and remyelination in the rat central nervous system following ethidium bromide injection. Lab Invest 41:385–392

Yang Y, Weiner J, Liu Y, Smith AJ, Huss DJ, Winger R, Peng H, Cravens PD, Racke MK, Lovett-Racke AE (2009) T-bet is essential for encephalitogenicity of both Th1 and Th17 cells. J Exp Med 206:1549–1564

Yasuda CL, Al-Sabbagh A, Oliveira EC, Diaz-Bardales BM, Garcia AA, Santos LM (1999) Interferon beta modulates experimental autoimmune encephalomyelitis by altering the pattern of cytokine secretion. Immunol Invest 28:115–126

Yednock TA, Cannon C, Fritz LC, Sanchez-Madrid F, Steinman L, Karin N (1992) Prevention of experimental autoimmune encephalomyelitis by antibodies against alpha 4 beta 1 integrin. Nature 356:63–66

Zhang X, Koldzic DN, Izikson L, Reddy J, Nazareno RF, Sakaguchi S, Kuchroo VK, Weiner HL (2004) IL-10 is involved in the suppression of experimental autoimmune encephalomyelitis by CD25 + CD4 + regulatory T cells. Int Immunol 16:249–256

Chapter 14
Modeling MS in Nonhuman Primates

Bert A. ’t Hart, S. Anwar Jagessar, Krista Haanstra, Yolanda S. Kap and Jon D. Laman

> Essentially, all models are wrong, but some are useful.
> *Quote from: Box G.E.P. & Draper N.R. Empirical Model-Building and Response Surfaces* (1987) p. 424.

14.1 Introduction

The classical role of the immune system is to detect and eliminate foreign organisms, such as microbial infection, while at the same time the system should not respond against the body itself (Mills 2011). This implies that the antigen-sensing and -presenting cells (APC) should have the capacity to detect a few foreign antigens within a sea of self-antigens. For this vital task, APC are equipped with conserved pattern-recognition receptor families (PRR), such as Toll-like receptors (TLR). TLR detect conserved molecular structures on pathogens, named pathogen-associated molecular patterns (PAMPS), and tissue-damage signals associated with self-antigens, named danger-associated molecular patterns (DAMPS, or alarmins). Nonresponsiveness is at least, in part, regulated by the interaction of C-type lectin receptors (CLR) with carbohydrates expressed on self-antigens. Conceptually, the integration of immune-activation signals received by dendritic cell

B. A. ’t Hart (✉) · S. A. Jagessar · Y. S. Kap
Department of Immunobiology, Biomedical Primate Research Centre, Lange Kleiweg 161, 2288 GJ RIJSWIJK Postbus 3306, 2280 GH RIJSWIJK, The Netherlands
e-mail: hart@bprc.nl

B. A. ’t Hart
Department of Neuroscience, University Medical Center Groningen, Groningen, The Netherlands

B. A. ’t Hart · Y. S. Kap
Department of Immunology, Erasmus Medical Center, Rotterdam, The Netherlands

MS center ErasMS, Rotterdam, The Netherlands

J. D. Laman
Department of Immunology, Erasmus Medical Center Rotterdam, The Netherlands
e-mail: j.laman@erasmusmc.nl

T. Yamamura, B. Gran (eds.), *Multiple Sclerosis Immunology,*
DOI 10.1007/978-1-4614-7953-6_14, © Springer Science+Business Media New York 2013

(DC) via TLR with immune-inhibitory signals received via CLR determines whether the DC will mature and induce immunity or remain immature and induce tolerance (Geijtenbeek et al. 2004; 't Hart and van Kooyk 2004). Although this theoretical model is likely wrong in its simplification, it has been useful for the modeling of MS in nonhuman primates.

14.2 Animal Models of MS

It is widely accepted that the risk to develop MS is determined by a combination of inherited and environmental factors, including bacterial or viral infection, which in susceptible individuals may induce the activation of autoreactive T and B cells. Genome-wide association (GWA) studies support an important influence of the immune system on MS as essentially all MS risk genes encode cellular immune functions, with the major histocompatibility complex (MHC) as strongest association. Three concepts for the infection–autoimmunity relationship prevail: (1) molecular mimicry, being cross-reaction of T and/or B cells activated by a pathogen with look-alike epitopes of self-antigens; (2) bystander activation, being induction of autoreactive T cells by pathogen-activated APC; and (3) pathogen persistence, as in the Theiler virus model of encephalitis (Fujinami et al. 2006). Although each of these mechanisms is supported by data from animal models, there is no undisputed evidence that they are indeed relevant for MS.

The elected animal model for MS, experimental autoimmune encephalomyelitis (EAE), has been seriously criticized (Sriram and Steiner 2005; Ransohoff 2006). Indeed, many therapies fail to reproduce the promising activity observed in EAE models, when they were tested in MS patients, illustrating the difficulty to extrapolate pathogenic mechanisms observed in EAE to MS. On the other hand, it cannot be ignored that the EAE model has helped the development of several treatments for relapsing-remitting MS (RRMS) (Steinman and Zamvil 2005, 2006). Well-known examples are the anti-$\alpha 4\beta 1$ integrin antibody natalizumab, the random polymer glatiramer acetate (copaxone), or the cytokine interferon-β (for review, see Lopez-Diego and Weiner 2008).

The use of only a few selected inbred and very clean (Specified Pathogen Free; SPF) mouse or rat strains at young-adult age and with limited antigenic experience, and often induced by immunization with only a single autoantigen in very strong adjuvant (CFA) to model a complex disease in the immunologically complex and genetically variable human population is understandable from a reductionist approach, but has obvious limitations. As discussed elsewhere ('t Hart et al. 2011), the EAE model can be a very useful experimental model of MS, but the Achilles' heel of the model seems the wide genetic, immunological, microbial, and anatomical gap between the laboratory mouse/rat and man. This problem is certainly not restricted to EAE, but applies to models for a wide range of immune-mediated inflammatory disorders ('t Hart et al. 2004). The extrapolation of data from EAE to MS can benefit from the usage of disease models in animals that are more closely related to humans than mice and rats, monkeys, for example. Monkeys are man's closest relatives in nature and the high degree of genetic, immunological, microbial, and anatomical similarity with humans has been well documented.

In this chapter, we will discuss established MS models in common laboratory primates, comprising two Old-World monkey species, the rhesus (*Macaca mulatta*) and cynomolgus (*Macaca fascicularis*) macaque, and one New-World monkey, the common marmoset (*Callithrix jacchus*). We will briefly summarize characteristic aspects of the models, which have been reviewed in more detail elsewhere (Brok et al. 2001a; 't Hart et al. 2005a; Kap et al. 2010), and highlight new insights into MS pathogenesis.

14.3 EAE in Old-World Monkeys

14.3.1 EAE in Rhesus and Cynomolgus Macaques

The first observations on autoimmune encephalomyelitis induced by sensitization against CNS antigens were made in humans vaccinated against rabies (Stuart and Krikorian 1933). Rivers et al. (1933) have used rhesus monkeys to analyze whether the fatal postvaccination encephalomyelitis observed in human vaccinees was induced by the virus or by components from the rabbit brain on which the virus was cultured. Although it could be shown that the disease was caused by the repeated injections of rabbit brain extract, the underlying mechanism was not understood. In a follow-up publication, the experiment was reproduced using repeated intramuscular injections (up to 85) with alcohol extract from normal rabbit brain giving essentially the same results (Rivers and Schwenkter 1935). The reported study also tested whether intracerebral injection of brain extract from a diseased monkey into two other monkeys would induce the same disease. As this was not observed, the investigators concluded that the neurological problems were most likely not caused by an infectious pathogen. More than a decade later, Kabat et al. observed that formulation of the rabbit brain extract with mycobacteria suspensions in oil strongly potentiated the immunogenicity, so that the number of injections needed to induce an acute type of EAE at high incidence could be substantially reduced (Kabat et al. 1947). The same publication reports that monkeys immunized with fetal rabbit brain, which contains only little myelin, did not develop the disease, proving for the first time that the encephalitogenic component in the rabbit brain extract is myelin. The subsequent work, from Alvord et al., for example (Alvord 1984), essentially followed observations collected in Lewis rat and guinea pig EAE models, identifying myelin basic protein (MBP) as an important encephalitogenic myelin component. Indeed, immunization of rhesus monkeys with MBP/CFA induced a similar type of acute EAE as was observed in monkeys injected with brain extracts.

It was well recognized that the acute clinical course and the destructive inflammatory pathology of the EAE model in rhesus monkeys more closely resembled acute disseminated encephalomyelitis (ADEM) than the most prevalent relapsing-remitting (RR) and secondary progressive (SP) forms of MS. Nevertheless, in the absence of a better alternative, the model has been used for immunogenetic and immunopathogenic research as well as for immunotherapy testing (van Lambalgen and Jonker 1987a, b; Slierendregt et al. 1995). These studies demonstrated a similar prominent pathogenic role of $CD4^+$ T cells as in rats and guinea pigs, whereas depletion of $CD8^+$ T cells had no detectable effect (Lambalgen and Jonker 1987b). Another study demonstrating a substantial suppressive effect of anti-CD18 antibody, which recognizes the integrin β2 chain of LFA-1 and Mac-1 and limits migration of leukocytes, emphasized the immunological basis of the model (Rose et al. 1997).

Attempts have been made to establish a more MS-like model in rhesus monkeys, such as by changing the immunizing antigen. However, it was observed that rhesus monkeys immunized with recombinant Oligodendrocyte-specific protein (OSP) (Bajramovic et al. 2008) or myelin/oligodendrocyte glycoprotein (MOG; Kerlero de Rosbo et al. 2000), or the immunodominant peptide $MOG_{34–56}$ (Brok et al. 2007) developed an equally acute onset EAE with necrotic brain lesions as was observed in the original model.

Others have tested EAE induction in another macaque species, i.e., long-tail/cynomolgus macaques (*Macaca fascicularis*). This showed some improvement as monkeys immunized with MBP/CFA were found to develop RR disease (Teitelbaum et al. 2004). Moreover, Massacesi et al. observed that monkeys immunized with human brain homogenate in CFA developed in part acute fatal and in part RR EAE (Massacesi et al. 1992).

14.3.2 Refinement of the Rhesus Macaque EAE Model

A large primate EAE model is definitely needed for studies of immunogenetic and immunopathogenic mechanisms that require large blood volumes or easy access to cerebrospinal fluid (CSF) as well as for immunotherapy evaluation. Macaques are more closely related to humans than marmosets and this is reflected by the higher genetic and immunological similarity. As an example, the percentage of candidate therapeutic monoclonal antibodies that cross-react with target molecules in macaques is higher than those in marmosets (approx. 90 % vs. 50–60 %). Also, brain-imaging studies with magnetic resonance imaging (MRI) or positron emission tomography (PET) will benefit from the anatomical similarities between the macaque and human brain. Finally, CSF analysis is more feasible in macaques than in the small-bodied marmoset, both with regard to the ease of CSF collection and the volume that can be collected. However, the establishment of a model in macaques that approximates the MS-like clinical and pathological presentation of the EAE model in marmosets remains a major challenge.

A possible explanation comes from the intriguing observation that rhesus monkeys consistently display a more vigorous response than marmoset monkeys in models of immune-mediated inflammatory disorder, such as EAE and collagen-induced arthritis (CIA) (Vierboom et al. 2005, 2010). Moreover, the ulcerative lesions developing at the intradermal injection sites of antigen/CFA emulsion are much more severe in rhesus monkeys than in marmosets (own unpublished observation). These observations suggest that the acute and destructive nature of the models may be due to a higher innate reactivity of rhesus monkeys against bacterial antigens present in the adjuvant, although this still needs to be proven.

Analogous to the situation in marmosets (see further), we have tested whether clinically evident EAE can be induced without usage of CFA. It was observed that in only two out of five tested rhesus monkeys, EAE could be induced by immunization with rhMOG in IFA, while similarly treated marmosets developed EAE in six out of six tested cases (Haanstra et al. 2013).

14.3.3 A Virus-Induced MS Model in Japanese Macaques

In a colony of Japanese macaques at the Oregon National Primate Research Center (Beaverton, OR), spontaneous outbreak of MS-like disease has been reported (Axthelm et al. 2011). The authors succeeded in isolating a new $\gamma 2$ herpes virus from acute central nervous system (CNS) white matter lesions. Further research showed that the virus could not be isolated from normal white matter from sick or healthy monkeys. This spontaneous disease may be very useful as a model for the viral etiology of MS.

14.4 EAE in New-World Monkey; the Common Marmoset (*Callithrix jacchus*)

14.4.1 What Is a Marmoset?

The common marmoset is a small-bodied Neotropical primate (approx. 350 g at maturity) that breeds well in captivity and adapts well to experimental procedures. A healthy female gives birth to two sets of twins or sometimes triplets per year, which are sexually mature after about 1.5 years (Tardif et al. 2003). Marmosets have been widely used in biomedical research (Abbott et al. 2003; Mansfield 2003). Twins usually have a shared placental blood stream creating chimerism at the level of bone marrow and hematopoietic lineages (Haig 1999). The chimerism therefore includes the immune systems of twin siblings, which are educated in the same thymic environment and are thus highly comparable.

The T and B cell receptor-encoding gene repertoires of the marmoset have been characterized and were found to be comparable with the human counterparts (Uccelli 1997; Budingen et al. 2001). It is not exactly known, however, which of the isotypes and subclasses defined for human Ig molecules are present in marmosets. Moreover, MHC class I and II regions have also been characterized. The MHC class I region of the marmoset does not encode equivalents of the human classical MHC class Ia molecules HLA-A and C, but genes encoding equivalents of HLA-B and the nonclassical MHC class Ib molecules HLA-E and -G have been identified (Cadavid et al. 1997; Shiina et al. 2011). Analysis of the natural killer receptor repertoire is in progress (Averdam et al. 2007). The MHC class II region of the common marmoset comprises two polymorphic (*Caja-DRB1*03* and *– DRB*W16*) and one monomorphic locus (*Caja-DRB*W1201*; Antunes et al. 1998). Later, it was found that only the *Caja-DRB*W1201* and – *DRB*W16* loci produce functional transcripts whereas the Caja-DRB1*03 locus encodes pseudogenes. However, *Caja-DRB1*03* exon 2 elements can be embedded within a Caja-DRB*W16 gene as a result of an exon shuffling event to form hybrid MHC class II molecules (Doxiadis et al. 2006).

14.4.2 Concise Overview of EAE Models in the Common Marmoset

The discovery that marmosets sensitized against human myelin formulated with a strong bacterial adjuvant (CFA) display MS-like disease has been a major breakthrough in the modeling of MS in nonhuman primates (Genain et al. 1994; Massacesi et al. 1995). After we reproduced the model from the original publication in our own laboratory ('t Hart et al. 1998), we have set out to refine and modify it as reviewed in detail elsewhere ('t Hart and Massacesi 2009).

We observed that immunization with myelin isolated from the CNS of wild-type C57BL/6 mice emulsified in CFA gave the same MS-like disease as immunization with MS patient myelin in five out of five monkeys. However, four out of five marmosets immunized with CNS myelin from C57BL/6 mice, in which the MOG gene was knocked out, failed to develop EAE (Jagessar et al. 2008). In the one case that did develop EAE, the disease was equally acute in both twin siblings. This observation suggests that acute EAE can be induced independent of MOG, whereas autoimmunity against MOG is essential for the induction of progressive disease. Essentially, the same results were obtained in the chronic relapsing EAE model in Biozzi ABH mice (Smith et al. 2005).

Genain et al. have pioneered the marmoset EAE model in great depth. Initially, they focused their research on the pathogenic contribution of two major myelin antigens (MBP and PLP), which were found to induce mainly inflammatory EAE when formulated with strong bacterial adjuvants, i.e., enriched CFA containing a high concentration of mycobacteria and intravenous *Bordetella pertussis* particles (Genain et al. 1995). However, extensive demyelination of white matter was observed only after additional injection of anti-MOG antibody (Genain et al. 1995). Similarly, McFarland et al. (1999) observed a critical role of anti-MOG autoimmunity in the development of clinically evident EAE in marmosets sensitized against a chimeric protein of MBP and PLP (MP4). Also, in our hands, immunization with MBP formulated with commercial CFA, containing a low dose of mycobacteria without intravenous administration of *Bordetella pertussis*, was much less effective in inducing clinical EAE than the quantitatively minor CNS myelin-constituent MOG (Brok et al. 2000).

These findings suggest the existence of a hierarchy in the pathogenic contribution of myelin antigens with a prominent role of MOG. We further explored the patterns of humoral and cellular anti-MOG autoimmune reactions relevant to the induction of lesion formation and neurological deficit. The EAE model for this research was induced by sensitization against the Ig-like extracellular domain of human MOG (amino acids 1–125; rhMOG) in CFA (Brok et al. 2000). Figure 14.1 shows the

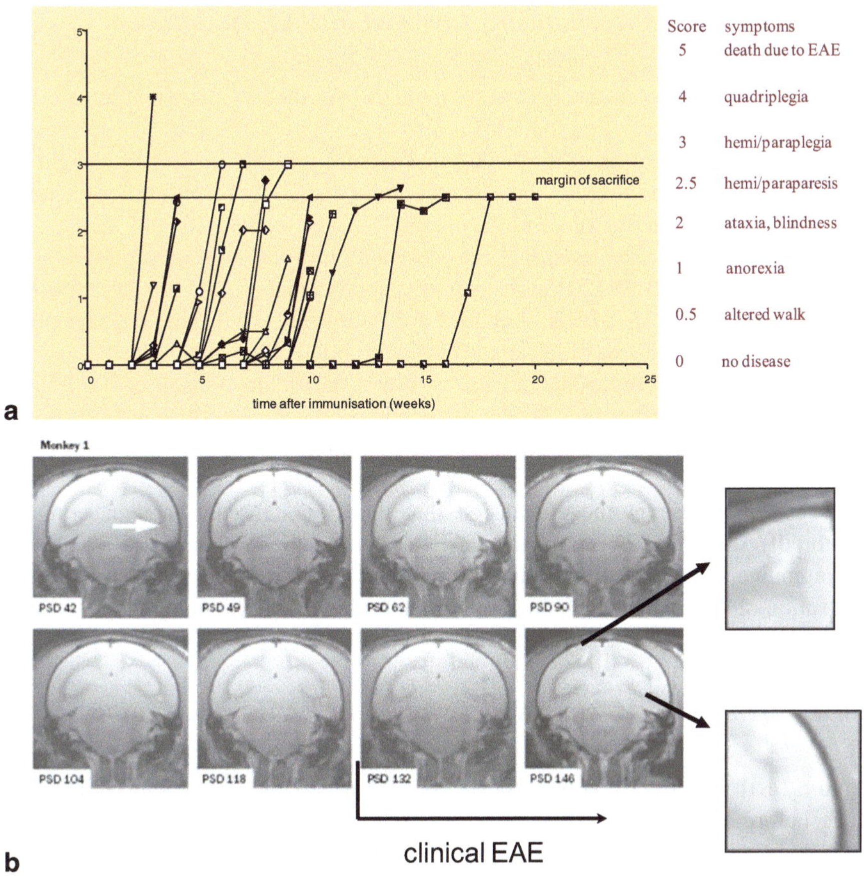

Fig. 14.1 Clinical and pathological development of the rhMOG/CFA EAE model. **a** A single immunization with 100 μg rhMOG in CFA suffices to induce clinical EAE in marmosets from an outbred population. The model is characterized by a 100 % incidence but variable time of onset. **b** Serial MRI (T2-weighted) shows that already after 6 weeks a white matter lesion is detectable whereas neurological deficits can be first observed about 3 months later. Around the presence of clinically evident EAE, spreading of lesions to the cortical gray matter can be found (*inserts*). The early and late phases of the disease in this model are likely driven by the two distinct pathogenic mechanisms depicted in Fig. 14.3

main characteristics of the EAE model induced with rhMOG/CFA. The model is characterized by 100 % disease incidence, but the time interval between EAE induction and onset of neurological deficit varies considerably between individual animals (Fig. 14.1a). Intriguingly, serial MRI of a late responder case shows that brain white matter T2 lesions are detectable long before neurological deficits are diagnosed (Fig. 14.1b). These observations led us to hypothesize that the initiation and perpetuation of the disease may involve distinct immunopathogenic mechanisms. In the following paragraphs, we will discuss data in support of this hypothesis.

14.4.3 Immune Mechanisms Involved in EAE Initiation

In MS as well as in mouse, rat, and rhesus monkey EAE models, disease susceptibility maps to the MHC class II region. This is also the case in marmosets. The specificity profiling of mononuclear cells (MNC) isolated from marmosets at the height of rhMOG/CFA-induced disease showed ubiquitous reactivity (proliferation) against two overlapping N-terminal peptides of rhMOG, i.e., MOG_{14-36} and MOG_{24-46}. It was subsequently confirmed that the presentation of the overlapping MOG_{24-36} peptide by Caja-DRB*W1201 molecules elicits inflammatory EAE by the activation of T helper 1 cells (Th1; Brok et al. 2000). Immunization with the longer peptide MOG_{14-36} indeed induced mild clinical EAE with small inflammatory lesions in four out of four monkeys. Independent from us, it was shown that transfer of T cell lines against the slightly elongated MOG_{21-40} peptide isolated from the naive marmoset immune repertoire induced a similar type of inflammatory EAE (Villoslada et al. 2001).

These data warrant the conclusion that the 100 % disease incidence in the (outbred!) rhMOG/CFA marmoset EAE model can be explained by a uniform autoimmune event in all marmosets, namely the Caja-DRB*W1201-restricted activation of Th1 cells, which cause inflammation in the CNS white matter.

14.4.4 Immune Mechanisms Involved in EAE Perpetuation

Figure 14.1b illustrates that formation of brain white matter lesions can be detected long before overt clinical signs are diagnosed. Interestingly, we observed in the depicted case that around the time that clinical signs appeared, several T2 lesions had spread into the cortical gray matter. This raised the question whether specific immunological changes can be observed around the time that neurological deficits appear.

The specificity profiling of MNC isolated from marmosets at the height of rhMOG/CFA-induced EAE also showed a variable reactivity against other MOG peptides, including MOG_{34-56} and the overlapping peptides MOG_{64-86}/MOG_{74-96} (Kap et al. 2008). Interestingly, marmosets with a short disease duration, i.e., fast progressors, displayed significantly more often a polyspecific proliferative response than monkeys with a longer disease duration, indicated as slow progressors (Kap et al. 2008). We have therefore tested in chimeric twins whether immunization with MOG_{34-56} or MOG_{74-96} formulated in CFA-induced EAE. It was observed that only monkeys immunized with MOG_{34-56}/CFA developed clinically evident EAE with widespread CNS inflammation and demyelination (Kap et al. 2008). In contrast, monkeys immunized with MOG_{74-96}/CFA displayed no detectable EAE symptoms, although small-sized abnormalities suggestive of inflammatory lesions were detected on postmortem T2W images. In these monkeys, a single booster immunization with MOG_{34-56} formulated with IFA induced clinically evident EAE within a few weeks (Kap et al. 2008). We concluded from this experiment that anti-MOG_{74-96} T cells are mildly encephalitogenic, inducing small-sized inflammatory lesions, which do not induce detectable neurological problems, whereas anti-$MOG_{34–56}$ T cells have a more potent encephalitogenic capacity.

As the induction of cross-reactive T cell responses between the nonoverlapping peptides $MOG_{34–56}$ and $MOG_{74–96}$ could be excluded, we hypothesized from this experiment that T cells activated by $MOG_{34–56}$ may exert a vigorous attack on small-sized lesions in the CNS white matter that have been induced by the autoimmune reactivity against $MOG_{74–96}$. This observation formed the basis of our "response-to-injury" paradigm for MS, which we would like to propose as an alternative for the classical "response-to-infection" model ('t Hart et al. 2009). We will discuss later that this new concept may also help understand immune mechanisms underlying secondary progressive MS.

14.4.5 The Heart of the Marmoset EAE Model

The most remarkable observation in the $MOG_{74–96}$/CFA-immunized monkeys was that sensitization with $MOG_{34–56}$/IFA was sufficient to elicit the complete clinical and pathological picture of the rhMOG/CFA model. This observation raised the question whether immunization of naive monkeys with $MOG_{34–56}$/IFA might also induce clinically evident EAE. It was indeed observed that essentially all tested monkeys ($N > 20$) developed overt clinical EAE, associated with widespread demyelination in brain and spinal cord affecting the white as well as gray matter (Jagessar et al. 2010). Representative examples of disease course and CNS pathology are depicted in Fig. 14.2. All this occurred without deliberate innate receptor-mediated activation of APC by microbial compounds in the adjuvant to a mature immunogenic state, which can break the immune regulatory mechanisms that maintain tolerance and in the absence of autoantibodies mediating demyelination. We thus concluded that the MS-like clinical and pathological features of this new model are directly induced by autoreactive memory-like T cells present in the naive marmoset repertoire.

Next, we investigated the nature of the autoreactive T cells and their mechanism of action in the $MOG_{34–56}$/IFA model. We used CFSE-vital dye dilution to identify in bulk suspensions of lymph nodes and spleen the in vivo-activated T cells, as these proliferate upon *ex vivo* restimulation with $MOG_{34–56}$ (Lyons 2000), and phenotyped them with a panel of preselected cross-reactive monoclonal antibodies (mAb; Brok et al. 2001b). It could be shown that the main peptide reactivity maps to $CD3^+CD4^+CD56^+$ cells predominating in the axillary lymph nodes that drain the immunization sites and $CD3^+CD4^+/CD8^+CD56^+$ predominating in the spleen. Immunostaining for additional markers showed that they are $CD27^+CD28^-CD45RO^-CCR7^-$. Functional characteristics relevant for the pathogenic role of T cells are the cytokine profile upon *ex vivo* stimulation with $MOG_{34–56}$, i.e., IL-$17A^{high}$, $IFN\gamma^{low}$, and $TNF\alpha^{low}$ and the specific cytotoxic activity towards target cell presenting the epitope $MOG_{40–48}$ via monomorphic Caja-E molecules (Jagessar et al. 2012b). Caja-E is the marmoset representative in a lineage of nonclassical MHC class Ib genes with a regulatory role of NK cells, also comprising HLA-E in humans and QA-1 in mice (Jensen et al. 2004).

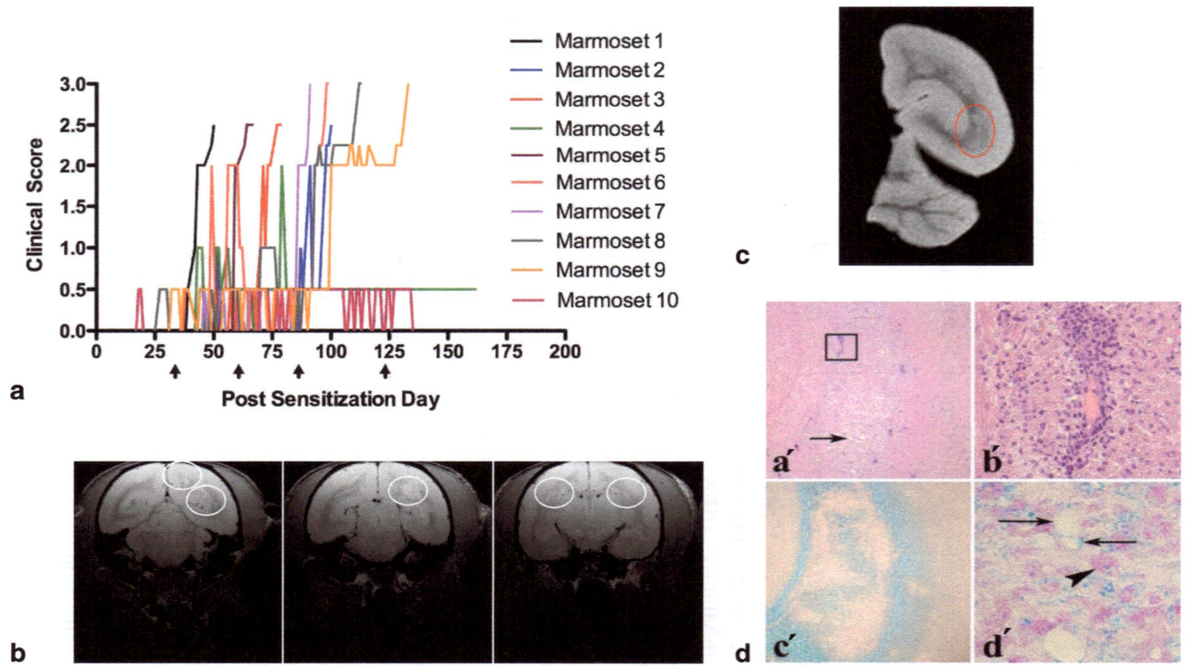

Fig. 14.2 Clinical and pathological development of the MOG_{34-56}/IFA EAE model. **a** Repeated immunization with MOG_{34-56} in IFA at 28 days interval induces clinical and pathological features of MS. In one case (monkey 4), the neurological deficit (score 2.0 = ataxia) is transient. **b** However, using T2W MRI, presence of large lesions could be detected. **c** A postmortem T2W MRI of a fixed hemisphere shows presence of large demyelinated areas within the white matter. The histology of the *encircled* lesion is depicted in **d**. **d** Klüver-Barrera staining shows intense primary demyelination (c′) with vacuolar structures (enlargement in d′). Within the lesion perivascular infiltrates of MNC are found (a′). The *boxed* infiltrate is shown enlarged in b′

14.5 Validation of the Models by Immunotherapy

We have used the marmoset EAE model for the preclinical evaluation of new immunotherapies. Such studies are of interest as they demonstrate which pathogenic mechanisms are equally important in MS and EAE and in this way serve as validation of the model. In this chapter, we will highlight three treatments that have been evaluated in the EAE model, namely the anti-IL12p40 antibody ustekinumab, the anti-CD20 antibody HuMab 7D8, which is clonally related to ofatumumab, and the cytokine interferon-γ.

Treatment 1 The discovery that distinct autoreactive T cell lineages exist with a different function in MS and that these can be distinguished on the basis of their cytokine profile has opened new avenues in EAE/MS research. Accumulating evidence, mainly coming from rodent EAE models, suggests that two T cell subtypes have a particularly important role in inducing CNS inflammation, i.e., Th1 cells, characterized by the signature cytokine IFNγ, and Th17 cells, characterized by the signature cytokine IL-17A (Axtell et al. 2010). The key cytokine for differentiation of Th0 cells to Th1 is the p35/p40 heterodimeric cytokine IL-12, whereas the p19/p40 heterodimeric cytokine IL-23 promotes differentiation to Th17. It was therefore expected that treatment with an antibody against the shared p40 subunit of IL-12 and IL-23 would inhibit the differentiation of both arms and that this would suppress neuroinflammation in MS.

We observed that early-stage treatment with a human IgG1κ antibody against human IL-12p40 (ustekinumab) in the marmoset EAE model, i.e., starting 1 day before the immunization, completely suppressed clinical and pathological features of EAE (Brok et al. 2002). However, late-stage treatment with the antibody, starting when brain white matter lesions had already been formed, was much less effective causing only a delayed disease onset ('t Hart et al. 2005b). Unexpectedly, the same antibody was found ineffective in a phase II clinical trial in RRMS (Segal et al. 2008). The discrepant efficacy of ustekinumab in MS and EAE justifies the question whether autoreactive Th1/Th17 cells have an equally important pathogenic role in MS as in the EAE model. The answer to this question suggested by the marmoset EAE model is that the T cells engaged in late-stage disease are committed effector memory T cells, which no longer require IL-12 or IL-23 for their activation and/or differentiation.

Treatment 2 The canonical role of B cells in the EAE model is to produce autoantibodies that support demyelination by opsonizing myelin. The findings by Genain and colleagues that anti-MOG antibodies are associated with CNS myelin pathology in MS and the marmoset EAE model (Genain et al. 1999; Raine et al. 1999) and that they amplify CNS demyelination when injected into a marmoset model with only inflammatory lesions (Genain et al. 1995) support this concept. The remarkable clinical effect of the B cell-depleting antibody rituximab, specific for human CD20, was therefore not completely unexpected (Hauser et al. 2008). However, as in clinical trials circulating antibody levels are usually not affected by treatment with anti-CD20 antibody, there is still uncertainty about a mechanistic explanation of the clinical effect (Barun and Bar-Or 2012). We have taken advantage of the availability of a clinically relevant anti-CD20 antibody that cross-reacts with marmoset CD20, HuMab 7D8, which is closely related to the fully human anti-CD20 antibody ofatumumab. A single intravenous injection of the antibody induced rapid and sustained systemic depletion of B cells in marmosets (Kap et al. 2008). The clinical efficacy of the antibody was tested in the rhMOG/CFA-induced EAE model, demonstrating that B cell depletion after the onset of autoantibody production (postsensitization day (psd) 21) led to complete abrogation of EAE development (Kap et al. 2008). Interestingly, the impressive clinical effect was associated with marked suppression of demyelination in white as well as gray matter (Kap et al. 2011). Importantly, we also observed impaired activation of MOG_{34-56}-specific T cells, which comprise a subset of T cells, engaged in the antibody-nondependent induction of CNS pathology and neurological deficits (Kap et al. 2008; Jagessar et al. 2010). This obviously raises the question whether the direct activation by B cells of an autoantibody-non-dependent pathway towards clinically evident EAE could provide a mechanistic explanation for the clinical effect of the anti-CD20 antibody. Thus, we repeated the experiment in the MOG_{34-56}/IFA model. Indeed, we observed complete suppression of EAE development as well as of CNS pathology (Jagessar et al. 2012c).

Treatment 3 Treatment with interferon-γ suppresses disease development in most Th1-driven rodent EAE models (Sanvito et al. 2010). However, we observed no clinical effect of the cytokine in the MOG_{34-56}/IFA model, neither as a prophylactic nor as a therapeutic treatment, although modulation of several Th1-associated autoimmune parameters was observed (Jagessar et al. 2012a).

14.6 A Paradigm Switch for MS: Response-to-Injury

According to a widely accepted concept, autoimmunity in MS is caused by the interaction of environmental and genetic factors. GWA studies show a dominant influence of genes involved in cellular immune mechanisms, such as the MHC class II region and polymorphisms, in the promoter regions of the cytokine receptors IL-2R and IL-7R (Sawcer et al. 2011). Suspected environmental factors comprise infections, smoking, and vitamin D insufficiency (van der Mei et al. 2011). Although no single pathogen has been definitively identified as a trigger of MS, the combination of *HLA-DRB*1501* positivity and infection with EBV seems to imply a markedly elevated risk of MS (De Jager et al. 2008). However, in the absence of undisputed evidence for an infectious cause of MS, for which we have coined the term "response-to-infection," other concepts deserve consideration ('t Hart et al. 2009).

The marmoset EAE model shows a disconnection between immune events operating in early- and late-stage disease. We observed that the expression of neurological deficit is associated with the activation of T cells that display characteristics of effector memory cells. These are present in the normal repertoire of primates, but not of EAE-susceptible mouse strains, such as Biozzi ABH and C57BL6, and can be activated by immunization with a single peptide in IFA (Jagessar et al. 2010).

Along another research line, we have shown in mouse and marmoset EAE models that in the course of EAE, CNS myelin degradation products are released from the CNS and appear in the cervical and lumbar lymph nodes, where they can be found within APC, some of which are DC-SIGN^{+}, localizing in T cell areas (de Vos et al. 2002; van Zwam et al. 2009a). We also showed (in the chronic relapsing Biozzi ABH mouse model) that surgical removal of cervical and lumbar lymph nodes after the acute phase impairs the subsequent relapse rate (van Zwam 2009b). These and other findings have led us to postulate that the autoimmunity in MS may not be a "response-to-infection" but rather a "response-to-injury" ('t Hart et al. 2009).

This latter concept essentially proposes that:

1. The primary cause of MS is an event within the CNS that causes myelin injury. This event can be pathological, such as ischemia or infection, or nonpathological, such as age-associated degeneration of myelin and oligodendrocytes (Bartzokis 2004).
2. The ensuing activation of cellular and humoral autoimmune mechanisms results from an immune hyperreaction against the self-antigens released from this primary CNS lesion. We hypothesize that the immune hyperreaction is caused by the interaction of genetic factors and infectious pathogens. The finding that the specific MOG_{34-56} epitope of cytotoxic T cells in marmosets (MOG_{40-48}; YRSPFSRV) and rhesus monkeys (MOG_{39-46}; WYRPPFSRV) share sequence similarity with peptide 986–993 of the immunodominant UL86 (WLRSPFSRV) antigen of primate cytomegalovirus (CMV) and that the peptide MOG_{34-56} and $UL86_{981-1003}$ induce a cross-reactive CD8 T cell response in rhesus monkeys has drawn our attention to CMV.

On the side of genetics, it is noteworthy that the peptide MOG_{35-55} is immunogenic in mice expressing the MS-associated DR2 allele HLA-DRB1*1501 (Rich et al. 2004) suggesting that this MHC allele selects encephalitogenic epitopes of the peptide for presentation to T cells. Human and mouse MOG_{35-55}, which only differ at position 42, where the mouse peptide is occupied by S and the human peptide by P, differ in encephalitogenic potential and HLA-DRB1*1501 binding, suggesting that position 42 is part of the encephalitogenic CD4 T cell epitope. This is in line with the identification of MOG_{37-48} as putative CD4^{+} T cell epitope in the marmoset EAE model (Jagessar et al. 2012b). It is thus conceivable that the mimicry epitope encompassed within the CD8^{+} T cell epitope MOG_{39-48} may be immunodominant in HLA-DRB1*1501 positive humans.

On the side of infection, it is of note that UL86 is an immunodominant antigen of CMV engaging an impressive proportion of the effector memory compartment, $\pm 1.5\,\%$ of CD4 and $\pm 0.5\,\%$ of CD8 (Sylwester et al. 2005). This may imply that HLA-DRB1*1501^{+} individuals have a high frequency of effector memory T cells specific for MOG_{34-56} in their repertoire. The data reported by Bielekova et al. (2004) point into that direction. The "response-to-injury paradigm" postulates that these T cells are activated by MOG draining from injured CNS white matter.

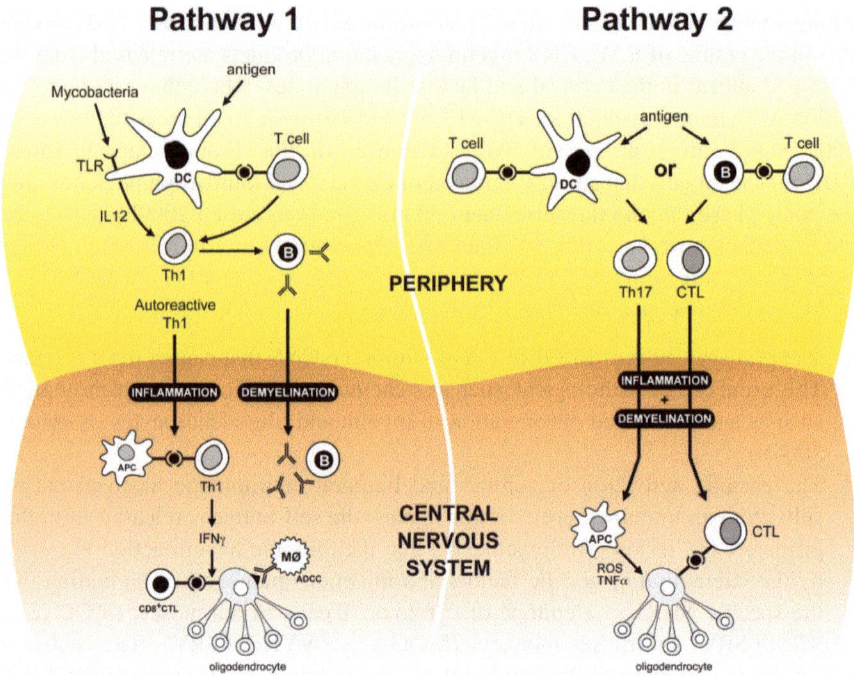

Fig. 14.3 Two pathogenic pathways operating in the marmoset EAE model. The development of EAE in marmosets immunized with rhMOG/CFA involves two separate pathways. Pathway 1 is active in the initiation of the disease as in classical mouse and rat EAE models, comprising the synergy of Th1 cells inducing inflammation and autoantibodies inducing demyelination. Pathway 2 is mediated by IL-17-producing and cytotoxic T cells, which induce demyelination of white and gray matter without support of autoantibodies. The model depicted in Fig. 14.2 is driven by pathway 2

14.7 Concluding Remarks

As discussed in more detail elsewhere, we postulate that the "response-to-injury paradigm" may help understand several open questions in MS, which are not explained by the "response-to-infection paradigm" ('t Hart and Weissert 2011). These issues include: (1) the notion that multiple factors may be responsible for triggering of MS rather than a single infection, (2) the observation that oligodendrogliopathy (Barnett and Sutton 2006) and focal activation of microglia (van der Valk and Amor 2009) precedes the CNS infiltration of immune cells, and (3) the poor efficacy of immunomodulatory treatment.

We believe that virus infections have an important role in MS, albeit not as an environmental trigger, but by creating a repertoire of cytotoxic effector memory T cells (CMV or other opportunistic infections) and by making B cells capable of activating these cytotoxic MHC-E-restricted T cells (EBV). In this concept, CNS infection can be a cause of the primary CNS injury, but other factors can be equally important.

The marmoset EAE model shows the existence of two distinct pathways leading to the same end point, i.e., demyelination of gray and white matter and irreversible neurological deficit (10; Fig. 14.3). One pathway includes a Th1-mediated pathogenic mechanism that starts with the activation of naive T cells by immunization with rhMOG or MOG_{34-56} in CFA. This classical autoantibody-dependent pathway develops more or less similarly in mice and marmosets. This is illustrated by similar beneficial effects of anti-IL-12p40 antibody.

There is, however, an alternative pathway where T cells mediate antibody-nondependent demyelination of white and gray matter. The pathogenic T cells are likely effector memory cells that are already committed to encephalitogenicity. This pathway is activated at a late stage in the rhMOG/CFA model, but is also directly activated in the MOG_{34-56}/IFA model. These T cells are relatively insensitive to treatments targeting their functional commitment, such as IFNγ (De Jager et al. 2008), IL-12/23 neutralization, or costimulation blockade (CD40; 't Hart et al. 2005c). It is tempting to speculate, albeit not proven, that these are the T cells operating in already established MS.

Acknowledgments The authors like to thank Mr. Henk van Westbroek for the artwork.

References

Abbott DH, Barnett DK, Colman RJ, Yamamoto ME, Schultz-Darken NJ (2003) Aspects of common marmoset basic biology and life history important for biomedical research. Comp Med 53:339–350

Alvord EC Jr (1984) Species-restricted encephalitogenic determinants. Prog Clin Biol Res 146:523–537

Antunes SG, Groot NG de, Brok H, Doxiadis G, Menezes AA, Otting N, Bontrop RE (1998) The common marmoset: a new world primate species with limited Mhc class II variability. Proc Natl Acad Sci U S A 95:11745–11750

Averdam A, Seelke S, Grutzner I, Rosner C, Roos C, Westphal N, Stahl-Hennig C, Muppala V, Schrod A, Sauermann U, Dressel R, Walter L (2007) Genotyping and segregation analyses indicate the presence of only two functional MIC genes in rhesus macaques. Immunogenetics 59:247–251

Axtell RC, Jong BA de, Boniface K, Voort LF van der, Bhat R, De Sarno P, Naves R, Han M, Zhong F, Castellanos JG, Mair R, Christakos A, Kolkowitz I, Katz L, Killestein J, Polman CH, Waal Malefyt R de, Steinman L, Raman C (2010) T helper type 1 and 17 cells determine efficacy of interferon-beta in multiple sclerosis and experimental encephalomyelitis. Nat Med 16:406–412

Axthelm MK, Bourdette DN, Marracci GH, Su W, Mullaney ET, Manoharan M, Kohama SG, Pollaro J, Witkowski E, Wang P, Rooney WD, Sherman LS, Wong SW (2011) Japanese macaque encephalomyelitis: a spontaneous multiple sclerosis-like disease in a nonhuman primate. Ann Neurol 70(3):362–373

Bajramovic JJ, Brok HP, Ouwerling B, Jagessar SA, Straalen L van, Kondova I, Bauer J, Amor S, Hart BA, Ben-Nun A (2008) Oligodendrocyte-specific protein is encephalitogenic in rhesus macaques and induces specific demyelination of the optic nerve. Eur J Immunol 38:1452–1464

Barnett MH, Sutton I (2006) The pathology of multiple sclerosis: a paradigm shift. Curr Opin Neurol 19:242–247

Bartzokis G (2004) Age-related myelin breakdown: a developmental model of cognitive decline and Alzheimer's disease. Neurobiol Aging 25:5–18; author reply 49–62

Barun B, Bar-Or A (2012) Treatment of multiple sclerosis with Anti-CD20 antibodies. Clin Immunol 142:31–37

Bielekova B, Sung MH, Kadom N, Simon R, McFarland H, Martin R (2004) Expansion and functional relevance of high-avidity myelin-specific CD4+ T cells in multiple sclerosis. J Immunol 172:3893–3904

Brok HP, Uccelli A, Kerlero De Rosbo N, Bontrop RE, Roccatagliata L, Groot NG de, Capello E, Laman JD, Nicolay K, Mancardi GL, Ben-Nun A, 't Hart BA (2000) Myelin/oligodendrocyte glycoprotein-induced autoimmune encephalomyelitis in common marmosets: the encephalitogenic T cell epitope pMOG24–36 is presented by a monomorphic MHC class II molecule. J Immunol 165:1093–1101

Brok HP, Bauer J, Jonker M, Blezer E, Amor S, Bontrop RE, Laman JD, 't Hart BA (2001a) Non-human primate models of multiple sclerosis. Immunol Rev 183:173–185

Brok HP, Hornby RJ, Griffiths GD, Scott LA, 't Hart BA (2001b) An extensive monoclonal antibody panel for the phenotyping of leukocyte subsets in the common marmoset and the cotton-top tamarin. Cytometry 45:294–303

Brok HP, Van Meurs M, Blezer E, Schantz A, Peritt D, Treacy G, Laman JD, Bauer J, 't Hart BA (2002) Prevention of experimental autoimmune encephalomyelitis in common marmosets using an anti-IL-12p40 monoclonal antibody. J Immunol 169:6554–6563

Brok HP, Boven L, Meurs M van, Kerlero de Rosbo N, Celebi-Paul L, Kap YS, Jagessar A, Hintzen RQ, Keir G, Bajramovic J, Ben-Nun A, Bauer J, Laman JD, Amor S, 't Hart BA (2007) The human CMV-UL86 peptide 981–1003 shares a crossreactive T-cell epitope with the encephalitogenic MOG peptide 34–56, but lacks the capacity to induce EAE in rhesus monkeys. J Neuroimmunol 182:135–152

Cadavid LF, Shufflebotham C, Ruiz FJ, Yeager M, Hughes AL, Watkins DI (1997) Evolutionary instability of the major histocompatibility complex class I loci in New World primates. Proc Natl Acad Sci U S A 94:14536–14541

De Jager PL, Simon KC, Munger KL, Rioux JD, Hafler DA, Ascherio A (2008) Integrating risk factors: HLA-DRB1*1501 and Epstein-Barr virus in multiple sclerosis. Neurology 70:1113–1118

de Vos AF, Meurs M van, Brok HP, Boven LA, Hintzen RQ, Valk P van der, Ravid R, Rensing S, Boon L, 't Hart BA, Laman JD (2002) Transfer of central nervous system autoantigens and presentation in secondary lymphoid organs. J Immunol 169:5415–5423

Doxiadis GG, Wiel MK van der, Brok HP, Groot NG de, Otting N, 't Hart BA, Rood JJ van, Bontrop RE (2006) Reactivation by exon shuffling of a conserved HLA-DR3-like pseudogene segment in a New World primate species. Proc Natl Acad Sci U S A 103:5864–5868

Fujinami RS, Herrath MG von, Christen U, Whitton JL (2006) Molecular mimicry, bystander activation, or viral persistence: infections and autoimmune disease. Clin Microbiol Rev 19:80–94

Geijtenbeek TB, Van Vliet SJ, Engering A, 't Hart BA, Van Kooyk Y (2004) Self- and nonself-recognition by C-type lectins on dendritic cells. Annu Rev Immunol 22:33–54

Genain CP, Lee-Parritz D, Nguyen MH, Massacesi L, Joshi N, Ferrante R, Hoffman K, Moseley M, Letvin NL, Hauser SL (1994) In healthy primates, circulating autoreactive T cells mediate autoimmune disease. J Clin Invest 94:1339–1345

Genain CP, Nguyen MH, Letvin NL, Pearl R, Davis RL, Adelman M, Lees MB, Linington C, Hauser SL (1995) Antibody facilitation of multiple sclerosis-like lesions in a nonhuman primate. J Clin Invest 96:2966–2974

Genain CP, Cannella B, Hauser SL, Raine CS (1999) Identification of autoantibodies associated with myelin damage in multiple sclerosis. Nat Med 5:170–175

Haanstra KG, Jagessar SA, Bauchet AL, Doussau M, Fovet CM, Heijmans N, Hofman SO, van Lubeek-Veth J, Bajramovic JJ, Kap YS, Laman JD, Touin H, Watroba L, Bauer J, Lachapelle F, Serguera C, 't Hart BA (2013) Induction of experimental autoimmune encephalomyelitis with recombinant human myelin oligodendrocyte glycoprotein in incomplete Freund's adjuvant in three non-human primate species. J Neuroimmune Pharmacol (in press)

Haig D (1999) What is a marmoset? Am J Primatol 49:285–296

Hauser SL, Waubant E, Arnold DL, Vollmer T, Antel J, Fox RJ, Bar-Or A, Panzara M, Sarkar N, Agarwal S, Langer-Gould A, and C. Smith H (2008) B-cell depletion with rituximab in relapsing-remitting multiple sclerosis. N Engl J Med 358:676–688

Jagessar SA, Smith PA, Blezer E, Delarasse C, Pham-Dinh D, Laman JD, Bauer J, Amor S, 't Hart BA (2008) Autoimmunity against myelin oligodendrocyte glycoprotein is dispensable for the initiation although essential for the progression of chronic encephalomyelitis in common marmosets. J Neuropathol Exp Neurol 67:326–340

Jagessar SA, Kap YS, Heijmans N, Driel N van, Brok HPM, Blezer ELA, Laman JD, Bauer J, 't Hart BA (2010) Induction of progressive demyelinating autoimmune encephalomyelitis in common marmoset monkeys using MOG34–56 peptide in incomplete Freund's adjuvant. J Neuropathol Exp Neurol 69:372–385

Jagessar SA, Gran B, Heijmans N, Bauer J, Laman JD, 't Hart BA, Constantinescu CS (2012a) Discrepant effects of human interferon-gamma on clinical and immunological disease parameters in a novel marmoset model for multiple sclerosis. J Neuroimmune Pharmacol 7(1):253–265

Jagessar SA, Heijmans N, Blezer EL, Bauer J, Blokhuis JH, Wubben JA, Drijfhout JW, den Elsen PJ van, Laman JD, Hart BA (2012b) Unravelling the T-cell-mediated autoimmune attack on CNS myelin in a new primate EAE model induced with MOG(34–56) peptide in incomplete adjuvant. Eur J Immunol 42:217–227

Jagessar SA, Heijmans N, Bauer J, Blezer ELA, Laman JD, Hellings N, 't Hart BA (2012c) B-cell depletion abrogates antibody nondependent CNS demyelination in the marmoset EAE model. J Immunol (resubmitted)

Jensen PE, Sullivan BA, Reed-Loisel LM, Weber DA (2004) Qa-1, a nonclassical class I histocompatibility molecule with roles in innate and adaptive immunity. Immunol Res 29:81–92

Kabat EA, Wolf A, Bezer AE (1947) The rapid production of acute disseminated encephalomyelitis in rhesus monkeys by injection of heterologous and homologous brain tissue with adjuvants. J Exp Med 85:117–130

Kap YS, Smith P, Jagessar SA, Remarque E, Blezer E, Strijkers GJ, Laman JD, Hintzen RQ, Bauer J, Brok HP, 't Hart BA (2008) Fast progression of recombinant human myelin/oligodendrocyte glycoprotein (MOG)-induced experimental autoimmune encephalomyelitis in marmosets is associated with the activation of MOG34–56-specific cytotoxic T cells. J Immunol 180:1326–1337

Kap YS, Laman JD, 't Hart BA (2010) Experimental autoimmune encephalomyelitis in the common marmoset, a bridge between rodent EAE and multiple sclerosis for immunotherapy development. J Neuroimmune Pharmacol 5:220–230

Kap YS, Bauer J, Driel NV, Bleeker WK, Parren PW, Kooi EJ, Geurts JJ, Laman JD, Craigen JL, Blezer E, 't Hart BA (2011) B-Cell Depletion Attenuates White and Gray Matter Pathology in Marmoset Experimental Autoimmune Encephalomyelitis. J Neuropathol Exp Neurol 70:992–1005

Kerlero de Rosbo N, Brok HP, Bauer J, Kaye JF, 't Hart BA, Ben-Nun A (2000) Rhesus monkeys are highly susceptible to experimental autoimmune encephalomyelitis induced by myelin oligodendrocyte glycoprotein: characterisation of immunodominant T- and B-cell epitopes. J Neuroimmunol 110:83–96

Lopez-Diego RS, Weiner HL (2008) Novel therapeutic strategies for multiple sclerosis–a multifaceted adversary. Nat Rev Drug Discov 7:909–925

Lyons AB (2000) Analysing cell division in vivo and in vitro using flow cytometric measurement of CFSE dye dilution. J Immunol Methods 243:147–154

Mansfield K (2003) Marmoset models commonly used in biomedical research. Comp Med 53:383–392

Massacesi L, Joshi N, Lee-Parritz D, Rombos A, Letvin NL, Hauser SL (1992) Experimental allergic encephalomyelitis in cynomolgus monkeys. Quantitation of T cell responses in peripheral blood. J Clin Invest 90:399–404

Massacesi L, Genain CP, Lee-Parritz D, Letvin NL, Canfield D, Hauser SL (1995) Active and passively induced experimental autoimmune encephalomyelitis in common marmosets: a new model for multiple sclerosis. Ann Neurol 37:519–530

McFarland HI, Lobito AA, Johnson MM, Nyswaner JT, Frank JA, Palardy GR, Tresser N, Genain CP, Mueller JP, Matis LA, Lenardo MJ (1999) Determinant spreading associated with demyelination in a nonhuman primate model of multiple sclerosis. J Immunol 162:2384–2390

Mills KH (2011) TLR-dependent T cell activation in autoimmunity. Nature reviews. Immunology 11:807–822

Ransohoff RM (2006) EAE: pitfalls outweigh virtues of screening potential treatments for multiple sclerosis. Trends Immunol 27:167–168

Rivers TM, Schwenkter FF (1935) Encephalomyelitis accompanied by myelin destruction experimentally produced in monkeys. J Exp Med 61:698–703

Raine CS, Cannella B, Hauser SL, Genain CP (1999) Demyelination in primate autoimmune encephalomyelitis and acute multiple sclerosis lesions: a case for antigen-specific antibody mediation. Ann Neurol 46:144–160

Rich C, Link JM, Zamora A, Jacobsen H, Meza-Romero R, Offner H, Jones R, Burrows GG, Fugger L, Vandenbark AA (2004) Myelin oligodendrocyte glycoprotein-35–55 peptide induces severe chronic experimental autoimmune encephalomyelitis in HLA-DR2-transgenic mice. Eur J Immunol 34:1251–1261

Rivers TM, Sprunt DH, Berry GP (1933) Observations on the attempts to produce acute disseminated allergic encephalomyelitis in primates. J Exp Med 58:39–53

Rose LM, Richards TL, Peterson J, Petersen R, Alvord EC Jr (1997) Resolution of CNS lesions following treatment of experimental allergic encephalomyelitis in macaques with monoclonal antibody to the CD18 leukocyte integrin. Mult Scler 2:259–266

Segal BM, Constantinescu CS, Raychaudhuri A, Kim L, Fidelus-Gort R, Kasper LH (2008) Repeated subcutaneous injections of IL12/23 p40 neutralising antibody, ustekinumab, in patients with relapsing-remitting multiple sclerosis: a phase II, double-blind, placebo-controlled, randomised, dose-ranging study. Lancet Neurol 7:796–804

Sanvito L, Constantinescu CS, Gran B, 't Hart BA (2010) The multifaceted role of interferon-γ in central nervous system autoimmune demyelination. Open Autoimmun J 2:151–159

Sawcer S, Hellenthal G, Pirinen M, Spencer CC, Patsopoulos NA, Moutsianas L, Dilthey A, Su Z, Freeman C, Hunt SE, Edkins S, Gray E, Booth DR, Potter SC, Goris A, Band G, Oturai AB, Strange A, Saarela J, Bellenguez C, Fontaine B, Gillman M, Hemmer B, Gwilliam R, Zipp F, Jayakumar A, Martin R, Leslie S, Hawkins S, Giannoulatou E, D'Alfonso S, Blackburn H, Boneschi FM, Liddle J, Harbo HF, Perez ML, Spurkland A, Waller MJ, Mycko MP, Ricketts M, Comabella M, Hammond N, Kockum I, McCann OT, Ban M, Whittaker P, Kemppinen A, Weston P, Hawkins C, Widaa S, Zajicek J, Dronov S, Robertson N, Bumpstead SJ, Barcellos LF, Ravindrarajah R, Abraham R, Alfredsson L, Ardlie K, Aubin C, Baker A, Baker K, Baranzini SE, Bergamaschi L, Bergamaschi R, Bernstein A, Berthele A, Boggild M, Bradfield JP, Brassat D, Broadley SA, Buck D, Butzkueven H, Capra R, Carroll WM, Cavalla P, Celius EG, Cepok S, Chiavacci R, Clerget-Darpoux F, Clysters K, Comi G, Cossburn M, Cournu-Rebeix I, Cox MB, Cozen W, Cree BA, Cross AH, Cusi D, Daly MJ, Davis E, Bakker PI de, Debouverie M, D'Hooghe BM, Dixon K, Dobosi R, Dubois B, Ellinghaus D, Elovaara I, Esposito F, Fontenille C, Foote S, Franke A, Galimberti D, Ghezzi A, Glessner J, Gomez R, Gout O, Graham C, Grant SF, Guerini FR, Hakonarson H, Hall P, Hamsten A, Hartung HP, Heard RN, Heath S, Hobart J, Hoshi M, Infante-Duarte C, Ingram G, Ingram W, Islam T, Jagodic M, Kabesch M, Kermode AG, Kilpatrick TJ, Kim C, Klopp N, Koivisto K, Larsson M, Lathrop M, Lechner-Scott JS, Leone MA, Leppa V, Liljedahl U, Bomfim IL, Lincoln RR, Link J, Liu J, Lorentzen AR, Lupoli S, Macciardi F, Mack T, Marriott M, Martinelli V, Mason D, McCauley JL, Mentch F, Mero IL, Mihalova T, Montalban X, Mottershead J, Myhr KM, Naldi P, Ollier W, Page A, Palotie A, Pelletier J, Piccio L, Pickersgill T, Piehl F, Pobywajlo S, Quach HL, Ramsay PP, Reunanen M, Reynolds R, Rioux JD, Rodegher M, Roesner S, Rubio JP, Ruckert IM, Salvetti M, Salvi E, Santaniello A, Schaefer CA, Schreiber S, Schulze C, Scott RJ, Sellebjerg F, Selmaj KW, Sexton D, Shen L, Simms-Acuna B, Skidmore S, Sleiman PM, Smestad C, Sorensen PS, Sondergaard HB, Stankovich J, Strange RC, Sulonen AM, Sundqvist E, Syvanen AC, Taddeo F, Taylor B, Blackwell JM, Tienari P, Bramon E, Tourbah A, Brown MA, Tronczynska E, Casas JP, Tubridy N, Corvin A, Vickery J, Jankowski J, Villoslada P, Markus HS, Wang K, Mathew CG, Wason J, Palmer CN, Wichmann HE, Plomin R, Willoughby E, Rautanen A, Winkelmann J, Wittig M, Trembath RC, Yaouanq J, Viswanathan AC, Zhang H, Wood NW, Zuvich R, Deloukas P, Langford C, Duncanson A, Oksenberg JR, Pericak-Vance MA, Haines JL, Olsson T, Hillert J, Ivinson AJ, De Jager PL, Peltonen L, Stewart GJ, Hafler DA, Hauser SL, McVean G, Donnelly P, Compston A (2011) Genetic risk and a primary role for cell-mediated immune mechanisms in multiple sclerosis. Nature 476:214–219

Shiina T, Kono A, Westphal N, Suzuki S, Hosomichi K, Kita YF, Roos C, Inoko H, Walter L (2011) Comparative genome analysis of the major histocompatibility complex (MHC) class I B/C segments in primates elucidated by genomic sequencing in common marmoset (*Callithrix jacchus*). Immunogenetics 63:485–499

Slierendregt BL, Hall M, 't Hart B, Otting N, Anholts J, Verduin W, Claas F, Jonker M, Lanchbury JS, Bontrop RE (1995) Identification of an Mhc-DPB1 allele involved in susceptibility to experimental autoimmune encephalomyelitis in rhesus macaques. Int Immunol 7:1671–1679

Smith PA, Heijmans N, Ouwerling B, Breij EC, Evans N, Noort JM van, Plomp AC, Delarasse C, Hart B, Pham-Dinh D, Amor S (2005) Native myelin oligodendrocyte glycoprotein promotes severe chronic neurological disease and demyelination in Biozzi ABH mice. Eur J Immunol 35:1311–1319

Sriram S, Steiner I (2005) Experimental allergic encephalomyelitis: A misleading model of multiple sclerosis. Ann Neurol 58:939–945

Steinman L, Zamvil SS (2005) Virtues and pitfalls of EAE for the development of therapies for multiple sclerosis. Trends Immunol 26:565–571

Steinman L, Zamvil SS (2006) How to successfully apply animal studies in experimental allergic encephalomyelitis to research on multiple sclerosis. Ann Neurol 60:12–21

Stuart G, Krikorian KS. (1933) Neuroparalytic accidents complicating antirabic treatment. Br Med J 1:501–504

Sylwester AW, Mitchell BL, Edgar JB, Taormina C, Pelte C, Ruchti F, Sleath PR, Grabstein KH, Hosken NA, Kern F, Nelson JA, Picker LJ (2005) Broadly targeted human cytomegalovirus-specific CD4 + and CD8 + T cells dominate the memory compartments of exposed subjects. J Exp Med 202:673–685

't Hart BA, van Y Kooyk. (2004) Yin-Yang regulation of autoimmunity by DCs. Trends Immunol 25:353–359

't Hart BA, Massacesi L (2009) Clinical, pathological, and immunologic aspects of the multiple sclerosis model in common marmosets (*Callithrix jacchus*). J Neuropathol Exp Neurol 68:341–355

't Hart BA, Bauer J, Muller HJ, Melchers B, Nicolay K, Brok H, Bontrop RE, Lassmann H, Massacesi L (1998) Histopathological characterization of magnetic resonance imaging-detectable brain white matter lesions in a primate model of multiple sclerosis: a correlative study in the experimental autoimmune encephalomyelitis model in common marmosets (*Callithrix jacchus*). Am J Pathol 153:649–663

't Hart B, Amor S, Jonker M (2004) Evaluating the validity of animal models for research into therapies for immune-based disorders. Drug Discov Today 9:517–524

't Hart BA, Bauer J, Brok HP, Amor S (2005a) Non-human primate models of experimental autoimmune encephalomyelitis: variations on a theme. J Neuroimmunol 168:1–12

't Hart BA, Brok HP, Remarque E, Benson J, Treacy G, Amor S, Hintzen RQ, Laman JD, Bauer J, Blezer EL (2005b) Suppression of ongoing disease in a nonhuman primate model of multiple sclerosis by a human-anti-human IL-12p40 antibody. J Immunol 175:4761–4768

't Hart BA, Blezer EL, Brok HP, Boon L, Boer M de, Bauer J, Laman JD (2005c) Treatment with chimeric anti-human CD40 antibody suppresses MRI-detectable inflammation and enlargement of pre-existing brain lesions in common marmosets affected by MOG-induced EAE. J Neuroimmunol 163:31–39

't Hart BA, Hintzen RQ, Laman JD (2009) Multiple sclerosis—a response-to-damage model. Trends Mol Med 15:235–244

't Hart BA, Gran B, Weissert R (2011) EAE: imperfect but useful models of multiple sclerosis. Trends Mol Med 17:119–125

Tardif SD, Smucny DA, Abbott DH, Mansfield K, Schultz-Darken N, Yamamoto ME (2003) Reproduction in captive common marmosets (*Callithrix jacchus*). Comp Med 53:364–368

Teitelbaum D, Aharoni R, Klinger E, Kreitman R, Raymond E, Malley A, Shofti R, Sela M, Arnon R (2004) Oral glatiramer acetate in experimental autoimmune encephalomyelitis: clinical and immunological studies. Ann N Y Acad Sci 1029:239–249

Uccelli A, Oksenberg JR, Jeong MC, Genain CP, Rombos T, Jaeger EE, Giunti D, Lanchbury JS, Hauser SL (1997) Characterization of the TCRB chain repertoire in the New World monkey *Callithrix jacchus*. J Immunol 158:1201–1207

van der Mei IA, Simpson S Jr, Stankovich J, Taylor BV (2011) Individual and joint action of environmental factors and risk of MS. Neurol Clin 29:233–255

van der Valk P, Amor S (2009) Preactive lesions in multiple sclerosis. Curr Opin Neurol 22:207–213

van Lambalgen R, Jonker M (1987a) Experimental allergic encephalomyelitis in rhesus monkeys: I. Immunological parameters in EAE resistant and susceptible rhesus monkeys. Clin Exp Immunol 68:100–107

van Lambalgen R, Jonker M (1987b) Experimental allergic encephalomyelitis in rhesus monkeys: II. Treatment of EAE with anti-T lymphocyte subset monoclonal antibodies. Clin Exp Immunol 68:305–312

van Zwam M, Huizinga R, Melief MJ, Wierenga-Wolf AF, Meurs M van, Voerman JS, Biber KP, Boddeke HW, Hopken UE, Meisel C, Meisel A, Bechmann I, Hintzen RQ, 't Hart BA, Amor S, Laman JD, Boven AL (2009a) Brain antigens in functionally distinct antigen-presenting cell populations in cervical lymph nodes in MS and EAE. J Mol Med 87:273–286

van Zwam M, Huizinga R, Heijmans N, Meurs M van, Wierenga-Wolf AF, Melief MJ, Hintzen RQ, 't Hart BA, Amor S, Boven LA, Laman DJ (2009b) Surgical excision of CNS-draining lymph nodes reduces relapse severity in chronic-relapsing experimental autoimmune encephalomyelitis. J Pathol 217:543–551

von Budingen HC, Hauser SL, Nabavi CB, Genain CP (2001) Characterization of the expressed immunoglobulin IGHV repertoire in the new world marmoset *Callithrix jacchus*. Immunogenetics 53:557–563

Vierboom MP, Jonker M, Bontrop RE, 't Hart BA (2005) Modeling human arthritic diseases in nonhuman primates. Arthritis Res Ther 7:145–154

Vierboom MP, Breedveld E, Kondova I, 't Hart BA (2010) Collagen-induced arthritis in common marmosets: a new nonhuman primate model for chronic arthritis. Arthritis Res Ther 12:R200

Villoslada P, Abel K, Heald N, Goertsches R, Hauser SL, Genain CP (2001) Frequency, heterogeneity and encephalitogenicity of T cells specific for myelin oligodendrocyte glycoprotein in naive outbred primates. Eur J Immunol 31:2942–2950

Chapter 15
A Novel Concept of Treatment in MS: Targeting Both Oligodendrocyte Death and Inflammatory Processes by Inhibiting Poly(Adp-Ribose) Polymerase

Zsolt Illes, Hans Lassmann and Ferenc Gallyas

15.1 Multiple Sclerosis: Mitochondrial Injury

The pathology of multiple sclerosis (MS) was originally defined by inflammation, focal primary demyelination in the white matter, and astrocytic gliosis. This plaque-centered view of MS pathology has been revised during the last years (Lassmann et al. 2007). It became clear that pathology is not restricted to focal white matter lesions, but that demyelination may also affect the gray matter, most prominently the cerebral and cerebellar cortex (Peterson et al. 2001; Kutzelnigg et al. 2005). In addition, there is a diffuse and global damage in the normal appearing white and gray matter, which increases with disease duration and age of the patients (Kutzelnigg et al. 2005). Both white and gray matter lesions can in part become repaired by remyelination (Patrikios et al. 2006; Albert et al. 2007). Pathological alterations within the MS brain are highly heterogeneous, depending in part on the activity and stage of evolution of focal demyelinated lesions (Lassmann 2011a), on their location within the brain gray or white matter (Geurts and Barkhof 2008), and on the stage of the disease when they arise (Kutzelnigg et al. 2005). In addition, an interindividual heterogeneity of active lesions can be seen between patients even when other contributing factors are excluded (Lucchinetti et al. 2000). Despite this

Z. Illes (✉)
Department of Neurology and Institute of Clinical Research, University of Southern Denmark, Odense, Denmark
e-mail: zsolt.illes@rsyd.dk

Department of Neurology, University of Pecs Medical School, Pecs, Hungary

H. Lassmann
Center for Brain Research, Medical University of Vienna, Vienna, Austria

F. Gallyas
Department of Biochemistry and Medical Chemistry, University of Pecs Medical School, Pecs, Hungary

Nuclear-Mitochondrial Interactions Research Group, Hungarian Academy of Sciences, Budapest, Hungary

T. Yamamura, B. Gran (eds.), *Multiple Sclerosis Immunology*,
DOI 10.1007/978-1-4614-7953-6_15, © Springer Science+Business Media New York 2013

profound heterogeneity in MS pathology, there are some general features, which are similar in all patients and all types of lesions. Inflammation is invariably dominated by CD8+ T cells, activated macrophages, and microglia (Babbe et al. 2000). In contrast to most other inflammatory diseases of the central nervous system (CNS), inflammation in MS is associated with primary demyelination and oligodendrocyte apoptosis (Barnett and Prineas 2004). Axons are destroyed in variable extent, but these are always the thin-caliber axons, which are predominantly affected (Evangelou et al. 2001; Trapp and Stys 2009). Remyelination may be extensive in some lesions, but it frequently fails in others (Patrikios et al. 2006) despite the presence of oligodendrocyte progenitor cells (OPCs; Chang et al. 2002). Finally, astrocytes in early lesions show increased cytoplasmic volume and expression of glial fibrillary acidic protein, which in patients with aggressive disease is associated with loss of cell polarity and cell processes as well as loss of molecules expressed in processes of the glia limitans (e.g., aquaporin 4; Sharma et al. 2010). These pathological alterations together are highly specific for MS. This raises the question whether they could be explained by a single pathogenetic mechanism. The data discussed here suggest that mitochondrial injury may reside in the center of the pathogenetic cascade in the MS brain.

The interest for mitochondria in MS pathogenesis was raised through several observations (Kalman 2006). In a subtype of patients with fulminate MS and highly active lesions, a type of pathology was found (Pattern III; Lucchinetti et al. 2000), which closely resembled that seen in acute white matter stroke lesions (Aboul Enein et al. 2003). Since this type of lesions occurred in the absence of vascular occlusions, it was assumed that histotoxic hypoxia due to mitochondrial injury may play a role. Another indication came from gene array studies of cortical tissue (Dutta et al. 2006), which showed a decreased expression for multiple mitochondrial genes. Furthermore, the selective destruction of thin-caliber axons in MS lesions suggested that energy deficiency subsequent to mitochondrial dysfunction may be involved in neurodegeneration (Stys 2005; Trapp and Stys 2009). Subsequent studies showed that the expression of certain mitochondrial proteins, in particular the COX1 molecule of Complex IV of the respiratory chain, is massively reduced in fulminate-active (Pattern III) MS lesions (Mahad et al. 2008), but that in chronic lesions mitochondrial numbers and enzyme activity in axons are increased (Mahad et al. 2009; Witte et al. 2009). The high number of mitochondria in demyelinated axons is reduced when remyelination occurs (Zambonin et al. 2011). The data suggest a complex scenario of mitochondrial injury in MS lesions. Mitochondrial damage is an important factor driving demyelination and neurodegeneration at sites of activity. However, in established lesions—in the absence of inflammation—the mitochondrial content in axons reflect their energy demand, which is highest in demyelinated fibers, lower in remyelination, and lowest in normal axons.

Interestingly, the molecular consequences of mitochondrial injury seem to be different for different cells and their processes. Using similar concentrations of mitochondrial toxins in vitro or by analyzing cell degeneration in lesions in vivo, mature oligodendrocytes (and their myelin sheaths) seem to be most susceptible followed in the order of magnitude by neurons and their processes, by OPCs, by astrocytes, and finally by macrophages and microglia. Energy deficiency seems to be a dominant trigger of axonal demise, leading to ionic imbalance, calcium influx, and activation of intra-axonal proteases (Trapp and Stys 2009). In nucleated cells, and in particular in oligodendrocytes, mitochondrial release of apoptosis- inducing factor (AIF) may trigger apoptotic cell death and secondary demyelination (Veto et al. 2010). In contrast, OPCs (and also astrocytes) survive mitochondrial toxin concentrations, which are sufficient to destroy mature oligodendrocytes, but the cells retract their cell processes and fail to myelinate in vitro (Ziabreva et al. 2010). Thus, most of the cardinal pathological features of MS lesions can be explained by a single mechanism: mitochondrial injury.

This raises the question on the cause of mitochondrial injury in MS lesions. In vitro studies have shown that oxygen and nitric oxide radicals or both together can induce mitochondrial injury in vitro and in vivo (Bolanos et al. 1997). In line with these data, profound oxidative modification of DNA, proteins, and lipids was reported in active MS lesions (Bizzozero et al. 2005; Vladimirova et al. 1998; Lu et al. 2000; Van Horssen et al. 2008), and it recently became clear that oxidized DNA and oxidized phospholipids label cells and axons in active MS plaques, which are in the process of being destroyed (Haider et al. 2011). Macrophages and microglia, which are activated in the course of the chronic inflammatory process, are likely to be the major source of radicals in active MS lesions. Active demyelination and neurodegeneration is invariably associated with inflammation in MS brains (Frischer et al. 2009). Activated microglia in (initial) active lesions express inducible nitric oxide synthase (Bagasra et al. 1995; Cross et al. 1998; Liu et al. 2001; Marik et al. 2007; Zeis et al. 2009), myeloperoxidase (Gray et al. 2008a, b; Marik et al. 2007), and NADPH oxidase complexes (NOX1 and NOX2; Fischer et al. 2012). However, radical production and toxicity can additionally be enhanced by the mitochondrial injury itself (Murphy 2009) as well as by the presence of divalent iron ions. Interestingly, iron accumulates in the human brain predominantly with age in oligodendrocytes (Hallgren and Sourander 1958) and will be liberated, when these cells are destroyed in the initial stages of plaque formation in MS brains. These amplification mechanisms may be particularly important in the progressive stage of the disease (Lassmann and van Horssen 2011).

15.2 Current Treatment Options of Multiple Sclerosis from the Point of Pathogenesis

Inflammation is present in the CNS of all patients with MS regardless of phenotype, duration, and other pathological characteristics. Inflammation is presumed to be autoimmune in origin, since in the inflammatory model of MS, experimental autoimmune encephalomyelitis (EAE), MS-like pathology and disease can be elicited by immunization with self-peptides of CNS myelin (Illes et al. 2004; Illes et al. 2005). Demyelination and loss of oligodendrocytes are partly related to the inflammation, but degenerative processes may be equally important

(Sriram 2011; Trapp and Nave 2008). Considering inflammation and oligodendrocyte loss, two main concepts have evolved. One emphasizes the heterogeneity of MS and indicates that either cellular (T cells and macrophages: pattern I) and humoral immune responses (antibodies and complement: pattern II) or profound oxidative injury associated with oligodendrocyte apoptosis (pattern III; Haider et al. 2011; Fischer et al. 2012) or oligodendrocyte dystrophy (pattern IV) are characteristic in different patients (Lucchinetti et al. 2000). This concept is supported by clinical experiences showing that all patients with pattern II, but none with pattern I or pattern III, achieved moderate to substantial functional neurological improvement after plasma exchange in fulminant CNS inflammatory demyelinating disease (Keegan et al. 2005). The other concept of MS pathogenesis suggests that every MS plaque starts with oligodendrocyte degeneration; in such scenario, the observed inflammation might be due to a secondary autoimmune phenomenon (Barnett and Prineas 2004). Nevertheless, we were unable to elicit such secondary autoimmune inflammation in MOG-specific TCR transgenic mice, where primary demyelination and oligodendrocyte loss was induced by cuprizone and complete Freund's adjuvant (CFA) was also given; in wild-type mice, administration of pertussis toxin and CFA during the peak of cuprizone-induced demyelination did not result in clinical signs of EAE and inflammatory alterations of the CNS either (*data not published*). Degenerative processes may be more important in the progressive types of MS, while inflammation predominates in the early phases; such dissection may be mirrored by reduction in number of relapses as the disease progresses (Vukusic and Confavreux 2007).

The current long-term treatment of MS aims to prevent both clinical relapses and progression of disability. Unfortunately, treatments used in the clinical practice have a modest impact on degenerative loss of axons, loss of oligodendrocytes, and demyelination, while profoundly influencing inflammation (Bates 2011). The first-line treatments, glatiramer acetate (GA), and interferon-β reduce the number of relapses by about one-third. But GA does not prevent disability progression (La Mantia et al. 2010), while the effect of interferon-β on disability progression is somewhat controversial, and the impact is minor at best (Bates 2011; La Mantia et al. 2012). Natalizumab, a humanized monoclonal antibody, prevents the transmigration of T cells to the CNS compartment and thus has a profound effect on inflammation, relapse rate, and active lesions on MRI (Pucci et al. 2011); nevertheless, short-term effect on disability progression is more modest (Weinstock-Guttman et al. 2011; Pucci et al. 2011). The oral fingolimod, which retains naive and central memory T cells within the lymph nodes due to downmodulation of sphingosine 1-phosphate (S1P) receptors, significantly reduces annualized relapse rate; but the risk of disability progression was not significant compared to placebo (Pinschewer et al. 2011; Devonshire et al. 2012). While much emphasis was put on the prevention of inflammation and degenerative axonal loss, prevention of demyelination and loss of oligodendrocytes were less explored. This would be important considering that pattern III and IV MS are characterized by profound loss of oligodendrocytes (Lucchinetti et al. 2000). Thus, treatments should target not only the inflammatory reaction but also aim to prevent oligodendrocyte loss and demyelination, or promote remyelination. The latter conception has already been addressed by the monoclonal antibody against lingo (Mi et al. 2007).

Ideally, treatments should target both inflammatory and primary/secondary degenerative processes, which may most probably improve the efficacy of treatments by both reducing relapses and preventing progression of disability. One possibility would be the combination of different therapies. On the other hand, one can target molecules, which are universally important in inflammation, cellular stress, degeneration, and apoptosis.

15.3 Role of Poly(ADP-ribose) Polymerase (PARP) and Mitochondria in Cell Death

Poly(ADP-ribose; PAR) polymerase-1 (PARP-1; EC 2.4.2.30) is a 116-kDa nuclear enzyme present in eukaryotes in high copy numbers. PARP-1 functions as a DNA damage sensor and signaling molecule binding to both single- and double-stranded DNA breaks. Upon binding to damaged DNA, PARP-1 forms homodimers and catalyzes the cleavage of NAD into nicotinamide and ADP-ribose using the latter to synthesize branched PAR polymers covalently attached to nuclear acceptor proteins including itself (de Murcia et al. 1986), histones (Tanuma et al. 1985), several transcription factors, DNA replication factors, and signaling molecules (Oliver et al. 1999; Kannan et al. 1999; Oei and Shi 2001; Cervellera and Sala 2000; Ariumi et al. 1999; Wesierska-Gadek et al. 1996). PAR polymers are rapidly degraded by PAR glycohydrolase and ADP-ribosyl protein lyase as it is indicated by their short ($\sim$ 1 min) half-life (Whitacre et al. 1995).

Biological effects of PARP-1 activation involve enhancement of DNA repair, maintenance of genomic integrity, replication, transcription, and proteasomal protein degradation (Burkle 2001). However, excessive DNA damage in oxidative stress induces overactivation of PARP-1 leading to depletion of its substrate NAD^+ that, in turn, causes ATP depletion because of the high energy demand of NAD^+ resynthesis, and results in necrotic cell death (Berger and Berger 1986). On the other hand, a mild-to-moderate level of oxidative stress and PARP-1 activation may initiate apoptosis via mitochondrial depolarization resulting in the release of cytochrome c, second mitochondria-derived activator of caspase/direct inhibitor of apoptosis-binding protein with low PI (Smac/Diablo), or AIF, and endonuclease G from the mitochondrial intermembrane space (Halmosi et al. 2001; Yu et al. 2002; Tapodi et al. 2005; van Wijk and Hageman 2005). AIF and endonuclease G translocation from mitochondria to the nucleus induces DNA fragmentation, which is considered an irreversible step in cell death and is caspase-independent (Yu et al. 2002; Li et al. 2001), while cytochrome c release induces caspase-dependent apoptotic cell death (Liu et al. 1996). In caspase-7- and caspase-3-mediated apoptosis, PARP-1 is cleaved by these caspases into p89 and p24 fragments (Tewari et al. 1995) resulting in the inactivation of the enzyme. The existence of this positive feedback regulation indicates the importance of blocking PARP-1 activation, thereby preserving cellular energy for ATP-dependent steps of apoptosis (Herceg and Wang 1999). Furthermore, cleavage-mediated inactivation of PARP-1 is necessary to release some elements of the apoptotic machinery, such as the human Ca^{2+}- or Mg^{2+}-dependent endonuclease, from PARylation-mediated inhibition (Boulares et al. 2001). However, depending on cell type, culture condition, and apoptosis inducers used, PARP-1 inhibitors attenuated, did not affect or augmented apoptosis indicating that PARP could be dispensable for most forms of apoptosis (Virag and Szabo 2002).

How PARP-1 activity is communicated to mitochondria is still obscure, although involvement of PAR-binding (Yu et al. 2006) protein kinase C (Sarker et al. 2001) and protein kinase B/Akt (Veres et al. 2003), the mitogen-activated protein kinases (MAPKs; O'Brien et al. 2001), and MAPK phosphatase-1 (Racz et al. 2010) was indicated. Regardless of the mechanism, the cross-talk between PARP-1 and mitochondria determines survival or death of the cells in various diseases.

15.4 The Cuprizone Model of Multiple Sclerosis

Cuprizone, oxalic acid bis(cyclohexylidene hydrazide) is a copper chelator, which can cause loss of weight, demyelination, astrogliosis, microglia infiltration, and hydrocephalus in the brain of C57BL/6 mice. In experiments, cuprizone is usually given in a diet at a concentration of 0.2–0.3 % to 6–9-week-old male mice. Higher concentration and younger age cause high mortality while older mice are more resistant. The pattern of demyelination depends on the strain and the toxic effects are different in distinct animal models (Taylor et al. 2009; Skripuletz et al. 2011). In the most widely used strain, C57BL/6 mice, demyelination and oligodendrocyte loss have been universally shown in the corpus callosum, the superior cerebellar peduncles, and anterior commissure while optic nerves, velum medullare anterior, the spinal cord, and the sciatic nerves remain unaffected (Kipp et al. 2009; Komoly 2005). Recent data indicated that the cerebellum, hippocampus, and the caudate-putamen might be also affected. Although there are differences in susceptibility between male and female mice in certain strains, de- and remyelination and glial reactions revealed no gender differences in C57BL/6 mice (Taylor et al. 2010).

The mechanism of oligodendrocyte loss and demyelination is not well understood. It seems that the primary targets are mature oligodendrocytes. Mitochondrial dysfunction and disturbed cellular respiration have been long suspected. Formation of mega-mitochondria in liver was an early observation (Tandler and Hoppel 1973). Similar giant mitochondria can be observed in oligodendrocytes as early as 3 days after cuprizone treatment along with downregulation of myelin genes (Komoly 2005). Indeed, cuprizone can induce changes in levels and function of a set of mitochondrial enzymes before myelin loss is apparent: activity of monoamine oxidase (MAO), cytochrome oxidase, and superoxide dismutase are reduced while activity of succinate dehydrogenase is increased (Venturini 1973; Russanov and Ljutakova 1980).

Carbonic anhydrase II (CA II), widely used as an immunohistochemical marker for oligodendrocytes, has an important function in maintaining the myelin sheath and maturation of oligodendrocytes (Cammer and Brion 2000; Cammer 1998). CA II also buffers acute changes in pH of the brain and oligodendrocytes and prevents acidosis (Kida et al. 2006; Ro and Carson 2004). A rapid decline in the activity of CA II can be observed in the brain of cuprizone- treated animals well before demyelination, similarly to MAO and cytochrome oxidase (Komoly et al. 1987). However, there is no explanation why a disturbed energy metabolism and mitochondrial dysfunction affects exclusively oligodendrocytes in the CNS and what is the reason of a preferential regional distribution of demyelination.

Since cuprizone is a copper chelator, copper deficiency has been considered to play a role in cuprizone toxicity. Although cuprizone induces copper deficiency in serum and brain, administration of copper could not protect against cuprizone-induced oligoendrocyte death (Carlton 1967). Chelating other heavy metals, such as Zn^{2+}, Fe^{2+}, or Mn^{2+} has also been considered (Venturini 1973; Zatta et al. 2005). Metabolites of cuprizone are unlikely to contribute since there is no evidence of metabolization.

The induced microglia activation may also impact demyelination by the production of proinflammatory cytokines, toxic metabolites, and enzymes (Pasquini et al. 2007). However, recent data indicate that microglia can already support remyelination at the onset of demyelination and it can express cytokines and chemokines, which activate and recruit endogenous oligodendrocyte precursors to the lesion site and deliver trophic support during remyelination (Olah et al. 2012; Mason et al. 2001; Arnett et al. 2001). At the onset of visible demyelination, week 3, microglia occur; they peak after 4.5 weeks and decline thereafter and become almost undetectable by week 6. Although microglia isolated from the demyelinated areas induced by cuprizone are potent antigen-presenting cells in vitro, T cells in such areas are not activated (Remington et al. 2007). Indeed, absence of T and B cells does not affect cuprizone-induced demyelination. In contrast to EAE, lymphocyte infiltration is controversial: B and T cells have been described to be missing, minor, or do not localize to demyelinating areas, and the blood–brain barrier remains intact (Remington et al. 2007; Hiremath et al. 2008). The vast number astrocytes in the demyelinating areas may also contribute to oligodendrocyte death (Kim et al. 2012). Astrocytes appear after 3 weeks and number of astrocytes peaks around week 5 (Skripuletz et al. 2011).

An interesting issue of the cuprizone model is spontaneous remyelination. The mRNA of myelin proteins produced by mature oligodendrocytes are downregulated after 3 days and decreased by 90 % after 3 weeks of cuprizone treatment, and increase afterward despite of exposure (Morell et al. 1998; Jurevics et al. 2002). Similar decline in proteins with different temporal patterns can be observed after 3 weeks reaching the maximum at 5 weeks: the compact myelin basic protein (MBP) is affected first and transmembrane protein PLP the last. Half of the mature oligodendrocytes disappear in the corpus callosum by week 2 and demyelination becomes evident after 3 weeks. Almost complete loss of mature oligodendrocytes can be observed after 4–5 weeks of cuprizone treatment. (Skripuletz et al. 2011). Nevertheless, during this period, a high number of new proliferating $Ng2^{+}$ oligodendrocyte precursor cells enter the corpus callosum, reaching a peak at weeks 4–4.5, suggesting that precursor recruitment and differentiation are not affected (Matsushima and Morell 2001; Gudi et al. 2009). Mature oligodendrocytes can be detected at low numbers at week 5 and reach more than 50 % by week 6. Expression of proteins during remyelination follows the same temporal profile as during demyelination. Thus, a partial remyelination is evident between 3 and 6 weeks with upregulation of promyelination factors IGF-1 and FGF-2 (Matsushima and Morell 2001; Mason et al. 2001). IGF-1 is produced by reactive astrocytes, while IGF-1 receptor is expressed by immature oligodendrocytes during early remyelination (Komoly et al. 1992). BDNF, GDNF, CNTF, and HGF may also play a role by regulating the numbers of progenitors and the abilities of demyelinating and differentiating cells to express myelin proteins (VonDran et al. 2011; Gudi et al. 2011). When cuprizone exposure is suspended, there is a rapid gain in body weight and the affected CNS areas completely remyelinate. However, despite completed remyelination, axonal degeneration continues to progress at a low level and becomes functionally apparent in the long term (Manrique-Hoyos et al. 2012).

15.5 The Role of Poly (ADP-Ribose) Polymerase in Oligodendrocyte Death and Callosal Demyelination Induced by Cuprizone and in Central Nervous System Plaques of Multiple Sclerosis

In MS patients, inflammation and demyelination, associated with oligodendrocyte loss, manifests in sporadic lesions that appear as hyperintensive spots on nuclear magnetic resonance (MR) images (Fig. 15.1a). It is very advantageous in the cuprizone model that demyelination mostly occurs in the corpus callosum, the superior cerebellar peduncles, and anterior commissure (Komoly 2005) enabling semiquantitative determination of its magnitude. T_2-weighted spin-echo MR serial sections (Fig. 15.1b) were analyzed and signal intensities were normalized to that of a tube of glycerol–water mixture providing a measure of demyelination in the corpus callosum of cuprizone-treated mice. Very intense demyelination occurred after 3 weeks of cuprizone exposure that was mostly prevented by cotreating the animals with the PARP inhibitor (Fig. 15.1b, c). Myelin loss was confirmed by immunoblotting utilizing antibody against MBP from excised corpus callosum samples (Fig. 15.1d). These results show that in the degenerative rodent model of MS, similar to its autoimmune model EAE (Scott et al. 2004), PARP inhibition effectively diminished the deleterious effect of the disease. Recently, PARP-1 inhibitors were found to reduce relapse incidence and severity, number of autoreactive Th17 cells, and epitope spreading even when applied after the first phase of disease (Cavone et al. 2011) further emphasizing the potential of PARP inhibition in MS therapy.

Mitochondrial dysfunction and consequently elevated reactive oxygen species (ROS) production was assumed to be involved in cuprizone- induced demyelination (Hemm et al. 1971; Ludwin 1978). Excessive ROS production triggers activation

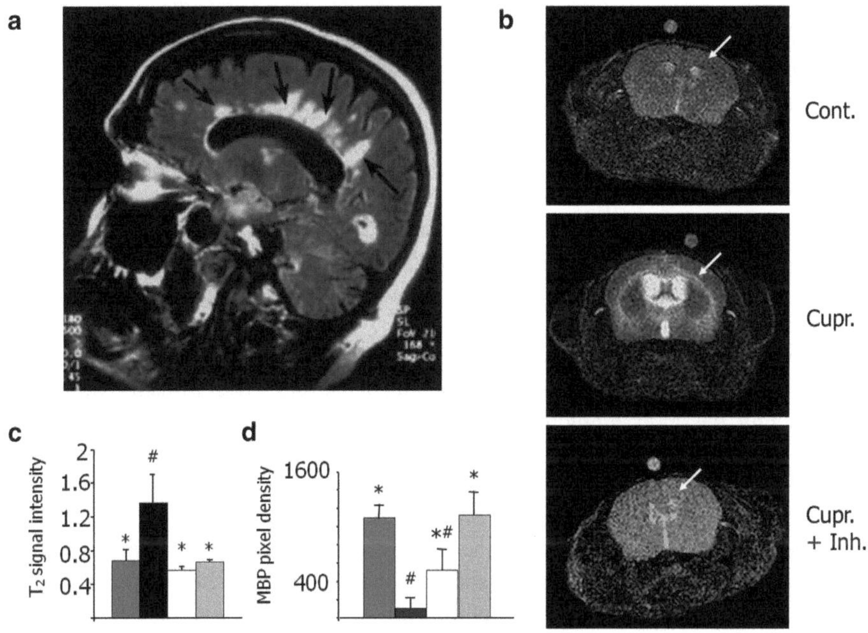

Fig. 15.1 Effect of cuprizone and Poly (ADP-ribose) polymerase (PARP) inhibitor treatment on demyelination in corpus callosum. Representative FLAIR MR image (**a**) of sagittal section of a sclerosis multiplex patient's brain is presented. *Black* arrows indicate SM lesions in the corpus callosum appearing as hyperintensive spots. Representative T_2-weighted spin-echo MR images (**b**) of brain coronal sections and quantification (**d**) of T_2 intensity changes in the corpus callosum of mice treated or not (Cont. and dark *gray* bars) for 4 weeks with cuprizone (Cupr. and *black* bars) and the PARP inhibitor 4-hydroxyquinazoline (Cupr.$^+$Inh. and open bars). Treatment with 4-hydroxyquinazoline alone did not affect the corpus callosum (data not shown and light *gray* bars). *White arrows* indicate hyperintensities (suggesting demyelination) or hypointensity (intact myelin status) in corpus callosum. Data are expressed as normalized mean signal intensities ± SD of three experiments. MBP expression in the dissected corpus callosum of mice treated for 5 weeks was detected by immunoblotting utilizing an anti-MBP antibody. Densitometric evaluation (D) mean pixel densities ± SD of three experiments are presented as a bar diagram (bar coloring is the same as in **c**). Mean pixel densities were normalized to those of the loading control actin. *$p < 0.001$ compared to cuprizone group. #$p < 0.001$ compared to control group

of PARP via generating DNA single-strand breaks, therefore, we assessed PARP activation by determining the end-product PAR using immunohistochemistry and immunoblotting. We found an increased activation of PARP in the corpus callosum, the specific region of cuprizone- induced oligodendrocyte death, indicating that PARP may contribute to oligodendrocyte depletion in this model. Similar to the cuprizone model, we observed PARP activation in oligodendrocytes of active pattern III MS lesions (Veto et al. 2010). This observation indicated that increased ROS production resulted from either the autoimmune inflammatory response or mitochondrial injury in oligodendrocytes caused PARP activation in the brain of MS patients. PAR-positive cells were defined as cells with strong PAR immunoreactivity within the nuclei as well as in the cytoplasm, including cell processes; in the majority of these cells, PAR-positive nuclei appeared condensed and in part fragmented suggesting apoptosis; in addition, cytoplasmic PAR reactivity revealed signs of cell degeneration consistent of in part fragmented cell processes and cytoplasmic vacuolization (Veto et al. 2010). In active pattern III MS lesions, a much higher number of PAR-positive nuclei were present suggesting a higher ROS production rate in developing lesions compared to those following other patterns of demyelination (Fischer et al. 2012; Haider et al. 2011). It is worth noting that in agreement with the short half-life of PAR polymers, only a fraction of the nuclei were PAR-positive.

Elevated ROS activate extracellular signal-regulated kinase (ERK) that phosphorylates Ser^{372} and Thr^{373} of PARP, thereby fully activating it (Kauppinen et al. 2006). Accordingly, we observed increased phosphorylation of ERK upon cuprizone treatment. Overactivation of PARP induces increased inflammatory response by elevating the expression of nuclear factor (NF)-κB-dependent genes (Oliver et al. 1999), promotes cell death by ATP depletion in the cell, and activation of p38 MAPK (O'Brien et al. 2001), and by destabilizing the mitochondria via c-Jun N-terminal kinase (JNK) activation and suppression of the phosphatidyl inositol 3 kinase (PI3 K)/Akt pathway (Tapodi et al. 2005). Destabilization of its outer membrane leads to release and nuclear translocation of AIF from mitochondria (Fig. 15.2a). Completely in agreement with the above scheme, we observed activation of all MAPKs and only a partial activation of the PI3 K/Akt pathway. The latter may reflect the combined effect of inhibition by PARP and activation by ROS via inactivation of the oxidation-sensitive phosphatase and tensin homologue deleted from chromosome 10 (PTEN) that inhibits the PI3 K/Akt pathway by dephosphorylation (Zhu et al. 2006). Nuclear translocation of AIF results in chromatin condensation, large-scale DNA fragmentation (> 50 kbp) and cell death in a caspase-independent manner (Lorenzo and Susin 2004). Indeed, we were not able to detect cleaved caspase-3 in the corpus callosum of cuprizone- treated mice by immunoblotting or measure caspase-3 activity by using fluorescent substrate in agreement with previous findings (Pasquini 2007; Copray et al. 2005). Similarly, caspase-3 activation is also not seen in apoptotic oligodendrocytes in MS (Aboul-Enein et al. 2003). In contrast, we observed nuclear translocation of AIF in several oligodendrocytes by immunohistochemistry in cuprizone-treated mice (Veto et al. 2010). All these results suggested that activation of PARP could significantly contribute to oligodendrocyte death and demyelination by a caspase-independent, AIF-mediated apoptosis in the cuprizone model. For quantification of AIF nuclear translocation in brain sections of MS patients, only those cells were counted, which showed unequivocal immunoreactivity within their nuclei. Similar to cuprizone- induced demyelination, in pattern III MS lesions, we observed AIF translocation to nucleus of oligodendrocytes, which showed elevated PARP activation (Veto et al. 2010). Therefore, we performed in vivo and in vitro experiments to investigate the effect of PARP inhibition in the cuprizone model.

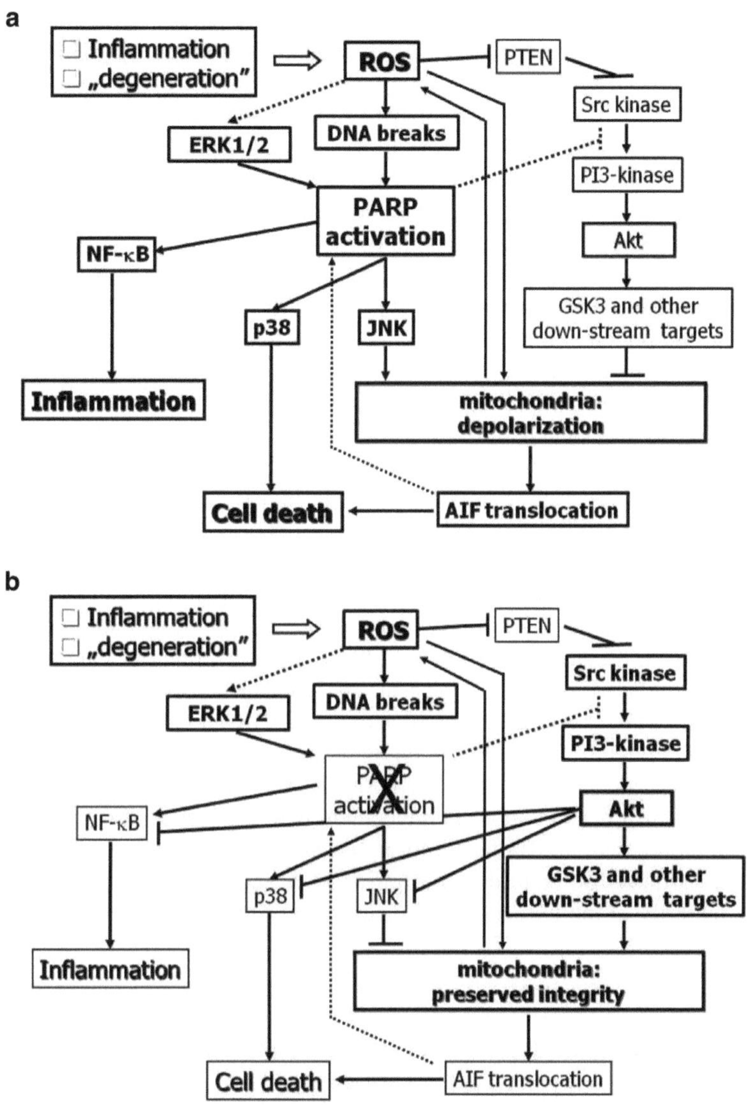

Fig. 15.2 Schematic diagram of the proposed molecular mechanism for the cytoprotective effect of PARP inhibition in the cuprizone model and SM. Well-documented effects are indicated by *solid* lines whereas effects involving yet unidentified mediator(s) or events are represented by a *dashed* line. Lines with a *pointed end* denote activation, whereas those with *flat end* indicate inhibition. Active processes are in *bold* while inhibited ones are in *regular*. PARP-1 activation in the cuprizone model and SM leads to NF-κB-mediated inflammatory response, JNK-mediated mitochondrial depolarization, and AIF- and p38-mediated cell death (**a**). The PI3 K/Akt pathway is inhibited by the PARP activation, therefore, fails to protect the mitochondria. Inhibition of PARP (large X) suppresses NF-κB, p38 and JNK activation, and relieves the PI3 K/Akt pathway from the inhibition shifting the balance to mitochondrial protection and cell survival (**b**)

The PARP inhibitor diminished demyelination and oligodendrocyte loss as it was revealed by serial in vivo nuclear MRI, semiquantitative histology, MBP immunohistochemistry, and MBP immunoblotting. Next, we explored the effect of the PARP inhibitor on kinase pathways, which may possibly regulate oligodendrocyte death in the corpus callosum. We observed that cuprizone-induced phosphorylation of JNK in the corpus callosum was attenuated by PARP inhibition suggesting the involvement of JNK in the AIF-dependent cuprizone-induced oligodendrocyte death. Similarly, activation of p38 MAPK in the corpus callosum upon the administration of cuprizone was also attenuated by the PARP inhibitor. Cuprizone- induced ERK1/2 activation in the corpus callosum was not affected by the PARP inhibitor, which is in agreement with the notion that ERK1/2 pathway is upstream to PARP activation (Tang et al. 2002; Kauppinen et al. 2006). In conclusion, all effects of PARP inhibition on the MAPK pathways, i.e., suppressing JNK and p38 activation while not affecting ERK, could promote OL survival. Cuprizone-induced Akt phosphorylation was further enhanced by coadministration of the PARP inhibitor. Furthermore, PARP inhibition alone caused phosphorylation of Akt in accordance with previous findings (Tapodi et al. 2005; Veres et al. 2003). Akt phosphorylates the BH3 domain protein Bad, preventing it from forming heterodimers with other proapoptotic BH3 domain proteins and destabilizing the mitochondrial membrane (Datta et al. 1997). Accordingly, activation of Akt prevented neuronal apoptosis by inhibiting translocation of AIF to the nucleus (Kim et al. 2007), by protection of oligodendrocytes against TNF-induced apoptosis (Pang et al. 2007) and by phosphorylating the respective upstream kinases and it decreased activity of JNK and p38 MAPK (Barthwal et al. 2003; Park et al. 2002). Based on these data, our results may suggest that in response to cuprizone, the cytoprotective PI-3 K/Akt pathway became activated, although it was insufficient to prevent oligodendrocyte death. Additional activation by PARP inhibition could be sufficient to protect oligodendrocytes against apoptosis, mediated partially by reduced activation of JNK and p38 MAPK and maintaining the integrity of the mitochondrial membrane systems, thus preventing nuclear translocation of AIF (Fig. 15.2b).

15.6 Inhibition of Poly (ADP-Ribose) Polymerase in Experimental Models and in the Clinical Practice; Poly (ADP-Ribose) Polymerase Inhibitors

The role of PARP activation and the effect of inhibition have been examined in several models of MS and partially in patients.

The role of PARP in inflammatory processes has been extensively studied. A number of studies implicate oxygen-derived free radicals such as superoxide and hydroxyl radical and high-energy oxidants such as peroxynitrite as mediators of inflammation and endotoxic shock. Elevated ROS induce DNA single-strand breaks that, in turn, activate PARP leading to eventual necrotic cell death. PARP inhibitors, as well as knocking out the PARP-1 gene, resulted in diminished inflammatory response and resistance against inflammatory damage in various cellular and animal models. This suggests an interaction between PARP-1 and NF-κB, the key transcription factor regulator of the expression of proinflammatory mediators as well as signaling and adhesion molecules. PARP-1-deficient mice were found to be resistant to bacterial lipopolysaccharide (LPS)-induced endotoxic shock, and PARP-1-deficient cells were defective in tumor necrosis factor α (TNFα)-induced expression of cytokines, chemokines, adhesion molecules, and inflammatory mediators such as inducible nitric oxide synthase and cyclooxygenase (Oliver et al. 1999). Together with reports utilizing various PARP inhibitors (Hauschildt et al. 1991, 1992; Pellat-Deceunynck et al. 1994; Szabo et al. 1998), these results clearly indicated that PARP protein and/or PARP activity is necessary for the expression of NF-κB- dependent genes. This mechanism was regarded as the molecular basis for the anti-inflammatory effect of PARP inhibitors and resistance of PARP-deficient mice against endotoxic shock. However, we have found that PARP inhibition activated the PI3 K/Akt pathway in lung, liver, and spleen and downregulated LPS-induced activation of ERK1/2 and p38 MAPK in a tissue-specific manner in a murine endotoxic shock model (Veres et al. 2003, 2004). In an oxidative stress model, we demonstrated that inhibition of the PI3 K/Akt pathway counteracted the cytoprotective effect of PARP inhibition (Tapodi et al. 2005). Furthermore, we showed that upregulation of MKP-1 expression by PARP-1 inhibition resulted in inactivation of the proinflammatory and proapoptotic JNK and p38 MAPK, and that this significantly contributed to the observed cytoprotection (Racz et al. 2010). These results suggest that regulation of these kinase signaling pathways by PARP inhibition could significantly contribute to its protective effects in the inflammatory models.

Recent data uniformly indicate that activation of PARP-1 is characteristic of several EAE models and EAE can be fundamentally altered by inhibition of PARP-1, suggesting its basic role in CNS autoimmune inflammation. Immunostaining for PAR, the enzymatic product of PARP-1, showed PARP-1 activation in plaque areas of EAE induced in the marmoset model of relapsing–remitting MS. Marked activation was found in astrocytes surrounding demyelinated EAE plaques and in scattered nearby microglia, oligodendrocytes, and neurons (Kauppinen et al. 2005). Cholesterol breakdown product 7-ketocholesterol-activated PARP-1 in microglial cells and induced neuronal damage via the activation and migration of microglial cells linking demyelination and progressive neuronal damage (Diestel et al. 2003). Higher serum concentrations of 15α-hydroxicholestene were found in patients with secondary progressive MS (SPMS) and in mice with secondary progressive EAE, which activated microglia, macrophages, and astrocytes through a pathway involving PARP-1 (Farez et al. 2009). Inhibition of PARP-1 ameliorated the clinical signs of EAE, postponed its onset, reduced the mortality, and suppressed the progression of EAE in several models (Scott et al. 2004; Farez et al. 2009; Cavone et al. 2011; Chiarugi 2002). Earlier, onset of EAE and a more severe course were observed in PARP-1-deficient mice characterized by B cell expansion, and $CD4^+$ T lymphocyte and macrophage infiltrated into the CNS, but cytokine profiles were not different (Selvaraj et al. 2009).

In MS, activation of PARP and the nuclear translocation of AIF were very similar to that observed in cuprizone- induced demyelination as discussed previously.

These data indicate that pattern III MS characterized by oligodendrocyte apoptosis and cuprizone-mediated toxic oligodendrocyte death share molecular pathways; cuprizone might be a degenerative model of MS, while EAE models autoimmune inflammation; and inhibition of PARP, which effectively ameliorated demyelination and prevented oligodendrocyte death, is a feasible therapy of MS (Veto et al. 2010). PARP-1 activity was higher in monocytes of patients with SPMS, suggesting that PARP-1 pathway is a potential new therapeutic target in SPMS (Farez et al. 2009). Altogether, these experimental and human data indicate that inhibition of PARP effectively targets basic aspects of MS: autoimmune inflammation, demyelination accompanied by oligodendrocyte death, and probably axonal degeneration responsible for secondary progression. Such an approach targeting several pathogenetic pathways by inhibiting a single enzyme may be an alternative of combining different compounds.

Numerous PARP-1 inhibitors, including iniparib (BiPar Sciences Inc./Sanofi-Aventis), olaparib (AstraZeneca plc), veliparib (Abbott Laboratories), PF-1367338 (Pfizer Inc.), MK-4827 (Merck & Co Inc.), and CEP-9722 (Cephalon Inc.), have already advanced into clinical trials. The major focus is primarily oncology, both as monotherapy in specific patient populations (e.g., BRCA-deficient) and as combination with other chemotherapeutics. The first phase I clinical trial was carried out between 2003 and 2005 in patients with advanced solid tumors, where PARP inhibitor was combined with the alkylating agent temozolomide. The 33 patients tolerated the treatment well (Plummer et al. 2008). At present, about 50 trials are registered including a phase III trial in patients with lung cancer (ECLIPSE). The majority of the trials combine a PARP inhibitor with a standard chemotherapeutic agent in patients with skin and solid tumors. Besides chemopotentiation, PARP inhibitors can also act as radiosensitizers. Enhanced response of tumor cells to radiation has been shown for several PARP inhibitors, and several phase I clinical trials have been started to examine the effect of combined radiation therapy and PARP inhibition in patients with primary and secondary brain tumors. Nevertheless, PARP inhibitors are also used as single agents based on the concept of "synthetic lethality": mutation in either of two genes has no effect but combination of the mutation results in cell death (Mégnin-Chanet et al. 2010). Accordingly, cells with insufficient double-strand break repairs caused by BRCA1 and BRCA2 deficiency are hypersensitive to PARP inhibition due to the blockade of single-strand repair (Bryant et al. 2005; Farmer et al. 2005). In the initial proof of concept study with the oral PARP1 inhibitor olaparib, 28 % of ovarian cancer patients with BRCA mutation achieved an objective response (Fong et al. 2009). Recently, responses have also been observed in patients without BRCA mutations but with a dysfunction of the homologous recombination system (e.g., PTEN mutations, ATM deficiency), which makes them more sensitive to the antitumor agents, which cause double-strand breaks of DNA (Sessa 2011).

While PARP inhibitors have never been examined in patients with MS, compounds with a PARP- inhibitory property and already in clinical practice have been tested in animal models of MS and in patients with MS. Tetracycline derivatives, including minocycline, have neuroprotective effects, which have been attributed to reduced inflammation and a direct effect on cell death. Neuronal cell death caused by excitotoxicity and ionizing radiation in vitro could be reduced by minocycline treatment. In addition, increased cell survival was obvious in animal models of degenerative neurological diseases after treatment (Yrjänheikki et al. 1998; Du et al. 2001; Chen et al. 2000; Zhu et al. 2002). Using primary cultures, minocycline was able to protect neurons against PARP-1-mediated toxicity at submicromolar concentrations. When different tetracycline derivatives were compared, the neuroprotective property directly correlated with the potency of PARP inhibition (Alano et al. 2006). Recently, the protective effect of minocycline on cardiac myocyte survival has also been attributed to the inhibition of PARP-1 activity (Tao et al. 2010). Many other effects of minocycline have been suggested to contribute to the antiapoptotic effects. For example, changes in mitochondrial functions favor cell survival (upregulation of bcl-2, reduced calcium uptake, scavenging of ROS, inhibition of MAPs). Minocycline also inhibits NF-kB in different cell types of the CNS, a transcription factor, which plays a central role in inflammation and cell death (Si et al. 2004; Orio et al. 2010; Cai et al. 2010). Effects of minocycline have been extensively studied in different animal models of MS and on human cell populations. The anti-inflammatory effects of minocycline are linked to inhibition of antigen processing, T cell proliferation, proinflammatory cytokine production, activation of MMPs, production of MMPs, reactivation of T cells within the CNS, and microglial activation; minocycline also promotes Th2 shifting. The antiapoptotic effects described in other models have also been found, including the induction of antiapoptotic intracellular signaling pathways, decreased glutamate excitotoxicity, decreased production of ROS and NOS, sequestration of excess calcium, and decreased iron deposition (Chen et al. 2011). Importantly, all these outcomes can be the result of PARP inhibition, which is a coactivator of NF-kB besides a number of other transcription factors; blocking such a central pathway of cell death, inflammation, and cellular stress could be responsible for all the observed results. Minocycline is able to exert its PARP-inhibitory effect at a far lower concentration than that required for the observed singular effects, nevertheless, it could trigger the same results through the inhibition of NF-kB and its downstream pathways (Ha et al. 2002; Alano et al. 2006).

Most of the experimental work and a few clinical trials in MS addressed the anti-inflammatory properties of minocycline, thus used the autoimmune animal model of MS, EAE. Several studies indicated that minocycline as monotherapy was able to prevent lethal EAE, decreased the severity of both mild and severe EAE, and optic neuritis in rats and mice (Popovic et al. 2002; Brundula et al. 2002; Maier et al. 2007; Nikodemova et al. 2010). Combination with immunomodulatory agents, such as interferon-β, GA, atorvastatin, and glucocorticosteroids was effective in decreasing clinical sores, improving MRI, and pathological outcomes in both acute and chronic phase of EAE (Giuliani et al. 2005a; Giuliani et al. 2005b; Chen et al. 2010; Luccarini et al. 2008).

Recently, the effect of minocycline on the degenerative aspects of MS and in degenerative MS models has been also examined. Intraperitoneal daily treatment with minocycline beginning on the day of cuprizone feeding had a beneficial effect on cortical and callosal demyelination, but the number of oligodendrocytes and precursor cells were not affected. Minocycline did not reduce astrogliosis and did not prevent microglia activation in the corpus callosum either (Skripuletz et al. 2010). In myelinating aggregating brain cell cultures treated simultaneously with interferon-γ and LPS, minocycline inhibited microglial activation, attenuated the increased phosphorylation of MAP kinases, and promoted remyelination by enhancing the differentiation of OPCs and immature oligodendrocytes (Defaux et al. 2011).

The first pilot study with minocycline was carried out in 2004 in 10 patients with relapsing-remitting MS (RRMS). The patients received 100 mg minocycline twice daily orally for 6 months. The trial was extended to 36 months (Metz et al. 2004; Zabad et al. 2007; Zhang et al. 2008). In contrast to four relapses during the 3-month period before minocycline therapy, only seven relapses occurred during the 3-year treatment, and six patients remained relapse-free. The number of enhancing lesions decreased by 93 % and local brain atrophy was also reduced. The treatment was well tolerated. Two additional trials examined the additive effect of minocycline in combination with GA. One in vitro study found that activation of myeloid peripheral blood monocyte-derived dendritic cells were affected by the combined treatment in both MS and healthy controls (Ruggieri et al. 2008). A multicenter, double-blind, placebo-controlled, phase II clinical trial examined the effect of add-on monocyline in 44 patients with RRMS, who had at least one enhancing lesion and were treated with GA. Twice daily 100 mg oral minocycline reduced the number of enhancing lesions by 63 %, new and enlarging T2 lesions by 65 %, and the total T2 disease burden; the risk of relapse was also lower. However, none of the differences were significant. No safety problem arose and the treatment was well tolerated (Metz et al. 2009).

15.7 Summary

The current treatment options in MS have a profound effect on inflammation, nevertheless, degenerative aspects of the disease are less targeted. To improve therapy, either a combination of treatments targeting inflammation and degenerative processes, or treatment with combined anti-inflammatory and antiapoptotic properties may be considered. As for demyelination, theoretically treatments preventing demyelination and oligodendrocyte loss or promoting remyelination could be applied; the latter strategy has been addressed by monoclonal antibody against lingo already in an ongoing clinical trial. Recently, we explored the other option and examined if a treatment with anti-inflammatory as well as antiapoptotic effects may influence oligodendrocyte loss in the CNS.

We chose to target the nuclear enzyme of PARP, which functions as a DNA damage sensor and signaling molecule binding to both single- and double-stranded DNA breaks.

Altogether, our data revealed several important issues regarding MS treatment and research: (1) indicated that activation of PARP and mitochondrial death pathways could be central of degenerative oligodendrocyte loss in MS; (2) based on the similar molecular mechanisms, indicated that the cuprizone model can be a model of MS regarding such processes, similarly as EAE can be a model of autoimmune inflammation; and (3) indicated for the first time that a strategy to target a single molecule involved in both inflammation and cell death, could be an alternative option to a combination of treatments. Since PARP activity is necessary for the expression of NF-κB- dependent genes, the anti-inflammatory effect of PARP inhibitors is not surprising and could well explain the profound effect on preventing EAE, ameliorating the clinical signs, mortality, and delayed onset of EAE.

Compounds with PARP-inhibitory properties have already been examined in MS. The tetracycline derivatives, including minocycline have neuroprotective effects; minocycline was able to protect neurons against PARP-1-mediated toxicity at submicromolar concentrations and the neuroprotective property directly correlated with the potency of PARP inhibition. Minocycline also inhibits NF-kB in different cell types of the CNS; this effect together with the other outcomes such as inhibition of matrix metalloproteinases could be all attributed to the upstream inhibition of PARP. Minocycline alone or in combination with GA suggested the possible efficacy of the treatment and potential to try in phase III clinical trials. In addition, the treatment was safe and well tolerated.

More importantly, numerous selective PARP-1 inhibitors, including iniparib (BiPar Sciences Inc./Sanofi-Aventis), olaparib (AstraZeneca plc), veliparib (Abbott Laboratories), PF-1367338 (Pfizer Inc.), MK-4827 (Merck & Co Inc.), and CEP-9722 (Cephalon Inc.), have already advanced into clinical trials. PARP inhibitors may thus prevent clinical relapses related to inflammation and progression of disability due to axonal and oligodendrocyte loss. Another interesting option concerning oligodendrocytes is the combination of PARP inhibition and antagonization of lingo: this could target both demyelination /oligodendrocyte loss and induce remyelination at the same time.

Acknowledgments This work was supported by TAMOP 4.2.1B-10/2KONV and 4.2.2B-10/1 as well as by 34039/KA-OTKA/11–06, OTKA K77892.

References

Aboul-Enein F, Rauschka H, Kornek B, Stadelmann C, Stefferl A, Brück W, Lucchinetti C, Schmidbauer M, Jellinger K, Lassmann H (2003) Preferential loss of myelin-associated glycoprotein reflects hypoxia-like white matter damage in stroke and inflammatory brain diseases. J Neuropathol Exp Neurol 62:25–33

Alano CC, Kauppinen TM, Valls AV, Swanson RA (2006) Minocycline inhibits poly(ADP-ribose) polymerase-1 at nanomolar concentrations. Proc Natl Acad Sci U S A 103(25):9685–90

Albert M, Antel J, Brück W, Stadelmann C (2007) Extensive cortical remyelination in patients with chronic multiple sclerosis. Brain Pathol 17:129–38

Ariumi Y, Masutani M, Copeland TD, Mimori T, Sugimura T, Shimotohno K, Ueda K, Hatanaka M, Noda M (1999) Suppression of the poly(ADP-ribose) polymerase activity by DNA-dependent protein kinase in vitro. Oncogene 18:4616–4625

Arnett HA, Mason J, Marino M, Suzuki K, Matsushima GK, Ting JP (2001) TNF alpha promotes proliferation of oligodendrocyteprogenitors and remyelination. Nat Neurosci 4:1116–1122

Babbe H, Roers A, Waisman A, Lassmann H, Goebels N, Hohlfeld R, Friese M, Schröder R, Deckert M, Schmidt S, Ravid R, Rajewsky K (2000) Clonal expansion of CD8+ T cells dominate the T cell infiltrate in active multiple sclerosis lesions as shown by micromanipulation and single cell polymerase chain reaction. J Exp Med 192:393–404

Bagasra O, Michaels FH, Zheng YM, Bobroski LE, Spitsin SV, Fu ZF, Tawadros R, Koprowski H (1995) Activation of the inducible form of nitric oxide synthase in the brains of patients with multiple sclerosis. Proc Natl Acad Sci U S A 92:12041–12045

Barnett MH, Prineas JW (2004) Relapsing and remitting multiple sclerosis: pathology of the newly forming lesion. Ann Neurol 55:458–468

Barthwal MK, Sathyanarayana P, Kundu CN, Rana B, Pradeep A, Sharma C, Woodgett JR, Rana A (2003) Negative regulation of mixed lineage kinase 3 by protein kinase B/AKT leads to cell survival. J Biol Chem 278:3897–3902

Bates D (2011) Treatment effects of immunomodulatory therapies at different stages of multiple sclerosis in short-term trials. Neurology 76(1 Suppl 1):S14–S25

Berger NA, Berger SJ (1986) Metabolic consequences of DNA damage: the role of poly (ADP-ribose) polymerase as mediator of the suicide response. Basic Life Sci 38:357–363

Bizzozero OA, Dejesus G, Callaha K, Pastuszyn A (2005) Elevated protein carbonylation in the brain white matter and grey matter of patients with multiple sclerosis. J Neurosci Res 81:687–695

Bolanos JP, Almeida A, Stewart V, Peuchen S, Land JM, Clark JB, Heales SJ (1997) Nitric oxide mediated mitochondrial damage in the brain: mechanisms and implication for neurdegenerative diseases. J Neurochem 68:2227–2240

Boulares AH, Zoltoski AJ, Contreras FJ, Yakovlev AG, Yoshihara K, Smulson ME (2001) Regulation of DNAS1L3 endonuclease activity by poly(ADPribosyl)ation during etoposide-induced apoptosis. Role of poly(ADP-ribose) polymerase-1 cleavage in endonuclease activation. J Biol Chem 277:372–378

Brundula V, Rewcastle NB, Metz LM, Bernard CC, Yong VW (2002) Targeting leukocyte MMPs and transmigration: minocycline as a potential therapy for multiple sclerosis. Brain 125 (Pt 6):1297–1308.

Bryant HE, Schultz N, Thomas HD, Parker KM, Flower D, Lopez E, Kyle S, Meuth M, Curtin NJ, Helleday T (2005) Specific killing of BRCA2-deficient tumours with inhibitors of poly(ADP-ribose) polymerase. Nature 434(7035):913–917

Burkle A (2001) Physiology and pathophysiology of poly(ADPribosyl)ation. Bioessays 23:795–806

Cai ZY, Yan Y, Chen R (2010) Minocycline reduces astrocytic reactivation and neuroinflammation in the hippocampus of a vascular cognitive impairment rat model. Neurosci Bull 26(1):28–36

Cammer W (1998) Glial-cell cultures from brains of carbonic anhydrase II-deficient mutant mice: delay in oligodendrocyte maturation. Neurochem Res 23:407–412

Cammer WB, Brion LP (2000) Carbonic anhydrase in the nervous system. EXS 90:475–489

Carlton WW (1967) Studies on the induction of hydrocephalus and spongy degeneration by cuprizone feeding and attempts to antidote the toxicity. Life Sci 6:11–19

Cavone L, Aldinucci A, Ballerini C, Biagioli T, Moroni F, Chiarugi A (2011) PARP-1 inhibition prevents CNS migration of dendritic cells during EAE, suppressing the encephalitogenic response and relapse severity. Mult Scler 17(7):794–807

Cervellera MN, Sala A (2000) Poly(ADP-ribose) polymerase is a B-MYB coactivator. J Biol Chem 275:10692–10696

Chang A, Tourtelotte WW, Rudick RA, Trapp BD (2002) Premyelinating oligodendrocytes in chronic lesions of multiple sclerosis. N Engl J Med 346:165–200

Chen M, Ona VO, Li M, Ferrante RJ, Fink KB, Zhu S, Bian J, Guo L, Farrell LA, Hersch SM, Hobbs W, Vonsattel JP, Cha JH, Friedlander RM (2000) Minocycline inhibits caspase-1 and caspase-3 expression and delays mortality in a transgenic mouse model of Huntington disease. Nat Med 6:797–801

Chen X, Ma X, Jiang Y, Pi R, Liu Y, Ma L (2011) The prospects of minocycline in multiple sclerosis. J Neuroimmunol 235(1–2):1–8
Chen X, Pi R, Liu M, Ma X, Jiang Y, Liu Y, Mao X, Hu X (2010) Combination of methylprednisolone and minocycline synergistically improves experimental autoimmune encephalomyelitis in C57 BL/6 mice. J Neuroimmunol 226(1–2):104–109
Chiarugi A (2002) Inhibitors of poly(ADP-ribose) polymerase-1 suppress transcriptional activation in lymphocytes and ameliorate autoimmune encephalomyelitis in rats. Br J Pharmacol 137(6):761–770
Copray JCVM, Küst BM, Mantingh-Otter I, Boddeke HWGM (2005) p75NTR independent oligodendrocyte death in cuprizone-induced demyelination in C57BL/6 mice 2005. Neuropath Appl Neuro 31:600–609.
Cross AH, Manning PT, Keeling RM, Schmidt RE, Misko TP (1998) Peroxynitrite formation within the central nervous system in active multiple sclerosis. J Neuroimmunol 88:45–56
Datta SR, Dudek H, Tao X, Masters S, Fu H, Gotoh Y, Greenberg ME (1997) Akt phosphorylation of BAD couples survival signals to the cell-intrinsic death machinery. Cell 91:231–241
de Murcia G, Huletsky A, Lamarre D, Gaudreau A, Pouyet J, Daune M, Poirier GG (1986) Modulation of chromatin superstructure induced by poly(ADP-ribose) synthesis and degradation. J Biol Chem 261:7011–7017
Defaux A, Zurich MG, Honegger P, Monnet-Tschudi F (2011) Minocycline promotes remyelination in aggregating rat brain cell cultures after interferon-γ plus lipopolysaccharide-induced demyelination. Neuroscience 187:84–92
Devonshire V, Havrdova E, Radue EW, O'Connor P, Zhang-Auberson L, Agoropoulou C, Häring DA, Francis G, Kappos L; for the FREEDOMS study group (2012) Relapse and disability outcomes in patients with multiple sclerosis treated with fingolimod: subgroup analyses of the double-blind, randomised, placebo-controlled FREEDOMS study. Lancet Neurol 11(5): 420–428
Diestel A, Aktas O, Hackel D, Hake I, Meier S, Raine CS, Nitsch R, Zipp F, Ullrich O (2003) Activation of microglial poly(ADP-ribose)-polymerase-1 by cholesterol breakdown products during neuroinflammation: a link between demyelination and neuronal damage. J Exp Med 198(11):1729–1740
Du Y, Ma Z, Lin S, Dodel RC, Gao F, Bales KR, Triarhou LC, Chernet E, Perry KW, Nelson DL, Luecke S, Phebus LA, Bymaster FP, Paul SM (2001) Minocycline prevents nigrostriatal dopaminergic neurodegeneration in the MPTP model of Parkinson's disease. Proc Natl Acad Sci U S A 98(25):14669–14674
Dutta R, McDonough J, Yin X, Peterson J, Chang A, Torres T, Gudz T, Macklin WB, Lewis DA, Fox RJ, Rudick R, Mirnics K, Trapp BD (2006) Mitochondrial dysfunction as a cause of axonal degeneration in multiple sclerosis patients. Ann Neurol 59:478–89
Evangelou N, Konz D, Esiri MM, Smith S, Palace J, Matthews PM (2001) Size-selective neuronal changes in the anterior optic pathways suggest a differential susceptibility to injury in multiple sclerosis. Brain 124:1813–1820
Farez MF, Quintana FJ, Gandhi R, Izquierdo G, Lucas M, Weiner HL (2009) Toll-like receptor 2 and poly(ADP-ribose) polymerase 1 promote central nervous system neuroinflammation in progressive EAE. Nat Immunol 10(9):958–964
Farmer H, McCabe N, Lord CJ, Tutt AN, Johnson DA, Richardson TB, Santarosa M, Dillon KJ, Hickson I, Knights C, Martin NM, Jackson SP, Smith GC, Ashworth A (2005) Targeting the DNA repair defect in BRCA mutant cells as a therapeutic strategy. Nature 434(7035):917–921
Fischer MT, Sharma R, Lim J, Haider L, Frischer J, Drexhage J, Mahad D, Bradl M, van Horssen J, Lassmann H (2012) NADPH oxidase expression in active multiple sclerosis lesions in relation to oxidative tissue damage and mitochondrial injury. Brain 135:886–899
Fong PC, Boss DS, Yap TA, Tutt A, Wu P, Mergui-Roelvink M, Mortimer P, Swaisland H, Lau A, O'Connor MJ, Ashworth A, Carmichael J, Kaye SB, Schellens JH, de Bono JS (2009) Inhibition of poly(ADP-ribose) polymerase in tumors from BRCA mutation carriers. N Engl J Med 361(2):123–34

Frischer JM, Bramow S, Dal Bianco A, Lucchinetti C, Rauschka H, Schmidbauer M, Laursen H, Sorensen PS, Lassmann H (2009) The relation between inflammation and neurodegeneration in multiple sclerosis. Brain 132:1175–1189

Geurts JJ, Brakhof F (2008) Grey matter pathology in multiple sclerosis. Lancet Neurol 7:841–851

Giuliani F, Fu SA, Metz LM, Yong VW (2005a) Effective combination of minocycline and interferon-beta in a model of multiple sclerosis. J Neuroimmunol 165(1–2):83–91

Giuliani F, Metz LM, Wilson T, Fan Y, Bar-Or A, Yong VW (2005b) Additive effect of the combination of glatiramer acetate and minocycline in a model of MS. J Neuroimmunol 158(1–2):213–21

Gray E, Thomas TL, Betmouni S, Scolding N, Love S (2008a) Elevated myeloperoxidase activity in white matter in multiple sclerosis. Neurosci Lett 442:195–198

Gray E, Thomas TL, Betmouni S, Scolding N, Love S (2008b) Elevated activity of microglial expression of myeloperoxidase in demyelinated cerebral cortex in multiple sclerosis. Brain Pathol 18:86–95

Gudi V, Škuljec J, Yildiz Ö, Frichert K, Skripuletz T, Moharregh-Khiabani D, Voss E, Wissel K, Wolter S, Stangel M (2011) Spatial and temporal profiles of growth factor expression during CNS demyelination reveal the dynamics of repair priming. PLoS One 6(7):e22623

Gudi V, Moharregh-Khiabani D, Skripuletz T, Koutsoudaki PN, Kotsiari A, Skuljec J, Trebst C, Stangel M (2009) Regional differences between grey and white matter in cuprizone induced demyelination. Brain Res 1283:127–138

Ha HC, Hester LD, Snyder SH (2002) Poly(ADP-ribose) polymerase-1 dependence of stress-induced transcription factors and associated gene expression in glia. Proc Natl Acad Sci U S A 99(5):3270–5

Haider L, Fischer MT, Frischer JM, Bauer J, Höftberger R, Botond G, Esterbauer H, Binder CJ, Witztum JL, Lassmann H (2011) Oxidative damage and neurodegeneration in multiple sclerosis lesions. Brain 134:1914–24

Hallgren B, Sourander P (1958) The effect of age on the non-haemin iron in the human brain. J Neurochem 3:41–51

Halmosi R, Berente Z, Osz E, Toth K, Literati-Nagy P, Sumegi B (2001) Effect of poly(ADP-ribose) polymerase inhibitors on the ischemia-reperfusion-induced oxidative cell damage and mitochondrial metabolism in Langendorff heart perfusion system. Mol Pharmacol 59: 1497–1505

Hauschildt S, Scheipers P, Bessler WG (1991) Inhibitors of poly (ADP-ribose) polymerase suppress lipopolysaccharide-induced nitrite formation in macrophages. Biochem Biophys Res Commun 179:865–871

Hauschildt S, Scheipers P, Bessler WG, Mulsch A (1992) Induction of nitric oxide synthase in L929 cells by tumour-necrosis factor alpha is prevented by inhibitors of poly(ADP-ribose) polymerase. Biochem J 288:255–600

Hemm RD, Carlton WW, Wesler JR (1971) Ultrastructural changes of cuprizone encephalopathy in mice. Toxicol Appl Pharm 28:869–882

Herceg Z, Wang ZG (1999) Failure of poly(ADP-ribose) polymerase cleavage by caspases leads to induction of necrosis and enhanced apoptosis. Mol Cell Biol 19:5124–5133

Hiremath MM, Chen VS, Suzuki K, Ting JP, Matsushima GK (2008) MHC class II exacerbates demyelination in vivo independently of T cells. J Neuroimmunol 203:23–32

Illes Z, Stern JN, Keskin DB, Reddy J, Brosnan CF, Waldner H, Santambrogio L, Kuchroo VK, Strominger JL (2005) Copolymer effects on microglia and T cells in the central nervous system of humanized mice. Eur J Immunol 35(12):3683–3693

Illes Z, Stern JN, Reddy J, Waldner H, Mycko MP, Brosnan CF, Ellmerich S, Altmann DM, Santambrogio L, Strominger JL, Kuchroo VK (2004) Modified amino acid copolymers suppress myelin basic protein 85–99-induced encephalomyelitis in humanized mice through different effects on T cells. Proc Natl Acad Sci U S A 101(32):11749–11754

Jurevics H, Largent C, Hostettler J, Sammond DW, Matsushima GK, Kleindienst A, Toews AD, Morell P (2002) Alterations in metabolism and gene expression in brain regions during cuprizone-induced demyelination and remyelination. J Neurochem 82:126–136

Kalman B (2006) Role of mitochondria in multiple sclerosis. Curr Neurol Neurosci Rep 6(3):244–52

Kannan P, Yu Y, Wankhade S, Tainsky MA (1999) PolyADP-ribose polymerase is a coactivator for AP-2-mediated transcriptional activation. Nucleic Acids Res 27:866–874

Kauppinen TM, Chan WY, Suh SW, Wiggins AK, Huang EJ, Swanson RA (2006) Direct phosphorylation and regulation of poly(ADP-ribose) polymerase-1 by extracellular signal-regulated kinases 1/2. Proc Natl Acad Sci U S A 103:7136–7141

Kauppinen TM, Suh SW, Genain CP, Swanson RA (2005) Poly(ADP-ribose) polymerase-1 activation in a primate model of multiple sclerosis. J Neurosci Res 81(2):190–198

Keegan M, König F, McClelland R, Brück W, Morales Y, Bitsch A, Panitch H, Lassmann H, Weinshenker B, Rodriguez M, Parisi J, Lucchinetti CF (2005) Relation between humoral pathological changes in multiple sclerosis and response to therapeutic plasma exchange. Lancet 366(9485):579–582.

Kida E, Palminiello S, Golabek AA, Walus M, Wierzba-Bobrowicz T, Rabe A, Albertini G, Wisniewski KE (2006) Carbonic anhydrase II in the developing and adult human brain. J Neuropathol Exp Neurol 65:664–674

Kim NH, Kim K, Park WS, Son HS, Bae Y (2007) PKB/Akt inhibits ceramide-induced apoptosis in neuroblastoma cells by blocking apoptosis-inducing factor (AIF) translocation. J Cell Biochem 102:1160–70

Kim S, Steelman AJ, Zhang Y, Kinney HC, Li J (2012) Aberrant upregulation of astroglial ceramide potentiates oligodendrocyte injury. Brain Pathol 22:41–57

Kipp M, Clarner T, Dang J, Copray S, Beyer C (2009) The cuprizone animal model: new insights into an old story. Acta Neuropathol 118:723–736

Komoly S (2005) Experimental demyelination caused by primary oligodendrocyte dystrophy. Clin Neurosi/Ideggy Szle 58:40–43

Komoly S, Jeyasingham MD, Pratt OE, Lantos PL (1987) Decrease in oligodendrocyte carbonic anhydrase activity preceding myelin degeneration in cuprizone induced demyelination. J Neurol Sci 79:141–148

Komoly S, Hudson LD, Webster HD, Bondy CA (1992) Insulin-like growth factor I gene expression is induced in astrocytes during experimental demyelination. Proc Natl Acad Sci U S A 89: 1894–1898

Kutzelnigg A, Lucchinetti CF, Stadelmann C, Bruck W, Rauschka H, Bergmann M, Schmidbauer M, Parisi JE, Lassmann H (2005) Cortical demyelination and diffuse white matter injury in multiple sclerosis. Brain 128:2705–2712

La Mantia L, Munari LM, Lovati R (2010) Glatiramer acetate for multiple sclerosis. Cochrane Database Syst Rev. 2010 May 12;(5):CD004678. doi: 10.1002/14651858.CD004678.pub2

La Mantia L, Vacchi L, Di Pietrantonj C, Ebers G, Rovaris M, Fredrikson S, Filippini G (2012) Interferon beta for secondary progressive multiple sclerosis. Cochrane Database Syst Rev 1:CD005181

Lassmann H (2011a) The Architecture of inflammatory demyelinating lesions: implications for studies on pathogenesis. J Neuropath Appl Neurobiol 37:698–710

Lassmann H, Brück W, Lucchinetti C (2007) The immunopathology of multiple sclerosis: an overview. Brain Pathol 17:210–218

Lassmann H, van Horssen J (2011) The molecular basis of neurodegeneration in multiple sclerosis. FEBS Let 585:3715–3732

Li LY, Luo X, Wang X (2001) Endonuclease G is an apoptotic DNase when released from mitochondria. Nature 412:95–99

Liu JSH, Zhao ML, Brosnan CF, Lee SC (2001) Expression of indicible nitric oxide synthase and nitrotyrosine in multiple sclerosis lesions. Amer J Pathol 158:2057–2066

Liu X, Kim CN, Yang J, Jemmerson R, Wang X (1996) Induction of apoptotic program in cell-free extracts: requirement for dATP and cytochrome c. Cell 86:147–157

Lorenzo HK, Susin SA (2004) Mitochondrial effectors in caspase-independent cell death. FEBS Lett 557:14–20

Lu F, Selak M, O'Connor J, Croul S, Lorenzana C, Butunoi C, Kalman B (2000) Oxidative damage to mitochondrial DNA and activity of mitochondrial enzymes in chronic active lesions of multiple sclerosis. J Neurol Sci 177:95–103

Luccarini I, Ballerini C, Biagioli T, Biamonte F, Bellucci A, Rosi MC, Grossi C, Massacesi L, Casamenti F (2008) Combined treatment with atorvastatin and minocycline suppresses severity of EAE. Exp Neurol 211(1):214–26

Lucchinetti C, Brück W, Parisi J, Scheithauer B, Rodriguez M, Lassmann H (2000) Heterogeneity of multiple sclerosis lesions: implications for the pathogenesis of demyelination. Ann Neurol 47:707–717

Ludwin SK (1978) Central nervous system demyelination and remyelination in the mouse: an ultrastructural study of cuprizone toxicity. Lab Invest 39:597–612

Mahad D, Ziabreva I, Lassmann H, Turnbull D (2008) Mitochondrial defects in acute multiple sclerosis lesions. Brain 131:1722–1735

Mahad DJ, Ziabreva I, Campbell G, Lax N, White K, Hanson PS, Lassmann H, Turnbull DM (2009) Mitochondrial changes within in multiple sclerosis. Brain 132:1161–1174

Maier K, Merkler D, Gerber J, Taheri N, Kuhnert AV, Williams SK, Neusch C, Bähr M, Diem R (2007) Multiple neuroprotective mechanisms of minocycline in autoimmune CNS inflammation. Neurobiol Dis 25(3):514–25

Manrique-Hoyos N, Jürgens T, Grønborg M, Kreutzfeldt M, Schedensack M, Kuhlmann T, Schrick C, Brück W, Urlaub H, Simons M, Merkler D (2012) Late motor decline after accomplished remyelination: impact for progressive multiple sclerosis. Ann Neurol 71(2):227–244. doi: 10.1002/ana.22681

Marik C, Felts P, Bauer J, Lassmann H, Smith KJ (2007) Lesion genesis in a subset of patients with multiple sclerosis: a role for innate immunity? Brain 130:2800–2815

Mason JL, Suzuki K, Chaplin DD, Matsushima GK (2001) Interleukin-1beta promotes repair of the CNS. J Neurosci 21:7046–7052

Matsushima GK, Morell P (2001) The neurotoxicant, cuprizone, as a model to study demyelination and remyelination in the central nervous system. Brain Pathol 11:107–116

Mégnin-Chanet F, Bollet MA, Hall J (2010) Targeting poly(ADP-ribose) polymerase activity for cancer therapy. Cell Mol Life Sci 67(21):3649–3662

Metz LM, Zhang Y, Yeung M, Patry DG, Bell RB, Stoian CA, Yong VW, Patten SB, Duquette P, Antel JP, Mitchell JR (2004) Minocycline reduces gadolinium-enhancing magnetic resonance imaging lesions in multiple sclerosis. Ann Neurol 55(5):756. (No abstract available)

LM, Li D, Traboulsee A, Myles ML, Duquette P, Godin J, Constantin M, Yong VW;GA/minocyclinestudyinvestigators (2009) Glatiramer acetate in combination with minocycline in patients with relapsing–remitting multiple sclerosis: results of a Canadian, multicenter, double-blind, placebo-controlled trial. Mult Scler 15(10):1183–1194

Mi S, Hu B, Hahm K, Luo Y, Kam Hui ES, Yuan Q, Wong WM, Wang L, Su H, Chu TH, Guo J, Zhang W, So KF, Pepinsky B, Shao Z, Graff C, Garber E, Jung V, Wu EX, Wu W (2007) LINGO-1 antagonist promotes spinal cord remyelination and axonal integrity in MOG-induced experimental autoimmune encephalomyelitis. Nat Med 13(10):1228–1233

Morell P, Barrett CV, Mason JL, Toews AD, Hostettler JD, Knapp GW, Matsushima GK (1998) Gene expression in brain during cuprizone-induced demyelination and remyelination. Mol Cell Neurosci 12:220–227

Murphy MP (2009) How mitochondria produce reactive oxygen species. Biochem J 417:1–13

Nikodemova M, Lee J, Fabry Z, Duncan ID (2010) Minocycline attenuates experimental autoimmune encephalomyelitis in rats by reducing T cell infiltration into the spinal cord. J Neuroimmunol 219(1–2):33–37

O'Brien KA, Muscarella DE, Bloom SE (2001) Differential induction of apoptosis and MAP kinase signaling by mitochondrial toxicants in drug-sensitive compared to drug-resistant B-lineage lymphoid cell lines. Toxicol Appl Pharmacol 74:245–256

Oei SL, Shi Y (2001) Poly(ADP-ribosyl)ation of transcription factor Yin Yang 1 under conditions of DNA damage. Biochem Biophys Res Commun 285:27–31

Olah M, Amor S, Brouwer N, Vinet J, Eggen B, Biber K, Boddeke HW (2012) Identification of a microglia phenotype supportive of remyelination. Glia 60(2):306–321. doi: 10.1002/glia.21266

Oliver FJ, Menissier deMJ, Nacci C, Decker P, Andriantsitohaina R, Muller S, de la RG, Stoclet JC, de Murcia G (1999) Resistance to endotoxic shock as a consequence of defective NF-kappaB activation in poly (ADP-ribose) polymerase-1 deficient mice. EMBO J 18:4446–4454

Orio L, Llopis N, Torres E, Izco M, O'Shea E, Colado MI (2010) A study on the mechanisms by which minocycline protects against MDMA ('ecstasy')-induced neurotoxicity of 5-HT cortical neurons. Neurotox Res 18(2):187–99

Pang Y, Zheng B, Fan LW, Rhodes PG, Cai Z (2007) IGF-1 protects oligodendrocyte progenitors against TNFα-induced damage by activation of PI3 K/Akt and interruption of the mitochondrial apoptotic pathway. Glia 55:1099–1107

Park HS, Kim M-S, Huh S-H, Park J, Chung J, Kang SS, Choi E-J (2002) Akt (protein kinase B) negatively regulates SEK1 by means of protein phosphorylation. J Biol Chem 277:2573–2578

Pasquini LA, Calatayud CA, Bertone UAL, Millet V, Pasquini JM, Soto EF (2007) The neurotoxic effect of cuprizone on oligodendrocytes depends on the presence of pro-inflammatory cytokines secreted by microglia. Neurochem Res 32:279–292

Patrikios P, Stadelmann C, Kutzelnigg A, Rauschka H, Schmidbauer M, Laursen H, Soelberg Sorensen P, Brück W, Lucchinetti C, Lassmann H (2006) Remyelination is extensive in a subset of multiple sclerosis patients. Brain 129:3165–3172

Pellat-Deceunynck C, Wietzerbin J, Drapier JC (1994) Nicotinamide inhibits nitric oxide synthase MRNA induction in activated macrophages. Biochem J 297:53–58

Peterson JW, Bo L, Mork S, Chang A, Trapp BD (2001) Transected neurites, apoptotic neurons, and reduced inflammation in cortical multiple sclerosis lesions. Ann Neurol 50:389–400

Pinschewer DD, Brinkmann V, Merkler D (2011) Impact of sphingosine 1-phosphate modulation on immune outcomes. eurology 76(8 Suppl 3):S15–S19

Plummer R, Jones C, Middleton M, Wilson R, Evans J, Olsen A, Curtin N, Boddy A, McHugh P, Newell D, Harris A, Johnson P, Steinfeldt H, Dewji R, Wang D, Robson L, Calvert H (2008) Phase I study of the poly(ADP-ribose) polymerase inhibitor, AG014699, in combination with temozolomide in patients with advanced solid tumors. Clin Cancer Res 14(23):7917–7923

Popovic N, Schubart A, Goetz BD, Zhang SC, Linington C, Duncan ID (2002) Inhibition of autoimmune encephalomyelitis by a tetracycline. Ann Neurol 51(2):215–23

Pucci E, Giuliani G, Solari A, Simi S, Minozzi S, Di Pietrantonj C, Galea I (2011) Natalizumab for relapsing remitting multiple sclerosis. Cochrane Database Syst Rev. 2011 Oct 5;(10):CD007621. doi: 10.1002/14651858.CD007621.pub2

Racz B, Hanto K, Tapodi A, Solti I, Kalman N, Jakus P, Kovacs K, Debreceni B, Gallyas F Jr, Sumegi B (2010) Regulation of MKP-1 expression and MAPK activation by PARP-1 in oxidative stress: a new mechanism for the cytoplasmic effect of PARP-1 activation. Free Radic Biol Med 49:1978–1988

Remington LT, Babcock AA, Zehntner SP, Owens T (2007) Microglial recruitment, activation, and proliferation in response to primary demyelination. Am J Pathol 170:1713–1724

Ro HA, Carson JH (2004) pH microdomains in oligodendrocytes. J Biol Chem 279:37115–37123

Ruggieri M, Pica C, Lia A, Zimatore GB, Modesto M, Di Liddo E, Specchio LM, Livrea P, Trojano M, Avolio C (2008) Combination treatment of Glatiramer Acetate and Minocycline affects phenotype expression of blood monocyte-derived dendritic cells in multiple sclerosis patients. J Neuroimmunol 197(2):140–146

Russanov EM, Ljutakova SG (1980) Effect of cuprizone on copper exchange and superoxide dismutase activity in rat liver. Gen Pharmacol 11:535–538

Sarker M, Ruiz-Ruiz C, López-Rivas A (2001) Activation of protein kinase C inhibits TRAIL-induced caspases activation, mitochondrial events and apoptosis in a human leukemic T cell line. Cell Death Differ 8:172–181

Scott GS, Kean RB, Mikheeva T, Fabis MJ, Mabley JG, Szabó C, Hooper DC (2004) The therapeutic effects of PJ34 [N-(6-oxo-5,6-dihydrophenanthridin-2-yl)-N, N-dimethylacetamide.HCl], a selective inhibitor of poly(ADP-ribose) polymerase, in experimental allergic encephalomyelitis are associated with immunomodulation. J Pharmacol Exp Ther 310:1053–1061

Selvaraj V, Soundarapandian MM, Chechneva O, Williams AJ, Sidorov MK, Soulika AM, Pleasure DE, Deng W (2009) PARP-1 deficiency increases the severity of disease in a mouse model of multiple sclerosis. J Biol Chem 284(38):26070–26084

Sessa C (2011) Update on PARP1 inhibitors in ovarian cancer. Ann Oncol 22(Suppl 8):viii72–76

Sharma R, Fischer MT, Bauer J, Felts PA, Smith KJ, Misu T, Fujihara K, Bradl M, Lassmann H (2010) Inflammation induced by innate immunity in the central nervous system leads to primary astrocyte dysfunction followed by demyelination. Acta Neuropathol 120:223–236

Si Q, Cosenza M, Kim MO, Zhao ML, Brownlee M, Goldstein H, Lee S (2004) A novel action of minocycline: inhibition of human immunodeficiency virus type 1 infection in microglia. J Neurovirol 10(5):284–92

Skripuletz T, Gudi V, Hackstette D, Stangel M (2011) De- and remyelination in the CNS white and grey matter induced by cuprizone: the old, the new, and the unexpected. Histol Histopathol 26:1585–97

Skripuletz T, Miller E, Moharregh-Khiabani D, Blank A, Pul R, Gudi V, Trebst C, Stangel M (2010 Beneficial effects of minocycline on cuprizone induced cortical demyelination. Neurochem Res 35(9):1422–1433

Sriram S (2011) Role of glial cells in innate immunity and their role in CNS demyelination. J Neuroimmunol 239(1–2):13–20

Stys PK (2005) General mechanisms of axonal damage and its prevention. J Neurol Sci 133:3–13

Szabo C, Virag L, Cuzzocrea S, Scott GS, Hake P, O'Connor MP, Zingarelli B, Salzman A, Kun E (1998) Protection against peroxynitrite-induced fibroblast injury and arthritis development by inhibition of poly(ADP-ribose) synthase. ProcNatl Acad Sci U S A 95:3867–3872

Tandler B, Hoppel CL (1973) Division of giant mitochondria during recovery from cuprizone intoxication. J Cell Biol 56:266–272

Tang D, Wu D, Hirao A, Lahti JM, Liu L, Mazza B, Kidd VJ, Mak TW, Ingram AJ (2002) ERK activation mediates cell cycle arrest and apoptosis after DNA damage independently of p53. J Biol Chem 277:12710–12717

Tanuma S, Yagi T, Johnson GS (1985) Endogenous ADP ribosylation of high mobility group proteins 1 and 2 and histone H1 following DNA damage in intact cells. Arch Biochem Biophys 237:38–42

Tao R, Kim SH, Honbo N, Karliner JS, Alano CC (2010) Minocycline protects cardiac myocytes against simulated ischemia–reperfusion injury by inhibiting poly(ADP-ribose) polymerase-1. J Cardiovasc Pharmacol 56(6):659–668

Tapodi A, Debreceni B, Hanto K, Bognar Z, Wittmann I, Gallyas F Jr, Varbiro G, Sumegi B (2005) Pivotal role of Akt activation in mitochondrial protection and cell survival by poly(ADP-ribose) polymerase-1 inhibition in oxidative stress. J Biol Chem 280:35767–35775

Taylor LC, Gilmore W, Matsushima GK (2009) SJL mice exposed to cuprizone intoxication reveal strain and gender pattern differences in demyelination. Brain Pathol 19:467–479

Taylor LC, Gilmore W, Ting JP, Matsushima GK (2010) Cuprizone induces similar demyelination in male and female C57BL/6 mice and results in disruption of the estrous cycle. J Neurosci Res 88:391–402

Tewari M, Quan LT, O'Rourke K, Desnoyers S, Zeng Z, Beidler DR, Poirier GG, Salvesen GS, Dixit VM (1995) Yama/CPP32 beta a mammalian homolog of CED-3, is a CrmA-inhibitable protease that cleaves the death substrate poly(ADPribose)polymerase. Cell 81:801–809

Trapp B, Stys P (2009) Virtual hypoxia and chronic necrosis of demyelinated axons in multiple sclerosis. Lancet Neurol 8:80–291

Trapp BD, Nave KA (2008) Multiple sclerosis: an immune or neurodegenerative disorder? Annu Rev Neurosci 31:247–269

Van Horssen J, Schreibelt G, Drexhage J, Hazes T, Dijkstra CD, van der Valk P, de Vires HE (2008) Severe oxidative damage in multiple sclerosis lesions coincides with enhanced antioxidant enzyme expression. Free Radical Biol Med 45:1729–1737

Van Wijk SJ, Hageman GJ (2005) Poly(ADP-ribose) polymerase-1 mediated caspase-independent cell death after ischemia/reperfusion. Free Radic Biol Med 39:81–90

Venturini G (1973) Enzymic activities and sodium, potassium and copper concentrations in mouse brain and liver after cuprizone treatment in vivo. J Neurochem 21:1147–1151
Veres B, Gallyas F Jr, Varbiro G, Berente Z, Osz E, Szekeres G, Szabo C, Sumegi B (2003) Decrease of the inflammatory response and induction of the Akt/protein kinase B pathway by poly-(ADP-ribose) polymerase 1 inhibitor in endotoxin-induced septic shock. Biochem Pharmacol 65:1373–1382
Veres B, Radnai B, Gallyas F Jr, Varbiro G, Berente Z, Osz E, Sumegi B (2004) Regulation of kinase cascades and transcription factors by a poly(ADP-ribose) polymerase-1 inhibitor, 4-hydroxyquinazoline, in lipopolysaccharide-induced inflammation in mice. J Pharmacol Exp Ther 310:247–255
Veto S, Acs P, Bauer J, Lassmann H, Berente Z, Setalo G Jr, Borgulya G, Sumegi B, Komoly S, Gallyas F Jr, Illes Z (2010) Inhibiting poly(ADP-ribose) polymerase: a potential therapy against oligodendrocyte death. Brain 133:822–834
Virag L, Szabo C (2002) The therapeutic potential of poly(ADP-ribose) polymerase inhibitors. Pharmacol Rev 54:375–429
Vladimirova O, O'Connor J, Cahill A, Alder H, Butunoi C, Kalman B (1998) Oxidative damage to DNA in plaques of MS brains. Mult Scler 4:413–418
VonDran MW, Singh H, Honeywell JZ, Dreyfus CF (2011) Levels of BDNF impact oligodendrocyte lineage cells following a cuprizone lesion. J Neurosci 31(40):14182–14190
Vukusic S, Confavreux C (2007) Natural history of multiple sclerosis: risk factors and prognostic indicators. Curr Opin Neurol 20:269–74
Weinstock-Guttman B, Galetta SL, Giovannoni G, Havrdova E, Hutchinson M, Kappos L, O'Connor PW, Phillips JT, Polman C, Stuart WH, Lynn F, Hotermans C (2011) Additional efficacy endpoints from pivotal natalizumab trials in relapsing-remitting MS. J Neurol. (Epub ahead of print)
Wesierska-Gadek J, Schmid G, Cerni C (1996) ADP-ribosylation of wild-type P53 in vitro: binding of P53 protein to specific P53 consensus sequence prevents its modification. Biochem Biophys Res Commun 224:96–102
Whitacre CM, Hashimoto H, Tsai ML, Chatterjee S, Berger SJ, Berger NA (1995) Involvement of NAD-poly(ADP-ribose) metabolism in P53 regulation and its consequences. Cancer Res 55:3697–3701
Witte ME, Bo L, Rodenburg R, Belien JA, Musters R, Hazes T, Wintjes L, Smeitink JA, Geurts JJ, de Vries HE, van der Valk P, van Horssen J (2009) Enhanced number and activity of mitochondria in multiple sclerosis lesions. J Pathol 2:193–204
Yrjänheikki J, Keinänen R, Pellikka M, Hökfelt T, Koistinaho J (1998) Tetracyclines inhibit microglial activation and are neuroprotective in global brain ischemia. Proc Natl Acad Sci U S A 95:15769–15774
Yu SW, Wang H, Poitras MF, Coombs C, Bowers WJ, Federoff HJ, Poirier GG, Dawson TM, Dawson VL (2002) Mediation of poly(ADP-ribose) polymerase-1-dependent cell death by apoptosis inducing factor. Science 297:259–263
Yu SW, Andrabi SA, Wang H, Kim NS, Poirier GG, Dawson TM, Dawson VL (2006) Apoptosis-inducing factor mediates poly(ADP-ribose) (PAR) polymer-induced cell death. Proc Natl Acad Sci U S A 103:18314–18319
Zabad RK, Metz LM, Todoruk TR, Zhang Y, Mitchell JR, Yeung M, Patry DG, Bell RB, Yong VW (2007) The clinical response to minocycline in multiple sclerosis is accompanied by beneficial immune changes: a pilot study. Mult Scler 13(4):517–526
Zambonin JL, Zhao C, Ohno N, Campbell GR, Engeham S, Ziabreva I, Schwarz N, Lee SE, Frischer JM, Turnbull DM, Trapp BD, Lassmann H, Franklin RJ, Mahad DJ (2011) Increased mitochondrial content in remyelinated axons: implications for multiple sclerosis. Brain 134:1901–1913
Zatta P, Raso M, Zambenedetti P, Wittkowski W, Messori L, Piccioli F, Mauri PL, Beltramini M (2005) Copper and zinc dismetabolism in the mouse brain upon chronic cuprizone treatment. Cell Mol Life Sci 62:1502–1513

Zeis T, Propst A, Steck AJ, Stadelmann C, Brück W, Schaeren-Wiemers N (2009) Molecular changes in white matter adjacent to an active demyelinating lesion in early multiple sclerosis. Brain Pathol 19:459–466

Zhang Y, Metz LM, Yong VW, Bell RB, Yeung M, Patry DG, Mitchell JR (2008) Pilot study of minocycline in relapsing-remitting multiple sclerosis. Can J Neurol Sci 35(2):185–191

Zhu S, Stavrovskaya IG, Drozda M, Kim BY, Ona V, Li M, Sarang S, Liu AS, Hartley DM, Wu DC, Gullans S, Ferrante RJ, Przedborski S, Kristal BS, Friedlander RM (2002) Minocycline inhibits cytochrome c release and delays progression of amyotrophic lateral sclerosis in mice. Nature 417(6884):74–78

Zhu Y, Hoell P, Ahlemeyer B, Krieglstein J (2006) PTEN: a crucial mediator of mitochondria-dependent apoptosis. Apoptosis 11:197–207

Ziabreva I, Campbell G, Rist J, Zambonin J, Rorbach J, Wydro MM, Lassmann H, Franklin RJ, Mahad D (2010) Injury and differentiation following inhibition of mitochondrial respiratory chain complex IV in rat oligodendrocytes. Glia 58:1827–1837

Chapter 16
Association of Multiple Sclerosis with Other Autoimmune Diseases

Ali Manouchehrinia, Laura J. Edwards and Cris S. Constantinescu

16.1 Multiple Sclerosis: An Immune-Mediated Disease

Since its first comprehensive clinico-pathological description by Charcot, multiple sclerosis (MS) has remained a mysterious clinical entity and has represented a fascination to scientists and clinicians of the most diverse disciplines. With an incompletely known pathogenesis and aetiology, it has given rise to numerous theories including the more plausible ones of infection (Ascherio and Munger 2007a, b), autoimmunity (Hafler and Weiner 1989) and primary neurodegenerative disease to the more daring ones of vascular disease (Zamboni 2006), psychological abnormality or even neurocristopathy (Behan and Chaudhuri 2010).

Over the years, however, it has become increasingly clear and substantiated by a wealth of data that MS is an immune-mediated disorder. As such, it is not surprising that the book aiming to summarise the newest knowledge of the key immunopathological mechanisms of MS is starting from the premise of MS as an immune-mediated disease. Arguments for this are strong and are reiterated at several points in this book and will not be discussed in this chapter outside of the context of autoimmunity.

Autoimmunity, thus, requires the next level of evidence. While many agree that MS has immune-mediated pathogenesis, whether primary or secondary, fewer may accept that MS is an autoimmune disease (AD). One of the frequent arguments in favour of this theory is its association with other ADs (Constantinescu and Gran 2010). In this chapter, we will briefly discuss the concept and mechanisms of autoimmunity, the pro and con arguments for MS being autoimmune, the evidence for association with ADs and the mechanistic insights and therapeutic implications.

C. S. Constantinescu (✉) · A. Manouchehrinia · L. J. Edwards
Division of Clinical Neurosciences, University of Nottingham, C Floor, South Block,
Queen's Medical Centre, Nottingham NG7 2UH, UK
e-mail: cris.constantinescu@nottingham.ac.uk

T. Yamamura, B. Gran (eds.), *Multiple Sclerosis Immunology*,
DOI 10.1007/978-1-4614-7953-6_16, © Springer Science+Business Media New York 2013

16.2 The Concept and General Mechanisms of Autoimmunity

Autoimmunity is the reaction of the organism's immune system against its own proteins, cells and tissues (Anaya 2012). While normal organisms have self-reactive immune cells and some aspects of autoimmunity may be protective (Schwartz et al. 2003; Schwartz and Kipnis 2005; Schwartz and Shechter 2010), AD occurs when this activity of the immune system produces damage to their target tissues or their surroundings (Antony et al. 2011).

There are several general mechanisms of autoimmunity and often a combination of these leads to the ADs. These include a primary failure of central and peripheral mechanisms of tolerance; the breakdown of the otherwise normal tolerance mechanism due to infection and inflammatory factors overriding the tissue homeostasis; or a genetic or acquired abnormality in the target tissue that makes it immunogenic or inappropriately activates danger signals from the innate immune system (Anaya 2010). As in many ADs, these mechanisms have been investigated in MS and roles for each or combinations of them have been postulated.

16.3 Autoimmune Diseases: Genes and Environment; Epidemiological Perspectives

With the exception of rare inherited monogenic ADs (e.g. IPEX syndrome; d'Hennezel et al. 2009), the most common ADs result from an interplay between genes and environment. Not only does the relative contribution of these factors vary, dependent on the individual AD, but it also tends to change over time, with the overall tendency of a significant increase over the last few decades, which cannot merely be attributed to ascertainment bias.

It has been estimated that around 5 % of the world's population suffers from forms of autoimmunity (Shoenfeld et al. 2008). Over the past decade several new developments and technological advances have clarified some of the mechanisms underlying ADs. Despite this and some well-known genetic factors (mainly in HLA region) (Zanelli et al. 2000; Thorsby and Lie 2005; 2006), most of the causal mechanisms remain to be identified.

One way to evaluate the association of ADs is to try to appropriately collect, correlate and assess epidemiologic evidence. Epidemiologic studies can never prove causation, although they can suggest a causal effect in conjunction with biological plausibility. It is essential to bear in mind that the concept underlying epidemiology is that diseases are not randomly distributed in a population and certain characteristics (e.g. environmental and/or genetic) make individuals susceptible or protected against them. Therefore, epidemiologic studies can not only identify at-risk populations but also direct us towards the association that determines the characteristics or factors (e.g. age and sex), which put these populations at greater risk.

The estimates of the association of MS and other ADs have been controversial. While some studies have shown higher susceptibility of MS patients to concurrent autoimmune or immune-mediated diseases, some suggested an inverse association. To clarify these, one needs a clear definition of the term "association". In a well-designed epidemiologic study, association means coincidental occurrence of a risk factor and the disease at a same time and does not necessarily mean the factor causes the disease. Determination of causation requires a series of evidence that considers epidemiology, biological mechanisms, etc. Nevertheless, it would be reasonable to say that whether this is a positive or negative association, it will not change the fact that certain characteristics make these individuals more or less susceptible to a condition.

16.3.1 General Demographic Characteristics

Recognising similarities and differences among diseases facilitates identifying the underlying pathways and may lead to identifying widespread and novel therapeutic approaches. The studies of many ADs, and in particular MS, encounter various epidemiologic difficulties, which makes it hard to accurately comment on their natural history and demographic characteristics. Significant time interval between the biological onset and clinical symptoms, the lack of pathologic evidence and the time interval between the first clinical manifestation and definite diagnosis are some examples of epidemiologic difficulties in the field of autoimmunity and particularly MS. Regardless of their shortcomings, our practice today (prognostication, diagnosis and therapy) relies heavily on population data acquired from case-control studies, clinical trials and emerging MS databases. One way to evaluate the association of MS and other ADs is to fully investigate their demographic differences and similarities. Some demographic characteristics in patients with MS and other ADs follow distinct patterns. This distributional similarity can be informative when genetic predisposition or environmental factor(s) are of interest. One subject that is found in nearly all of the researches in the field of autoimmunity is the increased risk of autoimmunity among females (Whitacre et al. 1999). The percentage of women varies in different age groups and different parts of the world but the majority of ADs disproportionately affect women, significantly more than men. It has previously been suggested that oestrogens, androgens and progesterone can influence both innate and adaptive immune responses, but our knowledge of the mechanisms leading to such disproportionality is far from clear. Age is also known to have some role in making individuals susceptible to the ADs. There are remarkable differences in the onset age distribution of ADs. While some are primarily seen in younger adults (such as autoimmune hepatitis; Gregorio et al. 1997), some mainly occur during the adulthood and some may have bimodal age distributional pattern suggesting the role of hormonal status or immunosenescence in the pathogenesis of these diseases. Since the biologic onset of the disease can occur years before the diagnosis or even symptom onset, there are question marks over reliability of the onset age data. Geography and ethnicity have also been shown to influence the incidence of ADs, although it is not clear which one is dominant. In recent years, there has been an increase in recognition of ethnic-specific

Table 16.1 Approximate female percentage and onset age of some selected autoimmune conditions are shown (except as referenced, female percentage from Jacobson et al. 1997)

	Approximate female percentage	Onset age (years)
Multiple sclerosis	65	20–40 (Ghezzi 2004)
Type 1 diabetes	age $\leq$ 15 years: 50 age $\geq$ 16 years: 40	Childhood onset: 5–9 and 10–14 (2000) Adulthood onset: 25–61 (Nishimura et al. 2000)
Graves' disease	>85	30–60 (Lantz et al. 2009)
Thyroiditis	95	20–40 (Furszyfer et al. 1972)
Systemic lupus erythematosus	88	65 % 16–55 (Ballou et al. 1982) 20 % <16 (Font et al. 1998) 15 % >55 (Font et al. 1998)
Rheumatoid arthritis	75	30–55 (Deal et al. 1985)
Crohn's disease	53 (Montgomery et al. 2003)	Bimodal onset age distribution Peak at 20 and 50 (Rose et al. 1988; Haug et al. 1989)
Uveitis	50	45–65 male >65 female (Gritz and Wong 2004)
Sjögren's syndrome	94	40–75 (Pillemer et al. 2001)

variations as being of major medical relevance. Studies have shown that geography is a better determinant of genetics than ethnicity (Manica et al. 2005), but our current understanding of human genetic traits is insufficient (Hirschhorn et al. 2002). In addition to demographic characteristics, there are similarities in the natural history of some ADs. For example, most of the ADs such as MS, rheumatoid arthritis (RA) and psoriasis are comparable in having episodes of exacerbations (flare ups, relapses, bouts). Table 16.1 shows female percentage and onset age of some selected ADs.

16.3.2 Concurrent MS and other ADs

Although the presence of one or more co-morbid diseases may result in less desirable clinical outcome, and, in the case of MS, has been shown to delay the diagnosis (Marrie et al. 2009), co-morbidity may facilitate identifying the at-risk population and underlying mechanisms more robustly, bearing in mind that diseases may not be randomly distributed. Studies have reported an association of MS with some ADs, such as an inverse association with RA not confirmed by other studies (see below) (Somers et al. 2006; Nielsen et al. 2008) and a positive association with autoimmune thyroid disease (Sloka et al. 2005; Munteis et al. 2007). Cases of patients with both MS and systemic sclerosis, autoimmune hepatitis or myasthenia gravis have also been reported at smaller scales in some case-control studies (Achari et al. 1976; de Seze et al. 2005; Pelidou et al. 2007). Accurately defining the association of MS and other ADs on the basis of the incidence and/or prevalence data can be limited because of possible sources of error in the rate calculation and the fact that the standards and criteria may vary significantly among different studies performed. A problem arises from variations in diagnostic criteria. One classic example of such a problem is clearly demonstrated in a study by O'Sullivan and Cathcart (1972) comparing the prevalence of RA using New York Rheumatoid Association and the American Rheumatoid Association (ARA) diagnosis criteria. The survey showed significant variation in the results of the population of Sudbury from 3.8 % for women and 1.3 % for men by ARA criteria to 0.5 % for women and 0.1 % for men by New York criteria. This notable variation in diagnostic criteria may also have significant effects on our evaluation of the associations of MS with other ADs. The second problem is related to the ascertainment errors given the fact that most of the diseases in the autoimmunity field are considered as being rare. Nevertheless, the problems with incidence and prevalence rates are not limited to numerator only. For a rate to have a meaningful sense, each individual in the control population (denominator) should have a certain potential to develop the disease. As a result, the main challenge arises when a control population needs to be chosen (ascertainment bias in the control group). In such circumstances, the main question would be: who is truly at risk of developing AD? Of course, there is no definite answer to this question, but there are partially effective ways, such as familial studies or matching for age, gender, ethnicity and possible confounders, to decrease the scale of the problem. Yet, these approaches cannot fully eliminate the errors.

In addition to the presence of publication bias, mainly affecting negative results, many of the studies investigating the association of MS with other ADs were conducted as population surveys and only some of the estimates in the current literature are drawn from MS-specific population-based cohorts. These have resulted in substantial differences in the rate estimated and significant between-study heterogeneity. There are also limitations in generalizability of the results due to factors such as geography. Therefore, most of our current estimations of the incidence and prevalence rates and consequently the association of MS and other ADs may be over- or underestimation of the real-world data.

Furthermore, treatment interventions may influence the rates greatly (see also later under therapeutic implications). One treatment may increase the risk of particular co-morbid AD and another treatment can keep the concurrent AD hidden in its preclinical stage. For example, interferon (IFN)-β has been shown to modify the clinical course of RA (Alsalameh et al. 1998). Cases of sclerosing skin disorder while receiving IFN-β have also been reported in MS patients (Hugle et al. 2009). It is well accepted that co-morbidity complicates the process of prescribing rational medicinal therapy, but information drawn from studies looking at treatment response can also be invaluably informative.

16.3.3 Some Examples of MS–AD Association Studies

A number of studies explored the coexistence of MS with ADs. As discussed earlier, all of them have inherent weaknesses: small sample sizes and clinic-based cohorts with unmatched, absent or historical control groups. Some of these biases are avoided in some studies using large databases, for example, large MS registers or collections such as those used for genetic studies (Barcellos et al. 2006; Ramagopalan et al. 2007a, b). The study of other, non-autoimmune co-morbidities may also help to reduce ascertainment bias. For genetic studies, spousal controls are often used, as they are often matched for many demographic characteristics, although this reverses the gender ratio.

In 2004, we carried out an analysis of co-morbidities of > 650 consecutive patients attending our specialist clinic, and compared them with known prevalence of the associated conditions in the closest geographical areas, in most cases, English Midlands or the UK (Edwards and Constantinescu 2004). We found an increased association of MS with asthma and all atopy, all inflammatory bowel disease, pernicious anaemia, autoimmune thyroid disease, seronegative spondyloarthropathy and uveitis. The results are interesting as they show coexistence of traditionally "Th1" and "Th2" diseases, which can now be explained through other shared immunopathological mechanisms (see below).

Barcellos et al. (2006) analysed a total of 176 families comprising 386 MS index cases and 1,107 first-degree relatives and found that 26 % of the index cases reported at least one coexisting autoimmune disorder. Autoimmune thyroid disease, psoriasis, inflammatory bowel disease and RA were the most common associations. Similar associations were found in first-degree relatives. Interestingly, there was a suggestion of a genetic segregation between index cases with association of other AD in their personal or family history, as these were strongly associated with a common variant of the CTLA4 gene.

The gender differences in MS and AD have been discussed earlier. Ramagopalan et al. (2007a, b), in a similar study, found that correcting for gender eliminates the higher than chance association of MS with other AD, and suggested that this simply represents the increased susceptibility of women to autoimmunity.

However, a subsequent study was performed on a large population database by Langer-Gould et al. (2010) who found an association between MS and AD even after correcting for gender. Thus, the association cannot be attributed entirely to the higher susceptibility of females to autoimmunity. There was an increased prevalence of uveitis, inflammatory bowel disease, Bell's palsy, Guillain–Barré syndrome (GBS), and bullous pemphigoid in MS patients. These results confirmed some of the previous findings and suggested that this association occurs more than expected by chance. Importantly, the authors distinguished between associated diseases occurring before or after the diagnosis of MS. Uveitis, inflammatory bowel disease and Bell's palsy tended to precede MS in this study. Previous clinic-based studies of uveitis and MS suggested a slightly higher frequency of MS preceding Uveitis. Since pathological evidence shows that uveitis and ocular inflammation is often widespread albeit pauci- or asymptomatic in MS (Green et al. 2010), the discovery of uveitis in patients with MS attending a specialist clinic may reflect increased awareness and ascertainment.

In conclusion, there is a certain degree of plausibility in asserting that MS and AD are associated. Because of the relative frequency of these disorders, their coexistence, even by chance, raises questions and has implications in terms of management.

16.4 Potentially Shared Immunological Mechanisms

Despite contradictory studies, there is now an increased number of studies showing that MS and atopy/asthma coexist, indicating that "Th1 and Th2" immune responses are not mutually exclusive. Thus, alternative immunopathogenic mechanisms are to be considered, and targeting these mechanisms may provide benefit both to MS and to the associated disease.

The most attractive common mechanism is an exaggerated Th17 response. IL-17 and Th17-associated cytokines have been implicated not only in MS but also in most ADs reported to be associated with MS. Although in experimental models, targeting IL-17 has not had dramatic effects (Hofstetter et al. 2005; Komiyama et al. 2006) and blocking IL-12/IL-23p40, which reduces both Th1 and Th17 expansion, has not had a significant effect in an MS clinical trial (Segal et al. 2008) (although a small effect was seen in another trial (Vollmer et al. 2011)), many successful interventions may reduce, directly or indirectly, Th17 cells.

Another possible factor is the platelet-activating factor (PAF). This inflammatory mediator is implicated in both allergy- and cell-mediated ADs including MS. We observed that PAF is involved in Th17 development (manuscript in preparation); therefore, PAF antagonism may suppress both MS and associated inflammatory diseases regardless of the definite phenotype of the inflammation (Edwards and Constantinescu 2009).

Another mechanism is defective immune regulation. In all these conditions, regulatory mechanisms, in particular regulatory T (Treg) cells, are deficient and modalities to enhance their function (and perhaps numbers) may be beneficial. We have shown that steroids, universal anti-inflammatory drugs, induce Treg cells in MS (Braitch et al. 2009), but less problematic and longer-active Treg-inducing interventions are likely to be necessary. Correale and Farez (2007) noted a favourable course of MS in people naturally infected with intestinal parasites. This protection was associated with a substantial increase in Treg cell function. Such mechanisms are explored in trials of MS, other ADs and atopic diseases, and they are likely to work in the same way if these diseases coexist in the same individual.

Deficient immunoregulatory mechanisms, common to a variety of ADs, including MS, type 1 diabetes, RA, etc., may be related to inadequate sun exposure, which explains the striking latitude gradient in MS (and other ADs). The mechanisms have implicated inadequate UVB exposure resulting in a deficit of vitamin D, a deficit which has been convincingly shown in MS and other ADs. Vitamin D deficiency is associated with increased susceptibility to MS (Ascherio and Munger 2007a). Data showing a month of birth effect in MS, diabetes mellitus, ulcerative colitis and systemic lupus erythematosus (SLE) also suggest a role for gestational vitamin D deficiency in the increased susceptibility to AD (Ramagopalan et al. 2009; Disanto et al. 2012). Vitamin D treatment may thus be an option for MS and other ADs, or when they exist in combination. Planned trials will prove whether this treatment, instituted after the disease has started, has a therapeutic effect. Experimental and some clinical data suggest an important role for the induction of Foxp3^{+} Treg cells and IL-10-secreting Treg cells (Tr1 cells) in the immunomodulatory effects of vitamin D (Taams et al. 2006).

Although vitamin D is the most studied factor involved in the latitude effect, other light-regulated factors such as melatonin or calcitonin gene-related peptide may be involved. Bright light or melatonin-suppressing therapy has previously been shown to suppress experimental autoimmune encephalomyelitis (EAE) (Stevens and Swanborg 1993), and light deprivation enhances experimental arthritis (Hansson et al. 1990). Light therapy has been advocated for MS treatment (Constantinescu 1995).

16.5 Negative Associations May Provide Hints to (Auto)Immune Mechanisms in MS

In addition to some coexisting conditions, there are some conditions that are less frequently encountered in people with MS than expected from the general population. Certain types of cancer are less frequent, which has been attributed to a more active immune surveillance (Bahmanyar et al. 2009). Although our study encountered some cases of gout (Edwards and Constantinescu 2004), this condition is thought to be very rare among people with MS, who have been reported to have lower levels of uric acid, a natural antioxidant and peroxinitrite inhibitor (Hooper et al. 1998). Treatment with inosine, which enhances the levels of uric acid, has been suggested in MS (Hooper et al. 1997).

In view of the increased evidence for the role of the Epstein–Barr virus (EBV) in MS (and other ADs), reports of a high association with other classical EBV-mediated disorders such as Hodgkin's and non-Hodgkin's lymphoma or nasopharyngeal carcinoma would be expected. Such reports, however, are merely anecdotal (Rolls et al. 2010), and lymphoma does not belong among the cancers reported to be increased in MS (Bahmanyar et al. 2009). The explanation for this could be that of a defective immunoregulation (e.g. induction of IL-10 or Treg) by EBV in MS, which would, however, provide benefits in terms of cancer immunosurveillance.

16.6 Diagnostic and Therapeutic Implications

Co-morbidity has an important influence on MS and other ADs. In addition to providing hints towards shared pathogenic pathways, it has diagnostic and therapeutic implications. For example, it has been shown that the presence of co-morbidity delays the diagnosis of MS (Marrie et al. 2009). Even coexistence of non-autoimmune conditions with MS may provide hints towards pathological mechanisms and therapeutic opportunities. The high prevalence of depression in MS, for example, and the recent experimental evidence of the role of serotonin reuptake inhibitors in immunomodulation and neuroprotection in EAE (Vollmar et al. 2009; Taler et al. 2011; Yuan et al. 2012) suggest the involvement of these pathways in MS and potential disease-modifying benefits of commonly used antidepressants in MS. Presence of hypertension in a person with MS may offer the opportunity of treating with an angiotensin-converting enzyme (ACE) inhibitor or an angiotensin receptor blocker (Constantinescu et al. 1995; Platten et al. 2009; Stegbauer et al. 2009), which may result in protective immunomodulation as shown in the EAE models.

Regardless of whether the coexisting AD represents shared pathology and susceptibility, and whether this coexistence is due to chance co-occurrence or a spectrum of poly-autoimmunity, there are important practical implications related to diagnosis and treatment. Classical diagnosis criteria preclude the diagnosis of MS in the presence of a condition that could explain the symptoms better. With inflammatory/autoimmune diseases that may affect the nervous system, this is not often possible. For example, SLE and MS can coexist (Hietaharju et al. 2001). It has been argued that a misdiagnosis of MS can be made in the presence of imitators such as anti-phospholipid syndrome, but these conditions can also coexist (Stosic et al. 2010). The presence of autoantibodies such as antinuclear antibodies (Collard et al. 1997) and anti-cardiolipin antibodies (Vilisaar et al. 2005) is not uncommon in MS, and need not raise suspicions of alternative diagnoses.

Although sarcoidosis is not strictly an AD, it is autoinflammatory and shares clinical and pathological features with ADs. ACE is elevated in serum and is a frequently used marker for sarcoidosis. A proportion of people with MS have an elevated serum ACE (Constantinescu et al. 1997), and this need not rule out MS. We have had patients with biopsy-proven non-neurological sarcoidosis who later went on to develop typical MS. An important therapeutic consideration is whether disease-modifying therapy (DMT) for MS would benefit or worsen the coexisting AD.

Berkovich et al. (2011) recently summarised these considerations. Briefly, hepatic dysfunction is relatively common in people treated with IFN-β and may have an autoimmune basis; thyroid dysfunction (autoimmune thyroid disease) can occur or be exacerbated in people with MS treated with IFN-β. Occurrence or exacerbation of psoriasis has also been reported in people receiving IFN-β for MS, as well as several cases of ulcerative colitis, panniculitis (also with glatiramer acetate (GA)) and vasculitis. At the case report level, GA has been associated with one case of urticarial vasculitis and one of autoimmune thyroid disease. One case of SLE and one of RA developed under treatment with IFN-β. These rare events are listed in the paper by Berkovich et al. (2011).

Although the first-line disease-modifying drugs act in part by inducing a Th1 to Th2 switch, none has been consistently associated with an exacerbation of coexisting Th2 diseases such as asthma and atopy. However, avoiding GA in people with asthma may help distinguish the post-injection reactions from asthma attacks.

As discussed earlier, in the cases of uveitis coexisting with MS, there is no indication that the DMTs have any negative effect on established uveitis nor is there evidence that they trigger it (Edwards et al. 2008). On the contrary, IFN has been advocated as a treatment for MS-associated uveitis (Becker et al. 2005).

Since type 1 IFN plays a pathogenic role in SLE (Elkon and Wiedeman 2012), in cases where features of SLE, mixed connective tissue diseases, Sjögren's syndrome and anti-phospholipid syndrome coexist with MS, IFN-β is probably best avoided. We have successfully treated two patients with coexisting MS and SLE, one with mixed connective tissue disease and one with anti-phospholipid syndrome with GA.

16.7 Considerations on the Relationship Between Anti-Tumour Necrosis Factor Biological Treatment and the Development of Demyelinating Disease

In 2001, a case series triggered by an index case and completed by interrogating an FDA database pointed to the appearance of demyelinating disease in patients with rheumatologic conditions receiving treatment with biological agents that block tumour necrosis factor (TNF) (Mohan et al. 2001). These included etanercept and infliximab, to which adalimumab was also added subsequently. This has been reviewed in Ramos-Casals et al. (2010).

Also, the use of anti-TNF agents in other inflammatory conditions, such as psoriatic arthritis, ankylosing spondylitis and inflammatory bowel disease, has been associated with rare and sporadic cases of demyelination.

This led to the conclusion that these treatments are contraindicated in MS. Reviewing the initial case series, some features argue against at least some of the reported cases being MS. The index case had a brain biopsy that showed spongiosis and was atypical for MS, the other patient undergoing biopsy had toxic encephalopathy changes without evidence of demyelination, and the one patient who underwent lumbar puncture had cerebrospinal fluid that was negative for oligoclonal bands.

This may mean that at least some of these neurological complications are not indicative of MS. In support of this is the fact that a substantial proportion of the reported cases are negative for oligoclonal bands and the abnormalities disappear upon discontinuation of anti-TNF treatment. Moreover, successful, uneventful rechallenge with anti-TNF agents after the development of such a demyelinating episode has been reported. Several studies estimating the risk of such demyelinating events argue against a true association between MS and TNF antagonists, beyond that expected between MS and the underlying inflammatory conditions that require the treatment (Magnano et al. 2004). An interesting study estimated the risk of demyelination under treatment with TNF antagonists for RA as not being higher than expected on the basis of chance occurrence of the conditions, and also not higher than that under treatment with anakinra, an IL-1 receptor antagonist (Bernatsky et al. 2010).

Based on the complex biology of TNF-α and its related cytokine TNF-β (lymphotoxin), there are rationales why TNF blockade may be detrimental in MS. Studies in the experimental model of EAE showed that TNF/lymphotoxin double knockout mice remain susceptible to autoimmune demyelination (Frei et al. 1997) and even have more severe disease. This was confirmed subsequently in studies by Liu et al. (1998) and Probert et al. (1997). Furthermore, in a cuprizone- induced demyelination model, the role of TNF was investigated using TNF knockout mice. While demyelination was more severe in wild-type mice, remyelination was significantly less complete in TNF−/− mice, suggesting a role for TNF in remyelination (Arnett et al. 2001).

Van Oosten et al. (1996) treated two patients with MS with anti-TNF agents and witnessed a worsening of the disease course including clinical relapses and an increase in gadolinium-enhancing lesions, suggesting a partially protective role for TNF. This was also confirmed in the lenercept MS trial, the results of which did not show a beneficial effect of anti-TNF agents (1999). Therefore, despite anecdotal reports of people with MS and associated ADs having been exposed to anti-TNF agents without complications, treatment of a coexisting AD in a patient with MS is currently discouraged.

However, going back to the case reports of demyelination during anti-TNF treatment and considering the bona fide MS cases among them, one needs to question the role of the anti-TNF agent itself or that of the likelihood of the AD being associated with MS by common pathogenetic mechanisms or by chance. It remains plausible, and supported by pharmacoepidemiology studies, that the occurrence of MS in people with anti-TNF treatment for another autoimmune inflammatory disorder is not higher than expected for MS in the general population.

We conducted a study showing no major differences in high-field (3 tesla) magnetic resonance imaging (MRI) in people who have received anti-TNF treatment compared with the general population. They had similar numbers and distribution of non-specific white matter changes as the healthy controls and showed no changes in quantitative MRI in the normal-appearing white and grey matter in contrast to the MS controls. A patient with ankylosing spondylitis who was in our study and had a normal MRI scan, who was receiving adalimumab and who developed MS later, had the typical MS lesions and positive oligoclonal bands, similar to the findings of the MS controls. An association of ankylosing spondylitis with MS has been reported and ~60 % of patients may have subtly abnormal evoked potentials (Hanrahan et al. 1988; Edwards and Constantinescu 2004). Thus, it is conceivable that MS developed independently of the anti-TNF treatment.

16.8 Alemtuzumab and Autoimmunity

Alemtuzumab is a promising monoclonal antibody against the CD52 molecule, which has shown excellent results in reducing the relapse rate and disability progression in MS (Coles et al. 2008; Jones and Coles 2009). Treatment with alemtuzumab is associated with the occurrence of ADs, with a cumulative risk of 22 % (Cossburn et al. 2011). The most common is the autoimmune thyroid disease, but there is a risk of idiopathic thrombocytopenic purpura, and a case of glomerular basement membrane disease has been reported. Other single cases of pulmonary hypersensitivity reactions, bullous skin disease and colitis have been reported in that series.

Since alemtuzumab induces significant immunosuppression and similar patterns of secondary autoimmunity are seen occasionally after haematopoietic stem cell transplantation (with or without use of alemtuzumab in vivo as part of the protocol), it is an opportunity to understand mechanisms of immune reconstitutions and homeostatic proliferation. In elegant studies, Coles et al. have demonstrated that the cytokine IL-21 is associated with the risk of autoimmune complications, as the pre-treatment IL-21 levels predicted (Jones et al. 2009). This not only completes the pathological picture of the cytokine network in MS but also underscores the complex relationship between MS, its treatment and autoimmunity.

In conclusion, MS is an immune-mediated disease, which coexists with other autoimmune or presumed autoimmune diseases. This coexistence may be the result of a chance association, an increased common predisposition of certain groups (such as women) to many autoimmune diseases, common pathogenic mechanisms, shared genetics or environmental risks, or in some cases, one disease is facilitated by the treatment for another. Finally, various combinations of the above may result in these associations. Nevertheless, these co-occurrences invite careful therapeutic considerations and may provide helpful insights into the pathophysiology of MS and the mechanisms of autoimmunity.

References

(1999) TNF neutralization in MS: results of a randomized, placebo-controlled multicenter study. The Lenercept Multiple Sclerosis Study Group and The University of British Columbia MS/MRI Analysis Group. Neurology 53(3):457–465

(2000) Variation and trends in incidence of childhood diabetes in Europe. EURODIAB ACE Study Group. Lancet 355(9207):873–876

(2006) Incidence and trends of childhood type 1 diabetes worldwide 1990–1999. Diabet Med 23(8):857–866

Achari AN, Trontelj JV et al (1976) Multiple sclerosis and myasthenia gravis. A case report with single fiber electromyography. Neurology 26(6 PT 1):544–546

Alsalameh S, Manger B et al (1998) New onset of rheumatoid arthritis during interferon beta-1B treatment in a patient with multiple sclerosis: comment on the case report by Jabaily and Thompson. Arthritis Rheum 41(4):754

Anaya JM (2010) The autoimmune tautology. Arthritis Res Ther 12(6):147

Anaya JM (2012) Common mechanisms of autoimmune diseases (the autoimmune tautology). Autoimmun Rev 11(11):781–784

Antony JM, Deslauriers AM et al (2011) Human endogenous retroviruses and multiple sclerosis: innocent bystanders or disease determinants? Biochim Biophys Acta 1812(2):162–176

Arnett HA, Mason J et al (2001) TNF alpha promotes proliferation of oligodendrocyte progenitors and remyelination. Nat Neurosci 4(11):1116–1122

Ascherio A, Munger KL (2007a) Environmental risk factors for multiple sclerosis. Part I: the role of infection. Ann Neurol 61(4):288–299

Ascherio A, Munger KL (2007b) Environmental risk factors for multiple sclerosis. Part II: noninfectious factors. Ann Neurol 61(6):504–513

Bahmanyar S, Montgomery SM et al (2009) Cancer risk among patients with multiple sclerosis and their parents. Neurology 72(13):1170–1177

Ballou SP, Khan MA et al (1982) Clinical features of systemic lupus erythematosus: differences related to race and age of onset. Arthritis Rheum 25(1):55–60

Barcellos LF, Kamdar BB et al (2006) Clustering of autoimmune diseases in families with a high-risk for multiple sclerosis: a descriptive study. Lancet Neurol 5(11):924–931

Becker MD, Heiligenhaus A et al (2005) Interferon as a treatment for uveitis associated with multiple sclerosis. Br J Ophthalmol 89(10):1254–1257

Behan PO, Chaudhuri A (2010) The sad plight of multiple sclerosis research (low on fact, high on fiction): critical data to support it being a neurocristopathy. Inflammopharmacology 18(6):265–290

Berkovich R, Subhani D et al (2011) Autoimmune comorbid conditions in multiple sclerosis. US Neurology 7(2):132–138

Bernatsky S, Renoux C et al (2010) Demyelinating events in rheumatoid arthritis after drug exposures. Ann Rheum Dis 69(9):1691–1693

Braitch M, Harikrishnan S et al (2009) Glucocorticoids increase CD4CD25 cell percentage and Foxp3 expression in patients with multiple sclerosis. Acta Neurol Scand 119(4):239–245
Coles AJ, Compston DA et al (2008) Alemtuzumab vs. interferon beta-1a in early multiple sclerosis. N Engl J Med 359(17):1786–1801
Collard RC, Koehler RP et al (1997) Frequency and significance of antinuclear antibodies in multiple sclerosis. Neurology 49(3):857–861
Constantinescu CS (1995) Melanin, melatonin, melanocyte-stimulating hormone, and the susceptibility to autoimmune demyelination: a rationale for light therapy in multiple sclerosis. Med Hypotheses 45(5):455–458
Constantinescu CS, Goodman DB et al (1997) Serum angiotensin-converting enzyme in multiple sclerosis. Arch Neurol 54(8):1012–1015
Constantinescu CS, Gran B (2010) Multiple sclerosis: autoimmune associations in multiple sclerosis. Nat Rev Neurol 6(11):591–592
Constantinescu CS, Ventura E et al (1995) Effects of the angiotensin converting enzyme inhibitor captopril on experimental autoimmune encephalomyelitis. Immunopharmacol Immunotoxicol 17(3):471–491
Correale J, Farez M (2007) Association between parasite infection and immune responses in multiple sclerosis. Ann Neurol 61(2):97–108
Cossburn M, Pace AA et al (2011) Autoimmune disease after alemtuzumab treatment for multiple sclerosis in a multicenter cohort. Neurology 77(6):573–579
d'Hennezel E, Ben-Shoshan M et al (2009) FOXP3 forkhead domain mutation and regulatory T cells in the IPEX syndrome. N Engl J Med 361(17):1710–1713
de Seze J, Canva-Delcambre V et al (2005) Autoimmune hepatitis and multiple sclerosis: a coincidental association? Mult Scler 11(6):691–693
Deal CL, Meenan RF et al (1985) The clinical features of elderly-onset rheumatoid arthritis. A comparison with younger-onset disease of similar duration. Arthritis Rheum 28(9):987–994
Disanto G, Chaplin G et al (2012) Month of birth, vitamin D and risk of immune mediated disease: a case control study. BMC Med 10(1):69
Edwards LJ, Constantinescu CS (2004) A prospective study of conditions associated with multiple sclerosis in a cohort of 658 consecutive outpatients attending a multiple sclerosis clinic. Mult Scler 10(5):575–581
Edwards LJ, Constantinescu CS (2009) Platelet activating factor/platelet activating factor receptor pathway as a potential therapeutic target in autoimmune diseases. Inflamm Allergy Drug Targets 8(3):182–190
Edwards LJ, Dua H et al (2008) Symptomatic Uveitis and multiple sclerosis. Neuro-Ophthalmology 32(2):49–54
Elkon KB, Wiedeman A (2012) Type I IFN system in the development and manifestations of SLE. Curr Opin Rheumatol 24(5):499–505
Font J, Cervera R et al (1998) Systemic lupus erythematosus (SLE) in childhood: analysis of clinical and immunological findings in 34 patients and comparison with SLE characteristics in adults. Ann Rheum Dis 57(8):456–459
Frei K, Eugster HP et al (1997) Tumor necrosis factor alpha and lymphotoxin alpha are not required for induction of acute experimental autoimmune encephalomyelitis. J Exp Med 185(12):2177–2182
Furszyfer J, Kurland LT et al (1972) Epidemiologic aspects of Hashimoto's thyroiditis and Graves' disease in Rochester, Minnesota (1935–1967), with special reference to temporal trends. Metabolism 21(3):197–204
Ghezzi A (2004) Clinical characteristics of multiple sclerosis with early onset. Neurol Sci 25 (Suppl 4):S336–S339
Green AJ, McQuaid S et al (2010) Ocular pathology in multiple sclerosis: retinal atrophy and inflammation irrespective of disease duration. Brain 133(Pt 6):1591–1601
Gregorio GV, Portmann B et al (1997) Autoimmune hepatitis in childhood: a 20-year experience. Hepatology 25(3):541–547
Gritz DC, Wong IG (2004) Incidence and prevalence of uveitis in Northern California; the Northern California epidemiology of Uveitis study. Ophthalmology 111(3):491–500. (discussion 500)

Hafler DA, Weiner HL (1989) MS: a CNS and systemic autoimmune disease. Immunol Today 10(3):104–107
Hanrahan PS, Russell AS et al (1988) Ankylosing spondylitis and multiple sclerosis: an apparent association? J Rheumatol 15(10):1512–1514
Hansson I, Holmdahl R et al (1990) Constant darkness enhances autoimmunity to type II collagen and exaggerates development of collagen-induced arthritis in DBA/1 mice. J Neuroimmunol 27(1):79–84
Haug K, Schrumpf E et al (1989) Epidemiology of Crohn's disease in western Norway. Study group of Inflammatory Bowel Disease in Western Norway. Scand J Gastroenterol 24(10):1271–1275
Hietaharju A, Peltola J et al (2001) The coexistence of systemic lupus erythematosus and multiple sclerosis in a mother and daughter. Scand J Rheumatol 30(2):120–122
Hirschhorn JN, Lohmueller K et al (2002) A comprehensive review of genetic association studies. Genet Med 4(2):45–61
Hofstetter HH, Ibrahim SM et al (2005) Therapeutic efficacy of IL-17 neutralization in murine experimental autoimmune encephalomyelitis. Cell Immunol 237(2):123–130
Hooper DC, Bagasra O et al (1997) Prevention of experimental allergic encephalomyelitis by targeting nitric oxide and peroxynitrite: implications for the treatment of multiple sclerosis. Proc Natl Acad Sci U S A 94(6):2528–2533
Hooper DC, Spitsin S et al (1998) Uric acid, a natural scavenger of peroxynitrite, in experimental allergic encephalomyelitis and multiple sclerosis. Proc Natl Acad Sci U S A 95(2):675–680
Hugle T, Gratzl S et al (2009) Sclerosing skin disorders in association with multiple sclerosis. Coincidence, underlying autoimmune pathology or interferon induced? Ann Rheum Dis 68(1):47–50
Jacobson DL, Gange SJ et al (1997) Epidemiology and estimated population burden of selected autoimmune diseases in the United States. Clin Immunol Immunopathol 84(3):223–243
Jones JL, Coles AJ (2009) Spotlight on alemtuzumab. Int MS J 16(3):77–81
Jones JL, Phuah CL et al (2009) IL-21 drives secondary autoimmunity in patients with multiple sclerosis, following therapeutic lymphocyte depletion with alemtuzumab (Campath-1 H). J Clin Invest 119(7):2052–2061
Komiyama Y, Nakae S et al (2006) IL-17 plays an important role in the development of experimental autoimmune encephalomyelitis. J Immunol 177(1):566–573
Langer-Gould A, Albers KB et al (2010) Autoimmune diseases prior to the diagnosis of multiple sclerosis: a population-based case-control study. Mult Scler 16(7):855–861
Lantz M, Abraham-Nordling M et al (2009) Immigration and the incidence of Graves' thyrotoxicosis, thyrotoxic multinodular goiter and solitary toxic adenoma. Eur J Endocrinol 160(2):201–206
Liu J, Marino MW et al (1998) TNF is a potent anti-inflammatory cytokine in autoimmune-mediated demyelination. Nat Med 4(1):78–83
Magnano MD, Robinson WH et al (2004) Demyelination and inhibition of tumor necrosis factor (TNF). Clin Exp Rheumatol 22(5 Suppl35):S134–S140
Manica A, Prugnolle F et al (2005) Geography is a better determinant of human genetic differentiation than ethnicity. Hum Genet 118(3–4):366–371
Marrie RA, Horwitz R et al (2009) Comorbidity delays diagnosis and increases disability at diagnosis in MS. Neurology 72(2):117–124
Mohan N, Edwards ET et al (2001) Demyelination occurring during anti-tumor necrosis factor alpha therapy for inflammatory arthritides. Arthritis Rheum 44(12):2862–2869
Montgomery SM, Wakefield AJ et al (2003) Sex-specific risks for pediatric onset among patients with Crohn's disease. Clin Gastroenterol Hepatol 1(4):303–309
Munteis E, Cano JF et al (2007) Prevalence of autoimmune thyroid disorders in a Spanish multiple sclerosis cohort. Eur J Neurol 14(9):1048–1052
Nielsen NM, Frisch M et al (2008) Autoimmune diseases in patients with multiple sclerosis and their first-degree relatives: a nationwide cohort study in Denmark. Mult Scler 14(6):823–829
Nishimura M, Obayashi H et al (2000) Association between type 1 diabetes age-at-onset and intercellular adhesion molecule-1 (ICAM-1) gene polymorphism. Hum Immunol 61(5):507–510

O'Sullivan JB, Cathcart ES (1972) The prevalence of rheumatoid arthritis. Follow-up evaluation of the effect of criteria on rates in Sudbury, Massachusetts. Ann Intern Med 76(4):573–577
Pelidou SH, Tsifetaki N et al (2007) Multiple sclerosis associated with systemic sclerosis. Rheumatol Int 27(8):771–773
Pillemer SR, Matteson EL et al (2001) Incidence of physician-diagnosed primary Sjogren syndrome in residents of Olmsted County, Minnesota. Mayo Clin Proc 76(6):593–599
Platten M, Youssef S et al (2009) Blocking angiotensin-converting enzyme induces potent regulatory T cells and modulates TH1- and TH17-mediated autoimmunity. Proc Natl Acad Sci U S A 106(35):14948–14953
Probert L, Akassoglou K et al (1997) TNF-alpha transgenic and knockout models of CNS inflammation and degeneration. J Neuroimmunol 72(2):137–141
Ramagopalan SV, Dyment DA et al (2007a) Clustering of autoimmune disease in families at high risk for multiple sclerosis? Lancet Neurol 6(3):206–207. (author reply 207)
Ramagopalan SV, Dyment DA et al (2007b) Autoimmune disease in families with multiple sclerosis: a population-based study. Lancet Neurol 6(7):604–610
Ramagopalan SV, Link J et al (2009) HLA-DRB1 and month of birth in multiple sclerosis. Neurology 73(24):2107–2111
Ramos-Casals M, Roberto PAetal (2010) Autoimmune diseases induced by biological agents: a double-edged sword? Autoimmun Rev 9(3):188–193
Rolls AE, Giovannoni G et al (2010) Multiple sclerosis, lymphoma and nasopharyngeal carcinoma: the central role of Epstein-Barr virus? Eur Neurol 63(1):29–35
Rose JD, Roberts GM et al (1988) Cardiff Crohn's disease jubilee: the incidence over 50 years. Gut 29(3):346–351
Schwartz M, Kipnis J (2005) Protective autoimmunity and neuroprotection in inflammatory and noninflammatory neurodegenerative diseases. J Neurol Sci 233(1–2):163–166
Schwartz M, Shaked I et al (2003) Protective autoimmunity against the enemy within: fighting glutamate toxicity. Trends Neurosci 26(6):297–302
Schwartz M, Shechter R (2010) Protective autoimmunity functions by intracranial immunosurveillance to support the mind: the missing link between health and disease. Mol Psychiatry 15(4):342–354
Segal BM, Constantinescu CS et al (2008) Repeated subcutaneous injections of IL12/23 p40 neutralising antibody, ustekinumab, in patients with relapsing-remitting multiple sclerosis: a phase II, double-blind, placebo-controlled, randomised, dose-ranging study. Lancet Neurol 7(9):796–804
Shoenfeld Y, Selmi C et al (2008) The autoimmunologist: geoepidemiology, a new center of gravity, and prime time for autoimmunity. J Autoimmun 31(4):325–330
Sloka JS, Phillips PW et al (2005). Co-occurrence of autoimmune thyroid disease in a multiple sclerosis cohort. J Autoimmune Dis 2:9
Somers EC, Thomas SL et al (2006) Autoimmune diseases co-occurring within individuals and within families: a systematic review. Epidemiology 17(2):202–217
Stegbauer J, Lee DH et al (2009) Role of the renin-angiotensin system in autoimmune inflammation of the central nervous system. Proc Natl Acad Sci U S A 106(35):14942–14947
Stevens DB, Swanborg RH (1993) Bromodeoxyuridine and light treatment deletes effector but not suppressor cells of autoimmune encephalomyelitis. J Neuroimmunol 44(2):177–184
Stosic M, Ambrus J et al (2010) MRI characteristics of patients with antiphospholipid syndrome and multiple sclerosis. J Neurol 257(1):63–71
Taams LS, Palmer DB et al (2006) Regulatory T cells in human disease and their potential for therapeutic manipulation. Immunology 118(1):1–9
Taler M, Gil-Ad I et al (2011) The immunomodulatory effect of the antidepressant sertraline in an experimental autoimmune encephalomyelitis mouse model of multiple sclerosis. Neuroimmunomodulation 18(2):117–122
Thorsby E, Lie BA (2005) HLA associated genetic predisposition to autoimmune diseases: genes involved and possible mechanisms. Transpl Immunol 14(3–4):175–182
van Oosten BW, Barkhof F et al (1996) Increased MRI activity and immune activation in two multiple sclerosis patients treated with the monoclonal anti-tumor necrosis factor antibody cA2. Neurology 47(6):1531–1534

Vilisaar J, Wilson M et al (2005) A comparative audit of anticardiolipin antibodies in oligoclonal band negative and positive multiple sclerosis. Mult Scler 11(4):378–380

Vollmar P, Nessler S et al (2009) The antidepressant venlafaxine ameliorates murine experimental autoimmune encephalomyelitis by suppression of pro-inflammatory cytokines. Int J Neuropsychopharmacol 12(4):525–536

Vollmer TL, Wynn DR et al (2011) A phase 2, 24-week, randomized, placebo-controlled, double-blind study examining the efficacy and safety of an anti-interleukin-12 and -23 monoclonal antibody in patients with relapsing-remitting or secondary progressive multiple sclerosis. Mult Scler 17(2):181–191

Whitacre CC, Reingold SC et al (1999) A gender gap in autoimmunity. Science 283(5406): 1277–1278

Yuan XQ, Qiu G et al (2012) Fluoxetine promotes remission in acute experimental autoimmune encephalomyelitis in rats. Neuroimmunomodulation 19(4):201–208

Zamboni P (2006) The big idea: iron-dependent inflammation in venous disease and proposed parallels in multiple sclerosis. J R Soc Med 99(11):589–593

Zanelli E, Breedveld FC et al (2000) HLA association with autoimmune disease: a failure to protect? Rheumatology (Oxford) 39(10):1060–1066

Chapter 17
Current and Future Treatments of Multiple Sclerosis

Aiden Haghikia and Ralf Gold

17.1 Introduction

For many years, treatment of multiple sclerosis (MS), as the most common, disabling neurological condition in young adults in the developed world (Compston and Coles 2008) has been hampered by a lack of understanding of its initiation and progression. However, accelerating progress in MS research on several fronts has led to numerous clinical trials with a range of drugs and therapeutic principles. The vast majority of these therapeutics target components of the immune system, as pathological, immunologic, and genetic studies point to the immune system as the primary driver of MS (Jager et al. 2009; Sawcer et al. 2011; Fugger et al. 2009; Popescu et al. 2012; Lucchinetti et al. 2011). While some of these drugs failed to show efficacy, others have revealed devastating side effects, and again others have proven to be beneficial. They have all shed more light on the pathogenesis of MS and contributed substantially to the understanding of this heterogeneous disease.

The introduction and approval of interferon beta (IFNβ)- 1b by the FDA in 1993 and glatiramer acetate (GLAT) 3 years later marked a line in the history of MS and its therapy. Despite limited beneficial effect in disease modulation, the invention of IFNβ and GLAT made MS a potentially treatable disease and gave rise to hope for more powerful therapeutic approaches or even thinking of curing the disease (Weiner 2009).

Within less than 20 years, eight drugs have emerged for the treatment of MS and at least another eight late-stage trial drugs are currently in the pipeline. Yet, at the same time these increasing therapeutic options add to the complexity of MS therapy and raise questions of how these therapeutics can be applied in a precise

A. Haghikia (✉) · R. Gold
Department of Neurology, St. Josef-Hospital Bochum, Ruhr-Universität, Bochum, Germany
e-mail: aiden.haghikia@ruhr-uni-bochum.de

R. Gold
e-mail: ralf.gold@ruhr-uni-bochum.de

A. Haghikia
Nuffield Department of Clinical Neurosciences and MRC Human Immunology Unit,
Weatherall Institute of Molecular Medicine, John Radcliffe Hospital,
University of Oxford, Oxford, UK

T. Yamamura, B. Gran (eds.), *Multiple Sclerosis Immunology*,
DOI 10.1007/978-1-4614-7953-6_17,

manner. Another unsolved issue that remains is the challenge on how to protect neuronal tissue from irreversible damage that is associated with the inflammatory process in MS. Until now the only option to prevent tissue damage has been early anti-inflammatory treatment. This notion has been a key driver of the significant reduction of time to diagnosis in patients who encounter first disease symptoms and the concomitant rapid improvement and availability of magnetic resonance imaging (MRI) techniques (Polman et al. 2011).

17.2 Current Multiple Sclerosis Treatments

17.2.1 First-Line Disease-Modifying Drugs for Relapsing–Remitting Multiple Sclerosis

Driven by the hypothesis that MS might be a virus-mediated disease and since interferons are involved in antiviral-immune responses, the rationale to treat MS patients with IFNβ was to supplement them with an agent that they were suspected to lack. Also, GLAT had a serendipitous path to MS therapy as it was initially designed to induce an MS-like disease in rodents, but it turned out to protect them from experimental autoimmune encephalomyelitis (EAE) instead.

Although still not completely understood, experimental studies have provided new insights into the mode(s) of action(s) of IFNβ and seem to converge on a common hypothesis that IFNβ acts via induction of anti-inflammatory genes and several cellular-immune functions that include: direct and indirect inhibition in function of autoreactive lymphocytes directed against the central nervous system (CNS) white matter (Prinz et al. 2008, Prinz and Kalinke 2010) and their mobility across the blood–brain barrier (BBB) by reducing the activity of matrix metalloproteinases (Fig. 17.1; Comabella et al. 2009a, b). Similar to IFNβ, the mode of action of GLAT has been only partially deciphered. Cumulative evidence suggests that GLAT impairs lymphocyte activity by inhibition/modulation of antigen-presenting cells and via regulatory T cells (Fig. 17.1) (Lalive et al. 2011).

Despite the limited efficacy of these so-called *first-line* DMDs over the last 20 years, their safety profile has been established by millions of patients' years of experience in relapsing remitting MS (RRMS) (Table 17.1). As there are no clear-cut differences concerning the indication of the IFNβ preparations or for GLAT in patients' use, many attempts have been made to show the advantages of the respective product over the others. However, even head-to-head studies that were conducted to test whether higher doses of IFNβ are more effective than the approved doses or to show the superiority over GLAT have failed. No major differences in the primary endpoints as defined by relapse rate and MRI disease activity were observed when high-dose subcutaneous IFNβ-1b was tested against GLAT in the BEYOND study (O'Connor et al. 2009) and high-dose subcutaneous IFNβ-1a over COP in the REGARD study (Mikol et al. 2008). The bottom line is that IFNβ and GLAT reduce disease activity by approximately 30 % in RRMS and up to 45 % in clinically

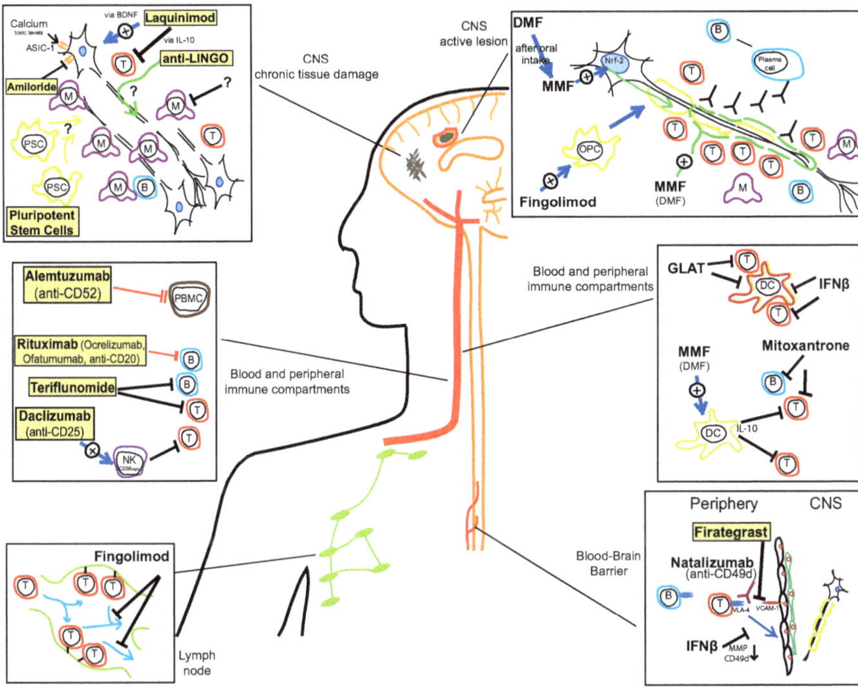

Fig. 17.1 Schematic summary of peripheral immunologic and central nervous compartments involved in MS including the known targets of approved drugs in use as well as experimental (*yellow* boxes) and late-stage trial drugs (*yellow* boxes). The compartments comprise the CNS with either acute lesions or chronically damaged CNS tissue, the blood–brain barrier, the periphery including blood, secondary immune compartments, e.g., lymph nodes. *T* T cells, *B* B cells, *PBMC* peripheral blood mononuclear cells (represent leukocytes), *NK* natural killer cells, *OPC* oligodendrocyte progenitor cells, *M* microglia/macrophages, *MMF* monomethyl fumarate (active metabolite of dimethyl fumarate after oral digestion), *Nrf-2* Nuclear factor (erythroid-derived 2)-like 2 (transcription factor that induces the expression of antioxidative proteins/enzymes), *IFNβ* interferon beta, *GLAT* glatiramer acetate; *DC* (*yellow*) regulatory dendritic cells, *DC* (*red/yellow*) inflammatory dendritic cells acting as antigen presenting cells, *IL-10* interleukin 10 (anti-inflammatory cytokine), *BDNF* brain-derived neurotrophic factor, *ASIC-1* acid sensing ion channels (upregulated during inflammatory process leading to toxic levels of inward rectifying calcium ions), *PSC* pluripotent stem cells, *VLA-4* very late antigen (integrin expressed by activated leukocytes), *VCAM-1* vascular cell adhesion molecule (cells with VLA-4 bind to VCAM-1 expressed on endothelial cells = in order to trespass the blood–brain barrier), *MMP* matrix metalloproteinase (is used by activated leukocytes to transmigrate through the blood–brain barrier)

isolated syndrome (CIS). The results of these studies, however, underline the importance of head-to-head studies and the incomparability of different studies due to differences in baseline demographics. Also, the long-term efficacy, in particular, on significantly delaying the time of conversion from CIS to clinically definitive MS (CDMS) has been shown to be fairly equal for all IFNβ preparations and GLAT (Kinkel et al. 2012, Kappos et al. 2009, Comi et al. 2009, Filippi et al. 2004).

Table 17.1 Currently approved multiple sclerosis (MS) therapeutics and drugs at late-stage development with their pivotal trials. For agents that are not approved yet, the results of the most recent clinical trials are summarized

Drug	Trial details	Outcome measures			Ref.
		MRI	Clinical	Adverse events	
IFNβ-1b s.c. 250 μg eod (Betaseron® in USA, Betaferon® in Europe, Bayer Healthcare, Leverkusen, Germany) FDA approval 1993	372 RRMS IFNβ-1b 250 μg (8 MIU) vs. IFNβ-1b 50 μg (1.6 MIU) vs. placebo 1: 1: 1	0·1 % decrease (IFNβ-1b s.c. 250 μg) vs. 20 % increase (placebo) in lesions area	ARR 0.84 (IFNβ-1b s.c. 250 μg) vs. 1.27 (placebo)	Flu-like symptoms, injection site reaction, allergic reaction, fatigue, emotional instability, reversible elevated liver enzymes, nAbs	(Paty and Li (1993; Group TIMSS 1993)
IFNβ-1a i.m. 30 μg weekly (Avonex®, Biogen Idec, Cambridge, USA) FDA approval 1996	301 RRMS IFNβ-1a 30 μg vs. placebo ~ 1: 1	Mean increase of 0.8 (IFNβ-1a) vs. 1.65 (placebo) Gd-lesions; no significant changes in T2-lesions	ARR 0.61 (IFNβ-1a) vs. 0.9 (placebo)	Flu-like symptoms, muscle ache, fever, chills	(Jacobs et al. 1996)
IFNβ-1a s.c. 22 μg and 44 μg 3 × /week (Rebif22®, Rebif44®, Merck Serono, Geneva, Switzerland) FDA approval 1998	560 RRMS IFNβ-1a 22 or 44 μg vs. placebo 1: 1: 1 (PRISMS study)	67 % (IFNβ-1a 22 μg) and 78 % (IFNβ-1a 44 μg) decrease in number of T2-lesions compared to placebo	Mean number of relapses decreased by 27 % (IFNβ-1a 22 μg) and 33 % (IFNβ-1a 44 μg) vs. placebo	Flu-like symptoms, injection site reaction, allergic reaction, emotional instability, reversible elevated liver enzymes, nAbs	(Group PS 1998)
GLAT s.c. 20 mg daily (Copaxone®, Teva Phamaceutical Industries, Netanya, Israel) FDA approval 1996	251 RRMS (clinical outcomes) (Johnson et al. 1995), 239 RRMS (MRI outcomes)(Comi et al. 2001), GLAT s.c. 20 mg vs. placebo 1: 1	29 % reduction of mean total number of Gd-lesions in the GLAT group as compared to placebo	29 % reduction in ARR or 0·59 (GLAT) vs. 0.84 (placebo)	Injection site reaction, self-limiting injection-related systemic reaction	(Johnson et al. 1995; Comi et al. 2001)

Table 17.1 (continued)

Drug	Trial details	Outcome measures			Ref.
		MRI	Clinical	Adverse events	
IFNβ-1b s.c. 500 μg eod (Betaseron® in USA, Betaferon® in Europe, Bayer Healthcare, Leverkusen, Germany)	2,244 RRMS IFNβ-1b s.c. 250 or 500 μg eod vs. GLAT s.c. 20 mg 2: 2: 1 (BEYOND study)	No significant differences in MRI outcomes	No significant differences in clinical outcomes	As for initial IFNβ-1b trial	(O'Connor et al. 2009)
IFNβ-1a s.c. 44 μg 3 × /week (Rebif22®, Rebif44®, Merck Serono, Geneva, Switzerland)	764 RRMS IFNβ-1a s.c. 44 μg 3 × /week vs. GLAT s.c. 20 mg daily 1: 1 (REGARD study)	No significant differences in number and volume of T2-lesions or volume of Gd-lesions, decreased number of gd + lesions	No significant differences in clinical outcomes	As for initial IFNβ-1a s.c. trial	(Mikol et al. 2008)
Mitoxantrone 12 mg/kg b.w. every 3 months (Novantrone® in the USA, EMD Serono, Darmstadt, Germany; Ralenova® in some European countries, Wyeth Pharma/Pfizer, New York, USA)	194 progressive RRMS and SPMS mitoxantrone 5 or 12 mg/kg b.w. vs. placebo every 3 months 1: 1: 1 (MIMS study)	No Gd-lesions in the mitoxantrone group vs. 16 % in the placebo group 0.29 mean increase of T2-lesions in the mitoxantrone group vs. 1.94 in the placebo group	Significant effect in 12 mg/kg b.w. for all clinical measures (EDSS, ambulation index, time to first relapse, and change in standardized neurological status)	Alopecia, nausea, mild infections, amenorrhea, leucopenia, elevated liver enzymes; from post hoc studies (Marriott et al. 2010; Le Page et al. 2011) 4.9–12 % for asymptomatic systolic dysfunction (LVEF < 50 %), 0.1–0.4 % for congestive cardiac failure, 0.25–0.8 % for TRAL, ~17 % irreversible amenorrhea (age-dependent)	(Hartung et al. 2002)

Table 17.1 (continued)

Drug	Trial details	Outcome measures			Ref.
		MRI	Clinical	Adverse events	
Natalizumab 300 mg i.v. every 4 weeks (Tysabri®, BiogenIdec Elan, Cambridge, MA, USA) First FDA approval 2004 (withdrawn from market 3 months later due to PML), reapproval 2006	942 RRMS natalizumab 300 mg i.v. every 4 weeks vs. placebo 2: 1 (AFFIRM study)	83 % less new or enlarged T2-lesions under natalizumab vs. placebo; 92 % less Gd-lesions under natalizumab vs. placebo	68 % less ARR under natalizumab vs. placebo, 42 % less risk of sustained disability progression under natalizumab vs. placebo	Allergic reactions and fatigue	(Polman et al. 2006)
	1,171 RRMS natalizumab 300 mg i.v. every 4 weeks plus weekly IFNβ-1a i.m. 30 μg vs. placebo plus weekly IFNβ-1a 30 μg 1: 1 (SENTINEL study)	Mean number of new or enlarging T-lesions decreased to 0.9 under combination therapy vs. 5.4 IFNβ-1a alone; no significant differences in Gd-lesions	ARR decreased under combination therapy to 0.34 as compared to 0.75 under IFNβ-1a alone; 24 % less risk of sustained disability progression under combination therapy vs. IFNβ-1a alone	Allergic reactions, anxiety, mild infections, IFN-related side effects, two cases of PML (one fatal)	(Rudick et al. 2006)

Table 17.1 (continued)

Drug	Trial details	Outcome measures			Ref.
		MRI	Clinical	Adverse events	
Fingolimod 0.5 mg daily (Gilenya®, Novartis, Basel Switzerland) FDA approval 2010	1,272 RRMS fingolimod 0.5 vs. 1·25 mg daily vs. placebo 1: 1: 1 (FREEDOMS study)	> 89 % under either dose of fingolimod were free of Gd-lesions vs. 65.1 % placebo; mean number of new or enlarged T2-lesions under either dose of fingolimod 2.5 vs. 9.8 under placebo	ARR reduction under fingolimod 53 % (0.5 mg) and 60 % (1.25 mg) vs. placbo; cumulative risk of disability progression less under fingolimod 17.7 % (0.5 mg) and 16.6 % vs. 24.1 % placebo	(Significantly more often than in the placebo group) infections of the upper respiratory tract, diarrhea, leukopenia, elevated liver enzymes, hypertension, bradycar-dia/bradyarrhythmia, atrioventricular block (1st degree)	(Kappos et al. 2006)
	1,272 RRMS fingolimod 0.5 mg vs. 1.25 mg daily vs. IFNβ-1a i.m. 30 μg 1: 1: 1 (TRANS-FORMS study)	Mean number of new or enlarged T2-lesions under fingolimod 1.7 (0.5 mg) and 1.5 (1.25 mg) vs. 2.6 under IFNβ-1a; mean number of new or Gd-lesions under fingolimod 0.23 (0.5 mg) and 0.14 (1.25 mg) vs. 0.51 under IFNβ-1a	ARR reduction under fingolimod 0.2 (0.5 mg) and 0.16 (1.25 mg) vs. 0.33 under IFNβ-1a; no significant differences in patients with no confirmed disability progression	Two fatal cases of encephalitis (varicella zoster and herpes simples), elevated liver enzymes, hypertension, bradycar-dia/bradyarrhythmia, atrioventricular block (1st and 2nd degree), macular edema, melanoma	(Cohen et al. 2010)

Table 17.1 (continued)

Drug	Trial details	Outcome measures			Ref.
		MRI	Clinical	Adverse events	
Dimethylfumarate 480 mg, 720 mg (Tecfidera®, BiogenIdec, Cambridge, MA, USA) EMA and FDA recommended approval in March 2013	1,237 RRMS BG-12 480 mg vs. 720 mg daily vs. placebo 1: 1: 1 (DEFINE study)	90 % (480 mg) and 73 % (720 mg) less Gd-lesions under BG-12 vs. placebo; 85 % (480 mg) and 74 % (720 mg) less new or enlarged T2-lesions under BG-12 vs. placebo	53 % ARR reduction under BG-12 (480 mg) and 48 % (720 mg) vs. placebo; ~40 % less cumulative risk of disability progression under BG-12 doses vs. placebo	Gastrointestinal side effects, such as mild and moderate diarrhea, flushing	(http://www.biogenidec.com/press_release_details.aspx?ID=5981&ReqId=1548648; http://www.biogenidec.com/press_release_details.aspx?ID=5981&ReqId=1621631)
	1,430 RRMS BG-12 480 mg vs. 720 mg daily vs. GLAT s.c. 20 mg daily vs. placebo 1: 1: 1: 1 (CONFIRM study)	71 % (480 mg) and 73 % (720 mg) less new or enlarged T2-lesions under BG-12 and 54 % by GLAT vs. placebo; 57 % (480 mg) and 65 % (720 mg) less T1-hypointense lesions under BG-12 and 41 % by GLAT vs. placebo	44 % ARR reduction under BG-12 (480 mg) and 51 % (720 mg) and 29 % GLAT vs. placebo; reduced risk of disability progression by 21 % (480 mg) and 24 % (720 mg) under BG-12 (not significant) and 7 % by GLAT (not significant) vs. placebo	As for DEFINE study	(http://www.biogenidec.com/press_release_details.aspx?ID=5981&ReqId=1548648; http://www.biogenidec.com/press_release_details.aspx?ID=5981&ReqId=1621631)

Table 17.1 (continued)

Drug	Trial details	Outcome measures			Ref.
		MRI	Clinical	Adverse events	
Teriflunomide 7, 14 mg daily Aubagio® (Genzyme/Sanofi, Cambridge, MA, USA) EMA approval March 2013	1,088 RRMS Teriflunomide 7 or 14 mg daily vs. placebo 1: 1: 1 (TEMSO study)	Mean volume (ml) of newly enlarged T2-lesions: 0.81 (7 mg) and 0·31 (14 mg) under teriflunomide vs. 1.67 under placebo; mean number of Gd-lesions: 0.57 (7 mg) and 0.26 (14 mg) under teriflunomide vs. 1.36 under placebo	~31 % relative risk reduction of ARR under either dose of teriflunomide vs. placebo ($p < 0{\cdot}001$); reduced risk of disability progression by 21.7 % (7 mg, not significant) and 20.2 % (14 mg) under teriflunomide vs. 27.3 % by placebo	Mild infections, headache, nausea, elevated liver enzymes, and hair thinning	(O'Connor et al. 2011a, b)
Rituximab 2 × 1,000 mg in 48 weeks (Mabthera®, Roche, Basel, Switzerland and Rituxan®, BiogenIdec, Cambridge, USA)	69 RRMS Rituximab 2 × 1,000 mg on days 1 and 15 in 48 weeks vs. placebo ~ 1: 1 (HERMES study)	91 % reduction of the relative risk of Gd-lesions under rituximab vs. placebo; mean changes of T-lesion volume (mm^3): – 175.4 under rituximab vs. + 417.8 under placebo	Relapses in 20.3 % of patients under rituximab vs. 40 % under placebo	Mild infections, infusion-related adverse events, such as chills, nausea, pruritus, rash, fatigue, and general pain	(Hauser et al. 2008)
Alemtuzumab 60 or 120 mg cumulative annual doses (Campath®, Genzyme, Cambridge, USA and BayerHealthcare, Leverkusen, Germany)	334 RRMS Alemtuzumab 60 or 120 mg cumulative annual doses vs. IFNβ-1a 44 μg 3x/week 1: 1: 1 (CAMMS223 study)	Reduction of T2-lesion load in up to 21.2 % of patients under alemtuzumab (60 mg, as compared to baseline after 24 months) vs. – 9.8 % under IFNβ-1a; increase in brain volume (T1-weighted MRI between 12 and 36 months) up 1.2 % under alemtuzumab (60 mg) vs. 0.2 % decrease under IFNβ-1a	Sustained disability reduced to 8.5 % of patients under alemtuzumab (60 mg) vs. 26.2 % under IFNβ-1a; up to 83.5 % under alemtuzumab free of relapses (120 mg) vs. 51.6 % under IFNβ-1a	Infusion-associated reactions in > 90 % of patients under alemtuzumab, infections (~4 % serious), autoimmune disorders: > 20 % thyroid-associated majority with hyperthyroidism, autoimmune nephritis; deaths—one due to immune thrombocytopenia	(Coles et al. 2008)

Table 17.1 (continued)

Drug	Trial details	Outcome measures			Ref.
		MRI	Clinical	Adverse events	
Daclizumab s.c. 6 mg (6 × 1) or 22 mg (11 × 1) per kg b.w. plus IFNβ (PDL Biopharma, Incline Village, USA and Biogen Idec, Cambridge, USA)	230 RRMS daclizumab s.c. 6 mg plus IFNβ vs. daclizumab s.c. 22 mg plus IFNβ vs. placebo plus IFNβ 1: 1: 1 (CHOICE study)	Mean number of new or enlarged Gd-lesions reduced to 72 % under daclizumab + IFNβ (22 mg) vs. placebo + IFNβ	ARR reduced up to 43 % under daclizumab + IFNβ (22 mg) vs. placebo + IFNβ	One fatal case due to dissemination of a local skin infection resulting in psoas empyema and mesenteric ischemia; otherwise no significant side effects as compared to placebo	(Wynn et al. 2010)
Laquinimod 0.6 mg daily (Teva Phamaceutical Industries, Netanya, Israel)	1,106 RRMS laquinimod 0.6 mg daily vs. placebo 1: 1 (ALLEGRO study)	Mean number of new or enlarged T2-lesions: 5.03 under laquinimod vs. 7.14 under placebo; mean number of Gd-lesions: 1.33 under laquinimod vs. 2.12 under placebo	ARR under laquinimod 0.3 vs. 0.39 under placebo, risk of sustained disability 11.1 % under laquinimod vs. 15.7 % under placebo	Gastrointestinal side effects, e.g., mild and moderate diarrhea, nausea, headache, vomiting, hypokalemia, back pain, arthralgia, and elevated liver enzymes	(Comi et al. 2012)

ARR annualized relapse rate, *eod* every other day, *Gd* gadolinium, *GLAT* glatiramer acetate, *IFNβ* interferon beta, *i.m.* intramuscularly, *MRI* magnetic resonance imaging, *RRMS* relapsing remitting MS, *s.c.* subcutaneously, *T1* T1-weighted MRI sequences, *T2* T2-weighted MRI sequences

In order to gain synergistic effects of available drugs, several combinations of first-line DMA with other agents have been tried. Some of these small open-label trials provided partly promising results, e.g., IFNβ or COP with mitoxantrone (see latter sections) (Jeffery et al. 2005; Vollmer et al. 2008), others showed no benefit from combination therapy, e.g., IFNβ combined with azathioprine (Havrdova et al. 2009a, b) or IFNβ with simvastatin (Sorensen et al. 2011b). Again, other combinations showed conflicting results, e.g., a trial in which IFNβ was more effective when applied together with oral methylprednisolone (Sorensen et al. 2009) but not with intravenous methylprednisolone (Ravnborg et al. 2010). The results of a large NIH-funded clinical trial (CombiRx) to evaluate the efficacy of combined IFNβ-1a plus GLAT versus either drug plus placebo with approximately 1,000 patients over 3 years did not reveal any significant improvement of the clnical endpoints by combination therapy (Lublin et al. 2013).

17.2.2 Escalation Therapy with the Immunosuppressant Mitoxantrone

The idea to test cytotoxic substances that suppress the immune system in MS goes back at least three decades, e.g., with cyclophosphamide and azathioprine. However, in 2000 mitoxantrone became the first immunosuppressant that was approved by the FDA, initially for the treatment of secondary progressive MS (SPMS) (Millac and Miller 1969; Hauser et al. 1983). Mitoxantrone is an anthracenedione that causes DNA strand breaks by intercalation and delays repair mechanisms by inhibiting the enzyme topoisomerase II, which ultimately leads to death of immune cells including T-lymphocytes and antibody-producing B-lymphocytes (Fig. 17.1). Mitoxantrone made its way to MS in the late 1990s from oncotherapy where it was first used in the beginning of that same decade (Bisteau et al. 1989; Gonsette and Demonty 1990). It was then a large phase III clinical trial (Table 17.1) that proved mitoxantrone to be significantly more effective over placebo by preventing EDSS progression and relapses (Hartung et al. 2002). These results led to extension of the FDA approval in 2002 also for escalation therapy in RRMS patients with high disease activity.

Unlike cyclophosphamide, the life-time dosage of mitoxantrone was limited to 140 mg/m^2 due to dose-dependent side effects that occurred during the clinical trials (Cohen and Mikol 2004). Besides reversible and potentially treatable side effects, like alopecia, nausea, and mild infections, the more severe and irreversible adverse events, namely cardiotoxicity and malignancies, still challenge the use of mitoxantrone. Depending on the dosages of mitoxantrone used and monitoring period in the follow-up, the numbers reported vary widely for asymptomatic systolic dysfunction as measured by left ventricular ejection fraction (LVEF) less than 50 %, congestive heart failure and therapy-related acute leukemia (TRAL) (Stroet et al. 2012). Two recent studies, one of which reviewing cases in the literature and the other reporting on the large French cohort treated with mitoxantrone, provided the following incidence rates: 4.9–12 % developed asymptomatic systolic dysfunction, 0.1–0.4 % congestive heart failure, and 0.25–0.8 % TRAL (Marriott et al. 2010; Le Page et al. 2011).

Furthermore, about 17 % of female MS patients treated with mitoxantrone developed irreversible amenorrhea, which has shown to be age-dependent (Le Page et al. 2011).

Despite the potentially severe and persisting adverse events, mitoxantrone remains a valuable therapeutic option in the MS armory, in particular, for SPMS where hardly any alternatives exist. New surrogate tools to identify patients at risk and to help individualize the mitoxantrone dosages for optimized treatment and maximum life-term dosages are needed for safer use of this drug. In this context, recently proposed gene polymorphisms in the so-called ATP-binding cassette transporters (*ABC* genes) might be a step towards a marker for mitoxantrone-associated side effects and help adjusting the mitoxantrone dosage needed for the individual MS patient (Cotte et al. 2009). Another feasible strategy to safe mitoxantrone dosages is the induction therapy followed by long-term first-line DMA treatment: several small clinical trials have shown with different induction regimen that initial high-dose mitoxantrone therapy was sufficient to calm down disease activity and the patients who had simultaneously started out COP or IFNβ injections were well off continuing the injections without further mitoxantrone for up to 15 months (Jeffery et al. 2005; Vollmer 2008).

17.2.3 Natalizumab—the New Era of Multiple Sclerosis Therapeutics with Monoclonal Antibodies

Natalizumab was the first therapeutic monoclonal antibody (mAb) approved for the use in RRMS. Its efficacy was shown clearly superior to first-line DMDs and it was developed from a pathomechanistic idea proven in the animal model of MS; it made its way to clinical use within a decade. Natalizumab binds specifically to the α4-subunit of the very late antigen (VLA-4), an anchor protein on the surface of activated immune cells that allows them to bind to the endothelial cells forming the BBB (Yednock et al. 1992). By blocking VLA-4, natalizumab prevents autoreactive inflammatory cells from accessing the CNS (Fig. 17.1). With the preliminary results of two large phase III clinical trials, AFFIRM and SENTINEL (Table 17.1), which were published later, natalizumab received a rapid FDA approval in November 2004, only 2 years after the trials had been launched (Polman et al. 2006; Rudick et al. 2006). While the AFFIRM study compared the efficacy of natalizumab with placebo, in SENTINEL natalizumab was combined with IFNβ-1a and compared to placebo. The robust effects of 4 weekly infusions of 300 mg natalizumab on relapse rate, MRI activity, and risk of disease progression were hampered by the occurrence of three cases of progressive multifocal leukoencephalopathy (PML); a JC virus (JCV)- mediated and potentially lethal infectious disease causing subacute demyelination throughout the CNS. Two PML cases were observed in the SENTINEL study and one in a trial to test natalizumab in patients with Crohn's disease (Assche et al. 2005; Langer-Gould et al. 2005; Kleinschmidt-DeMasters and Tyler 2005). As a consequence, natalizumab was withdrawn shortly after and only after a large reevaluation of over 3,000 patients, who had received natalizumab without further cases of PML, natalizumab was reapproved as second-line therapeutic for RRMS (Yousry et al. 2006).

PML was first suspected to occur when natalizumab was combined with another immunomodulatory agent such as IFN(. This hypothesis was repealed when the first two PML cases occurred under natalizumab monotherapy (Wenning et al. 2009; Linda et al. 2009). Meanwhile, over 100,000 MS patients have been treated with natalizumab and the risk of natalizumab- related PML is estimated 1:500 (www.biogenidec.com). Interestingly, one of the few reliable predisposing factors for natalizumab-associated PML seems to be the exposition time; PML risk increases up to 1:100 in patients treated for 24–26 months with natalizumab in patients who had previously been treated with immunosuppressants.

PML is caused by a harmless appearing virus that is—depending on the population screened—present in 60–90 % of healthy individuals. The question remains why a relatively small subgroup of MS patients is affected when PML otherwise only affects patients with major acquired immune defects such as HIV, which accounts for 80 % of all PML cases (Carson et al. 2009). However, despite conflicting data, there is consensus on a probable multistep process as a stochastic sequence of events for JCV to overcome several barriers to infect glial cells within the CNS (Major 2010; Berger 2011). The initial step is believed to be JCV infection during childhood, which is not apparently associated with a specific symptom(s). Hereafter, several tissues have been shown to host the virus in its latent state, among them the tonsils, bone marrow hematopoietic stem cells, and the kidneys. The virus in its native form is unable to infect oligodendrocytes and needs to undergo mutations in its noncoding region in order to become neuro- or gliopathogenic. This crucial step is one of the least understood although some data exist suggesting a role for (B-)cellular transcription factors being possibly involved in this process (Marshall et al. 2010). Another option is a (re)infection with a mutated JCV strain and the lack of immune response to the de novo infection in predisposed patients. Once the virus becomes neuropathogenic and enters the CNS, it is able to infect oligodendrocytes, if the local immune defense is impaired. This might be the case for natalizumab-treated MS patients where cerebrospinal immune cells are decreased after therapy initiation (Pilar et al. 2008). Unrestrained JCV replication destroys vast areas of CNS white matter and leads to the full clinical picture of PML, which frequently takes a fatal course. A major difference in natalizumab associated with other PML is the overall better outcome, especially if the antibody is removed by plasma exchange and/or immunoadsorption, the survival rate is more than 70 % (Vermersch et al. 2011).

Two further issues have accompanied natalizumab from the very first clinical trials: (1) persisting neutralizing antibodies (nAbs) that abolish the therapeutic effect of natalizumab and (2) the question of whether therapy cessation, e.g., during pregnancy or on patients' request, increases disease activity, the so-called *rebound* (Tubridy et al. 1999). The pivotal trials and a large postmarketing study evaluating the occurrence of nAbs in approximately 5,000 patients revealed that 3–6 % patients develop nAbs against natalizumab (Calabresi et al. 2007; Sorensen et al. 2011a); testing for nAbs routinely seems feasible during the first 6–12 months when the risk of developing them has been shown to be highest. The suspicion of postwithdrawal rebound in natalizumab-treated patients arose from the very first clinical and the post hoc analysis of a small subgroup of 21 patients from the phase III trials

(Tubridy et al. 1999; Vellinga et al. 2008). Smaller case series later supported or contradicted the occurrence of postwithdrawal rebound. However, the largest study so far evaluating the relapse rate in approximately 1,800 patients and MRI activity in 341 patients showed no increased disease activity above the pretreatment levels after natalizumab withdrawal (O'Connor et al. 2011b).

So far, several re-evaluations by the regulatory agencies have come to the conclusion that the therapeutic benefit of natalizumab overweighs its risks. Supporting this decision, a post hoc analysis showed that 60 % of natalizumab-treated MS patients were either free of clinical or MRI disease activity, and almost 40 % of them were free of any sign of disease (Havrdova et al. 2009a). New recommendations on the application of natalizumab in RRMS have been proposed to minimize the risk of PML, which include (Kappos et al. 2009): careful selection of eligible patients, application of the drug by experienced centers, clinical vigilance, and regular follow-up neurological/MRI surveys.

Whether the improved test (ELISA) to identify anti-JCV antibodies in MS patients further helps to reduce the risk of natalizumab-related PML will be answered by the monitoring programs TYGRIS and STRATA (Gorelik et al. 2010). Despite ongoing efforts to find the factor(s) that predisposes MS patients for developing PML, there are attempts to establish alternative drugs that have the same target as natalizumab—possibly without the risk of PML. Firategrast or the so-called "small anti-(4(-integrin molecule" has just been tested in a clinical trial (Miller et al. 2012). It is an oral drug with a short half-life time of approximately 5 h and is rapidly metabolized as opposed to natalizumab that has a biological half-life time of several months. The phase II clinical trial, testing four doses of firategrast (twice daily 150, 600, 900, or 1,200 mg) over 6 months showed a roughly 50 % decrease of Gd-enhancing lesions but no significant effect on relapse rate when compared to placebo.

17.2.4 A Switch from the Injectables to an Oral Drug for Multiple Sclerosis with Fingolimod

Fingolimod is the first approved oral drug for the treatment of RRMS at a daily dose of 0.5 mg. Via spingosine-1-phosphate receptor (S1P) fingolimod exerts its effects on peripheral immune cells and its therapeutic potential was first validated in transplant medicine (Schwab and Cyster 2007). The strong inhibitory effect of fingolimod on lymphocyte egress from secondary lymphoid organs via S1P1 (Fig. 17.1) is the predominant pharmacomechanism of fingolimod (Mandala et al. 2002); it prevents autoreactive immune cells from accessing their antigens and attenuates disease activity in autoimmunity. However, evidence from experimental works suggest a beneficial dual role of fingolimod (Fig. 17.1): a putative pathway within the CNS was shown to promote survival of oligodendrocytes and ultimately lead to remyelination in damaged white matter (Miron et al. 2008). This potentially regenerative feature needs further validation in MS patients, e.g., by newer MRI techniques that allow reliable monitoring of de- and remyelination over time.

Encouraged by positive results of the phase II clinical trial, two large phase III studies were initiated to evaluate the immunomodulatory effect of fingolimod in MS patients (Table 17.1), the FREEDOMS and the TRANSFORMS study (Kappos et al. 2006; Cohen et al. 2010; Kappos et al. 2010). While one study compared fingolimod with placebo, the second study was a head-to-head trial comparing fingolimod with IFNβ. Fingolimod proved to be superior over placebo and more interestingly also over IFNβ by reducing CNS disease activity by at least 50 %. The results of the 12-month extension study of TRANSFORMS provided further evidence for the stronger modulatory impact of fingolimod: patients formerly in the IFNβ control arm were switched to fingolimod (0.5 or 1.25 mg daily dose) and showed an estimated annual relapse rate (ARR) of 33 %, whereas ARR in the group continuing fingolimod treatment was decreased to approximately 20 % (Khatri et al. 2011). It awaits further evaluation whether the risk of developing relapses comes to equilibrium in long-term fingolimod treatment also for patients initially receiving first-line DMDs.

The occurrence of two cases with fatal virus encephalitis and several cases of bradycardia/bradyarrhythmia after first dose in the TRANSFORMS study led to restricted approval of fingolimod as escalation therapy in RRMS by the EMA; in the United States, fingolimod is used as a first-line DMD in MS. Monitoring programs, clinical alertness by treating neurologists, and the development of reliable markers to detect patients at risk for adverse events are needed for the use of fingolimod in MS.

17.2.5 Old Therapeutic Principles Revisited with Fumaric Acids

Dimethyl fumarate (DMF) or BG-12 is an enriched fumaric acid ester and the newest of the MS drugs that was recommended for approval by the EMA and the FDA in March 2013. Its history, however, goes back several decades: the chemist by whom it was presented in 1959 had treated his own psoriatic disease with it, under the assumption that fumaric acid as a component of the Krebs cycle would complement energy-deficient immune cells (Schweckendiek et al. 1959). Hereafter, DMF was mainly prescribed by dermatologists and approved by the German regulatory agency for the treatment of psoriasis in the 1990s accounting for its safety profile based on hundred thousands of patients' years of experience. DMF entered MS therapy by an open-label trial including 10 RRMS patients, which revealed a significant effect on Gd-enhancing MRI lesions with a reduction over 90 % after only 1 year of treatment (Schimrigk et al. 2006). Soon after, the results of a larger phase II clinical trial with DMF over 6 months confirmed its efficacy in RRMS (Kappos et al. 2008); the relatively short study duration has most likely been responsible for the comparably smaller effect. The new drug formulation of DMF showed less gastrointestinal side effects than the former fumaric acid that was used for psoriasis; diarrhea has been the major side effect of fumaric acids responsible for its restricted long-term application so far. The results of the two phase III clinical trials initiated hereafter with over 2,600 RRMS patients for over 2 years compared 240 mg BG-12 twice or three times daily to placebo in the DEFINE study and the same regimen for BG-12 to placebo versus COP in the CONFIRM trial (Table 17.1). While the trials resulted in slightly different conclusions for the efficacies of the two dosages, overall ARR was reduced up to 53 % and the mean number of Gd-enhancing MRI lesions up to 90 %. Concerning primary relapse end points, BG-12 was superior over COP by preventing at least 20 % more relapses. Apart from flushing and mild gastrointestinal side effects, no further adverse events were reported for BG-12 that exceeded adverse events also observed in the placebo group.

Although not fully understood, the suppressive effect on activated (T-)lymphocytes (Fig. 17.1) by fumaric acid has been known for quite some time (Treumer et al. 2003). New insights suggest that dendritic cells orchestrate a shift towards an anti-inflammatory environment in response to treatment with fumaric acid (Ghoreschi et al. 2011). Furthermore, the protective aspect of fumaric acid on neuronal cells, which had been assumed based on the clinical findings, was elucidated in an experimental setup (Linker et al. 2011). In vitro and in vivo experiments in an animal model of MS showed that fumaric acid activates a major regulator of antioxidative pathways ultimately protecting neuronal and glial cells from inflammation-induced cell death by nuclear factor E2-related factor2 (Nrf-2; Fig. 17.1; Linker et al. 2011). These observations are well supported by results of the clinical trials, especially by the secondary MRI endpoints. However, follow-up studies involving newer MRI technologies in the postmarketing phase are needed to further validate these results in MS patients.

17.3 Future Multiple Sclerosis Treatments

17.3.1 Multiple Sclerosis Drugs at Late-stage Development

The development and testing of new therapeutics for MS in clinical trials is proceeding at an accelerated pace. As for any chronic disease, the goal in MS is to establish therapeutics with higher efficacy, specificity, feasible application, and yet, at the same time a higher degree of safety and tolerability. The countless agents being currently at various stages of development allow only a brief roundup of selected drugs that are at late-stage clinical trials, including oral compounds and mAbs.

Teriflunomide and laquinimod are oral drugs that were given fast track status for approval by the FDA. However, after completion of their phase III clinical trials, two of them experienced a major setback: cladribine was rejected by the regulatory agency and laquinimod was put on hold as it was uncertain whether it would meet the primary endpoint of the study.

Laquinimod is a modified compound of linomide that had been withdrawn from use in MS patients despite efficacy because of severe cardiopulmonary side effects in the clinical trial (Noseworthy et al. 2000). In phase II trials, laquinimod showed promising results by significantly reducing MRI-measured disease activity in RRMS patients but failed to reduce the relapse rate in the first study and the second was not powered for this clinical outcome (Comi et al. 2008; Polman et al. 2005). Besides immunomodulatory effects, laquinimod was recently shown to possess some neuroprotective properties by stimulating the secretion of brain-derived neurotrophic factor (BDNF; Fig. 17.1; Thone et al. 2012). However, despite the positive safety profile and efficacy of clinical subanalyses in the phase III trials, the effect of laquinimod on ARR was modest (Table 17.1; Comi et al. 2012). The promising neuroprotective effect of laquinimod as an add-on therapeutic will be investigated in clinical trials.

Teriflunomide is, like its precursor molecule the antirheumatism drug leflunomide, an inhibitor of pyrimidine synthesis and its immunomodulatory effect is partially explained by reducing lymphocyte numbers (Fig. 17.1). Encouraged by the positive results of a phase II clinical trial, a total of five confirmatory trials were initiated (O'Connor et al. 2006) to validate its efficacy in MS. Teriflunomide proved to be effective by reducing ARR and several MRI endpoints (Table 17.1) (O'Connor et al. 2011a). With few gastrointestinal side effects, such as diarrhea, nausea, and reversible increased liver enzymes observed so far, it seems as teriflunomide might be safer than its precursor leflunomide for which a case of PML and fatal liver function failures have been reported. At the time of writing teriflunomide received recommendation of approval by the EMA as first-line therapy for RRMS in March 2013.

Since the approval of natalizumab, the emerging role of mAbs as therapeutic options for MS has become evident. MAbs appear to be particularly attractive as their ability to target specific structures promises high efficacy ("magic bullets"). However, unexpected side effects, such as natalizumab-related PML have lowered the enthusiasm and taught caution. Many mAbs have been tested as potential MS therapeutics in the past: some of them did not show the desired efficacy, e.g., ustekinumab that is directed against the subunit of both, the inflammatory cytokines IL-12 and IL-23 (Segal et al. 2008), although the failure could not be explained by pathophysiology; other mAbs led to disease exacerbating, e.g., the antibody-directed TNF-α therapies (Oosten et al. 1996); again others at the end of the spectrum caused unexpected severe side effects, e.g., anti-CD28 (TGN1412) that led a severe systemic inflammatory response syndrome or "cytokine storm" in a phase I trial in six healthy subjects. Still, mAbs remain an exciting option for therapeutic use in MS, as the mAbs presented here, some of which have come a long way and are likely to become part of the MS drug group.

The monoclonal anti-CD20 antibody *rituximab* has been in use for a long time not only for the treatment of malignancies, such as non-Hodgkin lymphoma, but also for the autoimmune disorder rheumatic arthritis. Furthermore, rituximab is applied off label for less common antibody-mediated autoimmune disorders in various medical disciplines, e.g., myasthenia gravis and some forms of vasculitis. To establish its efficacy in MS, rituximab has been employed in many trials. The anti-CD20 mAbs bind and cause a rapid depletion of all circulating cells belonging to the B cell lineage carrying the antigen CD20, and spare mature plasma cells and bone marrow stem cells (Fig. 17.1). The observed rapid effect of rituximab in RRMS patients, however, suggests an additional mechanism: the short-term impact of rituximab seems to be the abolition of B lymphocytes as direct supporters of T lymphocyte activation (Bar-Or et al. 2010). One of the major studies in MS showed the inefficacy of rituximab in primary progressive MS (PPMS), whereas it nearly halted disease in another trial, as measured by MRI and a decrease of relapses (Table 17.1; Hawker et al. 2009; Hauser et al. 2008). The occurrence of PML in patients with rheumatic arthritis gave reason for caution also in MS patients. Although PML was known in rituximab-treated patients with malignancies, so far the underlying disease had been held responsible (Carson et al. 2009; Fleischmann 2009). However, PML has not been observed in rituximab- treated MS patients. Together with infections, allergic reactions or infusions-related reactions are the most common adverse events reported so far in approximately 3 % of patients treated with rituximab (Tony et al. 2011). Allergic reactions and neutralizing host antibodies are a common phenomenon when foreign proteins are injected. Thus, the introduction of newer-generation anti-CD20 mAbs that are either humanized, such as ocrelizumab, or have a complete human structure, such as ofatumumab, give reason to expect high efficacy at a higher safety rate. Ocrelizumab has just completed a phase II clinical trial in RRMS patients in which both dosages used (600 and 2,000 mg) were clearly superior over placebo and the IFNβ-treated arm, by reducing the number of Gd-enhancing MRI lesions by almost 100 % (Kappos et al. 2011). According to unpublished data presented at Neurologic Meetings (ECTRIMS 2010), similar results have been expected for ofatumumab.

The therapeutic mAb *alemtuzumab* is presented in a separate chapter and is therefore only briefly summarized here. Alemtuzumab binds to the surface marker CD52 and depletes over 95 % of all circulating leukocytes (Fig. 17.1). As one of the first mAbs intended for the therapeutic use in MS patients, alemtuzumab or Campath was developed by the pathology department of the University of Cambridge in the United Kingdom and applied in a MS trial in the early 1990s (Moreau et al. 1994). The trial results suggested an overwhelmingly strong effect when therapy was initiated early in the course of disease but almost no effect when the disease had progressed revealing the degenerative aspect of MS. Although neuronal and axonal degeneration have been shown to occur early in the course of disease and no clear chronological line can be drawn between these two aspects, clinical observations deduced from the alemtuzumab studies clearly helped setting up the two-phase hypothesis of MS: while in RRMS the inflammatory aspect of the disease prevails later on during secondary progression MS (SPMS), it is the degenerative aspect, which causes long-term disability. So far, the results of only one controlled phase II study are available (Table 17.1) with participants either randomized to receive IFNβ-1a or alemtuzumab (Coles et al. 2008). The study was suspended after the second year due to the occurrence of six cases of immune thrombocytopenic purpura, one patient with a fatal course where the symptoms had been ignored by the patients. Despite the suspension, alemtuzumab-treated patients experienced up to 74 % less relapses and had over 70 % less progression probability when compared to IFNβ-1a, and remarkably, over 70 % of the patients treated with alemtuzumab were clinically free of disease. However, many questions have prompted after the rather surprising high rate of secondary autoimmune inflammatory syndromes of the thyroid gland in over 20 % of all alemtuzumab-treated patients, the majority of them suffering from hyperthyroidism. Increased levels of the inflammatory mediator IL-21 has been proposed for being responsible for the secondary autoimmunity in susceptible patients (Jones et al. 2009). As pretreatment serum levels of IL-21 in these patients were elevated, it might be a clinical surrogate marker that needs to be validated prospectively in a larger cohort. The preliminary results of the two completed phase III clinical trials CARE-MSSM I/II, including more than 1,500 RRMS patients, were presented at the annual meeting of the American Academy of Neurology (2012) and widely confirm previous findings; in CARE-MSSM II alemtuzumab also significantly reduced EDSS progression probability.

Daclizumab is an anti-CD25 mAb that has been in use since the end of the 1990s in transplant medicine to prevent kidney graft rejection, and is the first humanized mAb to be approved for therapeutic purposes (Vincenti et al. 1998; Soulillou et al. 1990). CD25 is a subunit of the Interleukin-2 receptor. Although the exact mechanism remains to be deciphered, binding of the mAb to CD25 has been shown to decrease T cell activity by cells of the innate immune system (Fig. 17.1): an increase of a subpopulation of natural killer cells, so-called CD56 (bright) cells as well as a decrease of dendritic cell activity have been implicated in this process (Bielekova et al. 2011; Wuest et al. 2011). Daclizumab initially entered MS clinical trials and was shown to be effective as add-on therapy in RRMS and SPMS patients who had sustained disease activity despite IFNβ therapy (Bielekova et al. 2004). A phase II clinical study included 230 patients who were randomized and received either high- or low-dose daclizumab plus IFNβ versus placebo plus IFNβ, each over 6 months (Wynn et al. 2010). Compared to IFNβ plus placebo, IFNβ plus daclizumab in both doses led to a significant relapse rate reduction and reduction of Gd-enhancing MRI lesions (Table 17.1). The results of the first randomized trials testing the efficacy of daclizumab monotherapy, the SELECT—a registrational phase II–III study, and DECIDE (phase III) trials, are outstanding as of April 2012. SELECT had enrolled 600 RRMS patients receiving either 150 or 300 mg daclizumab once monthly subcutaneous injections versus placebo in a 1:1:1 randomized fashion. Preliminary results presented at the annual AAN 2012 demonstrate that daclizumab reduces ARR in the high-dose arm by 50 and 54 % in the low-dose arm. In addition, Gd-enhancing MRI lesions are shown to be significantly reduced in the daclizumab-treated cohort (by 69 % in the low-dose and by 78 % in the high-dose arm). Concerning the safety profile of daclizumab, longitudinal data from transplant medicine suggest a good overall reliability with mild infections of the upper respiratory tract at an incidence rate comparable to IFNβ, nAbs (~8 %), and reversible skin rash (~15 %) as the most common side effects (Webster et al. 2010). However, one fatal case was reported in an MS patient treated with daclizumab who developed psoas empyema and mesenteric ischemia after dissemination of a local skin infection. The results of the multicenter DECIDE study that was initiated in May 2010 with 1,500 RRMS patients with the same treatment protocol as the SELECT study and a study period of 96–144 weeks will provide further insight on efficacy and tolerability of daclizumab.

17.3.2 Future Prospects

Research effort and clinical trials of the past decades have led to the current diagnostic and therapeutic advances in the field of MS. However, various issues on different levels remain unsolved. A reliable indicator for the ongoing search is the numerous agents currently tested in clinical trials. MS remains the most common chronic neurologic disabling disease of young adulthood, a period that is decisive in education, career, and family planning. The treatment options reviewed in this chapter have changed the field of MS within a relatively short time period. Which gaps need to be addressed now?

17.3.3 Personalized Therapy

One of the main goals in a heterogeneous disease as MS is to apply available drugs in an individualized fashion. A patient with a relatively aggressive form of disease will need different treatment than a young woman who has had mild relapses and is planning to have a child. Moreover, individualized therapy also means measuring the efficacy of the applied drug and quantifying its risks. In addition to thorough clinical monitoring, reliable surrogate markers consisting of serological, imaging, and also genetic testing are needed next to establish the best possible treatment for individual MS patients.

As reviewed for the approved drugs above, promising results from pharmacoimmunologic studies, polymorphisms of the *ABC* genes in mitoxantrone response and side effects are the first steps towards this direction (Cotte et al. 2009). Recent larger screening studies have revealed further genetic polymorphisms associated with therapy response to first-line DMA. They comprise polymorphisms in the MHC gene family (*HLA DRB1*1501*) as a predictor for positive GLAT response but also polymorphisms of multiple genes including not only IFN response pathways (*IFNAR2*) for IFNβ therapy but also "neurologic" genes as the glutamate receptor (*GRIA3*) (Gross et al. 2011; Comabella et al. 2009a, b). Associations with genetic polymorphisms have not only been reported for therapy response but also for therapy-related side effects. Several polymorphisms were found to be associated with an increased level of IL-21, which in turn was significantly increased in patients developing autoimmune thyroid inflammation under alemtuzumab (Jones et al. 2009). Yet, further HLA class II alleles have been shown to be significantly more often present in MS patients, who develop nAbs against IFNβ that are associated with efficacy loss in many patients (Hoffmann et al. 2008).

In addition to genetic and immunologic surrogate markers, MR imaging has become a rapidly developing field for monitoring disease course, therapy response, and also the occurrence of side effects. The MRI as a paraclinical measure of disease activity has been involved in MS therapy trials, ever since the first approval studies of IFNβ, and is now a key constituent of virtually every drug study (Paty and Li 1993). With newer sequence techniques and the development of machines that have stronger magnetic fields allowing higher spatial and temporal resolutions, the MRI has evolved to an irreplaceable tool. Many studies have manifested the predictive value of MRI in MS disease and disability progression, however, more recent studies show that MRI together with clinical measures over a period of 1 year entirely predict disease progression over 2 years (Barkhof et al. 2011; Sormani et al. 2011). The development of multivariate analyses that combine different surrogate markers including MRI has also revealed first interesting insights: polymorphisms of the MHC gene family together with distinct MRI sequences can predict clinical outcome, as shown for *HLA DRB1*1501* that is significantly more often present in MS patients with major motor function deficits and spinal cord damage; or *HLA B*44* that predicts a favorable outcome as quantified by the number of T2-weighted MRI lesions (Liguori et al. 2011; Sombekke et al. 2009). Despite the current routine use of 1.5 or 3 T MRI machines, in future sensitive images unraveling small cortical lesions can be expected, as experimental studies using ultrahigh field 7 T MRI promise (Pitt et al. 2010). Also, broadly available MRI technologies, currently applied in research, e.g., functional MRI studies and longitudinal studies evaluating brain atrophy have shown that functional cortical deficits reflective of neuronal damage occur early in disease and can be quantified (Deloire et al. 2011; Filippi et al. 2010; Colorado et al. 2012). Diffusion tensor imaging (DTI) MRI and double inversion recovery (DIR) MRI are MRI sequence techniques that have been employed to quantify early inflammatory cortical lesions and in areas in which the white matter appears normal on conventional MR images (Seewann et al. 2012; Moll et al. 2011). These MRI studies go well in line with established histopathological works that show early involvement of the brain cortex in the autoinflammatory process. Recent neuropathological data also display cortical lesions in pre-MS biopsies of individuals in whom MS became clinically apparent only later (Lucchinetti et al. 2011). These observations underline the need of early therapeutic intervention in MS to prevent irreversible tissue damage.

17.3.4 Neuroprotection—Therapies at Experimental Stages

However, once MS patients enter the stage of disease that is characterized by progressive neurodegeneration, as in SPMS, or more obvious in the disease course that only shows degenerative features, as in PPMS, the tools to save brain tissue become scarce. Although drugs that showed regenerative features for RRMS, such as fingolimod, are currently being tested in PPMS, the major challenge currently is how to protect from and to reverse the neurodegenerative process in MS. Many neurologic disciplines, e.g., Parkinson's, Alzheimer's, and amyotrophic lateral sclerosis, face similar challenges. Advances made in some of these disciplines have been successfully translated into the field of MS and vice versa: the blockade of a neuronal ion channel (ASIC-1) that transports neurotoxic calcium levels in a mouse model of stroke, successfully led to amelioration in the EAE (Xiong et al. 2004; Friese et al. 2007). Based on these findings, amiloride, a well-known antihypertensive drug that blocks several ion channels, is currently being investigated in a small exploratory trial in

PPMS patients (Ruiter et al. 2011). Antilingo, a drug that is currently being tested for its safety in phase I clinical settings has a similar background: the identification and blockade of factors that inhibit axonal outgrowth (Nogo and LINGO1) led to functional recovery in trauma-induced axonal damage (Prinjha et al. 2000; Merkler et al. 2001). Applying similar principles to EAE showed their regenerative potential also in inflammatory-mediated axonal injury (Mi et al. 2007). To investigate whether administered stem cells have the capacity to replace damaged neuronal tissue without causing neoplasms has long been a corporate question amid different neurodegenerative diseases. Various small studies have been undertaken to test their restorative potential (Uccelli et al. 2011). Besides the risk of undesired neoplasms, the question remains, what administration technique is the most adequate to place the stem cells at the site of damage. In an attempt to scrutinize the practicability and safety of stem cells in MS patients, in a recent study, autologous stem cells were injected intravenously in 10 patients with a progressive disease course (Connick et al. 2012). The authors did not observe any severe side effects during the monitoring period of 10 months. Although many of these studies have shown promising results, up to date, the question of whether the stem cells become functional neurons or myelin-forming oligodendrocytes has not been solved.

Eight approved MS therapeutics emerging within only two decades and at least another six at late-stage development demonstrate well the rapid translation from understanding some pathomechanisms of the disease to therapy. At this stage, further light needs to be shed on less well-understood aspects of MS, namely neurodegeneration, and to target them therapeutically in combination with effective immunomodulation.

References

Assche G Van, Ranst M Van, Sciot R et al (2005) Progressive multifocal leukoencephalopathy after natalizumab therapy for Crohn's disease. N Engl J Med 353:362–368

Barkhof F, Simon JH, Fazekas F et al (2011) MRI monitoring of immunomodulation in relapse-onset multiple sclerosis trials. Nat Rev Neurol 8:13–21

Bar-Or A, Fawaz L, Fan B et al (2010) Abnormal B-cell cytokine responses a trigger of T-cell-mediated disease in MS? Ann Neurol 67:452–461

Berger JR (2011) The basis for modeling progressive multifocal leukoencephalopathy pathogenesis. Curr Opin Neurol 24:262–267

Bielekova B, Richert N, Howard T et al (2004) Humanized anti-CD25 (daclizumab) inhibits disease activity in multiple sclerosis patients failing to respond to interferon beta. Proc Natl Acad Sci U S A 101:8705–8

Bielekova B, Richert N, Herman ML et al (2011) Intrathecal effects of daclizumab treatment of multiple sclerosis. Neurology 77:1877–86

Bisteau M, Devos G, Brucher JM, Gonsette RE (1989) Prevention of subacute experimental allergic encephalomyelitis in guinea-pigs with desferrioxamine, isoprinosine and mitoxantrone. Elsevier Science Publ B V, Amsterdam

Calabresi PA, Giovannoni G, Confavreux C et al (2007) The incidence and significance of anti-natalizumab antibodies: results from AFFIRM and SENTINEL. Neurology 69:1391–403

Carson KR, Focosi D, Major EO et al (2009) Monoclonal antibody-associated progressive multifocal leucoencephalopathy in patients treated with rituximab, natalizumab, and efalizumab: a Review from the Research on Adverse Drug Events and Reports (RADAR) Project. Lancet Oncol 10:816–24

Cohen BA, Mikol DD (2004) Mitoxantrone treatment of multiple sclerosis: safety considerations. Neurology 63:28–32

Cohen JA, Barkhof F, Comi G et al (2010) Oral fingolimod or intramuscular interferon for relapsing multiple sclerosis. N Engl J Med 362:402–415

Coles AJ, Compston DA, Selmaj KW et al (2008) Alemtuzumab vs. interferon beta-1a in early multiple sclerosis. N Engl J Med 359:1786–801

Colorado RA, Shukla K, Zhou Y, Wolinsky JS, Narayana PA (2012) Multi-task functional MRI in multiple sclerosis patients without clinical disability. NeuroImage 59:573–81

Comabella M, Craig DW, Morcillo-Suarez C et al (2009a) Genome-wide scan of 500,000 single-nucleotide polymorphisms among responders and nonresponders to interferon beta therapy in multiple sclerosis. Arch Neurol 66:972–978

Comabella M, Rio J, Espejo C et al (2009b) Changes in matrix metalloproteinases and their inhibitors during interferon-beta treatment in multiple sclerosis. Clin Immunol 130:145–150

Comi G, Filippi M, Wolinsky JS (2001) European/Canadian multicenter, double-blind, randomized, placebo-controlled study of the effects of glatiramer acetate on magnetic resonance imaging–measured disease activity and burden in patients with relapsing multiple sclerosis. European/Canadian Glatiramer Acetate Study Group. Ann Neurol 49:290–297

Comi G, Pulizzi A, Rovaris M et al (2008) Effect of laquinimod on MRI-monitored disease activity in patients with relapsing-remitting multiple sclerosis: a multicentre, randomised, double-blind, placebo-controlled phase IIb study. Lancet 371:2085–2092

Comi G, Martinelli V, Rodegher M et al (2009) Effect of glatiramer acetate on conversion to clinically definite multiple sclerosis in patients with clinically isolated syndrome (PreCISe study): a randomised, double-blind, placebo-controlled trial. Lancet 374:1503–1511

Comi G, Jeffery D, Kappos L et al (2012) Placebo-controlled trial of oral laquinimod for multiple sclerosis. N Engl J Med 366:1000–109

Compston A, Coles A (2008) Multiple sclerosis. Lancet 372:1502–1517

Connick P, Kolappan M, Crawley C et al (2012) Autologous mesenchymal stem cells for the treatment of secondary progressive multiple sclerosis: an open-label phase 2a proof-of-concept study. Lancet Neurol 11:150–156

Cotte S, Ahsen N von, Kruse N et al (2009) ABC-transporter gene-polymorphisms are potential pharmacogenetic markers for mitoxantrone response in multiple sclerosis. Brain 132:2517–2530

Deloire MS, Ruet A, Hamel D, Bonnet M, Dousset V, Brochet B (2011) MRI predictors of cognitive outcome in early multiple sclerosis. Neurology 76:1161–1167

Filippi M, Rocca MA, Benedict RH et al (2010) The contribution of MRI in assessing cognitive impairment in multiple sclerosis. Neurology 75:2121–128

Filippi M, Rovaris M, Inglese M et al (2004) Interferon beta-1a for brain tissue loss in patients at presentation with syndromes suggestive of multiple sclerosis: a randomised, double-blind, placebo-controlled trial. Lancet 364:1489–1496

Fleischmann RM (2009) Progressive multifocal leukoencephalopathy following rituximab treatment in a patient with rheumatoid arthritis. Arthritis Rheum 60:3225–3228

Friese MA, Craner MJ, Etzensperger R et al (2007) Acid-sensing ion channel-1 contributes to axonal degeneration in autoimmune inflammation of the central nervous system. Nat Med 13:1483–1489

Fugger L, Friese MA, Bell JI (2009) From genes to function: the next challenge to understanding multiple sclerosis. Nature Rev Immunol 9:408–417

Ghoreschi K, Bruck J, Kellerer C et al (2011) Fumarates improve psoriasis and multiple sclerosis by inducing type II dendritic cells. J Exp Med 208:2291–2303

Gonsette RE, Demonty L (1990) Immunosuppression with mitoxantrone in multiple sclerosis A pilot study for 2 years in 22 patients. Neurology 40:261

Gorelik L, Lerner M, Bixler S et al (2010) Anti-JC virus antibodies: implications for PML risk stratification. Ann Neurol 68:295–303

Gross R, Healy BC, Cepok S et al (2011) Population structure and HLA DRB1 1501 in the response of subjects with multiple sclerosis to first-line treatments. J Neuroimmunol 233:168–174

Group PS (1998) Randomised double-blind placebo-controlled study of interferon beta-1a in relapsing/remitting multiple sclerosis. PRISMS (Prevention of Relapses and Disability by Interferon beta-1a Subcutaneously in Multiple Sclerosis) Study Group. Lancet 352:1498–1504

Group TIMSS (1993) Interferon beta-1b is effective in relapsing-remitting multiple sclerosis. I. Clinical results of a multicenter, randomized, double-blind, placebo-controlled trial. The IFNB multiple sclerosis study group. Neurology 43:655–661

Hartung HP, Gonsette R, Konig N et al (2002) Mitoxantrone in progressive multiple sclerosis: a placebo-controlled, double-blind, randomised, multicentre trial. Lancet 360:2018–2025

Hauser SL, Dawson DM, Lehrich JR et al (1983) Intensive immunosuppression in progressive multiple sclerosis. A randomized, three-arm study of high-dose intravenous cyclophosphamide, plasma exchange, and ACTH. N Engl J Med 308:173–180

Hauser SL, Waubant E, Arnold DL et al (2008) B-cell depletion with rituximab in relapsing-remitting multiple sclerosis. N Engl J Med 358:676–688

Havrdova E, Galetta S, Hutchinson M et al (2009a) Effect of natalizumab on clinical and radiological disease activity in multiple sclerosis: a retrospective analysis of the Natalizumab Safety and efficacy in relapsing-remitting multiple sclerosis (AFFIRM) study. Lancet Neurol 2009 8:254–260

Havrdova E, Zivadinov R, Krasensky J et al (2009b) Randomized study of interferon beta-1a, low-dose azathioprine, and low-dose corticosteroids in multiple sclerosis. Mult Scler 15:965–976

Hawker K, O'Connor P, Freedman MS et al (2009) Rituximab in patients with primary progressive multiple sclerosis: results of a randomized double-blind placebo-controlled multicenter trial. Ann Neurol 66:460–471

Hoffmann S, Cepok S, Grummel V et al (2008) HLA-DRB1*0401 and HLA-DRB1*0408 are strongly associated with the development of antibodies against interferon-beta therapy in multiple sclerosis. Am J Hum Genet 83:219–227

www.Biogenidec.com

Jacobs LD, Cookfair DL, Rudick RA et al (1996) Intramuscular interferon beta-1a for disease progression in relapsing multiple sclerosis. The multiple sclerosis collaborative research group (MSCRG). Ann Neurol 39:285–294

Jager PL De, Jia XM, Wang J et al (2009) Meta-analysis of genome scans and replication identify CD6, IRF8 and TNFRSF1 A as new multiple sclerosis susceptibility loci. Nat Genet 41:776–782

Jeffery DR, Chepuri N, Durden D, Burdette J (2005) A pilot trial of combination therapy with mitoxantrone and interferon beta-1b using monthly gadolinium-enhanced magnetic resonance imaging. Mult Scler 11:296–301

Johnson KP, Brooks BR, Cohen JA et al (1995) Copolymer 1 reduces relapse rate and improves disability in relapsing-remitting multiple sclerosis: results of a phase III multicenter, double-blind placebo-controlled trial. The copolymer 1 multiple sclerosis study group. Neurology 1995 45:1268–1276

Jones JL, Phuah CL, Cox AL et al (2009) IL-21 drives secondary autoimmunity in patients with multiple sclerosis, following therapeutic lymphocyte depletion with alemtuzumab (Campath-1 H). J Clin Invest 119:2052–2061

Kappos L, Antel J, Comi G et al (2006) Oral fingolimod (FTY720) for relapsing multiple sclerosis. N Engl J Med 355:1124–1140

Kappos L, Gold R, Miller DH et al (2008) Efficacy and safety of oral fumarate in patients with relapsing-remitting multiple sclerosis: a multicentre, randomised, double-blind, placebo-controlled phase IIb study. Lancet 372:1463–1472

Kappos L, Freedman MS, Polman CH et al (2009) Long-term effect of early treatment with interferon beta-1b after a first clinical event suggestive of multiple sclerosis: 5-year active treatment extension of the phase 3 BENEFIT trial. Lancet Neurol 8:987–97

Kappos L, Radue EW, O'Connor P et al (2010) A placebo-controlled trial of oral fingolimod in relapsing multiple sclerosis. N Engl J Med 362:387–401
Kappos L, Li D, Calabresi PA et al (2011) Ocrelizumab in relapsing-remitting multiple sclerosis: a phase 2, randomised, placebo-controlled, multicentre trial. Lancet 378:1779–1787
Khatri B, Barkhof F, Comi G et al (2011) Comparison of fingolimod with interferon beta-1a in relapsing-remitting multiple sclerosis: a randomised extension of the TRANSFORMS study. Lancet Neurol 10:520–529
Kinkel RP, Dontchev M, Kollman C, Skaramagas TT, O'Connor PW, Simon JH (2012) Association between immediate initiation of intramuscular interferon beta-1a at the time of a clinically isolated syndrome and long-term outcomes: a 10-year follow-up of the controlled high-risk avonex multiple sclerosis prevention study in ongoing neurological surveillance. Arch Neurol 69(2):183–190
Kleinschmidt-DeMasters BK, Tyler KL (2005) Progressive multifocal leukoencephalopathy complicating treatment with natalizumab and interferon beta-1a for multiple sclerosis. N Engl J Med 353:369–374
Lalive PH, Neuhaus O, Benkhoucha M et al (2011) Glatiramer acetate in the treatment of multiple sclerosis: emerging concepts regarding its mechanism of action. CNS Drugs 25:401–414
Langer-Gould A, Atlas SW, Green AJ, Bollen AW, Pelletier D (2005) Progressive multifocal leukoencephalopathy in a patient treated with natalizumab. N Engl J Med 353:375–381
Le Page E, Leray E, Edan G (2011) Long-term safety profile of mitoxantrone in a French cohort of 802 multiple sclerosis patients: a 5-year prospective study. Mult Scler 17:867–875
Liguori M, Healy BC, Glanz BI et al (2011) HLA (A-B-C and -DRB1) alleles and brain MRI changes in multiple sclerosis: a longitudinal study. Genes Immun 12:183–190
Linda H, Heijne A von, Major EO et al (2009) Progressive multifocal leukoencephalopathy after natalizumab monotherapy. N Engl J Med 361:1081–1087
Linker RA, Lee DH, Ryan S et al (2011) Fumaric acid esters exert neuroprotective effects in neuroinflammation via activation of the Nrf2 antioxidant pathway. Brain 134:678–692
Lublin FD, Cofield SS, Cutter GR, Conwit R, Narayana PA, Nelson F, Salter AR, Gustafson T, Wolinsky JS, CombiRx Investigators (2013) Randomized study combining interferon and glatiramer acetate in multiple sclerosis. Ann Neurol 73(3):327-340. doi:10.1002/ana.23863
Lucchinetti CF, Popescu BF, Bunyan RF et al (2011) Inflammatory cortical demyelination in early multiple sclerosis. N Engl J Med 365:2188–197
Major EO (2010) Progressive multifocal leukoencephalopathy in patients on immunomodulatory therapies. Ann Rev Med 61:35–47
Mandala S, Hajdu R, Bergstrom J et al (2002) Alteration of lymphocyte trafficking by sphingosine-1-phosphate receptor agonists. Science 296:346–349
Marriott JJ, Miyasaki JM, Gronseth G, O'Connor PW (2010) Evidence report: the efficacy and safety of mitoxantrone (Novantrone) in the treatment of multiple sclerosis: report of the therapeutics and technology assessment subcommittee of the american academy of neurology. Neurology 74:1463–1470
Marshall LJ, Dunham L, Major EO (2010) Transcription factor Spi-B binds unique sequences present in the tandem repeat promoter/enhancer of JC virus and supports viral activity. J Gen Virol 91:3042–3052
Merkler D, Metz GA, Raineteau O, Dietz V, Schwab ME, Fouad K (2001) Locomotor recovery in spinal cord-injured rats treated with an antibody neutralizing the myelin-associated neurite growth inhibitor Nogo-A. J Neurosci 21:3665–3673
Mi S, Hu B, Hahm K et al (2007) LINGO-1 antagonist promotes spinal cord remyelination and axonal integrity in MOG-induced experimental autoimmune encephalomyelitis. Nat Med 13:1228–1233
Mikol DD, Barkhof F, Chang P et al (2008) Comparison of subcutaneous interferon beta-1a with glatiramer acetate in patients with relapsing multiple sclerosis (the REbif vs Glatiramer Acetate in Relapsing MS Disease [REGARD] study): a multicentre, randomised, parallel, open-label trial. Lancet Neurol 7:903–914

Millac P, Miller H (1969) Cyclophosphamide in multiple sclerosis. Lancet 1:783
Miller DH, Weber T, Grove R et al (2012) Firategrast for relapsing remitting multiple sclerosis: a phase 2, randomised, double-blind, placebo-controlled trial. Lancet Neurol 11(2):131–139
Miron VE, Jung CG, Kim HJ, Kennedy TE, Soliven B, Antel JP (2008) FTY720 modulates human oligodendrocyte progenitor process extension and survival. Annal Neurol 63:61–71
Moll NM, Rietsch AM, Thomas S et al (2011) Multiple sclerosis normal-appearing white matter: pathology-imaging correlations. Ann Neurol 70:764–73
Moreau T, Thorpe J, Miller D et al (1994) Preliminary evidence from magnetic resonance imaging for reduction in disease activity after lymphocyte depletion in multiple sclerosis. Lancet 344:298–301
Noseworthy JH, Wolinsky JS, Lublin FD et al (2000) Linomide in relapsing and secondary progressive MS: part I: trial design and clinical results. North American Linomide Investigators. Neurology 54:1726–1733
O'Connor PW, Li D, Freedman MS et al (2006) A Phase II study of the safety and efficacy of teriflunomide in multiple sclerosis with relapses. Neurology 66:894–900
O'Connor P, Filippi M, Arnason B et al (2009) 250 microg or 500 microg interferon beta-1b versus 20 mg glatiramer acetate in relapsing-remitting multiple sclerosis: a prospective, randomised, multicentre study. Lancet Neurol 8:889–97
O'Connor P, Wolinsky JS, Confavreux C et al (2011a) Randomized trial of oral teriflunomide for relapsing multiple sclerosis. N Engl J Med 365:1293–1303
O'Connor PW, Goodman A, Kappos L et al (2011b) Disease activity return during natalizumab treatment interruption in patients with multiple sclerosis. Neurology 76:1858–1865
Oosten BW van, Barkhof F, Truyen L et al (1996) Increased MRI activity and immune activation in two multiple sclerosis patients treated with the monoclonal anti-tumor necrosis factor antibody cA2. Neurology 47:1531–1534
Paty DW, Li DK (1993) Interferon beta-1b is effective in relapsing-remitting multiple sclerosis. II. MRI analysis results of a multicenter, randomized, double-blind, placebo-controlled trial. UBC MS/MRI Study Group and the IFNB Multiple Sclerosis Study Group. Neurology 43:662–667
Pilar MMdel, Cravens PD, Winger R et al (2008) Decrease in the numbers of dendritic cells and CD4 + T cells in cerebral perivascular spaces due to natalizumab. Arch Neurol 65:1596–1603
Pitt D, Boster A, Pei W et al (2010) Imaging cortical lesions in multiple sclerosis with ultra-high-field magnetic resonance imaging. Arch Neurol 67:812–818
Polman C, Barkhof F, Sandberg-Wollheim M, Linde A, Nordle O, Nederman T (2005) Treatment with laquinimod reduces development of active MRI lesions in relapsing MS. Neurology 64:987–991
Polman CH, O'Connor PW, Havrdova E et al (2006) A randomized, placebo-controlled trial of natalizumab for relapsing multiple sclerosis. N Engl J Med 354:899–910
Polman CH, Reingold SC, Banwell B et al (2011) Diagnostic criteria for multiple sclerosis: 2010 revisions to the McDonald criteria. Ann Neurol 69:292–302
Popescu BF, Lucchinetti CF (2012) Pathology of demyelinating diseases. Ann Rev Pathol 7:185–217
Prinjha R, Moore SE, Vinson M et al (2000) Inhibitor of neurite outgrowth in humans. Nature 403:383–384
Prinz M, Kalinke U (2010) New lessons about old molecules: how type I interferons shape Th1/Th17-mediated autoimmunity in the CNS. Trends Mol Med 16:379–386
Prinz M, Schmidt H, Mildner A et al (2008) Distinct and nonredundant in vivo functions of IFNAR on myeloid cells limit autoimmunity in the central nervous system. Immunity 28:675–686
Ravnborg M, Sorensen PS, Andersson M et al (2010) Methylprednisolone in combination with interferon beta-1a for relapsing-remitting multiple sclerosis (MECOMBIN study): a multicentre, double-blind, randomised, placebo-controlled, parallel-group trial. Lancet Neurol 9:672–680
Rudick RA, Stuart WH, Calabresi PA et al (2006) Natalizumab plus interferon beta-1a for relapsing multiple sclerosis. N Engl J Med 354:911–923
Ruiter MB de, Tomassini V, Arun T et al (2011) Acid-sensing ion channel 1 blockade preserves brain microstructural integrity in patients with multiple sclerosis. Mult Scler 17:S205

Sawcer S, Hellenthal G, Pirinen M et al (2011) Genetic risk and a primary role for cell-mediated immune mechanisms in multiple sclerosis. Nature 476:214–219

Schimrigk S, Brune N, Hellwig K et al (2006) Oral fumaric acid esters for the treatment of active multiple sclerosis: an open-label, baseline-controlled pilot study. Euro J Neurol 13:604–610

Schwab SR, Cyster JG (2007) Finding a way out: lymphocyte egress from lymphoid organs. Nat Immunol 8:1295–1301

Schweckendiek W (1959) [Treatment of psoriasis vulgaris]. Med Monatsschr 13:103–4

Seewann A, Kooi EJ, Roosendaal SD et al (2012) Postmortem verification of MS cortical lesion detection with 3D DIR. Neurology 78:302–308

Segal BM, Constantinescu CS, Raychaudhuri A, Kim L, Fidelus-Gort R, Kasper LH (2008) Repeated subcutaneous injections of IL12/23 p40 neutralising antibody, ustekinumab, in patients with relapsing-remitting multiple sclerosis: a phase II, double-blind, placebo-controlled, randomised, dose-ranging study. Lancet Neurol 7:796–804

Sombekke MH, Lukas C, Crusius JB et al (2009) HLA-DRB1*1501 and spinal cord magnetic resonance imaging lesions in multiple sclerosis. Arch Neurol 66:1531–1536

Sorensen PS, Jensen PE, Haghikia A et al (2011a) Occurrence of antibodies against natalizumab in relapsing multiple sclerosis patients treated with natalizumab. Mult Scler 17:1074–1078

Sorensen PS, Mellgren SI, Svenningsson A et al (2009) NORdic trial of oral Methylprednisolone as add-on therapy to Interferon beta-1a for treatment of relapsing-remitting Multiple Sclerosis (NORMIMS study): a randomised, placebo-controlled trial. Lancet Neurol 8:519–529

Sorensen PS, Lycke J, Eralinna JP et al (2011b) Simvastatin as add-on therapy to interferon beta-1a for relapsing-remitting multiple sclerosis (SIMCOMBIN study): a placebo-controlled randomised phase 4 trial. Lancet Neurol 10:691–701

Sormani MP, Li DK, Bruzzi P et al (2011) Combined MRI lesions and relapses as a surrogate for disability in multiple sclerosis. Neurology 77:1684–1690

Soulillou JP, Cantarovich D, Le MBetal (1990) Randomized controlled trial of a monoclonal antibody against the interleukin-2 receptor (33B3.1) as compared with rabbit antithymocyte globulin for prophylaxis against rejection of renal allografts. N Engl J Med 322:1175–1182

Stroet A, Gold R, Chan A, Martinelli V, Straffi L, Comi G (2012) Acute myeloid leukemia in italian patients with multiple sclerosis treated with mitoxantrone. Neurology 78:933–934

Thone J, Ellrichmann G, Seubert S et al (2012) Modulation of Autoimmune Demyelination by Laquinimod via Induction of Brain-Derived Neurotrophic Factor. Am J Pathol 180:267–274

Tony HP, Burmester G, Schulze-Koops H et al (2011) Safety and clinical outcomes of rituximab therapy in patients with different autoimmune diseases: experience from a national registry (GRAID). Arthritis Res Ther 13:R75

Treumer F, Zhu K, Glaser R, Mrowietz U (2003) Dimethylfumarate is a potent inducer of apoptosis in human T cells. J Invest Dermatol 121:1383–1388

Tubridy N, Behan PO, Capildeo R et al (1999) The effect of anti-alpha4 integrin antibody on brain lesion activity in MS. The UK Antegren Study Group. Neurology 53:466–472

Uccelli A, Laroni A, Freedman MS (2011) Mesenchymal stem cells for the treatment of multiple sclerosis and other neurological diseases. Lancet Neurol 10:649–656

Vellinga MM, Castelijns JA, Barkhof F, Uitdehaag BM, Polman CH (2008) Postwithdrawal rebound increase in T2 lesional activity in natalizumab-treated MS patients. Neurology 70:1150–1151

Vermersch P, Kappos L, Gold R et al (2011) Clinical outcomes of natalizumab-associated progressive multifocal leukoencephalopathy. Neurology 76:1697–1704

Vincenti F, Kirkman R, Light S et al (1998) Interleukin-2-receptor blockade with daclizumab to prevent acute rejection in renal transplantation. Daclizumab Triple Therapy Study Group. N Engl J Med 338:161–165

Vollmer T, Panitch H, Bar-Or A et al (2008) Glatiramer acetate after induction therapy with mitoxantrone in relapsing multiple sclerosis. Mult Scler 14:663–670

Webster AC, Ruster LP, McGee R et al (2010) Interleukin 2 receptor antagonists for kidney transplant recipients. Cochrane Database Syst Rev 1:CD003897

Weiner HL (2009) The challenge of multiple sclerosis: how do we cure a chronic heterogeneous disease? Ann Neurol 65:239–248

Wenning W, Haghikia A, Laubenberger J et al (2009) Treatment of progressive multifocal leukoencephalopathy associated with natalizumab. N Engl J Med 361:1075–1080

Wuest SC, Edwan JH, Martin JF et al (2011) A role for interleukin-2 trans-presentation in dendritic cell-mediated T cell activation in humans, as revealed by daclizumab therapy. Nat Med 17:604–609

Wynn D, Kaufman M, Montalban X et al (2010) Daclizumab in active relapsing multiple sclerosis (CHOICE study): a phase 2, randomised, double-blind, placebo-controlled, add-on trial with interferon beta. Lancet Neurol 9:381–390

Xiong ZG, Zhu XM, Chu XP et al (2004) Neuroprotection in ischemia: blocking calcium-permeable acid-sensing ion channels. Cell 118:687–698

Yednock TA, Cannon C, Fritz LC, Sanchez-Madrid F, Steinman L, Karin N (1992) Prevention of experimental autoimmune encephalomyelitis by antibodies against alpha 4 beta 1 integrin. Nature 356:63–66

Yousry TA, Major EO, Ryschkewitsch C et al (2006) Evaluation of patients treated with natalizumab for progressive multifocal leukoencephalopathy. N Engl J Med 354:924–933

Chapter 18
Targeting CD52 for the Treatment of Multiple Sclerosis

Alasdair Coles and Joanne Jones

18.1 Introduction

CD52 is the glycoprotein, of unknown function, that has been brought to prominence because it is the target of the monoclonal antibody, Campath-1H, which is now called alemtuzumab. Currently approved for the treatment of patients with advanced chronic lymphocytic leukaemia (CLL), alemtuzumab is likely to be licensed as a treatment for relapsing–remitting in 2013. This will be 22 years after it was first used in Cambridge, UK, as an experimental drug in multiple sclerosis. This long gestation is explained both by the time needed to understand the biological complexities of the drug and also its repeated shuffling between industrial and academic sponsorship.

18.1.1 First Uses of Alemtuzumab: From Laboratory to Clinic

Alemtuzumab was originally known as Campath-1H, because it was a humanised form of the first monoclonal antibody to be created for human use in the Pathology Department of the University of Cambridge, following the invention of the technology to make large quantities of monoclonal antibodies against almost any antigen by the Nobel laureates Cesar Milstein and George Kohler (Kohler and Milstein 1975). The original intention, by Herman Waldmann and colleagues, was to create a monoclonal capable of targeting and depleting human T cells from bone marrow in order to treat leukaemia and prevent graft-versus-host disease (Waldmann and Hale 2005). Soon, Martin Lockwood and other physicians at Addenbrooke's Hospital in Cambridge pursued its use in autoimmune diseases on the basis that T cell depletion would disable the inflammatory process, leading to tolerance and disease stabilisation (Lockwood et al. 2003; Dick et al. 2000; Isaacs et al. 1995,1996a, b; Newman et al. 1995).

A. Coles (✉) · J. Jones
Department of Clinical Neurosciences, University of Cambridge,
Addenbrooke's Hospital, Box 165, Cambridge, CB2 0QQ, UK
e-mail: ajc1020@medschl.cam.ac.uk

T. Yamamura, B. Gran (eds.), *Multiple Sclerosis Immunology*,
DOI 10.1007/978-1-4614-7953-6_18, © Springer Science+Business Media New York 2013

Initially, alemtuzumab was made in Cambridge by Geoff Hale and colleagues, who subsequently moved to the Oxford academic unit called the Therapeutic Antibody Centre. But, as European regulations around drug manufacture and trials tightened in the early 2000s, academic production of a drug became unfeasible, so all further development of alemtuzumab had to be done directly with industry. At first, British Technology Group® controlled the commercialisation of alemtuzumab. They handed this on to Burroughs Wellcome®, who soon discontinued development because of disappointing results in phase II rheumatoid arthritis trials. In 1997, Leukosite® licensed rights to Campath-1H from BTG and went into joint venture with ILEX Oncology®. In 1999, Millennium® purchased Leukosite and co-developed Campath-1H with ILEX Oncology and Schering AG®. In 2001, Campath-1H was licensed, as MabCampath©, for the treatment of chronic leukaemia in 2001. In 2004, Genzyme® acquired ILEX from Millennium. In 2009, Genzyme and Bayer® (previously Schering AG) agreed that Genzyme would take sole responsibility for further development of Campath-1H. In February 2011, Sanofi® acquired Genzyme.

18.1.2 Alemtuzumab and Its Antigen

Alemtuzumab is a humanised anti-CD52 monoclonal antibody with an approximate molecular weight of 150 kD. It is genetically engineered by grafting rat complementarity determining regions (CDRs) into human framework regions fused to human IgG1. CD52 is a cell-surface glycoprotein consisting of a short 12 amino acid peptide with a C-terminal GPI anchor (Hale 2001; Xia et al. 1993, 1991), CD52 is differentially expressed on peripheral blood mononuclear cell (PBMC) subsets, with memory B cells and myeloid dendritic cells (mDCs) showing highest surface expression, followed by T cell subsets. Natural killer (NK) cells, plasmacytoid dendritic cells (pDCs) and basophils show lowest expression. Importantly, CD52 is not expressed on haematological precursors. However it is produced by cells in the epididymis and seminal vesicle being (Kirchhoff et al. 1993). Despite its wide expression, its physiological role remains unclear; recent work suggests that surface-bound and soluble CD52 may regulate T cell activation (Bandala-Sanchez et al. 2013).

18.1.3 Biological Effects of Alemtuzumab

Within minutes of infusing a single dose of alemtuzumab, peripheral lymphocytes are undetectable in humans. This is associated with the induction of serum cytokines, including TNF-α, IL-6 and interferon gamma, which peak from 2 to 6 h after administration; this is likely to be due to cross-linking of NK cells rather than simply cell lysis (Wing et al. 1996). Cytokine release causes infusion-associated symptoms, which are successfully reduced or prevented by pre-treatment with corticosteroids and anti-histamines (Moreau et al. 1996).

In vitro, alemtuzumab is capable of depleting cells by complement-dependent cytotoxicity (CDC) and antibody-dependent cell-mediated cytotoxicity (ADCC) (Xia et al. 1993). The degree of CDC that occurs has been shown to correlate with CD52 surface density, apart from mDCs and monocytes, which, despite relatively high CD52 expression, are relatively resistant to depletion. These cells have been shown to express high levels of complement inhibitory proteins (CIPs), which may in part explain their resistance, demonstrating that, while important, CD52 density alone does not define susceptibility.

To circumvent the problems of studying the mechanism of depletion in vivo, the Kaplan group (Genzyme) created a transgenic mouse expressing human CD52, with comparable tissue distribution and immune cell subset levels of expression to those seen in humans (Hu et al. 2009). Treatment with alemtuzumab replicated the transient rise in serum cytokines and depletion of peripheral blood lymphocytes seen in patients. Lymphocyte depletion occurred in lymphoid tissue, but was not as complete as in blood. Both lymphocyte depletion and cytokine induction were found to be largely independent of complement and appeared to be mediated by neutrophils and NK cells, as deletion of these populations with antibodies to Gr-1 or asialo-GM-1 strongly inhibited alemtuzumab's activity; whereas removal of complement with cobra venom had little or no impact.

One explanation for alemtuzumab's efficacy as a treatment of multiple sclerosis is its ability to cause a long-lasting lymphopenia. However, the paucity of opportunistic infections and striking incidence of novel autoimmunity after treatment suggests that immune responses are very much intact post-alemtuzumab. For this and other reasons, we prefer the interpretation that the therapeutic effect of alemtuzumab is not due to lymphopenia per se, but rather due to the long-lasting immune changes it induces.

We have shown that the composition of the circulating lymphocyte pool is significantly altered after alemtuzumab. Simply in terms of numbers, T cells are under-represented; with CD8 and CD4 lymphocytes taking on average 20 and 35 months, respectively, to reach the lower limited of normal (LLN), with counts never returning to baseline for the majority of patients (only 30 and 21 % of patients, respectively). As CD8 cell recovery is more rapid than CD4, for the first 3–6 months the CD4:CD8 ratio is reversed. In contrast to T cells, B cells and monocytes recover rapidly. After alemtuzumab, B cell numbers return to baseline by 3 months, then typically continue to rise further reaching supra-normal levels by 12 months (particularly, after the first cycle of treatment). Monocytes recover to the LLN within days of treatment and are at 80 % of baseline by 3 months, then remain stable at this level.

Altered composition due to differential reconstitution is only part of the story, as phenotypic and functional changes are also observed. In particular, for the first 6 months or so, there is a predominance of memory T cells, particularly those with a regulatory phenotype ($CD4^+CD25hiFoxP3^+$), with reduced constitutive cytokine expression (Cox et al. 2005). During this time, the B cell compartment is largely naive, initially dominated by transitional type 1 cells ($CD19^+/CD23^-/CD27^-$), then after 3 months by "mature naive" cells ($CD19^+/CD23^+/CD27^-$), Memory B cells ($CD19^+/CD27^+$) are slow to return (Thompson et al. 2009; Hill-Cawthorne et al. 2012).

18.1.4 Dosing and Pharmacokinetics of Alemtuzumab

The dosing schedule for alemtuzumab in the phase III trials was an intravenous infusion of 12 mg/day for 5 consecutive days in the first cycle and 3 consecutive days in the second cycle. Evidence from the extension of the phase II trial suggests efficacy of two cycles is durable to 5 years of follow-up (Coles et al. 2012). Current practice in Cambridge, UK, therefore is to give two cycles of alemtuzumab electively, but to await a return of disease activity to trigger subsequent cycles.

Alemtuzumab has complex pharmacokinetics with non-linear elimination, and is probably different between autoimmune conditions and leukaemia, where the CD52 antigen may be present in vastly greater numbers (Le Page et al. 2008; Rebello et al. 2001; Rebello and Hale 2002). Clearance of the drug reduces with repeated administration due to loss of receptor-mediated clearance. Comparisons of the area under the curve in male and female patients have suggested that dose modification is not necessary. The pharmacokinetics of alemtuzumab has not been studied in paediatric patients or in those with hepatic or renal impairment.

Neutralising Antibodies Despite being humanised, alemtuzumab induces antialemtuzumab-binding and -neutralising antibodies in up to 30 and 70 % of patients 1 month after the first and second cycles, respectively. However, because the interval between treatment cycles is at least 1 year, such antibodies usually become undetectable before the next cycle (Somerfield et al. 2010). We anticipate that persistent neutralising antibodies may become problematic in patients who have received multiple alemtuzumab cycles. So to address this, in collaboration with Herman Waldmann and Geoff Hale, we tested the strategy of tolerising to alemtuzumab, by pretreatment with a high dose of a non-cell-binding variant called SM3 (Somerfield et al. 2010).

Classical "high-zone" tolerance experiments have shown that monomeric (deaggregated) antibodies, when given without adjuvants, can induce tolerance. T cell tolerance can be achieved with low doses, whereas combined T and B cell tolerance requires high doses. Antibodies that bind to cells aggregate and have enhanced immunogenicity, even at low doses; in addition, "danger signals" in the form of cytokines released during cytolysis would further undermine tolerance induction. So, it was reasoned that high doses of a non-cell-binding variant of alemtuzumab may be able to tolerise to all "wild-type" epitopes (both T and B cell).

SM3 was first shown to successfully tolerise to "wild-type" alemtuzumab in the CD52- expressing transgenic mouse (Gilliland et al. 1999). SM3 was constructed by making a point mutation in the H2 loop of the H chain (Lys53 to Asp53), a region of the antibody shown to be critical for CD52 binding. More recently, we have tested SM3 in humans (Somerfield et al. 2010). An infusion of high-dose SM3 prior to the first cycle of alemtuzumab reduced the percentage of patients with a detectable antiglobulin response to a second cycle of alemtuzumab (where SM3 was given) from 74 to 21 %. Furthermore, the concentration of anti-alemtuzumab antibodies was reduced by more than 300-fold. We do not know how long this tolerance, partial for some patients and complete for most, will persist. Only repeated cycles of alemtuzumab will clarify this. Nonetheless, this work has provided proof in principle that it may be possible to tolerise against biological agents intended to be given long term.

18.2 Clinical Trial Experience: Efficacy of Alemtuzumab

18.2.1 Early Days: Treatment of Progressive Multiple Sclerosis

In 1991, when the first patient with multiple sclerosis was treated using alemtuzumab, it was believed that this form of the disease was due to repeated waves of cerebral inflammation and was simply a more aggressive form of relapsing–remitting disease. So, the first group of patients to be treated with alemtuzumab for multiple sclerosis were 36 patients with progressive disease, with disease duration of 11 years, a mean EDSS score of 6.5 and an average of 0.7 relapses per year, whose disability had worsened by ≥ 1 EDSS point in the preceding year (Kurtzke 1983). After alemtuzumab, the mean relapse rate fell to 0.02 per annum, representing a 97 % reduction and new MRI lesion formation was also reduced by 90 % reduction was demonstrated. However, despite this potent anti-inflammatory activity, patients' disability continued to deteriorate at a mean of 0.2 EDSS points per patient per annum, which correlated with continued progressive cerebral atrophy. Those patients with greatest worsening of disability and brain atrophy had the highest MRI T2 lesion load at baseline. Remarkably, when these patients were re-examined by MRI 7 years later, there was no mean increase in T2 lesion volume, suggesting that there had been no new inflammatory events in the intervening years. However, there had been further brain atrophy (Coles et al. 2006) At latest follow-up, a median of 14 years post-treatment, the cohort's median disability had worsened to EDSS 7.5 (range 4.5–9; Hill-Cawthorne et al. 2012).

Our conclusions from this experience were that progressive disability is not due to inflammation, which is successfully suppressed by alemtuzumab, but due to progressive cerebral atrophy, which is due to non-inflammatory mechanisms conditioned by previous inflammation. We speculated that immunotherapies would be more effective if given earlier in the course of the disease.

18.2.2 Pilot Studies in Relapsing–Remitting Disease

The second group of patients to be treated with alemtuzumab had relapsing–remitting multiple sclerosis, with a mean disease duration of only 2.7 years but aggressive disease evidenced in the previous year by a mean relapse rate of 2.2 and an associated increase in their EDDS of 0–7.5 points. After alemtuzumab, their relapse rate fell to 0.14, a 94 % reduction. Unlike the progressive cohort, discussed above, mean disability scores fell after alemtuzumab (by a mean of 1.2 points at 2 years).

We concluded that disability accumulation early in multiple sclerosis is driven by inflammation and that anti-inflammatory treatments are effective if given early in the course of the disease. From this analysis emerged our suggestion that there is a "window of therapeutic opportunity" for immunotherapies in multiple sclerosis (Coles et al. 2006).

18.2.3 Industry-Sponsored Trials of Alemtuzumab

In collaboration, first with Ilex Oncology and then Genzyme, we designed a programme for the clinical trial development of alemtuzumab.

The principles behind this programme, which make it unique amongst multiple sclerosis clinical trials, were:

- That patients with early multiple sclerosis should be included. With the phase II trial, CAMMS223, we limited disease duration to 3 years from first symptom. This was loosened to 5 and 10 years for the phase III trials, CARE-MS1 (Coles et al. 2012) and CARE-MS2 (Cohen et al. 2012), respectively.
- That patients should not have acquired significant disability. For phase II, an inclusion criterion was EDSS ≤ 3.0, which was replicated in CARE-MS1 and extended to EDSS ≤ 5.0 in CARE-MS2.
- That patients should have above-average disease activity, represented by two relapses over the preceding 2 years. In the phase II trial, there was also a requirement for gadolinium-enhancing lesions to be present in one of at most four baseline MRI scans (MRI disease activity was not required for phase III trial inclusion).
- That alemtuzumab should be compared in all trials against an active drug. At the time of the design of these trials, the only disease-modifying therapies in routine use in multiple sclerosis in all regions were three types of interferon beta and glatiramer acetate. We elected to compare alemtuzumab against interferon beta-1a, given three times weekly.
- That disability should be a primary outcome in all trials. We chose to test the ability of alemtuzumab to reduce the number of patients whose EDSS Kurtzke score increased by at least one point, confirmed at 6 months. This was combined, in all three trials, with relapse rate as a co-primary endpoint.
- That alemtuzumab should be tested both as a first-line therapy (in the phase II trial and one of the phase III trials, CARE-MS1) and in patients who had experienced disease active on one of the licensed disease-modifying therapies (CARE-MS2). We did not include a population of patients who had "failed" such therapies. Rather, we selected a group of patients in whom there is considerable uncertainty about best management: those who may have had just one relapse whist on therapy whilst on therapy. Such a patient may not fulfil the criteria of "highly active disease" for licensed second-line therapy (such as natalizumab or fingolimod) and so may be encouraged to remain on their original therapy. However, they are at higher risk of accumulating fixed disability, even in the short term (Rudick et al. 2004; Prosperini et al. 2009; Rudick and Polman

Table 18.1 Baseline characteristics of patients in industry-sponsored studies

	Phase 2 CAMMS 223[a], $N=333$	Phase3 CARE-MS I, $N=581$	Phase 3 CARE-MS II[a], $N=637$
Age, years mean (SD)	32.3 (8.5)	33.0 (8.2)	35.1 (8.6)
Gender % female	64.3	64.7	66.9
EDSS score mean (SD)	2.0 (0.7)	2.0 (0.8)	2.7 (1.2)
Disease duration, years median (range)	1.3 (0.1–6.3)	1.7 (0.1–6.0)	3.8 (0.2–16.9)
Relapses in past 2 years, *n* mean (range)	2.3 (1–7)	2.4 (1–7)	2.7 (1–9)

[a] Just including here patients on the 12 mg/kg alemtuzumab arm

2009). When combined with increasing evidence that interferon beta has no long-term effect on disability (Ebers et al. 2010; Shirani et al. 2012), there is increasing pressure to augment therapy in such a patient.

Such considerations led to the selection of trial cohorts with the demographics and disease characteristics given in Table 18.1.

Table 18.2 summarises the clinical efficacy of data from these trials. We conclude that:

1. Alemtuzumab definitely reduces relapse rate compared with interferon beta-1a.
2. Alemtuzumab probably also reduces the accumulation of disability compared with interferon beta-1a. The evidence for this is less robust than for relapse rate reduction. In the phase II trial and CARE-MS2, the phase III trial in "treatment-experienced" patients, alemtuzumab also reduced the number of patients who acquired fixed disability during the trial. In CARE-MS1, fewer alemtuzumab patients accumulated disability than those on interferon beta-1a, but this difference was not statistically significant. One explanation for this apparently anomalous result is that, inadvertently, a cohort with particularly benign disease was recruited. The evidence for this is that the expectation, from prior experience, was that 20 % of patients would have a 6-month disability event on interferon beta-1a, but in fact only 11 % met this criterion.
3. In the phase II trial and CARE-MS2, not only did alemtuzumab lead to reduced proportions of people developing fixed disability, but mean disability of alemtuzumab-treated patients actually improved over 3 and 2 years, respectively. We described a novel outcome measure to capture this: "sustained reduction in disability" that is a fall in EDSS of ≥ 1 point confirmed at 6 months (Coles et al. 2011). Greater numbers of patients met this criteria after alemtuzumab treatment.

18.3 Safety of Alemtuzumab as a Treatment of Multiple Sclerosis

18.3.1 Infusion-Associated Symptoms

An infusion reaction, due to cytokine release, is common at the time of alemtuzumab treatment, with a rash, headache, influenza-like symptoms and less frequently

Table 18.2 Efficacy of alemtuzumab

	Phase 2 CAMMS 223[a], $N=223$ Over 3 years	Phase 3 CARE-MS1, $N=581$ Over 2 years	Phase 3 CARE-MS2, $N=637$ Over 2 years
Relapse rate			
Relapse rate reduction	69 %**	55 %***	49.4 %***
Annualised relapse rate (alem vs. IFNβ)	0.10 vs. 0.36	0.18 vs. 0.39	0.26 vs. 0.52
Proportion relapse free(alem vs. IFNβ)	77 vs. 52 %**	78 vs. 59 %***	65 vs. 47 %***
Disability			
% patients with sustained accumulation of disability at 6 months	7 vs. 26 %**	8 vs. 11 % Not significant	13 vs. 20%**
Change in mean EDSS from baseline	Improvement of 0.39 compared with deterioration of 0.38 on IFNβ1a**	No significant change	Improvement of 0.17 compared with deterioration of 0.24 on IFNβ1a***
Hazard ratio of patients with sustained reduction in disability	Not assessed	No significant change	2.57 (1.57, 4.2)**

[a] Just reporting here the results of the 12 mg/kg arm
** $p<0.01$; *** indicates $p<0.001$

transient recurrence of previous MS symptoms (Table 18.3). Pre-treatment with corticosteroids, an anti-histamine and paracetemol minimises these symptoms and they are generally well tolerated.

18.3.2 Infections

When we first used alemtuzumab, we anticipated that the lymphopenia it induced would predispose to opportunistic infections. But these have been striking by their absence; progressive multifocal leukoencephalopathy, cytomegalovirus and pneumocystis pneumonia have not been seen. Cases of infections, encountered in our open-label trials in Cambridge, that are potentially attributable to immune suppression are one case each of spirochaetal gingivitis, pyogenic granuloma and Listeria meningitis. Each of these patients went on to recover fully. The Listeria infection was contracted after eating unpasteurised cheese. Dietary advice is now included in the safety measures of alemtuzumab treatment.

In all trials, mild-to-moderate infections, especially of the respiratory and urinary tracts, were more frequent amongst patients receiving alemtuzumab than those receiving interferon beta-1a (Table 18.3).

Table 18.3 Safety profile of alemtuzumab

	Phase 2 CAMMS 223[a], $N=333$ Over 3 years	Phase 3 CARE-MS I, $N=581$ Over 2 years	Phase 3 CARE-MS II[a], $N=637$ Over 2 years
Deaths	1 due to ITP 1 due to myocardial infarct	1 due to motor accident	1 due to motor accident 1 due to aspiration pneumonia
Infusion-associated symptoms	98 %	90 %	92 %
Infections			
All	66 % mild to moderate (47 % on IFNβ)	67 % mild to moderate (46 % on IFNβ)	79 % mild to moderate (66 % on IFNβ)
Life-threatening	0	0	0
Autoimmunity			
Thyroid	26 %	18 %	17 %
ITP	0.9 %	0.8 %	1 %
Goodpastures' syndrome	0	1 case on extended follow-up	0
Neoplasia (alem vs. IFNβ)	2.8 vs. 0.9 %	0.5 % vs. 0	0.6 vs. 1.5 %
Details	1 colon cancer after IFNβ-1a, 1 cervical cancer, 1 breast cancer, and 1 non-EBV-associated Burkitt's lymphoma in patients receiving the 24-mg dose of alemtuzumab	2 cases of papillary thyroid cancer after alemtuzumab	1 basal cell carcinoma on IFNβ and 1 on alemtuzumab. 1 thyroid and 1 parathyroid tumour after alemtuzumab. 1 acute myeloid leukaemia on IFNβ

[a] Just reporting here the results of the 12 mg/kg arm

18.3.3 Malignancy

Cancers have not been statistically more frequent after alemtuzumab than interferon beta-1a in any of the trials (Table 18.3). But it should be recognised that these studies are not powered to pick up differences in low-frequency events. Malignancies of note are papillary thyroid cancer and one case of Burkitt's lymphoma. In the phase III trials, there were three cases of thyroid papillary carcinoma, all detected as a result of investigation of biochemical thyroid dysfunction. We do not suspect that alemtuzumab causes thyroid carcinoma, because the *incidence of papillary carcinoma* incidence of papillary carcinoma in patients with Graves' disease is estimated at 3–4 % (Kraimps et al. 2000; Kim et al. 2004), with a suggestion that thyroid evaluation or surgery in such patients may identify some cancers incidentally (Berker et al. 2011). In the extension of the phase II trial, one patient died from non-EBV-associated Burkitt's lymphoma, which is an unusual tumour usually seen in immunocompromised individuals, for which reason we suspect may have been caused by alemtuzumab. An additional patient developed Castleman's disease, a pre-lymphomatous condition, now in remission after R-CHOP (Somerfield et al. 2010).

18.3.4 Autoimmunity

The principal adverse effect of alemtuzumab is novel autoimmunity arising months to years after treatment. This is a recognised phenomenon of reconstitution from lymphopenia in a variety of different conditions (Hsiao et al. 2001; Gilquin et al. 1998). After treatment with alemtuzumab, the thyroid gland is the most common autoimmune target, being affected in –30 % of patients, most frequently with the development of Graves' disease. The predilection for the thyroid gland has not been explained predilection has not been explained although we suspect lymphopenia may have uncovered an inherited susceptibility to autoimmune thyroid disease in people with multiple sclerosis. Other evidence for this is the increased incidence in Graves' disease amongst relatives of people with multiple sclerosis (Broadley et al. 2000; Heinzlef et al. 2000).

Other autoimmune conditions have been seen after alemtuzumab (Table 18.3). Six patients (3 %) receiving alemtuzumab on the phase II trial developed immune thrombocytopenia. The index patient died of a brain haemorrhage. In retrospect, unreported cutaneous signs of a falling platelet count had been present for a number of weeks. Subsequent cases were identified by a risk management programme with education for patients and regular follow-up with specific discussion of the signs and symptoms of thrombocytopenia alongside monthly blood counts. This programme was carried through to the phase III trials in which other cases of immune thrombocytopenia (1–3 %) were identified and managed before any significant bleeding events occurred. Most have required corticosteroids; a number of patients have had intravenous immunoglobulin and some rituximab. All these patients are now well, most off treatment and with normal platelet counts.

Other autoimmune diseases have occurred at lower frequency after alemtuzumab: there have been three cases of Good-pastures' disease, in two of which renal transplant was required; the remaining case has stable renal function off treatment. These have been reported a number of times in the literature (Coles et al. 2006; Clatworthy et al. 2008). There have also been single cases of autoimmune neutropenia and autoimmune haemolytic anaemia.

18.3.5 Mechanism of Autoimmunity After Alemtuzumab

The paradoxical association between lymphopenia and autoimmunity is well recognised both experimentally and clinically (Gleeson et al. 1996; Khoruts and Fraser

2005; Zandman-Goddard and Shoenfeld 2002; King et al. 2004); indeed, more recently, the observation that lymphopenia leads to exaggerated anti-self responses has been exploited to enhance anti-tumour immunity (Dummer 2002; Wrzesinski et al. 2010; Gattinoni et al. 2005). Although why lymphopenia should promote self-reactivity is not fully understood, it is thought that changes in T cell differentiation and function induced by lymphopenia are permissive for breakdown in self-tolerance.

In a lymphopenic adult (with an atrophied thymus), early T cell reconstitution is dominated by the homeostatic expansion of T cells that have escaped depletion. This process relies on stimulation through self-peptide-self-MHC and non-self-peptides-self-MHC driven by homeostatic cytokines (Do et al. 2012; Kieper and Jameson 1999; Ge et al. 2004). The resulting T cell population is oligoclonal and short lived. Rapidly expanding cells acquire the phenotypic and functional characteristics of memory cells, including reduced dependence on co-stimulation, the ability to respond to lower doses of antigen than naive cells and the rapid secretion of inflammatory cytokines on re-stimulation (Cho et al. 2000; Goldrath et al. 2000; Murali-Krishna and Ahmed 2000). The group of Sarvetnik demonstrated in the nonobese diabetic (NOD) mouse (in which the mice are mildly lymphopenic) that onset of diabetes and destructed insulinitis strongly correlates with the fraction of rapidly dividing T cells; with $CD8^+$ "memory-like" cells playing a major role in disease pathogenesis (King et al. 2004). More recently, Le Saout et al. (2008) have shown that $CD8^+$ memory cells generated during lymphopenia cannot cause autoimmunity by themselves, but that self-tolerance can be overcome by the co-operation of memory-like $CD4^+$ and $CD8^+$ T cells under lymphopenic conditions. These studies point to lymphopenia as the trigger for autoimmunity, with memory-like T cells (CD4 and CD8) generated through homeostatic expansion acting as pathogenic effectors.

Following alemtuzumab, treatment of multiple sclerosis memory/memory-like $CD8^+$ and $CD4^+$ T cells dominate the reconstituting pool (Cox et al. 2005). These cells are highly proliferative and susceptible to apoptotic cell death; with rates of cell turnover and T cell death correlating with autoimmunity (Jones et al. 2009). King et al. demonstrated IL-21 levels to be four to seven fold higher in T cells from the NOD mouse (relative to B10H2g7 mice and congenic-B6.Idd3.NOD mice), with higher expression of the receptor for IL-21 (King et al. 2004). We have demonstrated that patients developing autoimmunity following alemtuzumab treatment of their MS have twofold higher circulating levels of IL-21 compared with the non-autoimmune group. Importantly, this difference was evident before treatment, leading us to suggest that Il-21 may serve as a biomarker for the risk of developing autoimmunity months to years after treatment (Jones et al. 2009).

18.4 Conclusion

With the success of alemtuzumab across a wide range of clinical indications, no doubt efforts are being made to develop monoclonal antibodies against other epitopes of the CD52 molecule, and indeed biosimilars of alemtuzumab. But for the present, the only data on the effects of targeting CD52 as a therapy for multiple sclerosis come from alemtuzumab, which we have been studying for 20 years.

Alemtuzumab is an unlicensed exploratory treatment for relapsing–remitting multiple sclerosis. A unique development programme has tested alemtuzumab against an active comparator in people with early disease in one phase II and two phase III trials. In each, alemtuzumab offers clinical efficacy superiority over interferon beta-1a. However, it has potentially serious adverse effects, particularly autoimmune diseases months or years after alemtuzumab. These require careful monitoring and a high degree of vigilance from patient and physician alike to institute timely therapy.

There is not yet a consensus on the place of alemtuzumab in the management of people with multiple sclerosis. Some will argue that, given the complex safety profile of alemtuzumab, it would be best to reserve it for patients who have failed other disease-modifying therapies. It is important that the potential downside of this strategy is recognised: the phase II alemtuzumab trial illustrated the disability advantage of treating early multiple sclerosis with first-line alemtuzumab. Others may use alemtuzumab as an "induction therapy" to induce disease remission, to be followed by either interferon beta or copaxone.

Important considerations for the future are the long-term safety of alemtuzumab, particularly for low-frequency events. If the provisional IL-21 findings are confirmed, then it may be possible to use serum IL-21 as a predictive biomarker of autoimmunity, the most concerning adverse effect of alemtuzumab identified to date. This would allow individual risk/benefit counselling for people considering alemtuzumab as a treatment. Furthermore, it would allow patients to be streamed into a "high-" and "low-"intensity monitoring programme after alemtuzumab treatment.

It is unclear whether subsequent cycles of therapy prolong or augment the established risks of two cycles of therapy. Nor is it yet known how frequently alemtuzumab should be given over the long term, and whether repeat cycles should be given at fixed intervals or only—as at present—when there is evidence for disease breakthrough. Options include: a fixed schedule of retreatment, retreatment only with no disease activity or retreatment with drugs such as interferon beta in an "induction" programme.

Acknowledgements Alasdair Coles is funded by the NIHR and has received honoraria and consulting fees and his department has received research grants from Ilex Oncology and Genzyme, both involved in the commercial development of alemtuzumab. Joanne Jones has received honoraria and consulting fees from Genzyme. She is funded by the NIHR.

References

Berker D, Isik S, Ozuguz U et al (2011) Prevalence of incidental thyroid cancer and its ultrasonographic features in subcentimeter thyroid nodules of patients with hyperthyroidism. Endocrine 39:13–20

Bandala-Sanchez E, Zhang Y, Reinwald S, Dromey JA, Lee BH, Qian J, Böhmer RM, Harrison LC (2013) T cell regulation mediated by interaction of soluble CD52 with the inhibitory receptor Siglec-10. Nat Immunol 14(7):741–748. doi: 10.1038/ni.2610

Broadley SA, Deans J, Sawcer SJ, Clayton D, Compston DAS (2000) Autoimmune disease in first-degree relatives of patients with multiple sclerosis—a UK survey. Brain 123:1102–1111
Cho BK, Rao VP, Ge Q, Eisen HN, Chen J (2000) Homeostasis-stimulated proliferation drives naive T cells to differentiate directly into memory T cells. J Exp Med 192:549–556
Clatworthy MR, Wallin EF, Jayne DR (2008) Anti-glomerular basement membrane disease after alemtuzumab. N Engl J Med 359:768–769
Cohen JA, Coles AJ, Arnold DL, Confavreux C, Fox EJ, Hartung HP, Havrdova E, Selmaj KW, Weiner HL, Fisher E, Brinar VV, Giovannoni G, Stojanovic M, Ertik BI, Lake SL, Margolin DH, Panzara MA, Compston DA (2012) CARE-MS I investigators. Alemtuzumab versus interferon beta 1a as first-line treatment for patients with relapsing-remitting multiple sclerosis: a randomised controlled phase 3 trial. Lancet 380(9856):1819–1828
Coles AJ, Cox A, Le Page E et al (2006) The window of therapeutic opportunity in multiple sclerosis: evidence from monoclonal antibody therapy. J Neurol 253:98–108
Coles AJ, Fox E, Vladic A et al (2011) Alemtuzumab versus interferon beta-1a in early relapsing-remitting multiple sclerosis: post-hoc and subset analyses of clinical efficacy outcomes. Lancet Neurol 10:338–348
Coles AJ, Fox E, Vladic A et al (2012) Alemtuzumab more effective than interferon beta-1a at 5-year follow-up of CAMMS223 Clinical Trial. Neurology 78(14):1069–1078
Coles AJ, Twyman CL, Arnold DL, Cohen JA, Confavreux C, Fox EJ, Hartung HP,Havrdova E, Selmaj KW, Weiner HL, Miller T, Fisher E, Sandbrink R, Lake SL, Margolin DH, Oyuela P, Panzara MA, Compston DA (2012) CARE-MS II investigators. Alemtuzumab for patients with relapsing multiple sclerosis after disease-modifying therapy: a randomised controlled phase 3 trial. Lancet 380(9856):1829–1839
Cox AL, Thompson SA, Jones JL et al (2005) Lymphocyte homeostasis following therapeutic lymphocyte depletion in multiple sclerosis. Eur J Immunol 35:3332–3342
Dick AD, Meyer P, James T et al (2000) Campath-1H therapy in refractory ocular inflammatory disease. Br J Ophthalmol 84:107–109
Do JS, Foucras G, Kamada N et al (2012) Both exogenous commensal and endogenous self antigens stimulate T cell proliferation under lymphopenic conditions. Cell Immunol 272:117–123
Dummer W (2002) T cell homeostatic proliferation elicits effective antitumor autoimmunity. J Clin Invest 110:185–192
Ebers GC, Traboulsee A, Li D et al (2010) Analysis of clinical outcomes according to original treatment groups 16 years after the pivotal IFNB-1b trial. J Neurol Neurosurg Psychiatry 81:907–912
Gattinoni L, Finkelstein SE, Klebanoff CA et al (2005) Removal of homeostatic cytokine sinks by lymphodepletion enhances the efficacy of adoptively transferred tumor-specific CD8+ T cells. J Exp Med 202:907–912
Ge Q, Bai A, Jones B, Eisen HN, Chen J (2004) Competition for self-peptide-MHC complexes and cytokines between naive and memory CD8+ T cells expressing the same or different T cell receptors. Proc Natl Acad Sci U S A 101:3041–3046
Gilliland LK, Walsh LA, Frewin MR et al (1999) Elimination of the immunogenicity of therapeutic antibodies. J Immunol 162:3663–3671
Gilquin J, Viard JP, Jubault V, Sert C, Kazatchkine MD (1998) Delayed occurrence of Graves' disease after immune restoration with HAART. Lancet 352:1907–1908
Gleeson PA, Toh BH, van Driel IR (1996) Organ-specific autoimmunity induced by lymphopenia. Immunol Rev 149:97–125
Goldrath AW, Bogatzki LY, Bevan MJ (2000) Naive T cells transiently acquire a memory-like phenotype during homeostasis-driven proliferation. J Exp Med 192:557–564
Hale G (2001) The CD52 antigen and development of the CAMPATH antibodies. Cyto Therapy 3:137–143
Heinzlef O, Alamowitch S, Sazdovitch V et al (2000) Autoimmune diseases in families of French patients with multiple sclerosis. Acta Neurol Scand 101:36–40

Hill-Cawthorne GA, Button T, Tuohy O et al (2012) Long term lymphocyte reconstitution after alemtuzumab treatment of multiple sclerosis. J Neurol Neurosurg Psychiatry 83:298–304
Hsiao LT, Liu JH, Yen CC et al (2001) Relapse of Graves' disease after successful allogeneic bone marrow transplantation. Bone Marrow Transplant 28:1151–1153
Hu Y, Turner MJ, Shields J et al (2009) Investigation of the mechanism of action of alemtuzumab in a human CD52 transgenic mouse model. Immunology 128:260–270
Isaacs JD, Hale G, Waldmann H et al (1995) Monoclonal antibody therapy of chronic intraocular inflammation using Campath-1H. Br J Ophthalmol 79:1054–1055
Isaacs JD, Hazleman BL, Chakravarty K, Grant JW, Hale G, Waldmann H (1996a) Monoclonal antibody therapy of diffuse cutaneous scleroderma with CAMPATH-1H. J Rheumatol 23:1103–1106
Isaacs JD, Manna VK, Rapson N et al (1996b) CAMPATH-1H in rheumatoid arthritis—an intravenous dose-ranging study. Br J Rheumatol 35:231–240
Jones JL, Phuah CL, Cox AL et al (2009) IL-21 drives secondary autoimmunity in patients with multiple sclerosis, following therapeutic lymphocyte depletion with alemtuzumab (Campath-1H). J ClinInvest 119:2052–2061
Khoruts A, Fraser J (2005) A causal link between lymphopenia and autoimmunity. Immunol Lett 98:23–31
Kieper WC, Jameson SC (1999) Homeostatic expansion and phenotypic conversion of naive T cells in response to self peptide/MHC ligands. Proc Natl Acad Sci U S A 96:13306–13311
Kim WB, Han S-M, Kim TY et al (2004) Ultrasonographic screening for detection of thyroid cancer in patients with Graves' disease. Clin Endocrinol 60:719–725
King C, Ilic A, Koelsch K, Sarvetnick N (2004) Homeostatic expansion of T cells during immune insufficiency generates autoimmunity. Cell 117:265–277
Kirchhoff C, Krull N, Pera I, Ivell R (1993) A major messenger-RNA of the human epididymal principal cells, HE5, encodes the leukocyte differentiation CDw52 antigen peptide backbone. Mol Reprod Dev 34:8-15
Kohler G, Milstein C (1975) Continuous cultures of fused cells secreting antibody of predefined specificity. Nature 256:495–497
Kraimps JL, Bouin-Pineau MH, Mathonnet M et al (2000) Multicentre study of thyroid nodules in patients with Graves' disease. Br J Surg 87:1111–1113
Kurtzke JF (1983) Rating neurologic impairment in multiple-sclerosis—an expanded disability status scale (EDSS). Neurology 33:1444–1452
Le Page E, Leray E, Taurin G et al (2008) Mitoxantrone as induction treatment in aggressive relapsing remitting multiple sclerosis: treatment response factors in a 5 year follow-up observational study of 100 consecutive patients. J Neurol Neurosurg Psychiatry 79:52–56
Le Saout C, Mennechet S, Taylor N, Hernandez J (2008) Memory-like CD8+ and CD4+ T cells cooperate to break peripheral tolerance under lymphopenic conditions. Proc Natl Acad Sci U S A 105:19414–19419
Lockwood CM, Hale G, Waldman H, Jayne DR (2003) Remission induction in Behcet's disease following lymphocyte depletion by the anti-CD52 antibody CAMPATH 1-H. Rheumatology (Oxford) 42:1539–1544
Moreau T, Coles A, Wing M et al (1996) Transient increase in symptoms associated with cytokine release in patients with multiple sclerosis. Brain 119(Pt 1):225–237
Murali-Krishna K, Ahmed R (2000) Cutting edge: naive T cells masquerading as memory cells. J Immunology 165:1733–1737
Newman DK, Isaacs JD, Watson PG, Meyer PA, Hale G, Waldmann H (1995) Prevention of immune-mediated corneal graft destruction with the anti-lymphocyte monoclonal antibody, CAMPATH-1H. Eye (Lond) 9(Pt 5):564–569
Prosperini L, Gallo V, Petsas N, Borriello G, Pozzilli C (2009) One-year MRI scan predicts clinical response to interferon beta in multiple sclerosis. Eur J Neurol 16:1202–1209
Rebello P, Hale G (2002) Pharmacokinetics of CAMPATH-1H: assay development and validation. J Immunol Methods 260:285–302

Rebello P, Cwynarski K, Varughese M, Eades A, Apperley JF, Hale G (2001) Pharmacokinetics of CAMPATH-1H in BMT patients. Cyto Therapy 3:261–267
Rudick RA, Polman CH (2009) Current approaches to the identification and management of breakthrough disease in patients with multiple sclerosis. Lancet Neurol 8:545–559
Rudick RA, Lee JC, Simon J, Ransohoff RM, Fisher E (2004) Defining interferon beta response status in multiple sclerosis patients. Ann Neurol 56:548–555
Shirani A, Zhao Y, Karim ME et al (2012) Association between use of interferon beta and progression of disability in patients with relapsing-remitting multiple sclerosis. JAMA 308:247–256
Somerfield J, Hill-Cawthorne GA, Lin A et al (2010) A novel strategy to reduce the immunogenicity of biological therapies. J Immunol 185:763–768
Thompson SA, Jones JL, Cox AL, Compston DA, Coles AJ (2009) B-Cell reconstitution and BAFF after alemtuzumab (Campath-1H) treatment of multiple sclerosis. J Clin Immunol 30(1):99–105
Waldmann H, Hale G (2005) CAMPATH: from concept to clinic. Philos Trans R Soc Lond B Biol Sci 360:1707–1711
Wing MG, Moreau T, Greenwood J et al (1996) Mechanism of first-dose cytokine-release syndrome by CAMPATH 1-H: involvement of CD16 (FcgammaRIII) and CD11a/CD18 (LFA-1) on NK cells. J Clin Invest 98:2819–2826
Wrzesinski C, Paulos CM, Kaiser A et al (2010) Increased intensity lymphodepletion enhances tumor treatment efficacy of adoptively transferred tumor-specific T cells. J Immunother 33:1–7
Xia MQ, Tone M, Packman L, Hale G, Waldmann H (1991) Characterization of the CAMPATH-1 (CDw52) antigen: biochemical analysis and cDNA cloning reveal an unusually small peptide backbone. Eur J Immunol 21:1677–1684
Xia MQ, Hale G, Lifely MR, Ferguson MA, Campbell D, Packman L, Waldmann H (1993) Structure of the CAMPATH-1 antigen, a glycosylphosphatidylinositol-anchored glycoprotein which is an exceptionally good target for complement lysis. Biochem J 293(Pt 3):633–640
Zandman-Goddard G, Shoenfeld Y (2002) HIV and autoimmunity. Autoimmun Rev 1:329–337

Chapter 19
Haematopoietic Stem Cells for the Treatment of MS

Sofia Abrahamsson, Miriam Mattoscio and Paolo A. Muraro

19.1 Introduction

The last decade of research has achieved unprecedented advances in our understanding of stem cell biology. Amongst the best characterised types of stem cells are haematopoietic stem cells (HSC). Starting from the morphological description of bone marrow (BM)-resident cells in the early 1900s, studies on the physiological function of haematopoietic precursor cells have caught momentum in the 1960s and 1970s and have expanded exponentially following the increased availability of reagents and molecular methodologies in the 1980s and 1990s. In parallel, the clinical application of BM— and peripherally mobilised HSC—transplantation for haematological indications has been studied intensively in trials and applied in clinical practice. Since the mid-1990s, treatment of autoimmune disorders, including multiple sclerosis (MS), with autologous haematopoietic transplantation has been explored in clinical trials. More recently, an integrin-blocking antibody approved for treatment of MS has been shown to exert an effect on HSC recirculation as well as the expected effects on leucocyte trafficking.

The aim of this chapter is to introduce essential elements of HSC biology, review the immunological basis and the clinical results of autologous haematopoietic stem cell transplantation (AHSCT) for treatment of MS and to discuss the evidence for and functional implications of HSC mobilisation during anti-α4 integrin treatment.

19.2 HSC Biology

HSC are the best characterised human adult stem cells, present in most self-renewing tissues including the skin, the intestinal epithelium as well as the haematopoietic system (Wilson and Trumpp 2006).

P. A. Muraro (✉) · S. Abrahamsson · M. Mattoscio
Division of Brain Sciences, Faculty of Medicine, Building 560/Burlington Danes, Room E415, Imperial College London, 160 Du Cane Road, London W12 0NN UK
e-mail: p.muraro@imperial.ac.uk

T. Yamamura, B. Gran (eds.), *Multiple Sclerosis Immunology*,
DOI 10.1007/978-1-4614-7953-6_19,

At the turn of the twentieth century, anatomists examining the BM macroscopically first noticed the presence of a variety of cells with different morphology corresponding to various lineages of blood cells, also possible at different stages of differentiation (Doulatov et al. 2012). HSC were then functionally identified by McCulloch and Till who were the first to perform a clonal in vivo repopulation assay in a mouse model demonstrating that blood lineages are derived from multipotent cells that form macroscopic colonies in the spleen following transplantation (Till and Mc 1961). Since then, the use of mouse models has been essential and has given fundamental inputs to the understanding of human haematopoiesis and HSC biology. In vitro, human BM cells were shown to be capable of generating colonies (colony forming units, CFU) when layered onto human peripheral blood (PB; Pike and Robinson 1970) and were then enriched in culture enabling the characterisation of long-term culture-initiating cells (LTC-IC) constituting the more primitive and long-term 'self-renewing' stem cell population in the BM, while short-term HSC were defined as having a limited self-renewal capacity (Sutherland et al. 1989).

Self-renewal is one of the unique abilities of stem cells through which cells retaining the stem cell fate are produced to ensure that stem cell reserves are maintained over time. The extraordinary developmental potential of HSC is also achieved by their capacity to differentiate giving rise to a defined population of mature downstream progeny that is able to maintain or repair the host tissue (Fuchs et al. 2004); in the mouse, even a single HSC can reconstitute the entire haematopoietic system (Osawa et al. 1996) and several humanised models have proven that human HSC can engraft immune-deficient mice (Weissman 2000) and repopulate the BM of the transplanted animal (Kamel-Reid and Dick 1988).

Regulation of human HSC activity and function in vivo is thought to depend on a specific microenvironment, which has been termed 'stem-cell niche'. A stem-cell niche, as first proposed by Schofield (Schofield 1978), can be defined like a spatial structure in which stem cells are housed and associated with other cell types that are responsible for HSC maintenance by allowing self-renewal and preventing differentiation.

The first evidence of how relevant the BM microenvironment is to HSC retention and function comes again from studies in a mouse model (Barker 1994, 1997). It is now well accepted that the HSC BM microenvironment comprises both an endosteal and a vascular niche (Fig. 19.1). The former consists of the endosteal bone surfaces, which are lined with stromal cells, and Spindle-shaped N-cadherin-expressing osteoblasts, which serve as niche cells to maintain quiescence and prevent differentiation of HSC (Zhang et al. 2003). The quiescent endosteal niche would maintain dormant HSC long term (Arai et al. 2004). In response to injury or treatments as well as during homeostasis, quiescent HSC can be activated and re-cruited to the vascular niche, where they would locate next to the osteoblasts and would attach to the fenestrated endothelium of the BM sinusoids (Kiel et al. 2005). This microenvironment would contain quiescent HSC intermingled with dividing HSC. Symmetrical divisions can indeed generate more HSC, thus an individual HSC would divide into two identical daughter cells maintaining the same stem cell fate and providing the vascular niche with new HSC. It remains to be determined

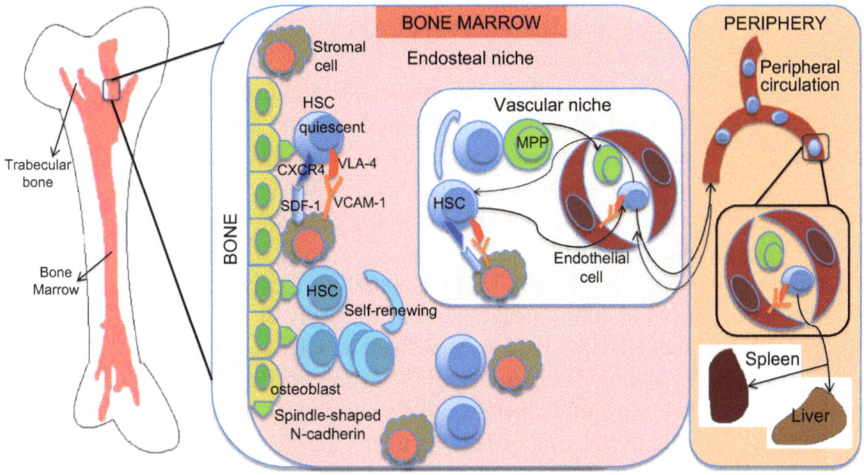

Fig. 19.1 Bone marrow niches and HSC mobilization to the peripheral compartment. Bone marrow (BM) niches, both endosteal and vascular, provide haematopoietic stem cells (HSC) with structural support as well as with cell-to-cell interactions and exposition to soluble factors, thus regulating HSC function. This schematic representation shows both quiescent and dividing HSC, the latest respectively self-renewing in the endosteal niche and going through asymmetric division in the vascular niche. In the endosteal niche, HSC are in firm contact with stromal cells and osteoblasts, while in the vascular niche they are located next to the BM sinusoids. Multipotent progenitors (MPP) and long term repopulating HSC can adhere to the endothelial cells of the BM sinusoids and access the peripheral circulation, subsequently migrating to the target organs and tissues. From the periphery, HSC can also home back to the BM through transendothelial migration to the vascular niche

whether HSC self-renewal can take place long term in the vascular niche; influx from the endosteal niches may be necessary to ensure prolonged haematopoietic cell production (Wilson et al. 2007; Wilson and Trumpp 2006). Also, self-renewing HSC activated by injury have the ability to return to quiescent status (Randall and Weissman 1997).

In the vascular niche, HSC can also produce multipotential progenitors (MPP) by asymmetric division, thus promoting differentiation and expansion of megakaryocytic and other myeloid cell lineages, particularly in response to injury. MPP can give rise to all haematopoietic lineages, including B cell precursors attached to randomly distributed CXC-chemokine ligand 12 (CXCL12)-expressing stromal cells, fundamental in the 'B cell niche'. T cell precursors would migrate to the thymus, whose unique microenvironment supports T cell maturation (Wilson et al. 2008; Wilson et al. 2007; Wilson and Trumpp 2006).

HSC can be defined not only by function but also by expression of specific surface markers. In humans, the recent characterisation of BM HSC has been enabled by the numerous informative studies that have been carried out in mice. Murine HSC were first isolated as a lineage-negative (Lin–), c-Kit+, Sca-1+(LSK) population (Harrer et al. 2012); cells possessing multilineage reconstitution and self-renewal capacities were then identified as CD34– (Osawa et al. 1996) and among those CD34−LSK cells, those expressing a CD150+CD48- SLAM phenotype were shown to have long-term-HSC activity (Doulatov et al.).

In humans, purification of BM HSC requires detection of CD34, which is expressed on less than 5 % of all blood cells and was first marker utilised to enrich products in human HSC and progenitors (Civin et al. 1984) since they express it on their surface in a proportion higher than 99 %. Human HSC also express FLT3 receptor (Sitnicka et al. 2003), not found on mouse cells, whereas they do not express CD150 (Larochelle et al. 2011).

However, among the total CD34+ population, only the small subset of CD34+Thy1+ cells has multilineage capacity (Murray et al. 1995); therefore, in recent years, human LT-HSC have been defined as CD34+CD38-Thy1+CD45RA- (or 'Thy1+' HSC) while CD45RA and CD38 expression has been used to identify more differentiated progenitors that negatively enrich HSC (Bhatia et al. 1997).

Another remarkable function of HSC is their motility (Fig. 19.1). As shown by several animal studies, in response to specific signals, HSC can both exit the BM, by a process named as 'mobilisation', and migrate through the peripheral circulation back to their niche, by a phenomenon known as 'homing' (Wilson and Trumpp 2006).

HSC mobilisation is mediated by changes in adhesion, mediated by changes in integrin expressions and activation status, modification of chemokine and growth factor receptor signalling and alteration of other less well-defined pathways. For example, deficiency of both Rho GPTases *Rac1* and *Rac2* was proven to lead to massive HSC mobilisation from the mouse BM and was also associated with ineffective haematopoiesis, both effects being reversed by re-expression of Rac1 (Jansen et al. 2005). Extensive HSC mobilisation is known to occur following treatment with granulocyte colony-stimulating factor (G-CSF) and/or cyclophosphamide; DNA-damaging agents by themselves can induce massive cell death of cycling HSC in the BM, spleen and blood and cause severe damage to the BM endothelium resulting into a dramatic increase in the levels of secreted chemokines, cytokines and proteolytic enzymes (Lapidot et al. 2005). The release of neutrophil proteases is a key mediator in the mobilisation process, which leads to the degradation of BM retention signals and adhesive connections such as membrane-bound SCF, adhesion molecules like P and E selectins and Very Late Antigen 4 (VLA-4), chemokines such as stromal derived factor-1 (SDF-1 or CXCL12) and IL-8 as well as for activation of proteolytic enzymes such as elastase and cathepsin G. Interaction of G-CSF with SDF-1 in the BM mediates mobilisation of human and murine stem cells, also causing reduction of SDF-1 levels on the surface of immature osteoblasts and upregulation of CXCR4 on the surface of HSC (Lapidot and Petit 2002). As for HSC activation processes within the niche, HSC release from the BM can also be observed during homeostasis, when a small number of HSC are constantly released into the circulation and constitute a rapidly accessible source of HSC to continuously repopulate the thymus and areas of damaged BM. On the other hand, HSC can also access the peripheral circulation subsequent to the physiological bone remodelling that causes constant destruction and re-formation of HSC niches (Wilson et al. 2008; Wilson and Trumpp 2006).

Stem cell release/mobilisation and homing are believed to be sequential events. Mobilised transplanted HSC can indeed be recruited from the peripheral circulation to the BM microvasculature and have the capacity to subsequently home back to the BM through transendothelial migration into its extravascular haematopoietic cords (Barker 1994; Wilson and Trumpp 2006). Homing is a rapid process, which can lead to transient retention and does not necessarily require cell division. HSC eventual engraftment in their niche is instead accompanied by the generation of a large number of haematopoietic progenitors and differentiated cells. Many cell types, including short-term repopulating progenitors and mature, specialised T cells and neutrophils, can home to the BM, but only long-term repopulating human CD34-/CD38- stem cells initiate long-term repopulation (Lapidot et al. 2005).

19.3 Use of HSC in AHSCT for MS

If MS is the final outcome of an immune system gone wrong, can we help it back on the right track? AHSCT is currently being explored as a treatment option for highly aggressive forms of MS. The basic principle of its use is to re-educate the immune system, first by depleting or reducing the pathogenic immune repertoire and then to regenerate a healthy immune system with the help of autologous HSC. 'Reprogramming', 'rebooting' or 'resetting' the immune system are all terms that have been used to describe this process. Does this treatment, as sometimes stated, provide a possibility to actually cure the disease?

Transplantation of HSC is a well-established treatment procedure for haematological malignancies and is aimed at restoring the depleted haematopoietic cell populations after high-intensity chemotherapy or radiotherapy. An estimated 55,000–60,000 haematopoietic stem cell transplantations (HSCT) are performed each year, most for the treatment of haematological malignancies such as lymphoproliferative diseases (54.5 %) and leukaemias (33.8 %; Gyurkocza et al. 2010; Li and Sykes 2012). As a treatment for autoimmune diseases, however, HSCT is currently under evaluation as an alternative for patients with aggressive disease course and who are refractory to standard therapies. The global survey by the Worldwide Network of Blood and Marrow Transplantation reports that an estimated 0.4 % of all HSCT, nearly all autologous, were applied to treat autoimmune diseases in 2006. AHSCT as a treatment option for autoimmune disease was first promoted in the mid-1990s (Burt et al. 1995; Marmont 1994). This proposition was based on the observation that patients with coincidental autoimmune disease often experienced a long-term remission of autoimmunity after undergoing AHSCT for malignancies and immune-mediated disorders (Marmont 2004). The use of AHSCT for MS was supported by work in animal models, which showed that the treatment could block or prevent autoimmune demyelination in the early stages after onset of clinical symptoms (Karussis et al. 1992a, b; van Gelder et al. 1993; van Gelder and van Bekkum 1996), but that advanced clinical damage could not be reversed (Burt et al. 1998a; Cassiani-Ingoni et al. 2007). Since the first pioneering studies took off (Burt et al. 1998b; Fassas et al. 1997), more than 600 patients with MS have been treated with AHSCT (Saccardi et al. 2012).

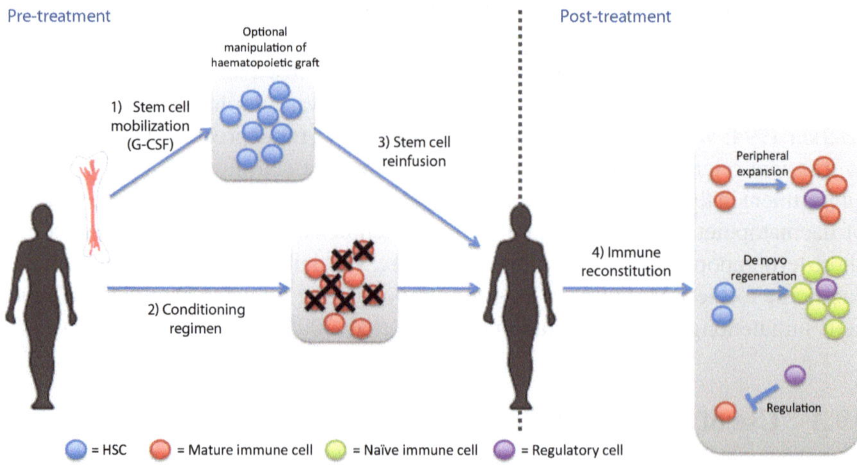

Fig. 19.2 AHSCT. The rationale for treating MS with AHSCT is to reprogramme the immune system. The treatment procedure consists of three basic steps: Mobilization of stem cells, lymphocyte depletion and stem cell reinfusion. Step 1: The most common source of HSCs (*blue cells*) are cells mobilized to the peripheral blood following mobilization with recombinant granulocyte colony-stimulating factor (G-CSF). The HSC-enriched blood can after immunosuppression be reinfused as an unmanipulated autograft, or immune cells are reduced by CD34− selection or lymphocyte depletion by antithymocyte globulin. Step 2: The immunosuppressive conditioning regimen consists of intense chemotherapy, biologics and/or radiation and aims at reducing the pre-existing immune cell repertoire (*red cells*). Intensities of immune suppression range from high-intensity, myeloablative protocols targeting all blood-forming cells, to non-myeloablative, reduced intensity schemes that more specifically target the immune system. Step 3: After immune depletion, the haematopoietic graft is reinfused into the patient. Step 4: Immune reconstitution commences after transplantation. The new immune system is regenerated by peripheral expansion of cells surviving the immune depletion (*red*), and is driven by cytokines or by antigens. De novo generated immune cells (*green*) diversifies the immune repertoire. Suppression of autoimmunity will depend on the balance between new cell specificities, pro-versus anti-inflammatory function of the cells in the regenerated immune system and reinstalled functional immune regulatory cells (*purple*)

19.4 Procedure of AHSCT

The basic rationale for treating MS with AHSCT is to reset the immune system, first by reducing the pathogenic cell repertoire and then by regenerating a healthy immune system. A schematic outline of the specific procedure is shown in Fig. 19.2. The autologous graft can be obtained directly from the BM in the iliac crest, however, the most common source of HSC are cells mobilised to the PB following treatment with recombinant G-CSF. Blood is generally preferred as a stem cell source since aphaeresis allows for collection of a larger numbers of HSC and may also allow for a faster engraftment. The HSC-enriched blood can be reinfused after immunosuppression as an unmanipulated autograft, however, is frequently manipulated in order to reduce the number of autoreactive cells (Farge et al. 2010). This manipulation usually consists of positive selection of CD34-expressing HSC or of lymphocyte depletion, achieved by in vivo or in vitro administration of anti-thymocyte globulin (ATG; Comi et al. 2000; Snowden et al. 2012).

The immunosuppressive conditioning regimen aimed at eliminating or reducing the pre-existing immune cell repertoire can consist either of intense chemotherapy, biologics and/or radiation. Intensities of immune suppression range from high-intensity, myeloablative protocols aimed at eliminating all blood-forming cells to non-myeloablative, reduced-intensity schemes that more specifically target the immune system. High-intensity conditionings such as total body irradiation (TBI) and chemotherapies including busulfan, were originally designed to maximise the killing of malignant cells and are highly cytotoxic. Transplantation of HSC in these cases is necessary for the BM to recover from aplasia. Intermediate-intensity regimens such as BEAM (carmustine, etoposide, cytarabine and melphalan) are combinations of reduced doses of cytoxins and are the most commonly used conditioning regimens in Europe. Reduced-intensity regimens generally consist of lymphodepleting antibodies, such as alemtuzumab (anti-CD52 mAb) and ATG.

19.5 Clinical Experience

Early clinical studies of AHSCT presented limitations to major conclusions about the clinical effects in that they were small, phase I–II uncontrolled trials that included heterogeneous patient populations and transplantation regimens. However, together they established some important points: (1) the clinical course of the disease stabilised for the majority of the treated patients through the duration of the follow-up in all but one study (Samijn et al. 2006) and (2) AHSCT typically suppressed inflammatory disease activity, measured by readouts such as acute clinical exacerbations, persistence of gadolinium-enhancing lesions at MRI of the brain or spinal cord or both (Mancardi et al. 2001; Mancardi et al. 2012; Saccardi et al. 2005; Saiz et al. 2001).

Table 19.1 summarises all major clinical trials and relevant retrospective studies since 2005. A retrospective large-scale analysis from the European Group for Blood and Marrow Transplantation (EBMT) in 2006 reported a progression-free survival (PFS) in 60–70 % of patients after 3 years and 50–60 % after 6–8 years (Saccardi et al. 2006). Several trials have reported a PFS in the range of 36–100 % after different lengths of follow-up (1.5–6 years) although a few recent studies with extended follow-up have reported that PFS decreases over time (Chen et al. 2011; Fassas et al. 2011; Krasulova et al. 2010). Despite this, it is believed that a high proportion of patients experience some form of stabilisation of their disease for long periods of time. A recent Italian multicentre study with a regimen including BEAM and ATG reports that 66 % of patients had improved or stabilised 5 years after treatment, compared to 44 % of the patients with a follow-up of 7 years or longer ($n = 8$). The disease progression was slower among the patients who relapsed (after a median of 3.5 years follow-up, $n = 10$; Mancardi et al. 2012). A retrospective study under the sponsorship of the Center for International Blood and Marrow Research (CIBMTR) and the EBMT, aimed at collecting long-term follow-up data in patients who received AHSCT between 1995 and 2006, is under way (PI: P Muraro).

Table 19.1 Recent trials or case series published since 2005 of autologous hematopoietic stem cell transplantation in patients with multiple sclerosis

Graft manipulation[a] (number of patients)	Conditioning regimen (number of patients)	Total number of patients treated	MS subtype (number of patients)	Range of EDSS at inclusion	Serious adverse events (number of patients)	Median follow-up (range)	Inflammatory lesion activity at MRI	Neurological disability[b]	Reference
No selection (19)	BEAM/ATG (19)	19	SPMS (15), RRMS (4)	5.0–6.5	Gastric ulcer bleeding requiring endoscopic intervention (1)	36 months (12–72)	No enhancing lesions in 18/19 (95 %) patients	18/19 (95 %) patients improved or stabilized	Saccardi et al. 2005
No selection (6), CD34+ selection (9)	Modified BEAM (etoposide substituted for teniposide) (15)	15	PPMS (3), SPMS (12)	4.5–7.5	Infections (4), mucositis (n/a), transient hepatotoxicity (n/a) and diarrhea (8), febrile episodes (3)	35 months (9–49)	No new lesions in 9 evaluated patients at 6 months	10/15 (67 %) patients improved or stabilized	Su et al. 2006
CD34+ selection (21)	CY/TBI (1) or BEAM/ATG (20)	21	SPMS (16), PPMS (2), PRMS (2), malignant (1) MS	5.0–9.5	Deaths from pneumonia (1) and from VZV hepatitis (1)	42 months (6–65)	No enhancing lesions in 18/21 (86 %) patients	2.1.1 16/19 (84 %) patients improved or stabilized	Ni et al. 2006

Table 19.1 (continued)

Graft manipulation[a] (number of patients)	Conditioning regimen (number of patients)	Total number of patients treated	MS subtype (number of patients)	Range of EDSS at inclusion	Serious adverse events (number of patients)	Median follow-up (range)	Inflammatory lesion activity at MRI	Neurological disability[b]	Reference
CD34+ selection (14)	CY/TBI/ATG (14)	14	SPMS (14)	5.5-6.5	EBV-related post-transplantation lymphoproliferative disorder (1), myelodysplastic syndrome (1) and death from respiratory infection 5 years after transplantation (1)	36 months (7-36)	No enhancing lesions in 14/14 (100 %) patients	5/14 (36 %) patients improved or stabilized	Samijn et al. 2006
CD34+ selection (77), other T cell depletion methods (20), unmanipulated (81)	BEAM+ATG (74), BEAM (30), BCNU+CY+/ATG (20), TBI/CY+ATG (16), Busulfan+ATG (10), others (19), unknown (9)	178[c]	SPMS (99), PPMS (32), RPMS (19), RRMS (22), unknown (11)	3.5–9.0	5.3 % TRM during the period 1995 to 2000; no mortality observed from 2000	41.7 months	Not available	90/142 (63 %) patients improved or stabilized	Saccardi et al. 2006

Table 19.1 (continued)

Graft manipulation[a] (number of patients)	Conditioning regimen (number of patients)	Total number of patients treated	MS subtype (number of patients)	Range of EDSS at inclusion	Serious adverse events (number of patients)	Median follow-up (range)	Inflammatory lesion activity at MRI	Neurological disability[b]	Reference
CD34+ selection (14)	Carmustine/CY/ATG (14)	14	SPMS (9), RRMS (5)	4.5–6.5	No long-term complications observed	At least 4.5 years for all (14) patients; 6 years for a subset of 9 patients	No enhancing lesions in 12/14 (85.7 %) patients	Progression-free survival in 10/14 (71 %) patients at 4.5 years	Saiz et al. 2008
No selection (50)	BEAM/hATG (50)	50	SPMS (28), PRMS (1), PPMS (10), RRMS (11)	1.5–8.0	Sepsis (1) neutropenic fever (51.6 %), hepatic toxicity grade I and II (48.1 %), transient neurological dysfunction (22.2 %), enteropathy (18.5 %)	19 months (6–90)	Data available for 37 patients; no enhancing lesions in 14/16 (87.5 %) patients with pre-treatment enhancement and in 20/21 (95.2 %) patients without pre-treatment enhancement	45/45 (100 %) patients stabilized or improved, 11/45 (24.4 %) of patients improved by 0.5 EDSS and 17/45 (37.7 %) patients improved by ≥ 1 EDSS	Shevchenko et al. 2008
No selection (9)	CY/ATG (1), BEAM/ATG (8)	9	Malignant (9)	6.5–9.0	Sepsis (2), serum sickness (2), temporary mucositis (n/a), herpes zoster (1)	29 months (23–47)	No enhancing lesions in 6/9 (66.7 %) patients	9/9 (100 %) patients stabilized and improved	Fagius et al. 2009

Table 19.1 (continued)

Graft manipulation[a] (number of patients)	Conditioning regimen (number of patients)	Total number of patients treated	MS subtype (number of patients)	Range of EDSS at inclusion	Serious adverse events (number of patients)	Median follow-up (range)	Inflammatory lesion activity at MRI	Neurological disability[b]	Reference
CD34+ selection (21)	CY/alemtuzumab (17), CY/ATG (4)	21	RRMS (21)	2.0–5.5	Dermatomal zoster (2), perforated peptic ulcer (1), neutropenic fever (4), rash (1), transaminitis (1), immune thrombocytopenia (2) and diarrhea caused by *Clostridium difficile* infection (1), haemorrhagic cystitis (1), deep vein thrombosis (1)	37 months (24–48)	No enhancing lesions in 17/21 (81 %)	21/21 (100 %) patients stabilized and 17/21 (81 %) improved by > 1 EDSS	Burt et al. 2009
No selection (41)	BEAM/hATG (21), CY/rATG (20)	14	SPMS (33), PPMS (4), RRMS (4)	4.5–7.0	Death following febrile neutropenia and sepsis (3; all in BEAM + hATG)	3 years for BEAM/-hATG and 2 years for CY/rATG (median and range unclear)	No enhancing lesions in 35/35 (100 %; only 8 patients had pre-enrollment disease activity)	No clinical progression in 10/18 (55.6 %) patients after 2 years from BEAM/hATG, 14/20 (70 %) patients 3 years from CY/rATG	Hamerschlak et al. 2010

Table 19.1 (continued)

Graft manipulation[a] (number of patients)	Conditioning regimen (number of patients)	Total number of patients treated	MS subtype (number of patients)	Range of EDSS at inclusion	Serious adverse events (number of patients)	Median follow-up (range)	Inflammatory lesion activity at MRI	Neurological disability[b]	Reference
T cell depletion (13/26)	BEAM (11), BEAM/ATG (15)	26	SPMS (15), RRMS (11)	2.5–7.5	Febrile neutropenia (14), sepsis (10), urinary tract infection (7), diarrhea (16) and severe mucositis grade II to III (11)	66 months (11–132): SPMS = 96 months (30–130); RRMS = 19 months (11–132)	MRI data not available, decrease in median annual relapse rate from 2 (year pre-AHSCT) to 0 (first 2 years post-AHSCT)	Progression-free survival in 84.4 % (actual number n/a) RRMS and 60 % SPMS patients	Krasulova et al. 2010
CD34+ selection (10)	BEAM/ATG (25), Busulfan (10)	35	SPMS (19), RPMS (3), Malignant (1), RRMS (1), PPMS (11)	4.5–8.0	Death following aspergillosis (1) and pulmonary haemorrhage (1)	11 years (2–15)	MRI data not available	Progression-free survival 25 % at 15 years (44 % in patients with active lesions and 10 % in patients without active lesions)	Fassas et al. 2011

Table 19.1 (continued)

Graft manipulation[a] (number of patients)	Conditioning regimen (number of patients)	Total number of patients treated	MS subtype (number of patients)	Range of EDSS at inclusion	Serious adverse events (number of patients)	Median follow-up (range)	Inflammatory lesion activity at MRI	Neurological disability[b]	Reference
CD34+ selection	BEAM/ATG (24), CY/TBI (1)	25	SPMS (19), RRMS (3), PPMS (1), PRMS (2)	3–9.5	Neutropenic fever (12), bacterial infections (13), hepatic toxicity (7), death due to severe pneumonia (1) and varicella-zoster virus hepatitis (1)	Mean 59.6 months (4.5–111)	7/12 with active lesions at pre-transplant were inactive at 5 years, 5/12 cases inactive at baseline: 3 progressed without further lesions and 2 had active MRI lesions	Progression-free survival in 74 % at 3 years, 65 % at 6 years and 48 % at 9 years, neurological improvement in 10 (40 %), disease stabilization in 7 (28 %)	Chen et al. 2011
Not available	BEAM/ATG	74	SPMS (41), RRMS (33)	3.5–9	Neutropenic fever (70 %), sepsis (30 %), urinary tract infections (25 %), diarrhoea and severe mucositis (15 %), reactivation of cytomegalovirus (5), late toxic effects (recurrent varicella zoster or urinary tract infections, 5 %), death due to engraftment failure and Actinomyces infection (1) and encephalopathy for unknown reasons(1)	48.3 months (0.8–126)	52/61 (85 %) relapse-free at 5 years, no enhancing lesions in 45/45 (100 %) at 1 year, no enhancing lesions in 22/24 (92 %) at 2 years	Progression-free survival in 66 % at 5 years (87 % in patients with enhancing lesions at baseline and 46 % in patients without, 71 % in RRMS and 61 % of SPMS), progression-free survival in 44 % at 10 years	Mancardi et al. 2012

Table 19.1 (continued)

Graft manipulation[a] (number of patients)	Conditioning regimen (number of patients)	Total number of patients treated	MS subtype (number of patients)	Range of EDSS at inclusion	Serious adverse events (number of patients)	Median follow-up (range)	Inflammatory lesion activity at MRI	Neurological disability[b]	Reference
Unmanipulated	BCNU/CCNU +mephalan (60), reduced dose 'mini-BEAM-like' (35)	95	SPMS (35), PPMS (15), PRMS (3), RRMS (42)	1.5–8.5	Thrombocytopenia (100 %), neutropenia (100 %), fatigue (100 %), anaemia (80 %), alopecia (80 %), neutropenic fever (31.6 %), hepatic toxicity grade I and II (42.1 %), transient neurological dysfunction (27.4 %), enteropathy (7.4 %), skin allergy (8.4 %), pneumonia (2.1 %), oral candidiasis (1.05 %), nasal haemorrhage (1.05 %), uterine bleeding (2.1 %), oral herpes (1.05 %), genital herpes (1.05 %), sepsis (3)	Mean 46 months (10–66)	No enhancing lesions in 39/40 RRMS patients	12m: 53 % stable and 43 % improved (of 90), 46 months: 28 patients improved 31 patients stable, progression-free survival in 82 % at 5 years	Shevchenko et al. 2012

ATG Antithymocyte globulin, *BEAM* carmustine, etoposide, cytosine-arabinoside and melphalan, *CY* cyclophosphamide, *hATG* horse ATG, *AHSCT* hematopoietic stem cell transplantation, *MP* melphalan, *MS* multiple sclerosis, *PFS* progression-free survival, *PPMS* primary-progressive multiple sclerosis, *PRMS* progressive-relapsing multiple sclerosis, *rATG* rabbit ATG, *RRMS* relapsing–remitting multiple sclerosis, *SPMS* secondary progressive multiple sclerosis

[a]Haematopoietic graft was peripheral blood stem cells for all studies except in the study by Samijn et al., in which bone marrow was used

[b]Neurological disability was assessed using the Expanded Disability Status Scale (EDSS) scale. The definition of stabilization differed among studies, with some requiring no EDSS change and others allowing an increase of 0.5 EDSS

[c]Retrospective multicenter observational analysis. The survey by Saccardi et al. includes data from European studies that were previously reported independently, as well as data from the earlier retrospective report by Fassas et al.

Treatment with AHSCT has a more favourable outcome in patients with active inflammatory disease, while patients with chronic disease associated with high and established disability (EDSS of 6 and over) often continue to progress (Saccardi et al. 2006). Three recently reported AHSCT trials confirm a higher PFS in patients with a relapsing–remitting as opposed to secondary progressive disease course (Krasulova et al. 2010; Mancardi et al. 2012; Shevchenko et al. 2012). In accordance with these observations, two studies report a significantly lower PFS in patients with inflammatory activity at baseline (Chen et al. 2011; Mancardi et al. 2012). Mancardi et al. (2012) found that a significantly higher percentage of patients with gadolinium-enhancing lesions at baseline scans had stabilised or improved at 5 years as opposed to patients without inflammatory activity. In addition to several other studies, they also identified young age and short disease duration as factors that may determine a more favourable outcome of AHSCT (Krasulova et al. 2010; Mancardi et al. 2012; Saccardi et al. 2006; Shevchenko et al. 2008).

AHSCT seems particularly promising as potential treatment for young patients with malignant MS, characterised by a relapsing–remitting disease course with poor prognosis, recurrent inflammatory events and severe disability (Fagius et al. 2009; Kimiskidis et al. 2008). The relapse rate was dramatically reduced from 61 in 82 patient months pre-AHCST to 1 in 289 patient months after transplantation (Fagius et al. 2009).

Safety of AHSCT is mainly determined by the conditioning regimen, patient selection and the experience of transplant for MS within the centre (Farge et al. 2010). A recent review of the EBMT database reported that the treatment-related mortality rate has decreased to 1.3 % for patients treated during 2001–2007, indicating that increased experience with MS in transplantation and more appropriate patient selection has led to improved safety.

To identify the optimal treatment regimens is a remaining challenge that can only be met after carefully considering the risk-to-efficacy profile of the conditioning schemes and their application to specific patient groups. For example, high-intensity conditionings are more efficient in depleting the pre-existing immune repertoire and associated with a better clinical outcome in animals, but are also highly toxic to the patient. The study of the European database found that treatment-related mortality was linked to the use of regimens containing busulfan (Saccardi et al. 2006), although there was no difference in neurological result between high- and intermediate-intensity schemes without manipulation of the autograft. Conditioning regimens including TBI resulted in continued brain atrophy at a significantly increased rate and unremitting neurological progression (Burt et al. 2003; Nash et al. 2003; Samijn et al. 2006), suggesting that radiation can be specifically harmful to the central nervous system (CNS). These observations suggest that prudence needs to be adopted with the use of radiotherapy in future trials. However, recent trials have shown that toxicity of the high-intensity regimen Cy and busulfan can be reduced, suggesting that high-intensity conditionings may be a treatment option for the future (Atkins and Freedman 2009).

Intermediate-intensity transplantation regimens with BEAM are currently deemed to involve acceptable toxicities (Saccardi et al. 2012, 2006). In the cases reported to the European database until 2005, no TRM was observed after intermediate-intensity transplantation regimen with BEAM and ATG, indicating different toxicities between high- and intermediate-conditioning schemes (Saccardi et al. 2006). Mancardi et al. recently reported the results from a large multicentre study using AHSCT with BEAM and ATG. The treatment-related mortality was 2.7 % and 66 % of the patients had stabilised or improved 5 years after transplantation ($n = 74$; Mancardi et al. 2012).

The use of reduced-intensity conditioning regimens has been proposed in order to reduce the toxicities and risks of AHSCT (Burt et al. 2003). A recent comparative Brazilian study of intermediate (BEAM and ATG) and reduced-intensity (CY and ATG) conditioning regimens suggested a higher toxicity of intermediate as compared to reduced-intensity treatments, with the intermediate scheme resulting in higher mortality and longer hospital stays. The results from one prospective trial with non-myeloablative AHSCT scheme show minimal toxicity, with stabilisation of disease in 100 % of the patients and 81 % patients experiencing improvement of neurological disability after a median of 3 years of follow-up (Burt et al. 2009). Inclusion of alemtuzumab as in vivo lymphodepleting agent in the original conditioning regimen in this trial was associated with some cases of secondary autoimmunity and was replaced with ATG in order to reduce the risk of immune thrombocytopenia (Loh et al. 2007).

Animal studies seem to suggest that an unmanipulated graft can increase the risk of disease recurrence (Euler et al. 1996; van Gelder and van Bekkum 1996), however, no association with graft manipulation and outcome has been demonstrated in MS patients (Saccardi et al. 2006). T cell depletion can, however, slow down the quantitative reconstitution of cells, especially the CD4 T cells (Bomberger et al. 1998; Rutella et al. 2000), which could significantly increase the risk of opportunistic infections during the lymphopenia succeeding the immunosuppressive conditioning.

19.6 Allogeneic HSCT (allo-HSCT) for MS

Allo-HSCT as treatment option for severe MS is theoretically attractive because the procedure may correct the genetic predisposition to autoimmunity by substituting the patient's pathogenic immune system with that of a healthy donor and it may establish control of the disease by a putative mechanism known as graft-versus-autoimmunity effect (Van Wijmeersch et al. 2007). Patients with aggressive MS who failed AHSCT and have a fully matched available donor have been suggested as suitable candidates for small tentative clinical trials of allo-HSCT (Griffith et al. 2005). It is, however, generally agreed that the outlook of greater efficacy of allogeneic over autologous transplantation for MS does not compensate for the increased morbidity and mortality risks. A recent report showed that allo-HSCT did not only fail to completely suppress inflammation in MS patients, but also that patients without MS who received allo-HSCT for other indications had inflammation in the CNS following treatment (Lu et al. 2010).

19.7 Ongoing and Future Clinical Trials

In 2004, the EBMT launched a prospective, randomised phase II trial, the Autologous Stem cell Transplantation International Multiple Sclerosis Trial (ASTIMS; www.astims.org) in which the transplantation arm consisted of BEAM-ATG and no graft manipulation and the control arm of mitoxantrone. The trial was closed to recruitment in November 2009 and the follow-up analysis is currently ongoing.

The multicentre US phase II trial, High-Dose Immunosuppression and Autologous Transplantation for Multiple Sclerosis (HALT MS; ClinicalTrials.gov Identifier: NCT00288626) was closed to accrual in August 2009. The first preliminary results have reported a 77 % event-free survival at 2 years post-AHSCT in 25 patients with highly active, treatment-refractory RRMS (Nash et al. 2013). Preliminary results from the Canadian MS/BMT trial (NCT01099930) report that AHSCT with BEAM and ATG completely suppressed relapse and inflammation by MRI in 23 evaluated patients over a median follow-up of 5 years (Freedman et al. 2007; Atkins and Freedman 2009).

The ongoing Multiple Sclerosis International Stem cell Transplant (MIST) randomises patients with two or more steroid-treated relapses within 12 months despite first-line therapy with interferon or copaxone to either AHSCT with cyclophosphamide and ATG or best available approved second-line therapy (ClinicalTrials.gov Identifier: NCT00273364). Patient recruitment is ongoing in Chicago, Sweden and Brazil.

A large international phase III randomised trial where patients are treated either with AHSCT or an appropriate non-AHSCT comparator, with a clinical endpoint, is currently needed and discussions are ongoing amongst several European and North American centres. Type of study, patient selection, treatment regimen and outcome measures are currently under discussion (Burt et al. 2012; Saccardi et al. 2012).

19.8 Mechanisms of AHSCT in MS

MS is believed to occur as a result of multiple environmental immune challenges throughout the life of an individual with a susceptible genetic background. Although AHSCT cannot correct the underlying genetic component, the treatment can partly erase the immunological history of an individual and provide the immune system a second opportunity. This 'rebooting', 'resetting' or 'reprogramming' may not yield a cure for the disease, but has the potential to delay the re-emergence of autoimmunity for several years at minimum.

Current knowledge indicates that the mechanisms that contribute to reinstalling self-tolerance after AHSCT likely include: (1) the reduction of the pathogenic lymphocyte population, (2) de novo regeneration of naive immune cells and (3) a new balance of pro- and anti-inflammatory cell populations after treatment (Fig. 19.2). The degree of contribution of each mechanism is determined both by the immune conditioning scheme and the patient characteristics, such as their age and disease stage.

The extreme lymphopenia following intense immune ablation induces homeostatic signals that support the recovery of the lymphocyte pool by both central and peripheral expansion. Central expansion of naive cells arising from the primary lymphoid organs is an important component of immune tolerance, resulting in a diversification of lymphocyte specificities. Peripheral expansion of cells that survived the immune conditioning may favour the rapid expansion of any residual cells that have survived the immune conditioning or in the graft (Kieper et al. 2005), both by homeostatic proliferation induced by cytokines in profound lymphopenia or by antigen-driven proliferation.

19.9 Immune Renewal Beyond Immune Suppression

Studies on immune reconstitution after AHSCT are scarce and have generally been performed on patients receiving a myeloablative conditioning regimen. The early studies demonstrated that the first 1–2 years following immunosuppression and AHSCT are characterised by a profound reduction of the peripheral lymphocyte populations. The various lymphocyte populations are replenished at different pace: The recovery of the lymphocyte population is generally accompanied by an increase in CD4 T cell numbers, whereas B cells, natural killer cells and CD8 T cells normally reconstitute completely to pre-transplantation levels within 3 months (Burt et al. 2003; Carreras et al. 2003; Koehne et al. 1997; Nash et al. 2003; Saccardi et al. 2005). The notion that the clinical effects of AHSCT persist even after numerical recovery of the lymphocyte populations supports that, not merely quantitative but also qualitative changes take place in the reconstituted immune system and can suppress inflammation.

Somewhat contradictory to the idea that AHSCT induced immune renewal, peripherally expanded memory cells predominate during the early T cell reconstitution. Extensive immune renewal with expansion of naive T cells and thymic reactivation was shown to take place in patients only 1–2 years after TBI and AHSCT for MS (Muraro et al. 2005) and cancer (Hakim et al. 2005). A detailed T cell receptor analysis showed the regeneration of a different and more diverse repertoire post-transplant in patients with MS (Muraro et al. 2005). Thymic rebound, expansion of naive T cells and diversifications of the repertoire were recently confirmed after AHSCT also in patients with systemic lupus erythematosus (SLE; Alexander et al. 2009).

The efficiency of immune ablation and the various cell populations and immune compartments that are targeted by the conditioning regimen are determined both by the intensity of the scheme and the specific chemical or biological compound used for immunosuppression. However, while a total depletion of the pre-transplant clonal repertoire is not feasible even with an intense radiotherapy conditioning (Dubinsky et al. 2010), a complete renewal is probably not required for remission of inflammatory activity (Muraro et al. 2005). In fact, reduced-intensity conditionings, which by definition are non-myeloablative and less lymphodepleting, also induce suppression of inflammation for several years. T cell diversity also appears to be near-to-normal despite incomplete depletion even before thymic reactivation (Storek et al. 2008). The re-emergence of autoreactive T cells in the absence of clinical relapse after AHSCT (Sun et al. 2004) suggests that newly installed qualitative differences such as pro- versus anti-inflammatory cell balance, avidity for the antigen (Bielekova et al. 2004) or reinstalled immunoregulatory functions (de Kleer et al. 2006; Zhang et al. 2009) could contribute to control autoimmunity after treatment.

The effect of AHSCT on the B cell compartment has been less investigated in MS, however, some data are available from the use of AHSCT in other autoimmune diseases. A study in patients with SLE found that B cell homeostasis was reinstalled after AHSCT, resulting in the expansion of the naive cells and the elimination of plasma cells resident in the BM (Alexander et al. 2009). Studies on antibody responses to foreign antigens such as after vaccination or revaccination preceding or following AHSCT, have shown that immunoablative conditioning and AHSCT purged immunological memory for a neoantigen given after the graft harvest, and reduced the immunological memory for a recall antigen boosted before harvest, following nonrigorous T cell depletion of the autograft (Brinkman et al. 2007). The attenuation of antibody immunological memory therefore suggests that the B cell compartment may also undergo a renewal. Again, the immunosuppressive conditioning could play a role in how efficiently B cell depletion is accomplished. Plasma cells are inefficiently deleted by TBI and B cell-depleting anti-CD20 Ab (Anolik et al. 2004; Radbruch et al. 2006); however, ATG, included in the protocol in both the German and the Dutch studies, contains polyclonal antibodies and can deplete both activated B cells and plasma cells in vitro (Zand et al. 2005).

A number of studies have concentrated on the effect of AHSCT on the renewal of the peripheral immune system; however, the goal is ultimately to deplete the self-reactive cells not only from the periphery but also, and most importantly, from the target organ. Studies performed on the CNS indicate the persistence of lymphocytes post-AHSCT. Intrathecal lymphocyte activation measured by soluble CD27 and the persistence of oligoclonal IgG in the cerebrospinal fluid (CSF; Mondria et al. 2008) indicate an inefficient depletion of plasma cells from the CNS after AHSCT. Postmortem studies on brains after autologous (Metz et al. 2007) and allogeneic (Lu et al. 2010) stem cell infusion have shown the presence of T cells in tissue for up to 8 months after treatment. A case study on allo-HSCT confirmed infiltrated T cells of recipient origin (Lu et al. 2009) arguing for, in this specific case, an incomplete depletion of intrathecal cells as opposed to infiltration of T cells through a damaged blood–brain barrier. These postmortem studies have severe limitations given the selection of cases with worst possible outcome and studies addressing the trafficking of immune cells to the CNS in vivo after HSCT are needed.

19.10 Immune Regulation After AHSCT

Immunoregulatory CD25-high Foxp3+CD4 T cells play an essential role in regulating autoimmune responses and are described as functionally compromised in MS patients (Venken et al. 2008; Viglietta et al. 2004). The idea that AHSCT may reinstall regulatory circuits was first suggested from animal experiments. Syngeneic BM transplantation in experimental autoimmune encephalomyelitis (EAE) rats resulted in attenuation of active disease and protection from induced relapses, which was associated with an increase of CD4+CD25+ T cells (Herrmann et al. 2005). In MS, data on regulatory mechanisms after AHSCT are scarce, but a few clinical studies in other autoimmune disease may be revealing. In juvenile idiopathic arthritis, a higher frequency of CD4+CD25^{high} T cells after AHSCT with high-intensity immune suppression correlated with clinical remission of disease (de Kleer et al. 2006). Also, in SLE, AHSCT caused an increase of Foxp3-expressing CD4 cells after conditioning with CY/melphalan/ATG (Alexander et al. 2009) and after reduced-intensity AHSCT (Zhang et al. 2009). The latter study also identifies a regulatory CD8 cell population that is inducible to express Foxp3 and produces the immunoregulatory cytokine TGF-β (Zhang et al. 2009). Regulatory CD25+Foxp3+CD4+ T cells were reported to be more resistant to irradiation than effector cells and mediated the amelioration of experimental graft-versus-host disease (Anderson et al. 2004). CD4 Tregs have also been described to present a faster reconstitution than effector T cells (de Kleer et al. 2006; Zhang et al. 2005) and their presence at the time of new antigenic priming could help to establish control of autoimmunity (O'Gorman et al. 2009). Regulatory CD4 cells can prevent antigen-induced, as opposed to homeostatic, proliferation in lymphopenic mice and their presence during the reconstitution of the immune system preserves the TCR diversity of the conventional T cell repertoire (Winstead et al. 2008, 2010). Taken together, the evidence suggests that AHSCT exerts significant effects on immunoregulatory cell pool, which may be relevant to its treatment effect in autoimmune disease.

19.11 HSC-mobilising Effects of Natalizumab Treatment in MS

Natalizumab is a recombinant humanised IgG4 monoclonal antibody that binds to the α4 integrin subunit and has been approved in recent years for treatment of active relapsing–remitting MS based on results of trials that have shown reduced brain-inflammatory activity as determined by MRI and reduction in the frequency of relapses (Muraro and Bielekova 2007; Polman et al. 2006); postmarketing studies have also confirmed its efficacy (Sangalli et al. 2011).

The α4 integrin family includes the VLA-4 or α4β1 integrin that plays a key role in T cell transmigration across the vascular endothelia. The α4β1-integrin is indeed expressed at moderate-to-high levels on almost all lymphocytes, monocytes and eosinophils and enables their capture from the circulation by interaction with the vascular cell adhesion molecule-1 (VCAM-1); captured leucocytes consequently adhere firmly to the endothelium and then transmigrate across the endothelial cell layer towards the site of inflammation (Davenport and Munday 2007). The VCAM-1 has been shown to be upregulated by inflammatory cytokines on the endothelium of MS patients (Rose et al. 2007) suggesting that α4β1 signalling pathway may be involved in the pathogenesis of the disease. It has also been shown that transcriptional downmodulation of adhesion molecules during interferon-β therapy contributes to the treatment mode of action in MS (Muraro et al. 2000, 2004).

The α4 integrin-blocking treatment with natalizumab results in specific rearrangements of the immune cells number in the peripheral circulation as well as in the CNS in both treated MS patients and EAE; indeed, a significant elevation of leucocyte and lymphocyte numbers was reported in the PB of treated MS patients, this effect confirming evidence from the preclinical studies on animals and constituting the most robust biomarker of successful α4 integrin antagonism. Also, the PB ratio CD4+/CD8+ was found to decrease significantly with increasing numbers of natalizumab doses, but remaining within normal limits (Stuve 2008). A significant decrease in detectability of the α4 integrin subunit was shown on all lymphocyte subsets during natalizumab treatment in parallel to the increase of lymphocyte-bound drug, indicating a therapy-induced reduction of a4 (Harrer et al. 2012). Interestingly, a significant decrease of β-1 surface levels was also observed in natalizumab-treated MS patients on T cells, B cells, natural killer cells and natural killer T cells, but not on monocytes (Harrer et al. 2011). Moreover, in the CNS compartment, a decrease in the numbers of CD4+and CD8+ T lymphocytes, CD19+ B cells and CD138+ plasma cells was demonstrated in the CSF of patients with MS on natalizumab therapy; such an increase was also shown to be sustained in time with the cell numbers remaining unchanged in the CSF even 6 months after cessation of the treatment (Stuve et al. 2009).

Antagonising α4 integrin also has an impact on the BM compartment, thus VLA-4, as described earlier in the chapter, is expressed by HSC and via interaction with VCAM-1-expressing stromal cells both contributing to HSC retention within the endosteal stem-cell niche and allowing HSC self-renewal in the absence of differentiation (Wilson and Trumpp 2006). Several studies on animals have shown that VLA-4 integrin plays a fundamental role in the HSC migration process to and from the BM: a dramatic inhibition of homing (> 90 %) was demonstrated when β_2- or selectin-null donor stem cells were additionally treated with anti-α_4 integrin antibodies before their transplantation to normal or selectin-deficient recipients; only 35–40 % of homing inhibition was instead seen when transferring the β_2- or selectin-null donor stem cells by themselves (Papayannopoulou et al. 2001). The β1-integrin-deficient HSC were also shown to fail to migrate to the BM after transfer (Wilson et al. 2008, 2009). Both the studies are suggesting that the α4β1/VCAM-1 pathway is possibly capable alone of providing effective capture of cells within the BM. Moreover, studies in primates have provided fundamental insights onto the VLA4-integrin involvement in HSC trafficking in vivo, showing that HSC peripheralisation can occur in these animals after a single injection of anti-α4; the treatment was also able to further augment HSC numbers in primates who had undergone a preceding course of G-CSF (Papayannopoulou and Nakamoto 1993).

In accordance with the animal studies, natalizumab treatment has been shown in recent years to result in significant and protracted increase of circulating HSC in treated MS patients (Bonig et al. 2008; Zohren et al. 2008). It was also observed that natalizumab- treated patients had 5.5-fold elevated levels of circulating CD34+ cells median concentration compared to healthy subjects and sevenfold elevated values compared to untreated MS patients; also, a threefold increase was achieved within 72 h following the first infusion (Zohren et al. 2008). Furthermore, natalizumab-mobilised HSC have been shown to have a different phenotype to that of G-CSF-mobilised HSC, thus expressing lower levels of VLA-4 integrin and higher concentration of CXCR-4, which associates with more than double migration capacity towards a chemokine stimulus; natalizumab-mobilised HSC have also been found to express lower levels of the stem cell marker CD133 compared to healthy subjects and untreated MS patients circulating HSC (Jing et al. 2010).

In contrast to the strong evidence provided by the numerous studies mentioned before, a single report has recently described that natalizumab treatment causes reduced adhesion and migration capacity of PB-isolated HSC compared to BM HSC in MS patients, which have been interpreted by the same authors as indicating a natalizumab-mediated impaired homing of HSC to the BM (Saure et al. 2011). However, the extensively demonstrated increased migration profile of natalizumab-induced HSC compared to G-CSF-mobilised HSC strongly supports the HSC mobilisation capacity of natalizumab.

A study from our group has confirmed the natalizumab-induced HSC mobilisation effect previously described (Mattoscio et al. 2012). We have also detected clear interindividual differences in circulating HSC count among natalizumab-treated MS patients with only approximately half of the subjects having a significant increase of HSC in the blood after natalizumab treatment. This observation enabled the definition of a 'Non-Mobiliser' group of subjects as those who failed to show such an increase. We have also determined that during natalizumab treatment, the proportion of quiescent HSC increases, suggesting an augmented rate of egress from the BM, as previously shown (Jing et al. 2010). The CD4 and CD8 T cells proportion were shown to increase transiently while the proportion of CD19 B cells increased preferentially, according to a previous report of particular interest that has shown how natalizumab is able to increase more significantly the number of circulating pre-B cells and B mature cells compared to other progenitors and mature lymphocytes and monocytes in MS patients (Krumbholz et al. 2008); in our study, the B cell proportion increased even more significantly in the Mobiliser group of patients. Moreover, the proportion of CD103+CD8 T cells, described as regulatory (Ho et al. 2008; Uss et al. 2006), was found to increase gradually in the first 12 months on treatment, again more significantly in the Mobiliser cohort. Therefore, both the natalizumab-induced effects on circulating B cells and CD8 Tregs correlated with the HSC mobilisation status in our studied population and could be consistent with further anti-inflammatory mechanisms of the drug. Moreover, an upgrowing trend in the number of T2 and T1 gadolinium-enhanced lesions was observed in the non-Mobiliser group of subjects and not in the Mobiliser one when analysing the MRI performed at 6 months on treatment and those patients who relapsed during the first year on natalizumab were found to be only among the non-Mobiliser cohort, suggesting that HSC mobilisation failure correlates with lack of treatment response (Mattoscio et al. 2013).

The evidence from the literature strongly suggests that natalizumab induced an augmented rate of egress of HSC from the BM and that, contrary to some claims, natalizumab-mobilised CD34+ HSC are not a relevant reservoir for JC virus (Warnke et al. 2011). Contributions from our group have suggested a variable HSC mobilisation response to natalizumab among treated MS patients and demonstrated a clinical and radiological disease activity in the Nonmobiliser group of subjects despite treatment, supporting the use of circulating HSC count as biomarker for response to natalizumab.

Furthermore, the rearrangements in the proportion of B mature and progenitor cells as well as regulatory T cells that have been clearly described in the literature to follow natalizumab treatment in MS patients, together with the drug-induced increase of HSC, suggest further anti-inflammatory and immune reconstitution-like effect of the drug, similar to the one described post-transplant in patients affected by SLE (Zhang et al. 2009).

19.12 Future Perspectives and Conclusions

Studies of AHSCT and anti-integrin treatment of MS indicate a central role of the haematopoietic system and of BM as well as circulating HSC in the generation and maintenance of the immune system. Transient numeric depletion of immune cells fails to explain the prolonged remissions observed after AHSCT in MS. Clinical effects on brain inflammation are better explained by qualitative changes in the reconstituted immune repertoire. AHSCT indeed induces substantial post-transplant modifications in the adaptive immune system. Nevertheless, further studies are required to establish whether and to what extent the suppression of inflammation observed post-therapy depends on the eradication of disease-associated T and/or B cell populations or on their functional regulation.

Several studies have shown natalizumab-induced increase of circulating HSC (Bonig 2008, p. 6; Zohren 2008, p. 1410) and suggested that this is due to a true mobilisation effect of the drug rather than to natalizumab-induced impedance of HSC homing (Jing 2010, p. 145). Evidence from our group has confirmed HSC mobilisation following natalizumab and also suggested widely different mobilisation responses in individual MS patients correlating with radiological and clinical anti-inflammatory response to the treatment, supporting the possible use of circulating HSC count as biomarker of response to natalizumab. Furthermore, the reported preferential effect of natalizumab in redistributing the B cell precursor pool among the total HSC population (Krumbholz et al. 2008) strongly supports further investigations on the already widely accepted fundamental role of B cells in MS pathogenesis (Disanto et al. 2012a, b). Furthermore, the tissue-regenerating potential of mobilised HSC, suggested by several studies reporting evidence of their potential for differentiation and integration into tissues including the CNS (Eglitis and Mezey 1997; Gordon et al. 2006; Mallet et al. 2002; Mezey and Chandross 2000; Mezey et al. 2000, 2003; Sigurjonsson et al. 2005), might contribute to the drug efficacy, perhaps actively contributing to neural tissue repair or indirectly promoting spontaneous tissue through paracrine secretion of neurotrophic factor, recruitment of neural precursors, or both.

Taken together, current knowledge on HSC biology highlights the interdependence of the haematopoietic and immune system for maintenance of immune competence and tolerance and provides great opportunities for therapeutic targeting in autoimmune disease including MS.

Acknowledgments This work was supported by grants from the UK MS Society (Ref. 938/10) and the Italian MS Society (FISM; ref. no. 2010/R/24; and ref. no. 2010/B/10).

References

Alexander T, Thiel A, Rosen O, Massenkeil G, Sattler A et al (2009) Depletion of autoreactive immunologic memory followed by autologous hematopoietic stem cell transplantation in patients with refractory SLE induces long-term remission through de novo generation of a juvenile and tolerant immune system. Blood 113:214–223

Anderson BE, McNiff JM, Matte C, Athanasiadis I, Shlomchik WD, Shlomchik MJ (2004) Recipient CD4+ T cells that survive irradiation regulate chronic graft-versus-host disease. Blood 104:1565–1573

Anolik JH, Barnard J, Cappione A, Pugh-Bernard AE, Felgar RE et al (2004) Rituximab improves peripheral B cell abnormalities in human systemic lupus erythematosus. Arthritis Rheum 50:3580–3590

Arai F, Hirao A, Ohmura M, Sato H, Matsuoka S et al (2004) Tie2/angiopoietin-1 signaling regulates hematopoietic stem cell quiescence in the bone marrow niche. Cell 118:149–161

Atkins H, Freedman M (2009) Immune ablation followed by autologous hematopoietic stem cell transplantation for the treatment of poor prognosis multiple sclerosis. Methods Mol Biol 549:231–246

Barker JE (1994) Sl/Sld hematopoietic progenitors are deficient in situ. Exp Hematol 22:174–177

Barker JE (1997) Early transplantation to a normal microenvironment prevents the development of Steel hematopoietic stem cell defects. Exp Hematol 25:542–547

Bhatia M, Wang JC, Kapp U, Bonnet D, Dick JE (1997) Purification of primitive human hematopoietic cells capable of repopulating immune-deficient mice. Proc Natl Acad Sci U S A 94:5320–5325

Bielekova B, Sung MH, Kadom N, Simon R, McFarland H, Martin R (2004) Expansion and functional relevance of high-avidity myelin-specific CD4+ T cells in multiple sclerosis. J Immunol 172:3893–3904

Bomberger C, Singh-Jairam M, Rodey G, Guerriero A, Yeager AM et al (1998) Lymphoid reconstitution after autologous PBSC transplantation with FACS-sorted CD34+ hematopoietic progenitors. Blood 91:2588–2600

Bonig H, Wundes A, Chang KH, Lucas S, Papayannopoulou T (2008) Increased numbers of circulating hematopoietic stem/progenitor cells are chronically maintained in patients treated with the CD49d blocking antibody natalizumab. Blood 111:3439–3441

Brinkman DM, de Kleer IM, ten Cate R, van Rossum MA, Bekkering WP et al (2007) Autologous stem cell transplantation in children with severe progressive systemic or polyarticular juvenile idiopathic arthritis: long-term follow-up of a prospective clinical trial. Arthritis Rheum 56:2410–2421

Burt RK, Burns W, Hess A (1995) Bone marrow transplantation for multiple sclerosis. Bone Marrow Transplant 16:1–6

Burt RK, Padilla J, Begolka WS, Canto MC, Miller SD (1998a) Effect of disease stage on clinical outcome after syngeneic bone marrow transplantation for relapsing experimental autoimmune encephalomyelitis. Blood 91:2609–2616

Burt RK, Traynor AE, Cohen B, Karlin KH, Davis FA et al (1998b) T cell-depleted autologous hematopoietic stem cell transplantation for multiple sclerosis: report on the first three patients. Bone Marrow Transplant 21:537–541

Burt RK, Cohen BA, Russell E, Spero K, Joshi A et al (2003) Hematopoietic stem cell transplantation for progressive multiple sclerosis: failure of a total body irradiation-based conditioning regimen to prevent disease progression in patients with high disability scores. Blood 102:2373–2378

Burt RK, Loh Y, Cohen B, Stefoski D, Balabanov R et al (2009) Autologous non-myeloablative haemopoietic stem cell transplantation in relapsing-remitting multiple sclerosis: a phase I/II study. Lancet Neurol 8:244–253

Burt RK, Balabanov R, Voltarelli J, Barreira A, Burman J (2012) Autologous hematopoietic stem cell transplantation for multiple sclerosis–if confused or hesitant, remember: 'treat with standard immune suppressive drugs and if no inflammation, no response'. Mult Scler 18:772–775

Carreras E, Saiz A, Marin P, Martinez C, Rovira M et al (2003) CD34+ selected autologous peripheral blood stem cell transplantation for multiple sclerosis: report of toxicity and treatment results at one year of follow-up in 15 patients. Haematologica 88:306–314

Cassiani-Ingoni R, Muraro PA, Magnus T, Reichert-Scrivner S, Schmidt J et al (2007) Disease progression after bone marrow transplantation in a model of multiple sclerosis is associated with chronic microglial and glial progenitor response. J Neuropathol Exp Neurol 66:637–649

Chen B, Zhou M, Ouyang J, Zhou R, Xu J et al (2011) Long-term efficacy of autologous haematopoietic stem cell transplantation in multiple sclerosis at a single institution in China. Neurol Sci 33(4):881–886

Civin CI, Strauss LC, Brovall C, Fackler MJ, Schwartz JF, Shaper JH (1984) Antigenic analysis of hematopoiesis. III. A hematopoietic progenitor cell surface antigen defined by a monoclonal antibody raised against KG-1a cells. J Immunol 133:157–165

Comi G, Kappos L, Clanet M, Ebers G, Fassas A et al (2000) Guidelines for autologous blood and marrow stem cell transplantation in multiple sclerosis: a consensus report written on behalf of the European Group for Blood and Marrow Transplantation and the European Charcot Foundation. BMT-MS Study Group. J Neurol 247:376–382

Davenport RJ, Munday JR (2007) Alpha4-integrin antagonism—an effective approach for the treatment of inflammatory diseases? Drug Discov Today 12:569–576

De Kleer I, Vastert B, Klein M, Teklenburg G, Arkesteijn G et al (2006) Autologous stem cell transplantation for autoimmunity induces immunologic self-tolerance by reprogramming autoreactive T cells and restoring the CD4+ CD25+ immune regulatory network. Blood 107:1696–1702

Disanto G, Morahan JM, Barnett MH, Giovannoni G, Ramagopalan SV (2012a) The evidence for a role of B cells in multiple sclerosis. Neurology 78:823–832

Disanto G, Sandve GK, Berlanga-Taylor AJ, Morahan JM, Dobson R et al (2012b) Genomic regions associated with multiple sclerosis are active in B cells. PloS one 7:e32281

Doulatov S, Notta F, Laurenti E, Dick JE (2012) Hematopoiesis: a human perspective. Cell stem. Cell 10:120–136

Dubinsky AN, Burt RK, Martin R, Muraro PA (2010) T-cell clones persisting in the circulation after autologous hematopoietic SCT are undetectable in the peripheral CD34+ selected graft. Bone Marrow Transplant 45:325–331

Eglitis MA, Mezey E (1997) Hematopoietic cells differentiate into both microglia and macroglia in the brains of adult mice. Proc Natl Acad Sci U S A 94:4080–4085

Euler HH, Marmont AM, Bacigalupo A, Fastenrath S, Dreger P et al (1996) Early recurrence or persistence of autoimmune diseases after unmanipulated autologous stem cell transplantation. Blood 88:3621–3625

Fagius J, Lundgren J, Oberg G (2009) Early highly aggressive MS successfully treated by hematopoietic stem cell transplantation. Mult Scler 15:229–237

Farge D, Labopin M, Tyndall A, Fassas A, Mancardi GL et al (2010) Autologous hematopoietic stem cell transplantation for autoimmune diseases: an observational study on 12 years' experience from the European Group for Blood and Marrow Transplantation Working Party on Autoimmune Diseases. Haematologica 95:284–292

Fassas A, Anagnostopoulos A, Kazis A, Kapinas K, Sakellari I et al (1997) Peripheral blood stem cell transplantation in the treatment of progressive multiple sclerosis: first results of a pilot study. Bone Marrow Transplant 20:631–638

Fassas A, Kimiskidis VK, Sakellari I, Kapinas K, Anagnostopoulos A et al (2011) Long-term results of stem cell transplantation for MS: a single-center experience. Neurology 76:1066–1070

Freedman MS, Atkins HL, Arnold DL, Bar-Or A on behalf of the Canadian BMT group (2007) Immune ablation and autologous stem cell transplantation for aggressive multiple sclerosis: interim 5-year report. Mult Scler 13 (Suppl 2):22(abstr)

Fuchs E, Tumbar T, Guasch G (2004) Socializing with the neighbors: stem cells and their niche. Cell 116:769–778

Gordon MY, Levicar N, Pai M, Bachellier P, Dimarakis I et al (2006) Characterization and clinical application of human CD34+ stem/progenitor cell populations mobilized into the blood by granulocyte colony-stimulating factor. Stem Cells 24:1822–1830

Gratwohl A, Baldomero H, Aljurf M, Pasquini MC, Bouzas LF et al (2010) Hematopoietic stem cell transplantation: a global perspective. JAMA 303:1617–1624

Griffith LM, Pavletic SZ, Tyndall A, Bredeson CN, Bowen JD et al (2005) Feasibility of allogeneic hematopoietic stem cell transplantation for autoimmune disease: position statement from a National Institute of Allergy and Infectious Diseases and National Cancer Institute-Sponsored International Workshop, Bethesda, MD, March 12 and 13, 2005. Biol Blood Marrow Transplant 11:862–870

Gyurkocza B, Rezvani A, Storb RF (2010) Allogeneic hematopoietic cell transplantation: the state of the art. Expert Rev Hematol 3:285–299

Hakim FT, Memon SA, Cepeda R, Jones EC, Chow CK et al (2005) Age-dependent incidence, time course, and consequences of thymic renewal in adults. J Clin Invest 115:930–939

Hamerschlak N, Rodrigues M, Moraes DA, Oliveira MC, Stracieri AB et al (2010) Brazilian experience with two conditioning regimens in patients with multiple sclerosis: BEAM/horse ATG and CY/rabbit ATG. Bone Marrow Transplant 45:239–248

Harrer A, Wipfler P, Einhaeupl M, Pilz G, Oppermann K et al (2011) Natalizumab therapy decreases surface expression of both VLA-heterodimer subunits on peripheral blood mononuclear cells. J Neuroimmunol 234:148–154

Harrer A, Pilz G, Einhaeupl M, Oppermann K, Hitzl W et al (2012) Lymphocyte subsets show different response patterns to in vivo bound natalizumab—a flow cytometric study on patients with multiple sclerosis. PloS one 7:e31784

Herrmann MM, Gaertner S, Stadelmann C, van den BJ, Boscke R et al (2005) Tolerance induction by bone marrow transplantation in a multiple sclerosis model. Blood 106:1875–1883

Ho J, Kurtz CC, Naganuma M, Ernst PB, Cominelli F, Rivera-Nieves J (2008) A CD8+/CD103high T cell subset regulates TNF-mediated chronic murine ileitis. J Immunol 180:2573–2580

Jansen M, Yang FC, Cancelas JA, Bailey JR, Williams DA (2005) Rac2-deficient hematopoietic stem cells show defective interaction with the hematopoietic microenvironment and long-term engraftment failure. Stem Cells 23:335–346

Jing D, Oelschlaegel U, Ordemann R, Holig K, Ehninger G et al (2010) CD49d blockade by natalizumab in patients with multiple sclerosis affects steady-state hematopoiesis and mobilizes progenitors with a distinct phenotype and function. Bone Marrow Transplant 45:1489–1496

Kamel-Reid S, Dick JE (1988) Engraftment of immune-deficient mice with human hematopoietic stem cells. Science 242:1706–1709

Karussis DM, Slavin S, Ben-Nun A, Ovadia H, Vourka-Karussis U et al (1992a) Chronic-relapsing experimental autoimmune encephalomyelitis (CR-EAE): treatment and induction of tolerance, with high dose cyclophosphamide followed by syngeneic bone marrow transplantation. J Neuroimmunol 39:201–210

Karussis DM, Slavin S, Lehmann D, Mizrachi-Koll R, Abramsky O, Ben-Nun A (1992b) Prevention of experimental autoimmune encephalomyelitis and induction of tolerance with acute immunosuppression followed by syngeneic bone marrow transplantation. J Immunol 148:1693–1698

Kiel MJ, Yilmaz OH, Iwashita T, Terhorst C, Morrison SJ (2005) SLAM family receptors distinguish hematopoietic stem and progenitor cells and reveal endothelial niches for stem cells. Cell 121:1109–1121

Kieper WC, Troy A, Burghardt JT, Ramsey C, Lee JY et al (2005) Recent immune status determines the source of antigens that drive homeostatic T cell expansion. J Immunol 174:3158–3163

Kimiskidis V, Sakellari I, Tsimourtou V, Kapina V, Papagiannopoulos S et al (2008) Autologous stem-cell transplantation in malignant multiple sclerosis: a case with a favorable long-term outcome. Mult Scler 14:278–283

Koehne G, Zeller W, Stockschlaeder M, Zander AR (1997) Phenotype of lymphocyte subsets after autologous peripheral blood stem cell transplantation. Bone Marrow Transplant 19:149–156

Krasulova E, Trneny M, Kozak T, Vackova B, Pohlreich D et al (2010) High-dose immunoablation with autologous haematopoietic stem cell transplantation in aggressive multiple sclerosis: a single centre 10-year experience. Mult Scler 16:685–693

Krumbholz M, Meinl I, Kumpfel T, Hohlfeld R, Meinl E (2008) Natalizumab disproportionately increases circulating pre-B and B cells in multiple sclerosis. Neurology 71:1350–1354

Lapidot T, Petit I (2002) Current understanding of stem cell mobilization: the roles of chemokines, proteolytic enzymes, adhesion molecules, cytokines, and stromal cells. Exp Hematol 30:973–81

Lapidot T, Dar A, Kollet O (2005) How do stem cells find their way home? Blood 106:1901–1910

Larochelle A, Savona M, Wiggins M, Anderson S, Ichwan B et al (2011) Human and rhesus macaque hematopoietic stem cells cannot be purified based only on SLAM family markers. Blood 117:1550–1554

Li HW, Sykes M (2012) Emerging concepts in haematopoietic cell transplantation. Nat Rev Immunol 12:403–416

Loh Y, Oyama Y, Statkute L, Quigley K, Yaung K et al (2007) Development of a secondary autoimmune disorder after hematopoietic stem cell transplantation for autoimmune diseases: role of conditioning regimen used. Blood 109:2643–2548

Lu JQ, Storek J, Metz L, Yong VW, Stevens AM et al (2009) Continued disease activity in a patient with multiple sclerosis after allogeneic hematopoietic cell transplantation. Arch Neurol 66:116–120

Lu JQ, Joseph JT, Nash RA, Storek J, Stevens AM et al (2010) Neuroinflammation and demyelination in multiple sclerosis after allogeneic hematopoietic stem cell transplantation. Arch Neurol 67:716–722

Mallet VO, Mitchell C, Mezey E, Fabre M, Guidotti JE et al (2002) Bone marrow transplantation in mice leads to a minor population of hepatocytes that can be selectively amplified in vivo. Hepatology 35:799–804

Mancardi GL, Saccardi R, Filippi M, Gualandi F, Murialdo A et al (2001) Autologous hematopoietic stem cell transplantation suppresses Gd-enhanced MRI activity in MS. Neurology 57:62–68

Mancardi GL, Sormani MP, Di Gioia M, Vuolo L, Gualandi F et al (2012) Autologous haematopoietic stem cell transplantation with an intermediate intensity conditioning regimen in multiple sclerosis: the Italian multi-centre experience. Mult Scler 18:835–842

Marmont AM (1994) Immune ablation followed by allogeneic or autologous bone marrow transplantation: a new treatment for severe autoimmune diseases? Stem Cells 12:125–135

Marmont AM (2004) Stem cell transplantation for autoimmune disorders. Coincidental autoimmune disease in patients transplanted for conventional indications. Best Pract Res Clin Haematol 17:223–232

Mattoscio M, Nicholas R, Malik O, Dazzi F, Lee J, Waldman A et al (2012) Differential increase of circulating haematopoietic stem cells (HSC) following therapeutic alpha 4-integrin blockade in multiple sclerosis: correlation between HSC mobilization status and response to treatment (IN8-1.006). Neurology. April 22, 78(Meeting Abstracts 1):IN8-1.006

Mattoscio M, Nicholas R, Malik O, Muraro P (2013) Circulating Hematopoietic Stem Cell Numbers during Natalizumab Treatment in Patients with Multiple Sclerosis: Association with Clinical and MRI Variables (P05.194). Neurology. February 14, 2013;80(Meeting Abstracts 1):P05.194

Metz I, Lucchinetti CF, Openshaw H, Garcia-Merino A, Lassmann H et al (2007) Autologous haematopoietic stem cell transplantation fails to stop demyelination and neurodegeneration in multiple sclerosis. Brain 130:1254–1262

Mezey E, Chandross KJ (2000) Bone marrow: a possible alternative source of cells in the adult nervous system. Eur J Pharmacol 405:297–302

Mezey E, Chandross KJ, Harta G, Maki RA, McKercher SR (2000) Turning blood into brain: cells bearing neuronal antigens generated in vivo from bone marrow. Science 290:1779–1782

Mezey E, Key S, Vogelsang G, Szalayova I, Lange GD, Crain B (2003) Transplanted bone marrow generates new neurons in human brains. Proc Natl Acad Sci U S A 100:1364–1369

Mondria T, Lamers CH, te Boekhorst PA, Gratama JW, Hintzen RQ (2008) Bone-marrow transplantation fails to halt intrathecal lymphocyte activation in multiple sclerosis. J Neurol Neurosurg Psychiatry 79:1013–1015

Muraro PA, Bielekova B (2007) Emerging therapies for multiple sclerosis. Neurother 4:676–692

Muraro PA, Leist T, Bielekova B, McFarland HF (2000) VLA-4/CD49d downregulated on primed T lymphocytes during interferon-b therapy in multiple sclerosis. J Neuroimmunol 111:186–194

Muraro PA, Liberati L, Bonanni L, Pantalone A, Caporale CM et al (2004) Decreased integrin gene expression in patients with MS responding to interferon-beta treatment. J Neuroimmunol 150:123–131

Muraro PA, Douek DC, Packer A, Chung K, Guenaga FJ et al (2005) Thymic output generates a new and diverse TCR repertoire after autologous stem cell transplantation in multiple sclerosis patients. J Exp Med 201:805–816

Murray L, Chen B, Galy A, Chen S, Tushinski R et al (1995) Enrichment of human hematopoietic stem cell activity in the CD34+ Thy-1+Lin- subpopulation from mobilized peripheral blood. Blood 85:368–378

Nash RA, Bowen JD, McSweeney PA, Pavletic SZ, Maravilla KR et al (2003) High-dose immunosuppressive therapy and autologous peripheral blood stem cell transplantation for severe multiple sclerosis. Blood 102:2364–2372

Nash R, Hutton GJ, Racke M, Popat U, Devine SM, Georges G, Griffith L, Muraro PA et al (2013) Treatment of severe relapsing-remitting multiple sclerosis with high-dose immunosuppressive therapy and autologous hematopoietic cell transplantation: 2-year follow-up results of the HALT MS clinical trial (Immune Tolerance Network: ITN033AI). BMT Tandem Meetings, 13 Feb 2013–17 Feb 2013. Biol Blood Marrow Transplant 19(2):S 129

Ni XS, Ouyang J, Zhu WH, Wang C, Chen B (2006) Autologous hematopoietic stem cell transplantation for progressive multiple sclerosis: report of efficacy and safety at three yr of follow up in 21 patients. Clin Transplant 20:485–489

O'Gorman WE, Dooms H, Thorne SH, Kuswanto WF, Simonds EF et al (2009) The initial phase of an immune response functions to activate regulatory T cells. J Immunol 183:332–339

Osawa M, Hanada K, Hamada H, Nakauchi H (1996) Long-term lymphohematopoietic reconstitution by a single CD34-low/negative hematopoietic stem cell. Science 273:242–245

Papayannopoulou T, Nakamoto B (1993) Peripheralization of hemopoietic progenitors in primates treated with anti-VLA4 integrin. Proc Natl Acad Sci U S A 90:9374–9378

Papayannopoulou T, Priestley GV, Nakamoto B, Zafiropoulos V, Scott LM (2001) Molecular pathways in bone marrow homing: dominant role of alpha(4)beta(1) over beta(2)-integrins and selectins. Blood 98:2403–2411

Pike BL, Robinson WA (1970) Human bone marrow colony growth in agar-gel. J Cell Physiol 76:77–84

Polman CH, O'Connor PW, Havrdova E, Hutchinson M, Kappos L et al (2006) A randomized, placebo-controlled trial of natalizumab for relapsing multiple sclerosis. N Engl J Med 354:899–910

Radbruch A, Muehlinghaus G, Luger EO, Inamine A, Smith KG et al (2006) Competence and competition: the challenge of becoming a long-lived plasma cell. Nat Rev Immunol 6:741–750

Randall TD, Weissman IL (1997) Phenotypic and functional changes induced at the clonal level in hematopoietic stem cells after 5-fluorouracil treatment. Blood 89:3596–3606

Rose DM, Alon R, Ginsberg MH (2007) Integrin modulation and signaling in leukocyte adhesion and migration. Immunol Rev 218:126–134

Rutella S, Rumi C, Laurenti L, Pierelli L, Sora F et al (2000) Immune reconstitution after transplantation of autologous peripheral CD34+ cells: analysis of predictive factors and comparison with unselected progenitor transplants. Br J Haematol 108:105–115

Saccardi R, Mancardi GL, Solari A, Bosi A, Bruzzi P et al (2005) Autologous HSCT for severe progressive multiple sclerosis in a multicenter trial: impact on disease activity and quality of life. Blood 105:2601–2607

Saccardi R, Kozak T, Bocelli-Tyndall C, Fassas A, Kazis A, Havrdova E, Carreras E, Saiz A, Löwenberg B, te Boekhorst PA, Gualandio F, Openshaw H, Longo G, Pagliai F, Massacesi L, Deconink E, Ouyang J, Nagore FJ, Besalduch J, Lisukov IA, Bonini A, Merelli E, Slavino S, Gratwohl A, Passweg J, Tyndall A, Steck AJ, Andolina M, Capobianco M, Martin JL, Lugaresi A, Meucci G, Sáez RA, Clark RE, Fernandez MN, Fouillard L, Herstenstein B, Koza V, Cocco E, Baurmann H, Mancardi GL, Autoimmune Diseases Working Party of EBMT (2006) Autologous stem cell transplantation for progressive multiple sclerosis: update of the European Group for Blood and Marrow Transplantation autoimmune diseases working party database. Mult Scler 12(6):814–823

Saccardi R, Freedman M, Sormani M, Atkins H, Farge D et al (2012) A prospective, randomized, controlled trial of autologous haematopoietic stem cell transplantation for aggressive multiple sclerosis: a position paper. Mult Scler 18:825–834

Saiz A, Carreras E, Berenguer J, Yague J, Martinez C et al (2001) MRI and CSF oligoclonal bands after autologous hematopoietic stem cell transplantation in MS. Neurology 56:1084–1089

Saiz A, Blanco Y, Berenguer J, Gomez-Choco M, Carreras E et al (2008) Clinical outcome 6 years after autologous hematopoietic stem cell transplantation in multiple sclerosis. Neurologia 23:405–407

Samijn JP, te Boekhorst PA, Mondria T, van Doorn PA, Flach HZ et al (2006) Intense T cell depletion followed by autologous bone marrow transplantation for severe multiple sclerosis. J Neurol Neurosurg Psychiatry 77:46–50

Sangalli F, Moiola L, Bucello S, Annovazzi P, Rizzo A et al (2011) Efficacy and tolerability of natalizumab in relapsing-remitting multiple sclerosis patients: a post-marketing observational study. Neurol Sci 31(Suppl 3):299–302

Saure C, Warnke C, Zohren F, Schroeder T, Bruns I et al (2011) Natalizumab and impedance of the homing of CD34+ hematopoietic progenitors. Arch Neurol 68:1428–1431

Schofield R (1978) The relationship between the spleen colony-forming cell and the haemopoietic stem cell. Blood Cells 4:7–25

Shevchenko YL, Novik AA, Kuznetsov AN, Afanasiev BV, Lisukov IA et al (2008) High-dose immunosuppressive therapy with autologous hematopoietic stem cell transplantation as a treatment option in multiple sclerosis. Exp Hematol 36:922–928

Shevchenko JL, Kuznetsov AN, Ionova TI, Melnichenko VY, Fedorenko DA et al (2012) Autologous haematopoietic stem cell transplantation with reduced intensity conditioning in multiple sclerosis. Exp Hematol 40(11):892–898

Sigurjonsson OE, Perreault MC, Egeland T, Glover JC (2005) Adult human hematopoietic stem cells produce neurons efficiently in the regenerating chicken embryo spinal cord. Proc Natl Acad Sci U S A 102:5227–5232

Sitnicka E, Buza-Vidas N, Larsson S, Nygren JM, Liuba K, Jacobsen SE (2003) Human CD34+ hematopoietic stem cells capable of multilineage engrafting NOD/SCID mice express flt3: distinct flt3 and c-kit expression and response patterns on mouse and candidate human hematopoietic stem cells. Blood 102:881–886

Snowden JA, Saccardi R, Allez M, Ardizzone S, Arnold R et al (2012) Haematopoietic SCT in severe autoimmune diseases: updated guidelines of the European Group for Blood and Marrow Transplantation. Bone Marrow Transplant 47:770–790

Storek J, Zhao Z, Liu Y, Nash R, McSweeney P, Maloney DG (2008) Early recovery of CD4T cell receptor diversity after "lymphoablative" conditioning and autologous CD34 cell transplantation. Biol Blood Marrow Transplant 14:1373–1379

Stuve O (2008) The effects of natalizumab on the innate and adaptive immune system in the central nervous system. J Neurol Sci 274:39–41

Stuve O, Cravens PD, Frohman EM, Phillips JT, Remington GM et al (2009) Immunologic, clinical, and radiologic status 14 months after cessation of natalizumab therapy. Neurology 72:396–401

Su L, Xu J, Ji BX, Wan SG, Lu CY et al (2006) Autologous peripheral blood stem cell transplantation for severe multiple sclerosis. Int J Hematol 84:276–281

Sun W, Popat U, Hutton G, Zang YC, Krance R et al (2004) Characteristics of T-cell receptor repertoire and myelin-reactive T cells reconstituted from autologous haematopoietic stem-cell grafts in multiple sclerosis. Brain 127:996–1008

Sutherland HJ, Eaves CJ, Eaves AC, Dragowska W, Lansdorp PM (1989) Characterization and partial purification of human marrow cells capable of initiating long-term hematopoiesis in vitro. Blood 74:1563–1570

Till JE, Mc CE (1961) A direct measurement of the radiation sensitivity of normal mouse bone marrow cells. Radiat Res 14:213–222

Uss E, Rowshani AT, Hooibrink B, Lardy NM, van Lier RA, ten Berge IJ (2006) CD103 is a marker for alloantigen-induced regulatory CD8+ T cells. J Immunol 177:2775–2783

van Gelder M, van Bekkum DW (1996) Effective treatment of relapsing experimental autoimmune encephalomyelitis with pseudoautologous bone marrow transplantation. Bone Marrow Transplant 18:1029–1034

van Gelder M, Kinwel-Bohre EP, van Bekkum DW(1993) Treatment of experimental allergic encephalomyelitis in rats with total body irradiation and syngeneic BMT. Bone Marrow Transplant 11:233–241

Van Wijmeersch B, Sprangers B, Rutgeerts O, Lenaerts C, Landuyt W et al (2007) Allogeneic bone marrow transplantation in models of experimental autoimmune encephalomyelitis: evidence for a graft-versus-autoimmunity effect. Biol Blood Marrow Transplant 13:627–637

Venken K, Hellings N, Thewissen M, Somers V, Hensen K et al (2008) Compromised CD4+ CD25(high) regulatory T-cell function in patients with relapsing-remitting multiple sclerosis is correlated with a reduced frequency of FOXP3-positive cells and reduced FOXP3 expression at the single-cell level. Immunology 123:79–89

Viglietta V, Baecher-Allan C, Weiner HL, Hafler DA (2004) Loss of functional suppression by CD4+ CD25+ regulatory T cells in patients with multiple sclerosis. J Exp Med 199:971–979

Warnke C, Smolianov V, Dehmel T, Andree M, Hengel H et al (2011) CD34+ progenitor cells mobilized by natalizumab are not a relevant reservoir for JC virus. Mult Scler 17:151–156

Weissman IL (2000) Stem cells: units of development, units of regeneration, and units in evolution. Cell 100:157–168

Wilson A, Trumpp A (2006) Bone-marrow haematopoietic-stem-cell niches. Nat Rev Immunol 6:93–106

Wilson A, Oser GM, Jaworski M, Blanco-Bose WE, Laurenti E et al (2007) Dormant and self-renewing hematopoietic stem cells and their niches. Ann N Y Acad Sci 1106:64–75

Wilson A, Laurenti E, Oser G, van der Wath RC, Blanco-Bose W et al (2008) Hematopoietic stem cells reversibly switch from dormancy to self-renewal during homeostasis and repair. Cell 135:1118–1129

Wilson A, Laurenti E, Trumpp A (2009) Balancing dormant and self-renewing hematopoietic stem cells. Curr Opin Genet Dev 19:461–468

Winstead CJ, Fraser JM, Khoruts A (2008) Regulatory CD4+CD25+Foxp3+ T cells selectively inhibit the spontaneous form of lymphopenia-induced proliferation of naive T cells. J Immunol 180:7305–7317

Winstead CJ, Reilly CS, Moon JJ, Jenkins MK, Hamilton SE et al (2010) CD4+CD25+Foxp3+ regulatory T cells optimize diversity of the conventional T cell repertoire during reconstitution from lymphopenia. J Immunol 184:4749–4760

Zand MS, Vo T, Huggins J, Felgar R, Liesveld J et al (2005) Polyclonal rabbit antithymocyte globulin triggers B-cell and plasma cell apoptosis by multiple pathways. Transplantation 79:1507–1515

Zhang H, Chua KS, Guimond M, Kapoor V, Brown MV et al (2005) Lymphopenia and interleukin-2 therapy alter homeostasis of CD4+CD25+ regulatory T cells. Nat Med 11:1238–1243

Zhang J, Niu C, Ye L, Huang H, He X et al (2003) Identification of the haematopoietic stem cell niche and control of the niche size. Nature 425:836–841

Zhang L, Bertucci AM, Ramsey-Goldman R, Burt RK, Datta SK (2009) Regulatory T cell (Treg) subsets return in patients with refractory lupus following stem cell transplantation, and TGF-beta-producing CD8+ Treg cells are associated with immunological remission of lupus. J Immunol 183:6346–6358

Zohren F, Toutzaris D, Klarner V, Hartung HP, Kieseier B, Haas R (2008) The monoclonal anti-VLA-4 antibody natalizumab mobilizes CD34+ hematopoietic progenitor cells in humans. Blood 111:3893–3895

Chapter 20
Mesenchymal Stem Cells for the Treatment of Multiple Sclerosis

Laura Lovato, Nicole Kerlero de Rosbo and Antonio Uccelli

Although currently approved therapies, mostly directed towards downregulating inflammation, can help patients with multiple sclerosis (MS), in particular those with the relapsing–remitting form of MS, they are unsatisfactory for a significant number of patients. Indeed, patients with aggressive disease do not always respond to these therapies; patients can be faced with tolerability issues, and/or be at risk of serious adverse events. Most importantly, at present there is no therapy that can trigger repair of the irreversible neuronal damage, a hallmark of the disease, which leads to a progressive accumulation of disability in most affected subjects and is observed clinically in the secondary progressive phase of the disease. Similarly, no treatment has yet been approved for the primary progressive variant of the disease. The unmet need for a therapy that could reverse permanent disability and lead to recovery of neurological functions has boosted the search by the scientific community for an innovative treatment of MS that is safe and well tolerated, potentially able to control the inflammatory activity leading to neurodegeneration and, more importantly, to promote repair of the damaged central nervous system (CNS).

So far, the development of such treatments has been hampered by the impracticality of in vivo regeneration of neural cells and the inability to reestablish the complex neural network supporting neurological functions. Although these challenges might be met with therapies that promote remyelination, no agents are available with proven remyelinating action. In addition, remyelination by itself would be insufficient unless it could be accompanied by restored order in the damaged neural networks through either cell replacement or fostering of endogenous neurogenesis (Franklin and Ffrench-Constant 2008).

A. Uccelli (✉) · L. Lovato · N. Kerlero de Rosbo
Department of Neurology, Rehabilitation, Ophthalmology, Genetics,
Maternal and Child Health (DINOGMI), University of Genoa, Largo Paolo Daneo 3,
16132 Genoa, Italy
e-mail: auccelli@neurologia.unige.it

A. Uccelli
Center of Excellence for Biomedical Research, University of Genoa, Italy

Advanced Biotechnology Center, Genoa, Italy

T. Yamamura, B. Gran (eds.), *Multiple Sclerosis Immunology*,
DOI 10.1007/978-1-4614-7953-6_20, © Springer Science+Business Media New York 2013

At present, stem cells represent the most promising approach to try and achieve such tissue repair because of their therapeutic plasticity. Accordingly, they have recently entered the scenario of MS therapies based on a robust amount of preclinical data suggesting that they could be of clinical value through immunomodulation, trophic actions, and neuroprotection.

Though different types of stem cells have been considered (see further), this chapter will focus on the rationale for, and state of the art of, the clinical use of bone marrow-derived mesenchymal stem cells (MSC) in MS treatment.

20.1 Types of Stem Cells Considered for Therapy in MS

20.1.1 Embryonic Stem Cells

Studies of embryonic stem cells, which, in contrast to stem cells isolated from adult or even fetal tissues, retain the ability to differentiate into cell types of all lineages (multipotentiality), have been carried out in animal models of neurological diseases including MS (Aharonowiz et al. 2008; Ben-Hur et al. 2004; Joannides and Chandran 2008). However, such studies and their translation into clinical practice are greatly impeded by ethical issues and national legislation limits (Abbott 2011).

20.1.2 Neural Precursor Cells (NPC)

Although not endowed with the multipotentiality of embryonic stem cells, NPC still have outstanding therapeutic plasticity because of their ability to survive as undifferentiated cells in ectopic perivascular niches in the inflamed CNS. These cells release factors that foster survival and proliferation of nearby neural (progenitor) cells, and they interact with CNS-infiltrating immune cells and the local microenvironment. Intravenous or intrathecal infusion of NPC showed therapeutic effect in several animal models of neurological disorders (Abematsu et al. 2010; Bacigaluppi et al. 2009; Pluchino et al. 2003), including experimental autoimmune encephalomyelitis (EAE), the model for MS. However, as NPC are isolated from fetal brain tissue, clinical translation of these promising results faces great difficulties related to obtaining fetal neural tissues as well as technical problems in expanding to large-scale yields under good manufacturing practice conditions and injecting cells into non-MHC-compatible hosts, which might require preconditioning and maintenance with immunosuppressive agents (Pluchino et al. 2009).

20.1.3 Induced Pluripotent Stem Cells (iPSC)

The demonstration that pluripotent stem cells could be derived from human somatic cells has raised the hope that these induced pluripotent stem cells (iPSC) could achieve extensive tissue repair, while circumventing the problems related to the use of stem cells derived from embryonic and fetal tissue (Cundiff and Anderson 2011). The iPSC can differentiate into glial and neuronal cells (Czepiel et al. 2011; Lebonvallet et al. 2012), and disease-relevant cell types and disease-specific iPSC have been generated from patients with neurological diseases (Saporta et al. 2011), including MS (Song et al. 2012). However, this technology is still in its infancy, and safety, either in the short or long term, has yet to be established. Consequently, the use of several other types of adult stem cells has been explored.

20.1.4 Hematopoietic Stem Cells (HSC)

Adult stem cells of hemopoietic origin, mostly isolated from cord blood or adult bone marrow, have been used in MS (Mancardi and Saccardi 2008), mainly with the aim of reconstituting and possibly resetting a functional immune system after intense immunosuppression (Muraro et al. 2005). The state of the art and possible therapeutic translation of these cells in MS is discussed in another chapter.

20.1.5 Mesenchymal Stem Cells (MSC)

Together with NPC, MSC have been tested most consistently in animal models of neurological disease, including MS (Uccelli et al. 2011). MSC are a heterogeneous subset of stromal progenitors of mesodermal cells that have been isolated from almost every connective tissue, but characterized mainly upon isolation from bone marrow and adipose tissue. MSC can provide therapeutic effects similar to NPC, irrespective of the tissue from which they are isolated. MSC appear to have properties that allow them to escape immune rejection and have been successfully used in xenogeneic settings (human MSC in mice; Gordon et al. 2008) and, more importantly, allogeneically in human disorders (Le Blanc et al. 2008). It should be noted, however, that some studies have shown the possibility that MSC might be rejected by the host immune system (Eliopoulos et al. 2005); nevertheless, the added possibility that in an allogeneic environment MSC exert their effect acutely before rejection is of utmost relevance in a therapeutic approach with adult stem cells.

20.2 General Features of Bone Marrow-Derived MSC

MSC can be isolated from several tissues, but those derived from the bone marrow are the most characterized for their physiological and potentially therapeutic features. MSC, first isolated in the stromal compartment of bone marrow and described as colony-forming-unit fibroblasts by Friedenstein and colleagues in the

1960s (Friedenstein et al. 1974, 1968), constitute an essential component of the hematopoietic stem cell niche (Mendez-Ferrer et al. 2010).

20.2.1 Plasticity

MSC have self-renewal capability (Caplan 1991; Mendez-Ferrer et al. 2010) and proliferate in vitro as plastic-adherent cells of fibroblast-like morphology that form colonies and support hematopoiesis (Muguruma et al. 2006; Uccelli et al. 2008). Being the common predecessors of mesenchymal tissues, MSC can differentiate into adipocytes, chondrocytes, and osteocytes, even after transfer in vivo (Friedenstein et al. 1974, 1968). They also have endodermic and neuroectodermic differentiation potential, but such transdifferentiation into cells from unrelated germline lineages is controversial in vivo (Kopen et al. 1999; Pittenger et al. 1999).

20.2.2 Phenotype

Although they have no known specific markers, MSC that are cultured in vitro are phenotypically identified by the expression of variable levels of stromal markers, including CD105, CD73, CD44, CD90, CD71, the ganglioside GD2, and CD271, together with the lack of hematopoietic markers such as CD45, CD34, and CD14, or the costimulatory molecules CD80, CD86, and CD40 (Chamberlain et al. 2007; Horwitz et al. 2005).

20.2.3 Role in Homeostasis of HSC in Bone Marrow

In culture, MSC produce a number of cytokines and extracellular matrix proteins and express cell adhesion molecules, all of which are involved in the regulation of hematopoiesis (Conget and Minguell 1999; Majumdar et al. 1998; Mendez-Ferrer et al. 2010; Muguruma et al. 2006). In vivo, MSC are spatially associated with HSC and adrenergic nerve fibers. In these structurally unique niches made of MSC–HSC pairings, MSC play a crucial role in the regulation of the hematopoietic lineage, while local input from the surrounding microenvironment and long-distance cues from hormones and the autonomic nervous system can modulate MSC proliferation and differentiation, as well as HSC maintenance (Mendez-Ferrer et al. 2010). MSC highly express HSC maintenance genes and other genes triggering osteoblastic differentiation, which are selectively downregulated during enforced HSC mobilization or sympathetic nervous system activation (Mendez-Ferrer et al. 2010). Moreover, depletion of MSC from the bone marrow rapidly reduces the HSC content in the bone marrow. Thus, MSC provide a sheltering environment that supports the maintenance and self-renewal of HSC by shielding them from differentiation and apoptotic stimuli that would otherwise challenge stem cell reserves. Indeed, bone marrow stromal cells are responsible for the maintenance of HSC in the G0 phase of the cell cycle in the endosteal niche, and for the control of HSC proliferation, differentiation, and recruitment in the vascular niche (Kiel and Morrison 2008).

20.3 Mechanisms of Action of MSC

In addition to their physiological role in the bone marrow, MSC can exert a variety of actions that represent the rational basis for their clinical use in MS. MSC can interact with cells of both the innate and adaptive immune systems, leading to the modulation of several effector functions (immunomodulatory effect); MSC can release antiapoptotic and neurotrophic molecules that provide a neuroprotective effect in the presence of neuronal damage (neuroprotective effect); and, despite little or no engraftment in the CNS, MSC can apparently mediate CNS tissue repair to some extent (regenerative effect). All these actions contribute to define the so-called "therapeutic plasticity" of MSC.

20.3.1 Immunomodulation

The immunomodulatory effect of MSC has been described in the last decade, following the observation that bone marrow-derived MSC suppressed T cell proliferation (Bartholomew et al. 2002; Di Nicola et al. 2002). These studies paved the way for the characterization of the broad immunoregulatory activities of MSC, demonstrating that they are able to modulate several effector functions of T and B cells, dendritic cells (DC), and cells of the innate immune system, which have a role in pathogenesis of autoimmune diseases (Uccelli et al. 2008). In vitro studies have shown that soluble factors are involved in MSC-mediated immunomodulation, either produced constitutively by MSC or released upon cross-talk with target cells.

T cells Autologous and allogeneic MSC can inhibit the mitogenic, allogeneic, or antigen-specific proliferation of both $CD4^+$ and $CD8^+$ T cells (Aggarwal and Pittenger 2005; Benvenuto et al. 2007; Chabannes et al. 2007; Di Nicola et al. 2002; Glennie et al. 2005; Krampera et al. 2003; Meisel et al. 2004; Sato et al. 2007; Tse et al. 2003; Zappia et al. 2005) by supporting their survival in a quiescent state, an effect dependent on the arrest of T cells in the G0/G1 phase of the cell cycle (Benvenuto et al. 2007; Glennie et al. 2005) and which can be partially reversed by IL-2 stimulation (Zappia et al. 2005). Inhibition of T cell proliferation by MSC apparently leads to a shift in T cells from a proinflammatory to an anti-inflammatory state with decreased IFNγ production and increased IL-4 production (Aggarwal and Pittenger 2005; Zappia et al. 2005). Transwell experiments, in which cell–cell contact between MSC and effector cells is prevented, result in a significant inhibition of

T cell proliferation, suggesting the involvement of soluble factors; in this context, transforming growth factor β1 and hepatocyte growth factor (HGF) have been identified as mediators of T cell suppression by MSC (Di Nicola et al. 2002). Among other such molecules, the nonclassic human leukocyte antigen class I molecule HLA-G (Selmani et al. 2008) was also shown to be involved in MSC-mediated suppression of effector T cells. The study showed that MSC secrete the soluble isoform HLA-G5 through an IL-10-dependent mechanism and that cell–cell contact was required for full HLA-G5 secretion and, thereby, full modulation by MSC (Selmani et al. 2008). The production of indoleamine 2,3-dioxygenase (IDO), which is required to inhibit the proliferation of IFNγ-producing Th1 cells, is only released by MSC after triggering by IFNγ produced by the T cells (Krampera et al. 2006).

Regulatory T cells MSC exert both indirect and direct effect on regulatory T cells, a specialized subpopulation of T cells that help to maintain homeostasis and tolerance to self-antigens. MSC induce the production of IL-10 by plasmacytoid DC, which, themselves, trigger the generation of regulatory T cells (Aggarwal and Pittenger 2005; Maccario et al. 2005). MSC can also directly induce the proliferation of regulatory T cells, while suppressing effector T cells, through release of HLA-G5, upon coculture with antigen-specific T cells (Selmani et al. 2008).

Although these findings indicate that MSC can modulate the intensity of an immune response by inhibiting antigen-specific T cell proliferation and cytotoxicity and promoting the generation of regulatory T cells, such activity, which is obviously of great value in treatment of autoimmune inflammatory diseases such as MS, could become deleterious. Indeed, from a clinical perspective, excessive inhibition of T cell responses by MSC would render the host vulnerable to infectious agents. However, fail-safe mechanisms might exist, in particular through the expression by MSC of functional Toll-like receptors (TLR) that, upon interaction with pathogen-associated ligands, induce the proliferation, differentiation, and migration of MSC and their secretion of chemokines and cytokines (Pevsner-Fischer et al. 2007; Tomchuck et al. 2008); in addition, after triggering of TLR3 and TLR4, MSC lose their T cell modulatory activity through impairment of signaling to Notch receptors in T cells (Liotta et al. 2008). Thus, pathogen-associated molecules might reverse the suppressive effects of MSC on T cells, thereby restoring efficient T cell responses in the course of infections; it is also possible that tissue stromal cells can instruct local immune responses after pathogen infections (Svensson and Kaye 2006).

B cells The general consensus is that MSC inhibit B cell proliferation in vitro (Augello et al. 2005; Corcione et al. 2006; Glennie et al. 2005). These effects seem to depend on the release of soluble factors (Augello et al. 2005; Corcione et al. 2006) and on cell–cell contact, possibly mediated by interactions between programmed cell death 1 (PD1) and its ligands (Augello et al. 2005). MSC can also inhibit B cell differentiation and the constitutive expression of chemokine receptors (Corcione et al. 2006). However, possibly as a result of differences in the experimental conditions used, other in vitro studies have shown that MSC could support the survival, proliferation, and differentiation to antibody-secreting cells of B cells isolated from normal individuals or from pediatric patients with systemic lupus erythematosus (Rasmusson et al. 2007; Traggiai et al. 2008). Regardless of the controversial in vitro effects, it should be emphasized that, as B cell responses are mainly T cell-dependent, the final outcome of the interaction between MSC and B cells in vivo might be significantly influenced by MSC-mediated inhibition of T cell functions.

Dendritic cells MSC have been shown in vitro to have different actions on DC that could lead to downregulation of the inflammatory process by precluding efficient antigen presentation and thereby expansion of effector T cells. Thus, MSC could inhibit DC maturation via soluble factors (Djouad et al. 2007; Jiang et al. 2005; Nauta et al. 2006), affect the antigen-presenting function of mature DC by decreasing their cell-surface expression of MHC class II molecules, CD11c, CD83, and costimulatory molecules (Chiesa et al. 2011; Djouad et al. 2007; Nauta et al. 2006; Zhou et al. 2009), as well as their production of IL-12 (Chiesa et al. 2011; Nauta et al. 2006), and decrease the proinflammatory potential of mature DC by inhibiting their production of tumor necrosis factor and increasing their production of IL-10 (Aggarwal and Pittenger 2005). The in vivo effect of MSC on DC functions has been elegantly demonstrated following their intravenous administration in mice. In this experimental condition, MSC led to inhibition of T cell priming associated with a rapid arrest of DC migration into lymph nodes (Chiesa et al. 2011).

Innate immune cells MSC can also affect cells of the innate immune system, such as natural killer (NK) cells and neutrophils. In vitro, MSC inhibit the cytotoxic activity of resting NK cells by downregulating expression of activating receptors that are involved in NK cell activation and target cell killing (Spaggiari et al. 2006), and by abrogating their proliferation and IFNγ production induced by IL-2 or IL-15 (Spaggiari et al. 2008, 2006). Similar to resting NK cells, preactivated NK cells had decreased proliferation, IFNγ production, and cytotoxicity after in vitro culture with MSC (Aggarwal and Pittenger 2005; Poggi et al. 2005; Selmani et al. 2008; Spaggiari et al. 2008, 2006). However, the significance of these in vitro observations in relation to MSC treatment in MS is unclear. Indeed, animal models of MS have provided evidence for both disease-accelerating and disease-protective effects of NK cells, and NK cells were shown to be less frequent in MS patients and to expand during effective immunotherapy (reviewed in Lunemann and Munz 2008). Although these observations suggest that these innate lymphocytes exert beneficial functions, the mechanisms that could mediate such immunoregulatory NK cell functions in MS are, however, poorly understood. It should be noted that cytokine-activated NK cells can themselves kill both autologous and allogeneic MSC in vitro (Poggi et al. 2005; Spaggiari et al. 2008, 2006) and that MSC are partially protected from NK cell-mediated cytotoxicity upon exposure to IFNγ (Spaggiari et al. 2006). Thus, in a microenvironment rich in IFNγ, such as would occur in vivo in inflamed CNS, NK cell function could be inhibited by MSC, whereas in the absence of IFNγ, the balance would be tilted towards the elimination of MSC by activated NK cells.

Due to their indiscriminate histotoxic potential, neutrophil activation is tightly regulated through a complex mechanism called "priming" that precedes full activation. There is evidence of neutrophil priming in inflammatory autoimmune disease, such as rheumatoid arthritis (Wright et al. 2010), and, while the role of neutrophils has not been examined extensively in MS, a recent study indicated that neutrophils from MS patients are increased in number and show a priming signature, including reduced apoptosis, and enhanced degranulation and oxidative burst (Naegele et al. 2012). In this context, MSC were shown to dampen the respiratory burst and to delay the spontaneous apoptosis of resting and activated neutrophils in vitro through an IL-6 dependent mechanism (Raffaghello et al. 2008). MSC-mediated preservation of resting neutrophils might be important in those anatomical sites where large numbers of mature and functional neutrophils are stored, such as the bone marrow and lungs.

It should be noted that in vitro inhibition of any one of the MSC-derived soluble immunosuppressive factors does not fully abrogate the immunomodulatory activity of MSC, and their relative contribution to the immunosuppressive effects varies between different studies. Therefore, it is clear that MSC-mediated immunoregulation is a redundant system that involves several molecules.

20.3.2 Neuroprotection

Downregulation of the inflammatory process by MSC can halt or at least delay immune damage to the CNS, thereby resulting in sparing of axons (Gerdoni et al. 2007; Kassis et al. 2008; Zhang et al. 2006). MSC could also exert a potent neuroprotective effect in neurological diseases such as MS through different mechanisms, such as paracrine release of neuroprotective molecules, without the need for cell–cell contact with the target cells. Thus, MSC secrete brain-derived neurotrophic factor and nerve growth factor (β-NGF), which promote neuronal survival in vitro (Crigler et al. 2006; Wilkins et al. 2009). MSC also promote neurite outgrowth within dorsal root ganglion explants despite secreting a much lower level of β-NGF required exogenously to produce a similar effect (Crigler et al. 2006). Several groups have demonstrated in vitro that MSC can rescue neurons from apoptosis (Scuteri et al. 2006; Wilkins et al. 2009), and coculture of dorsal root ganglia sensory neurons with MSC led to long-lasting survival and maturation of the neurons instead of commitment to die (Scuteri et al. 2006). In this latter study, cellular contact was seen to be mandatory for the supporting function of MSC on neuronal survival and maturation, and the long-lasting survival promoting effect observed during the coculture of MSC was exclusively due to the direct interaction of MSC with neurons, and not due to the differentiation of MSC or to the release of neurotrophic factors (Scuteri et al. 2006).

A recent study has shown that i.v. administration of MSC does not lead to a consistent CNS engraftment, but is sufficient to protect hippocampal neurons from kainic acid glutamate-mediated excitotoxicity in a mouse model of temporal lobe epilepsy (Voulgari-Kokota et al. 2012). This effect relies on the ability of MSC to secrete molecules that can protect mouse cortical neurons from N-Methyl-D-Aspartate (NMDA)-induced increase of calcium influx and subsequent excitotoxicity. These results are in line with the ability of MSC to inhibit glutamatergic excitotoxicity in the spinal cord of SOD1/G93A mice, a transgenic mouse model of amyotrophic lateral sclerosis, upon i.v. administration, resulting in a significant increase in animal survival (Uccelli et al. 2012).

In vivo, the neuroprotective effect of MSC may occur through an action on local neural cells, as supported by in vitro experiments addressing the interaction between MSC and microglia, where MSC were seen to increase expression and release of neuroprotective molecules by microglia, in particular fractalkine receptor CX3CR1, nuclear receptor 4 family NURR1, CD200 receptor, and insulin growth factor 1 (Giunti et al. 2012). The effects on CX3CR1-expressing microglia were shown to be due to the release of the CX3CR1 ligand, CX3CL1 (fractalkine), by MSC, and exogenous CX3CL1 induced phenotypic and functional changes in microglia similar to those induced by the MSC themselves (Giunti et al. 2012). MSC can also have a direct neuroprotective effect on neurons, as shown by their protective effect from oxidative stress damage on neuroblastoma cells; the increase in oxidative stress-associated proteins in neurons exposed to H_2O_2 was abrogated in these cells upon in vitro coculture with MSC (Lanza et al. 2009).

20.3.3 Neuroregeneration

There is evidence in vitro to suggest that MSC are a promising approach to achieve neuroregeneration. An early study showed that bone marrow stromal cells induced neuronal differentiation of rat mesencephalic neural stem cells through soluble factors (Lou et al. 2003). More recent studies showed that MSC can instruct NPC in vitro to enter an oligodendrogenic program while inhibiting their ability to differentiate into astrocytes (Rivera et al. 2006). Thus, interaction between MSC and NPC through soluble factors induced an increase in cells expressing the oligodendroglial markers, galactocerebroside and myelin basic protein; a reduction in glial fibrillary acidic protein-expressing cells; and an enhanced expression of the oligodendrogenic transcription factors Olig1, Olig2, and Nkx2.2, with diminished expression of Id2, an inhibitor of oligodendrogenic differentiation (Rivera et al. 2006). Similarly, in vitro neurospheres from MSC-treated EAE mice gave rise to more oligodendrocytes and less astrocytes than nontreated neurospheres, suggesting that MSC modulate CNS responses to injury in part through suppression of astrogliosis (Bai et al. 2009).

The potent anti-inflammatory capacity, the direct release of antiapoptotic and neurotrophic factors, the ability to induce other cells, such as microglia, to acquire a protective phenotype and to induce proliferation of local neural progenitor cells possibly leading to remyelination, are likely to sustain the protective effects observed in preclinical EAE models upon treatment with MSC.

20.4 Preclinical Studies

Studies in EAE, as well as in models of other neurological diseases, have clearly shown that immunomodulatory, neuroprotective, and neuroregenerative effects of MSC in vitro can translate in vivo (Table 20.1). Thus, upon administration in laboratory animals, MSC induced peripheral tolerance and, in some cases, migrated

Table 20.1 Preclinical studies of bone marrow-derived MSC in EAE

Mouse strain	EAE model[a]	MSC Source	MSC Number	MSC Route	Immune cell affected	MSC infiltration/engraftment in CNS	Neuroprotection	Neuroregeneration (cell marker)	Reference
C57Bl/6J	Chronic	Syngeneic	1×10^6 (2x or 3x)	i.v.	T cell	Yes/No	⇓ Inflammation, ⇓ demyelination	ND	Zappia et al. 2005
SJL/J	RR	Human	0.5–3 $\times 10^6$ (1x)	i.v.	?	Yes/±	⇓ Inflammation, ⇓ demyelination	NG2	Zhang et al. 2005
SJL/J	RR	Human	2×10^6 (1x)	i.v.	?	Yes/±	⇑ Axonal density, ⇑ NGF	NG2	Zhang et al. 2006
SJL/J	RR	Allogeneic	1×10^6 (1x)	i.v.	T cell, B cell	Yes/No	⇓ Inflammation, ⇓ demyelination, ⇓ axonal damage	ND	Gerdoni et al. 2007
SJL/J	RR	Syngeneic	2×10^6 (1x)	i.v.	T cell, DC	±/No	⇓ Inflammation, ⇓ demyelination	ND	Matysiak et al. 2008
C57Bl/6J	Chronic	Syngeneic	1×10^6 (1x)	i.v., i.vt.	T cell	Yes/Yes	⇓ Inflammation, ⇓ axonal damage	β-tubulin III, GFAP, GalC	Kassis et al. 2008
C57Bl/6J	Chronic	Human	1×10^6 (1x)	i.p.	?	No/?	?	ND	Gordon et al. 2008
C57Bl/6J	Chronic	Syngeneic	2×10^6 (1x)	i.p.	Th17 cell	?	⇓ Inflammation	?	Rafei et al. 2009
C57Bl/6J, SJL/J	Chronic, RR	Human	3×10^6(2x), 3×10^6(1x)	i.v.	⇓ Th1 cell, ⇑ Th2 cell	Yes/?	⇓ Inflammation, ⇓ demyelination, ⇓ axonal damage	⇑ PLP, ⇑ NG2	Bai et al. 2009
C57Bl/6J	Chronic	Syngeneic	1×10^6 (1x)	i.v.	?	?	⇓EAE-dependent oxidative stress	?	Lanza et al. 2009
C57Bl/6J	Chronic	Syngeneic	1×10^6 (2x)	i.p.	T cell	?	?	?	Lanz et al. 2010
C57Bl/6J	Chronic	Human	1×10^6 (1x)	i.v.	?	Yes/±	⇓ Inflammation, ⇓ demyelination	±Nestin, ±β-tubulin III	Gordon et al. 2010
C57Bl/6J	Chronic	hMSC-CM	0.5 mg	i.v.	–	–	⇓ Demyelination	–	Bai et al. 2012

ND not detected, ? not described, *i.vt.* intraventricular, *b-tubulin III* neuronal marker, *GFAP (glial fibrillary protein)* astrocytic marker, *GalC (galactocerebroside)* oligodendrocyte marker, *NG2* oligodendrocyte progenitor marker, *PLP* proteolipid protein, oligodendrocyte marker, *Nestin* neural stem cell marker, *hMSC-CM* conditioned growth medium from human MSC

[a] Chronic, MOG-induced; relapsing-remitting (RR), PLP-induced

to injured tissues, reducing the release of proinflammatory cytokines and promoting the survival of damaged cells. In most of these studies, the beneficial effect of MSC on the injured tissue occurred despite limited levels of engraftment and transdifferentiation, suggesting that the multipotentiality of these cells is not essential for their clinical effect, but that the therapeutic plasticity of MSC is exploited mainly in a paracrine fashion rather than in a cell–cell contact-mediated mechanism. In both chronic and relapsing–remitting EAE models of MS, induced with encephalitogenic peptides of myelin oligodendrocyte glycoprotein (MOG_{35-55}) and proteolipid protein ($PLP_{139-151}$), respectively, MSC could improve the clinical course of the disease, decrease demyelination, and promote tissue repair (Bai et al. 2012; Bai et al. 2009; Constantin et al. 2009; Gerdoni et al. 2007; Gordon et al. 2008; Rafei et al. 2009; Zappia et al. 2005; Zhang et al. 2006). Only a few studies provided some evidence, mainly by histological staining, that a small number of MSC engrafted in the CNS, possibly acquiring a neural phenotype (Zhang et al. 2006), particularly if injected directly in the CNS (Kassis et al. 2008).

In the first study of the effect of MSC administration on EAE, Zappia et al. (2005) showed that preventive treatment (i.v. infusion before disease onset) decreased severity of chronic EAE induced with MOG_{35-55} and led to a reduction in demyelination and CNS infiltration by T cells, B cells, and macrophages. Therapeutic treatment (i.v. infusion after disease onset) was also effective, albeit if administered early during disease course or at peak of disease and not in the chronic progressive phase (Zappia et al. 2005). Analysis with GFP-MSC showed that some cells may migrate to lymphoid organs where they are likely to interact with activated T cells and DC and exert their immunoregulatory activity, inducing peripheral T cell tolerance to the immunizing antigen (Zappia et al. 2005). A similar effect of MSC on encephalitogenic T cells was shown in the study of Gerdoni et al. (2007), where, upon adoptive transfer, encephalitogenic T cells activated in vitro with $PLP_{139-151}$ in the presence of MSC induced a milder relapsing–remitting disease compared with that induced by untreated activated encephalitogenic T cells. This study also demonstrated that MSC treatment can inhibit antigen-specific B cell response in vivo (Gerdoni et al. 2007). Rafei et al. (2009) have proposed that the immunomodulatory effect of MSC is related to blockade of IL-17-driven inflammation and cellular infiltration of the CNS, through their secretion of the antagonist form of CCL2 as ligand for CCR2 expressed by pathogenic Th17 $CD4^+$ T cells. They found that i.p. administration of wild-type MSC in ongoing disease significantly reduced severity, whereas MSC isolated from CCL2-knockout mice had no significant impact akin to the vehicle control group, and showed that the effect was probably mediated at least in part through upregulation of B7H-1, which blocks proliferation, on MOG-specific T cells (Rafei et al. 2009). On the basis of in vitro studies (see previous discussion), Lanz et al. (2010) addressed the role of IDO1-mediated tryptophan catabolism, a major immunosuppressive effector pathway, in the suppression of antigen-specific T cell responses by mouse MSC in EAE; in contrast to expectations from in vitro studies, mouse MSC, unlike human MSC, did not display IDO1-mediated suppression of antigen-specific T cell responses. These data, however, contrast with those of Matysiak et al. (2008) who reported that MSC ameliorate EAE via an IDO- mediated mechanism. Whether or not the differences in data obtained are related to the different EAE models used in both studies (chronic MOG-induced vs. relapsing–remitting PLP-induced) remains to be determined.

Although all studies so far concur on the immunomodulatory effect of syngeneic or allogeneic MSC on EAE (Table 20.1), there is controversy as to the ability of these cells to engraft and/or transdifferentiate. Regardless, the neuroprotective effect of MSC has been clearly demonstrated. In chronic and relapsing–remitting EAE studies, syngeneic and allogeneic MSC were seen to enter the CNS but did not transdifferentiate noticeably (Gerdoni et al. 2007, 2010; Zappia et al. 2005). Thus, Zhang et al. (2005) reported that upon treatment of PLP-induced EAE with human MSC, a small proportion (less than 5 %) of injected cells expressing NG2, an oligodendrocyte progenitor marker, could be seen in the CNS of EAE–affected mice, suggesting some degree of neural differentiation; the neuroprotective effect they observed was apparently associated with increased expression of brain-derived nerve factor in the CNS upon treatment. Kassis et al. (2008) also observed putative transdifferentiation ability of MSC, mostly when administered intraventricularly, with detection of cells expressing neuronal, astrocytic, and oligodendrocytic markers in inflamed CNS of mice with MOG-EAE; they report a strong neuroprotective effect of the treatment with prevention of axonal damage apparently more effective upon intraventricular administration. Although Gordon et al. (2008) confirmed the therapeutic potential of human MSC on EAE with a different route of administration, that is intraperitoneally, they did not detect significant presence of human MSC in the CNS, possibly due to the mode of delivery (Gordon et al. 2010). Bai et al. (2009) reported similar immunomodulatory and neuroprotective effects on both chronic and relapsing–remitting EAE upon treatment with human MSC to those reported in previous studies with mouse MSC (Gerdoni et al. 2007; Zappia et al. 2005); they suggested that the recovery of myelination they observed reflects a combination of suppression of the autoimmune response and induction of proliferation or enhanced differentiation of endogenous progenitor cells, as shown by the increase in density of $NG2^{+}$ cells and oligodendrocytes in the CNS of treated animals (Bai et al. 2009). A similar observation of increased endogenous oligodendrocyte progenitors, albeit with MSC derived from adipose tissue rather than bone marrow, was made by Constantin et al. (Constantin et al. 2009). A possible mechanism for the neuroprotective effects played by MSC in EAE was proposed by Lanza et al. (2009) who showed that MSC are endowed with a potent antioxidant effect in vivo, as demonstrated by the remarkable reduction in CNS levels/activities of antioxidant molecules involved in the defense against EAE-induced oxidative stress and tissue damage.

As clearly demonstrated by in vitro studies, MSC mediate their immunomodulatory and neuroprotective effects mainly through the release of soluble factors. The idea that such an action could translate in vivo was recently demonstrated by the study of Bai et al. (2012) who demonstrated that conditioned growth medium from human MSC promotes functional recovery in MOG- induced EAE; the effect, associated with remyelination and stimulation of neural development, is apparently mediated by HGF probably through its receptor cMet, which is expressed on both immune and neural lineage cells.

Recent studies have also focused on the possibility of enhancing the neuroprotective effect of MSC by differentiating them towards neural progenitors (Harris et al. 2012; Matysiak et al. 2011, 2008), or by engineering them to express, and thereby secrete, neuroprotective molecules to synergize MSC-mediated immunosuppression and neuroprotection (Lu et al. 2009). However, the results of these studies are somewhat contradictory and further investigations are necessary.

Overall, preclinical studies of MSC in EAE (Table 20.1) indicate that the three different mechanisms at play in disease amelioration, namely peripheral modulation of pathogenic immune responses, neuroprotection, and neuroregeneration, albeit the latter as yet poorly studied, provide a strong rationale for the use of MSC in therapeutic trials for neurological diseases characterized by inflammation and neural damage, such as MS.

20.5 Clinical Studies in MS

The robust amount of data in the preclinical studies demonstrating the therapeutic properties of MSC in the EAE models as well as in other neurological diseases (Uccelli et al. 2011), has opened the way to the clinical translation of MSC in MS.

Four small phase I open-label studies have yielded preliminary results on the safety of clinical application of MSC in MS (Connick and Li 2012; Karussis et al. 2010; Mohyeddin Bonab et al. 2007; Yamout et al. 2010), and the International Mesenchymal Stem Cells Transplantation (IMSCT) study group recently started an international multicenter phase II clinical trial in order to clearly define the safety and the efficacy of an established protocol on a large cohort of patients.

20.5.1 Source, Route of Administration, and Dose of MSC

Autologous MSC for the treatment of MS patients present advantages over xenogeneic or allogeneic cells. First, while xenogeneic (Zhang et al. 2005) and allogeneic (Eliopoulos et al. 2005; Le Blanc et al. 2008) MSC have proven effective in some preclinical (Zhang et al. 2005) and clinical studies (Le Blanc et al. 2008), other studies have shown that they might be rejected by the host immune system (Eliopoulos et al. 2005). Second, the use of autologous MSC minimizes the risk of transmission of infectious disease. Thus, as MSC isolated from MS patients display a normal phenotype and are fully functional in terms of proliferation, in vitro differentiation, and immunosuppressive ability (Mallam et al. 2010), autologous MSC seem to be the best choice for transplantation in MS patients. Accordingly, to date, all pilot clinical studies on MS have been conducted with autologous MSC (Connick and Li 2012; Karussis et al. 2010; Mohyeddin Bonab et al. 2007; Yamout et al. 2010).

As clearly shown in the preclinical studies on EAE, intravenous administration suffices to obtain most of the beneficial effect of MSC in terms of immune modulation and neuroprotection/neuroregeneration (Table 20.1). Indeed, local MSC administration did not provide significant advantage when compared with systemic infusion in EAE (Morando et al. 2012). It can be argued that intrathecal administration could overcome the limited amount of cells engrafted in the CNS that is usually obtained when MSC are infused intravenously, with local release by MSC of molecules favoring neuroprotection and neuroregeneration further promoting repair of damaged CNS areas. However, whether or not MSC will disseminate to all relevant areas of damage and engraft in the CNS upon intrathecal administration is unclear and, most importantly, intrathecal administration is invasive and may be associated with side effects such as transient acute encephalopathy and meningeal irritation observed in recent pilot clinical studies (Karussis et al. 2010; Mohyeddin Bonab et al. 2007; Yamout et al. 2010). These considerations should favor intravenous infusion as the route of administration in clinical trials of MSC in MS patients.

Different amount of MSC have been used in the recent pilot clinical trials in MS (Connick and Li 2012; Karussis et al. 2010; Mohyeddin Bonab et al. 2007; Yamout et al. 2010). The mean dose was about 1–2 $\times$ 10^6 MSC/kg of body weight, as similarly utilized in clinical trials for hematological disease and other autoimmune diseases (Duijvestein et al. 2011; Le Blanc et al. 2008). It has to be noted that MSC doses in clinical trials have been considerably lower than those of the preclinical studies, and must per force be so. The doses of 1–3 $\times$ 10^6 MSC per mouse utilized in EAE studies are not at present translatable to human treatment; indeed, it is almost impossible to recover and expand human MSC in vitro from a standard bone marrow aspiration to equivalent quantities.

20.5.2 Safety and Efficacy

MSC have been used clinically for over a decade and many trials were recently started to provide evidence for the safety and efficacy of their clinical use in neurological diseases (Uccelli et al. 2011). Results of the pilot trials in MS suggest that MSC treatment is well tolerated and generally safe, albeit with data only available for short-term periods. Nevertheless, it should be noted that some adverse events have been recorded associated with intrathecal injection. Thus, in their pilot study of intrathecal MSC injection in ten progressive MS patients, Mohyeddin et al. (2007) reported mild side effects of meningeal irritation and one case of iatrogenic meningitis due to the invasive procedure, with no further adverse event through the 13–26-month follow-up; in their subsequent study, they reported a major adverse event, transient encephalopathy with seizure that occurred a few days after MSC infusion, in one of the seven patients treated (Yamout et al. 2010). In contrast Karussis et al. (2010) observed only fever and headache at the time of intrathecal injection in their study on 15 MS patients and reported an acceptable short-term safety profile of the intrathecal route of administration of MSC at doses of up to 70 $\times$ 10^6 cells per injection per patient. In the only trial conducted to date in MS patients treated with

MSC exclusively by i.v. infusion, none of the ten patients experienced a significant adverse event through the 7-month follow-up (Connick and Li 2012).

However, long-term safety issues of MSC are still unresolved. Only a few clinical trials with long-term follow-up have been conducted in chronic diseases, such as stroke and amyotrophic lateral sclerosis (Bang et al. 2005; Mazzini et al. 2012); they showed no adverse long-term side effect following MSC infusion. In addition, the concern that MSC might induce tumor cell growth has not yet been resolved, and in vitro and in vivo data are inconsistent (Ame-Thomas et al. 2007; Bergfeld and DeClerck 2010; Bruno and Smith 2012; Djouad et al. 2003; Hass and Otte 2012; Karnoub and Weinberg 2006; Khakoo et al. 2006; Ramasamy et al. 2007), perhaps due to the heterogeneous nature of the MSC populations and the different experimental tumor models used in which the microenvironment probably influences the behavior of the MSC (Bergfeld and DeClerck 2010). Nevertheless, irrespective of the possible interactions between cancer cells, immune cells, and MSC, the potential risk of stimulating the growth of a previously undetected cancer in the long term upon treatment with MSC must be taken into consideration.

Of the four clinical studies published so far, only one aimed at assessing efficacy of MSC treatment. In their open-label phase IIa proof-of-concept study, Connick et al. measured visual parameters in ten patients with secondary progressive MS and visual pathway involvement who had received MSC i.v.; they report improvement in visual acuity and visual evoked response latency, with an increase in optic nerve area (Connick and Li 2012). The other three studies report anecdotal improvement in some clinical and radiological outcomes (Karussis et al. 2010; Mohyeddin Bonab et al. 2007; Yamout et al. 2010).

Obviously, large and long-term controlled clinical studies are needed to clearly assess safety along with efficacy, in terms of immune modulation and neuroprotection for this therapeutic strategy. Nevertheless, preclinical and clinical studies altogether suggest that MSC are likely to find a place among the therapies for MS patients with clinical or radiological evidence of inflammation, and who are refractory to first-line treatments. It is also reasonable to expect that in these patients, the therapeutic plasticity of MSC might foster tissue repair, delaying the progression of disability. The latter aspects have to be evaluated by specific MRI measures (Giacomini and Arnold 2008) and robust techniques will need to be developed to track the homing of exogenously infused MSC into the CNS (Karp and Leng Teo 2009).

20.5.3 Perspectives

To clearly dissect the potential of MSC as treatment for MS, properly controlled clinical studies on a cohort of patients are urgently needed (Martino et al. 2010). Safety and efficacy in terms of immune modulation and, more interestingly, repair of the CNS damage have to be addressed adequately in the framework of rigorous controlled clinical trials. On the basis of these considerations, the IMSCT study group has been established, which includes scientists and clinicians from several centers in

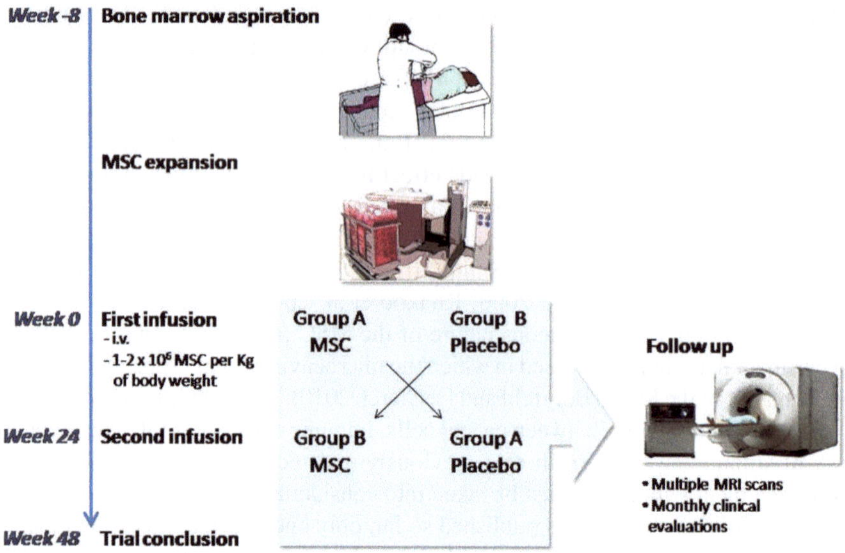

Fig. 20.1 The MESEMS protocol

Europe, Canada, and Australia. In 2010, the IMSCT study group reached a consensus to guide a large international phase II clinical trial of MSC for the treatment of MS, based on a protocol termed Mesenchymal Stem cells for MS (MESEMS; Freedman et al. 2010; Fig. 20.1). This trial is to be conducted as a randomized, double-blind, cross-over study of intravenous treatment with autologous MSC compared with suspension medium in MS patients with active disease, including relapsing–remitting, secondary progressive with relapses and/or enhancing lesions, and primary progressive with enhancing lesions. After bone marrow harvesting, MSC will be isolated, expanded under good manufacturing procedures, and cryopreserved. Randomized patients will be infused i.v. with $1–2 \times 10^6$ MSC/kg of body weight or suspension medium and, 6 months later, subjected to another infusion, where patients who had been treated with MSC will be treated with suspension medium and vice versa, in a double-blinded manner (Fig. 20.1). The primary objectives of the study will be to assess the safety of the treatment and its efficacy by clinical evaluation and frequent MRI scans (Fig. 20.1). Secondary objectives include efficacy of treatment evaluated by cumulative MRI activity and brain atrophy, evidence of remyelination measured by magnetization transfer ratio, effect on clinical parameters, visual functions, neuropsychological tests, and immunological responses.

It is expected that current clinical trials will answer fundamental questions concerning the efficacy of MSC, and whether these can play a role in the future armamentarium of treatments for MS, hopefully as one of the first steps towards tissue repair.

Acknowledgments We gratefully acknowledge the financial support of the Italian MS Foundation (FISM, project grant No. 2012/S/4), the Italian Ministry of Health (Ricerca Finalizzata, grant No. RF-LIG-2008–1221276/CUP G35J11000180001), the Italian Ministry of the University and Scientific Research (MIUR, grant No. 2009JN7SCN_003), the Liguria Region, and the CARIGE Foundation. L. Lovato is supported by an FISM Senior Research Fellowship (2010/B/10).

References

Abbott A (2011) Europe rules against stem-cell patents. Nature 471(7338):280

Abematsu M, Tsujimura K, Yamano M, Saito M, Kohno K, Kohyama J, Namihira M, Komiya S, Nakashima K (2010) Neurons derived from transplanted neural stem cells restore disrupted neuronal circuitry in a mouse model of spinal cord injury. J Clin Invest 120(9):3255–3266

Aggarwal S, Pittenger MF (2005) Human mesenchymal stem cells modulate allogeneic immune cell responses. Blood 105(4):1815–1822

Aharonowiz M, Einstein O, Fainstein N, Lassmann H, Reubinoff B, Ben-Hur T (2008) Neuroprotective effect of transplanted human embryonic stem cell-derived neural precursors in an animal model of multiple sclerosis. PLoS One 3(9):e3145

Ame-Thomas P, Maby-El Hajjami H, Monvoisin C, Jean R, Monnier D, Caulet-Maugendre S, Guillaudeux T, Lamy T, Fest T, Tarte K (2007) Human mesenchymal stem cells isolated from bone marrow and lymphoid organs support tumor B-cell growth: role of stromal cells in follicular lymphoma pathogenesis. Blood 109(2):693–702

Augello A, Tasso R, Negrini SM, Amateis A, Indiveri F, Cancedda R, Pennesi G (2005) Bone marrow mesenchymal progenitor cells inhibit lymphocyte proliferation by activation of the programmed death 1 pathway. Eur J Immunol 35(5):1482–1490

Bacigaluppi M, Pluchino S, Peruzzotti-Jametti L, Kilic E, Kilic U, Salani G, Brambilla E, West MJ, Comi G, Martino G, Hermann DM (2009) Delayed post-ischaemic neuroprotection following systemic neural stem cell transplantation involves multiple mechanisms. Brain 132(Pt 8):2239–2251

Bai L, Lennon DP, Eaton V, Maier K, Caplan AI, Miller SD, Miller RH (2009) Human bone marrow-derived mesenchymal stem cells induce Th2-polarized immune response and promote endogenous repair in animal models of multiple sclerosis. Glia 57(11):1192–1203

Bai L, Lennon DP, Caplan AI, Dechant A, Hecker J, Kranso J, Zaremba A, Miller RH (2012) Hepatocyte growth factor mediates mesenchymal stem cell-induced recovery in multiple sclerosis models. Nat Neurosci 15(6):862–870

Bang OY, Lee JS, Lee PH, Lee G (2005) Autologous mesenchymal stem cell transplantation in stroke patients. Ann Neurol 57(6):874–882

Bartholomew A, Sturgeon C, Siatskas M, Ferrer K, McIntosh K, Patil S, Hardy W, Devine S, Ucker D, Deans R, Moseley A, Hoffman R (2002) Mesenchymal stem cells suppress lymphocyte proliferation in vitro and prolong skin graft survival in vivo. Exp Hematol 30(1):42–48

Ben-Hur T, Idelson M, Khaner H, Pera M, Reinhartz E, Itzik A, Reubinoff BE (2004) Transplantation of human embryonic stem cell-derived neural progenitors improves behavioral deficit in Parkinsonian rats. Stem Cells 22(7):1246–1255

Benvenuto F, Ferrari S, Gerdoni E, Gualandi F, Frassoni F, Pistoia V, Mancardi G, Uccelli A (2007) Human mesenchymal stem cells promote survival of T cells in a quiescent state. Stem Cells 25(7):1753–1760

Bergfeld SA, DeClerck YA (2010) Bone marrow-derived mesenchymal stem cells and the tumor microenvironment. Cancer Metastasis Rev 29(2):249–261

Bruno RD, Smith GH (2012) Reprogramming non-mammary and cancer cells in the developing mouse mammary gland. Semin Cell Dev Biol 23(5):591–598

Caplan AI (1991) Mesenchymal stem cells. J Orthop Res 9(5):641–650

Chabannes D, Hill M, Merieau E, Rossignol J, Brion R, Soulillou JP, Anegon I, Cuturi MC (2007) A role for heme oxygenase-1 in the immunosuppressive effect of adult rat and human mesenchymal stem cells. Blood 110(10):3691–3694

Chamberlain G, Fox J, Ashton B, Middleton J (2007) Concise review: mesenchymal stem cells: their phenotype, differentiation capacity, immunological features, and potential for homing. Stem Cells 25(11):2739–2749

Chiesa S, Morbelli S, Morando S, Massollo M, Marini C, Bertoni A, Frassoni F, Bartolome ST, Sambuceti G, Traggiai E, Uccelli A (2011) Mesenchymal stem cells impair in vivo T-cell priming by dendritic cells. Proc Natl Acad Sci U S A 108(42):17384–17389

Conget PA, Minguell JJ (1999) Phenotypical and functional properties of human bone marrow mesenchymal progenitor cells. J Cell Physiol 181(1):67–73

Connick P, Kolappan M, Crawley C, Webber DJ, Patani R, Michell AW, Du MQ, Luan SL, Altmann DR, Thompson AJ, Compston A, Scott MA, Miller DH, Chandran S (2012) Autologous mesenchymal stem cells for the treatment of secondary progressive multiple sclerosis: an open-label phase 2a proof-of-concept study. Lancet Neurol 11(2):150–156

Constantin G, Marconi S, Rossi B, Angiari S, Calderan L, Anghileri E, Gini B, Bach SD, Martinello M, Bifari F, Galie M, Turano E, Budui S, Sbarbati A, Krampera M, Bonetti B (2009) Adipose-derived mesenchymal stem cells ameliorate chronic experimental autoimmune encephalomyelitis. Stem Cells 27(10):2624–2635

Corcione A, Benvenuto F, Ferretti E, Giunti D, Cappiello V, Cazzanti F, Risso M, Gualandi F, Mancardi GL, Pistoia V, Uccelli A (2006) Human mesenchymal stem cells modulate B-cell functions. Blood 107(1):367–372

Crigler L, Robey RC, Asawachaicharn A, Gaupp D, Phinney DG (2006) Human mesenchymal stem cell subpopulations express a variety of neuro-regulatory molecules and promote neuronal cell survival and neuritogenesis. Exp Neurol 198(1):54–64

Cundiff PE, Anderson SA (2011) Impact of induced pluripotent stem cells on the study of central nervous system disease. Curr Opin Genet Dev 21(3):354–361

Czepiel M, Balasubramaniyan V, Schaafsma W, Stancic M, Mikkers H, Huisman C, Boddeke E, Copray S (2011) Differentiation of induced pluripotent stem cells into functional oligodendrocytes. Glia 59(6):882–892

Di Nicola M, Carlo-Stella C, Magni M, Milanesi M, Longoni PD, Matteucci P, Grisanti S, Gianni AM (2002) Human bone marrow stromal cells suppress T-lymphocyte proliferation induced by cellular or nonspecific mitogenic stimuli. Blood 99(10):3838–3843

Djouad F, Plence P, Bony C, Tropel P, Apparailly F, Sany J, Noel D, Jorgensen C (2003) Immunosuppressive effect of mesenchymal stem cells favors tumor growth in allogeneic animals. Blood 102(10):3837–3844

Djouad F, Charbonnier LM, Bouffi C, Louis-Plence P, Bony C, Apparailly F, Cantos C, Jorgensen C, Noel D (2007) Mesenchymal stem cells inhibit the differentiation of dendritic cells through an interleukin-6-dependent mechanism. Stem Cells 25(8):2025–2032

Duijvestein M, Wildenberg ME, Welling MM, Hennink S, Molendijk I, van Zuylen VL, Bosse T, Vos AC, de Jonge-Muller ES, Roelofs H, van der Weerd L, Verspaget HW, Fibbe WE, te Velde AA, van den Brink GR, Hommes DW (2011) Pretreatment with interferon-gamma enhances the therapeutic activity of mesenchymal stromal cells in animal models of colitis. Stem Cells 29(10):1549–1558

Eliopoulos N, Stagg J, Lejeune L, Pommey S, Galipeau J (2005) Allogeneic marrow stromal cells are immune rejected by MHC class I- and class II-mismatched recipient mice. Blood 106(13):4057–4065

Franklin RJ, Ffrench-Constant C (2008) Remyelination in the CNS: from biology to therapy. Nat Rev Neurosci 9(11):839–855

Friedenstein AJ, Petrakova KV, Kurolesova AI, Frolova GP (1968) Heterotopic of bone marrow. Analysis of precursor cells for osteogenic and hematopoietic tissues. Transplantation 6(2):230–247

Friedenstein AJ, Chailakhyan RK, Latsinik NV, Panasyuk AF, Keiliss-Borok IV (1974) Stromal cells responsible for transferring the microenvironment of the hemopoietic tissues. Cloning in vitro and retransplantation in vivo. Transplantation 17(4):331–340

Freedman MS, Bar-Or A, Atkins HL, Karussis D, Frassoni F, Lazarus H, Scolding N, Slavin S, Le Blanc K, Uccelli A, Group MS (2010) The therapeutic potential of mesenchymal stem cell transplantation as a treatment for multiple sclerosis: consensus report of the International MSCT Study Group. Mult Scler 16(4):503–510

Gerdoni E, Gallo B, Casazza S, Musio S, Bonanni I, Pedemonte E, Mantegazza R, Frassoni F, Mancardi G, Pedotti R, Uccelli A (2007) Mesenchymal stem cells effectively modulate pathogenic immune response in experimental autoimmune encephalomyelitis. Ann Neurol 61(3):219–227

Giacomini PS, Arnold DL (2008) Non-conventional MRI techniques for measuring neuroprotection, repair and plasticity in multiple sclerosis. Curr Opin Neurol 21(3):272–277

Giunti D, Parodi B, Usai C, Vergani L, Casazza S, Bruzzone S, Mancardi G, Uccelli A (2012) Mesenchymal stem cells shape microglia effector functions through the release of CX3CL1. Stem Cells 30(9):2044–2053

Glennie S, Soeiro I, Dyson PJ, Lam EW, Dazzi F (2005) Bone marrow mesenchymal stem cells induce division arrest anergy of activated T cells. Blood 105(7):2821–2827

Gordon D, Pavlovska G, Glover CP, Uney JB, Wraith D, Scolding NJ (2008) Human mesenchymal stem cells abrogate experimental allergic encephalomyelitis after intraperitoneal injection, and with sparse CNS infiltration. Neurosci Lett 448(1):71–73

Gordon D, Pavlovska G, Uney JB, Wraith DC, Scolding NJ (2010) Human mesenchymal stem cells infiltrate the spinal cord, reduce demyelination, and localize to white matter lesions in experimental autoimmune encephalomyelitis. J Neuropathol Exp Neurol 69(11):1087–1095

Harris VK, Yan QJ, Vyshkina T, Sahabi S, Liu X, Sadiq SA (2012) Clinical and pathological effects of intrathecal injection of mesenchymal stem cell-derived neural progenitors in an experimental model of multiple sclerosis. J Neurol Sci 313(1–2):167–177

Hass R, Otte A (2012) Mesenchymal stem cells as all-round supporters in a normal and neoplastic microenvironment. Cell Commun Signal 10(1):26

Horwitz EM, Le Blanc K, Dominici M, Mueller I, Slaper-Cortenbach I, Marini FC, Deans RJ, Krause DS, Keating A (2005) Clarification of the nomenclature for MSC: the International Society for Cellular Therapy position statement. Cytotherapy 7(5):393–395

Jiang XX, Zhang Y, Liu B, Zhang SX, Wu Y, Yu XD, Mao N (2005) Human mesenchymal stem cells inhibit differentiation and function of monocyte-derived dendritic cells. Blood 105(10):4120–4126

Joannides AJ, Chandran S (2008) Human embryonic stem cells: an experimental and therapeutic resource for neurological disease. J Neurol Sci 265(1–2):84–88

Karnoub AE, Weinberg RA (2006) Chemokine networks and breast cancer metastasis. Breast Dis 26:75–85

Karp JM, Leng Teo GS (2009) Mesenchymal stem cell homing: the devil is in the details. Cell Stem Cell 4(3):206–216

Karussis D, Karageorgiou C, Vaknin-Dembinsky A, Gowda-Kurkalli B, Gomori JM, Kassis I, Bulte JW, Petrou P, Ben-Hur T, Abramsky O, Slavin S (2010) Safety and immunological effects of mesenchymal stem cell transplantation in patients with multiple sclerosis and amyotrophic lateral sclerosis. Arch Neurol 67(10):1187–1194

Kassis I, Grigoriadis N, Gowda-Kurkalli B, Mizrachi-Kol R, Ben-Hur T, Slavin S, Abramsky O, Karussis D (2008) Neuroprotection and immunomodulation with mesenchymal stem cells in chronic experimental autoimmune encephalomyelitis. Arch Neurol 65(6):753–761

Khakoo AY, Pati S, Anderson SA, Reid W, Elshal MF, Rovira II, Nguyen AT, Malide D, Combs CA, Hall G, Zhang J, Raffeld M, Rogers TB, Stetler-Stevenson W, Frank JA, Reitz M, Finkel T (2006) Human mesenchymal stem cells exert potent antitumorigenic effects in a model of Kaposi's sarcoma. J Exp Med 203(5):1235–1247

Kiel MJ, Morrison SJ (2008) Uncertainty in the niches that maintain haematopoietic stem cells. Nat Rev Immunol 8(4):290–301

Kopen GC, Prockop DJ, Phinney DG (1999) Marrow stromal cells migrate throughout forebrain and cerebellum, and they differentiate into astrocytes after injection into neonatal mouse brains. Proc Natl Acad Sci U S A 96(19):10711–10716

Krampera M, Glennie S, Dyson J, Scott D, Laylor R, Simpson E, Dazzi F (2003) Bone marrow mesenchymal stem cells inhibit the response of naive and memory antigen-specific T cells to their cognate peptide. Blood 101(9):3722–3729

Krampera M, Cosmi L, Angeli R, Pasini A, Liotta F, Andreini A, Santarlasci V, Mazzinghi B, Pizzolo G, Vinante F, Romagnani P, Maggi E, Romagnani S, Annunziato F (2006) Role for interferon-gamma in the immunomodulatory activity of human bone marrow mesenchymal stem cells. Stem Cells 24(2):386–398

Lanz TV, Opitz CA, Ho PP, Agrawal A, Lutz C, Weller M, Mellor AL, Steinman L, Wick W, Platten M (2010) Mouse mesenchymal stem cells suppress antigen-specific TH cell immunity independent of indoleamine 2,3-dioxygenase 1 (IDO1). Stem Cells Dev 19(5):657–668

Lanza C, Morando S, Voci A, Canesi L, Principato MC, Serpero LD, Mancardi G, Uccelli A, Vergani L (2009) Neuroprotective mesenchymal stem cells are endowed with a potent antioxidant effect in vivo. J Neurochem 110(5):1674–1684

Le Blanc K, Frassoni F, Ball L, Locatelli F, Roelofs H, Lewis I, Lanino E, Sundberg B, Bernardo ME, Remberger M, Dini G, Egeler RM, Bacigalupo A, Fibbe W, Ringden O (2008) Mesenchymal stem cells for treatment of steroid-resistant, severe, acute graft-versus-host disease: a phase II study. Lancet 371(9624):1579–1586

Lebonvallet N, Boulais N, Le Gall C, Cheret J, Pereira U, Mignen O, Bardey V, Jeanmaire C, Danoux L, Pauly G, Misery L (2012) Characterization of neurons from adult human skin-derived precursors in serum-free medium: a PCR array and immunocytological analysis. Exp Dermatol 21(3):195–200

Liotta F, Angeli R, Cosmi L, Fili L, Manuelli C, Frosali F, Mazzinghi B, Maggi L, Pasini A, Lisi V, Santarlasci V, Consoloni L, Angelotti ML, Romagnani P, Parronchi P, Krampera M, Maggi E, Romagnani S, Annunziato F (2008) Toll-like receptors 3 and 4 are expressed by human bone marrow-derived mesenchymal stem cells and can inhibit their T-cell modulatory activity by impairing Notch signaling. Stem Cells 26(1):279–289

Lou S, Gu P, Chen F, He C, Wang M, Lu C (2003) The effect of bone marrow stromal cells on neuronal differentiation of mesencephalic neural stem cells in Sprague-Dawley rats. Brain Res 968(1):114–121

Lu Z, Hu X, Zhu C, Wang D, Zheng X, Liu Q (2009) Overexpression of CNTF in mesenchymal stem cells reduces demyelination and induces clinical recovery in experimental autoimmune encephalomyelitis mice. J Neuroimmunol 206(1–2):58–69

Lunemann JD, Munz C (2008) Do natural killer cells accelerate or prevent autoimmunity in multiple sclerosis? Brain 131(Pt 7):1681–1683

Maccario R, Podesta M, Moretta A, Cometa A, Comoli P, Montagna D, Daudt L, Ibatici A, Piaggio G, Pozzi S, Frassoni F, Locatelli F (2005) Interaction of human mesenchymal stem cells with cells involved in alloantigen-specific immune response favors the differentiation of CD4+ T-cell subsets expressing a regulatory/suppressive phenotype. Haematologica 90(4):516–525

Majumdar MK, Thiede MA, Mosca JD, Moorman M, Gerson SL (1998) Phenotypic and functional comparison of cultures of marrow-derived mesenchymal stem cells (MSCs) and stromal cells. J Cell Physiol 176(1):57–66

Mallam E, Kemp K, Wilkins A, Rice C, Scolding N (2010) Characterization of in vitro expanded bone marrow-derived mesenchymal stem cells from patients with multiple sclerosis. Mult Scler 16(8):909–918

Mancardi G, Saccardi R (2008) Autologous haematopoietic stem-cell transplantation in multiple sclerosis. Lancet Neurol 7(7):626–636

Martino G, Franklin RJ, Baron VEvercoorenA, Kerr DA (2010) Stem cell transplantation in multiple sclerosis: current status and future prospects. Nat Rev Neurol 6(5):247–255

Matysiak M, Stasiolek M, Orlowski W, Jurewicz A, Janczar S, Raine CS, Selmaj K (2008) Stem cells ameliorate EAE via an indoleamine 2,3-dioxygenase (IDO) mechanism. J Neuroimmunol 193(1–2):12–23

Matysiak M, Orlowski W, Fortak-Michalska M, Jurewicz A, Selmaj K (2011) Immunoregulatory function of bone marrow mesenchymal stem cells in EAE depends on their differentiation state and secretion of PGE2. J Neuroimmunol 233(1–2):106–111

Mazzini L, Mareschi K, Ferrero I, Miglioretti M, Stecco A, Servo S, Carriero A, Monaco F, Fagioli F (2012) Mesenchymal stromal cell transplantation in amyotrophic lateral sclerosis: a long-term safety study. Cytotherapy 14(1):56–60

Meisel R, Zibert A, Laryea M, Gobel U, Daubener W, Dilloo D (2004) Human bone marrow stromal cells inhibit allogeneic T-cell responses by indoleamine 2,3-dioxygenase-mediated tryptophan degradation. Blood 103(12):4619–4621

Mendez-Ferrer S, Michurina TV, Ferraro F, Mazloom AR, Macarthur BD, Lira SA, Scadden DT, Ma'ayan A, Enikolopov GN, Frenette PS (2010) Mesenchymal and haematopoietic stem cells form a unique bone marrow niche. Nature 466(7308):829–834

Mohyeddin Bonab M, Yazdanbakhsh S, Lotfi J, Alimoghaddom K, Talebian F, Hooshmand F, Ghavamzadeh A, Nikbin B (2007) Does mesenchymal stem cell therapy help multiple sclerosis patients? Report of a pilot study. Iran J Immunol 4(1):50–57

Morando S, Vigo T, Esposito M, Casazza S, Novi G, Principato MC, Furlan R, Uccelli A (2012) The therapeutic effect of mesenchymal stem cell transplantation in experimental autoimmune encephalomyelitis is mediated by peripheral and central mechanisms. Stem Cell Res Ther 3(1):3

Muguruma Y, Yahata T, Miyatake H, Sato T, Uno T, Itoh J, Kato S, Ito M, Hotta T, Ando K (2006) Reconstitution of the functional human hematopoietic microenvironment derived from human mesenchymal stem cells in the murine bone marrow compartment. Blood 107(5):1878–1887

Muraro PA, Douek DC, Packer A, Chung K, Guenaga FJ, Cassiani-Ingoni R, Campbell C, Memon S, Nagle JW, Hakim FT, Gress RE, McFarland HF, Burt RK, Martin R (2005) Thymic output generates a new and diverse TCR repertoire after autologous stem cell transplantation in multiple sclerosis patients. J Exp Med 201(5):805–816

Naegele M, Tillack K, Reinhardt S, Schippling S, Martin R, Sospedra M (2012) Neutrophils in multiple sclerosis are characterized by a primed phenotype. J Neuroimmunol 242(1–2):60–71

Nauta AJ, Kruisselbrink AB, Lurvink E, Willemze R, Fibbe WE (2006) Mesenchymal stem cells inhibit generation and function of both CD34+ -derived and monocyte-derived dendritic cells. J Immunol 177(4):2080–2087

Pevsner-Fischer M, Morad V, Cohen-Sfady M, Rousso-Noori L, Zanin-Zhorov A, Cohen S, Cohen IR, Zipori D (2007) Toll-like receptors and their ligands control mesenchymal stem cell functions. Blood 109(4):1422–1432

Pittenger MF, Mackay AM, Beck SC, Jaiswal RK, Douglas R, Mosca JD, Moorman MA, Simonetti DW, Craig S, Marshak DR (1999) Multilineage potential of adult human mesenchymal stem cells. Science 284(5411):143–147

Pluchino S, Quattrini A, Brambilla E, Gritti A, Salani G, Dina G, Galli R, Del Carro U, Amadio S, Bergami A, Furlan R, Comi G, Vescovi AL, Martino G (2003) Injection of adult neurospheres induces recovery in a chronic model of multiple sclerosis. Nature 422(6933):688–694

Pluchino S, Gritti A, Blezer E, Amadio S, Brambilla E, Borsellino G, Cossetti C, Del Carro U, Comi G, t Hart B, Vescovi A, Martino G (2009) Human neural stem cells ameliorate autoimmune encephalomyelitis in non-human primates. Ann Neurol 66(3):343–354

Poggi A, Prevosto C, Massaro AM, Negrini S, Urbani S, Pierri I, Saccardi R, Gobbi M, Zocchi MR (2005) Interaction between human NK cells and bone marrow stromal cells induces NK cell triggering: role of NKp30 and NKG2D receptors. J Immunol 175(10):6352–6360

Rafei M, Campeau PM, Aguilar-Mahecha A, Buchanan M, Williams P, Birman E, Yuan S, Young YK, Boivin MN, Forner K, Basik M, Galipeau J (2009) Mesenchymal stromal cells ameliorate experimental autoimmune encephalomyelitis by inhibiting CD4 Th17T cells in a CC chemokine ligand 2-dependent manner. J Immunol 182(10):5994–6002

Raffaghello L, Bianchi G, Bertolotto M, Montecucco F, Busca A, Dallegri F, Ottonello L, Pistoia V (2008) Human mesenchymal stem cells inhibit neutrophil apoptosis: a model for neutrophil preservation in the bone marrow niche. Stem Cells 26(1):151–162

Ramasamy R, Lam EW, Soeiro I, Tisato V, Bonnet D, Dazzi F (2007) Mesenchymal stem cells inhibit proliferation and apoptosis of tumor cells: impact on in vivo tumor growth. Leukemia 21(2):304–310

Rasmusson I, Le Blanc K, Sundberg B, Ringden O (2007) Mesenchymal stem cells stimulate antibody secretion in human B cells. Scand J Immunol 65(4):336–343

Rivera FJ, Couillard-Despres S, Pedre X, Ploetz S, Caioni M, Lois C, Bogdahn U, Aigner L (2006) Mesenchymal stem cells instruct oligodendrogenic fate decision on adult neural stem cells. Stem Cells 24(10):2209–2219

Saporta MA, Grskovic M, Dimos JT (2011) Induced pluripotent stem cells in the study of neurological diseases. Stem Cell Res Ther 2(5):37

Sato K, Ozaki K, I Oh, Meguro A, Hatanaka K, Nagai T, Muroi K, Ozawa K (2007) Nitric oxide plays a critical role in suppression of T-cell proliferation by mesenchymal stem cells. Blood 109(1):228–234

Scuteri A, Cassetti A, Tredici G (2006) Adult mesenchymal stem cells rescue dorsal root ganglia neurons from dying. Brain Res 1116(1):75–81

Selmani Z, Naji A, Zidi I, Favier B, Gaiffe E, Obert L, Borg C, Saas P, Tiberghien P, Rouas-Freiss N, Carosella ED, Deschaseaux F (2008) Human leukocyte antigen-G5 secretion by human mesenchymal stem cells is required to suppress T lymphocyte and natural killer function and to induce CD4+CD25highFOXP3+ regulatory T cells. Stem Cells 26(1):212–222

Song B, Sun G, Herszfeld D, Sylvain A, Campanale NV, Hirst CE, Caine S, Parkington HC, Tonta MA, Coleman HA, Short M, Ricardo SD, Reubinoff B, Bernard CC (2012) Neural differentiation of patient specific iPS cells as a novel approach to study the pathophysiology of multiple sclerosis. Stem Cell Res 8(2):259–273

Spaggiari GM, Capobianco A, Becchetti S, Mingari MC, Moretta L (2006) Mesenchymal stem cell-natural killer cell interactions: evidence that activated NK cells are capable of killing MSCs, whereas MSCs can inhibit IL-2-induced NK-cell proliferation. Blood 107(4):1484–1490

Spaggiari GM, Capobianco A, Abdelrazik H, Becchetti F, Mingari MC, Moretta L (2008) Mesenchymal stem cells inhibit natural killer-cell proliferation, cytotoxicity, and cytokine production: role of indoleamine 2,3-dioxygenase and prostaglandin E2. Blood 111(3):1327–1333

Svensson M, Kaye PM (2006) Stromal-cell regulation of dendritic-cell differentiation and function. Trends Immunol 27(12):580–587

Tomchuck SL, Zwezdaryk KJ, Coffelt SB, Waterman RS, Danka ES, Scandurro AB (2008) Toll-like receptors on human mesenchymal stem cells drive their migration and immunomodulating responses. Stem Cells 26(1):99–107

Traggiai E, Volpi S, Schena F, Gattorno M, Ferlito F, Moretta L, Martini A (2008) Bone marrow-derived mesenchymal stem cells induce both polyclonal expansion and differentiation of B cells isolated from healthy donors and systemic lupus erythematosus patients. Stem Cells 26(2):562–569

Tse WT, Pendleton JD, Beyer WM, Egalka MC, Guinan EC (2003) Suppression of allogeneic T-cell proliferation by human marrow stromal cells: implications in transplantation. Transplantation 75(3):389–397

Uccelli A, Moretta L, Pistoia V (2008) Mesenchymal stem cells in health and disease. Nat Rev Immunol 8(9):726–736

Uccelli A, Laroni A, Freedman MS (2011) Mesenchymal stem cells for the treatment of multiple sclerosis and other neurological diseases. Lancet Neurol 10(7):649–656

Uccelli A, Milanese M, Principato MC, Morando S, Bonifacino T, Vergani L, Giunti D, Voci A, Carminati E, Giribaldi F, Caponnetto C, Bonanno G (2012) Intravenous mesenchymal stem cells improve survival and motor function in experimental amyotrophic lateral sclerosis. Mol Med 18(1):794–804

Voulgari-Kokota A, Fairless R, Karamita M, Kyrargyri V, Tseveleki V, Evangelidou M, Delorme B, Charbord P, Diem R, Probert L (2012) Mesenchymal stem cells protect CNS neurons against glutamate excitotoxicity by inhibiting glutamate receptor expression and function. Exp Neurol 236(1):161–170

Wilkins A, Kemp K, Ginty M, Hares K, Mallam E, Scolding N (2009) Human bone marrow-derived mesenchymal stem cells secrete brain-derived neurotrophic factor which promotes neuronal survival in vitro. Stem Cell Res 3(1):63–70

Wright HL, Moots RJ, Bucknall RC, Edwards SW (2010) Neutrophil function in inflammation and inflammatory diseases. Rheumatology 49(9):1618–1631

Yamout B, Hourani R, Salti H, Barada W, El-Hajj T, Al-Kutoubi A, Herlopian A, Baz EK, Mahfouz R, Khalil-Hamdan R, Kreidieh NM, El-Sabban M, Bazarbachi A (2010) Bone marrow mesenchymal stem cell transplantation in patients with multiple sclerosis: a pilot study. J Neuroimmunol 227(1–2):185–189

Zappia E, Casazza S, Pedemonte E, Benvenuto F, Bonanni I, Gerdoni E, Giunti D, Ceravolo A, Cazzanti F, Frassoni F, Mancardi G, Uccelli A (2005) Mesenchymal stem cells ameliorate experimental autoimmune encephalomyelitis inducing T-cell anergy. Blood 106(5):1755–1761

Zhang J, Li Y, Chen JL, Cui YS, Lu M, Elias SB, Mitchell JB, Hammill L, Vanguri P, Chopp M (2005) Human bone marrow stromal cell treatment improves neurological functional recovery in EAE mice. Exp Neurol 195(1):16–26

Zhang J, Li Y, Lu M, Cui Y, Chen J, Noffsinger L, Elias SB, Chopp M (2006) Bone marrow stromal cells reduce axonal loss in experimental autoimmune encephalomyelitis mice. J Neurosci Res 84(3):587–595

Zhou C, Zhang C, Chi S, Xu Y, Teng J, Wang H, Song Y, Zhao R (2009) Effects of human marrow stromal cells on activation of microglial cells and production of inflammatory factors induced by lipopolysaccharide. Brain Res 1269:23–30

[illegible]

Index

T. Yamamura, B. Gran (eds.), *Multiple Sclerosis Immunology*,
DOI 10.1007/978-1-4614-7953-6, © Springer Science+Business Media New York 2013

FSC
www.fsc.org
MIX
Papier aus verantwortungsvollen Quellen
Paper from responsible sources
FSC® C105338

If you have any concerns about our products,
you can contact us on
ProductSafety@springernature.com

In case Publisher is established outside the EU,
the EU authorized representative is:
Springer Nature Customer Service Center GmbH
Europaplatz 3, 69115 Heidelberg, Germany

Printed by Libri Plureos GmbH
in Hamburg, Germany